Melatonin and Melatonergic Drugs in Clinical Practice

V. Srinivasan
Amnon Brzezinski • Sukru Oter
Samuel D. Shillcutt
Editors

Melatonin and Melatonergic Drugs in Clinical Practice

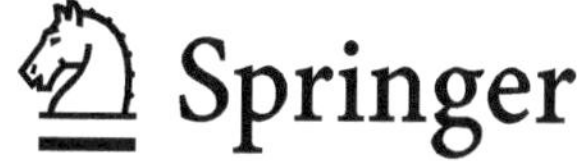

Editors
V. Srinivasan, MSc, PhD, MAMS
Sri Sathya Sai Medical Educational and Research Foundation
An International Medical Sciences Research Study Center
Coimbatore, TN
India

National Health Service,
Department of Mental Health
Psychiatric Service of Diagnosis and Treatment, Hospital "G. Mazzini"
Teramo
Italy

Department of Neuroscience and Imaging
University "G.D' Annunzio"
Chieti
Italy

Amnon Brzezinski, MD
Department of Obstetrics and Gynecology
Hadassah Hebrew-University Medical Center
Jerusalem
Israel

Sukru Oter, MD, PhD
Department of Physiology
Gulhane Military Medical Academy
Ankara
Turkey

Samuel D. Shillcutt, PharmD, PhD
Department of Psychiatry and Behavioral Sciences
Mercer University School of Medicine
Macon, GA
USA

ISBN 978-81-322-0824-2 ISBN 978-81-322-0825-9 (eBook)
DOI 10.1007/978-81-322-0825-9
Springer New Delhi Heidelberg New York Dordrecht London

Library of Congress Control Number: 2013956613

Printed on acid-free paper

Springer is part of Springer Science+Business Media (www.springer.com)

Preface

Melatonin is a ubiquitous molecule that is widely distributed in nature and is synthesized by most of the living organisms including unicellular organisms, fungi, plants, and animals. Melatonin synthesis in human beings is unique as this hormone is synthesized in many areas of the body in much higher concentration than that is produced by the pineal gland, which is considered as the major site of its production. Melatonin displays multiplicity of actions that ranges from chronobiotic, hypnotic, antioxidative, oncostatic, immune regulating, to controlling reproduction including the timing of puberty. In addition to these, its participation in the control of human mood and behavior has attained clinical significance. Deficiencies in melatonin production, or melatonin receptor expression, or changes in its rhythm and amplitude of secretion have been shown to be primary causes in breast cancer; neurodegenerative diseases like Parkinson's disease and Alzheimer's disease; certain neurological disorders seen in children; and conditions like chronic insomnia and circadian rhythm sleep disorders. Melatonin's involvement in neuropsychiatric illnesses like major depressive disorders deserves special attention due to the discovery and use of melatonergic antidepressant agomelatine. Since melatonin has a short half-life, its use as a therapeutic agent for treatment of insomnia has not been successful and has given conflicting results. To overcome this problem, newly developed melatonergic agonist ramelteon with more potency and duration of action has been introduced for treating chronic and primary insomnias, and this has found to be beneficial. With regard to mood disorders, the recently introduced melatonergic antidepressant agomelatine with 5-HT_{2c} antagonism has been found more beneficial, since this drug has rapid onset of action with fewer side effects when compared to other antidepressants that are in clinical use today.

This book, first of its kind, focuses more on the therapeutic use of melatonergic drugs for treating insomnias and depressive disorders and at the same time also presents chapters that discuss melatonin's involvement in important functions of the body like regulation of reproduction, sleep, circadian rhythms, immune function, antioxidative mechanisms, cancer, and jet lag. Much importance has also been given to melatonin's therapeutic application in treating neurodegenerative disorders like Alzheimer's and Parkinson's disease. This book will be useful not only for scientists engaged in melatonin research but also to graduate students, psychopharmacologists, psychiatrists, neurologists, oncologists, and other clinicians treating neurological, psychiatric, and cancer patients.

Acknowledgements

We are immensely indebted to all authors who have contributed for this book despite their busy academic and professional work schedule, whom have greatly helped to complete the book project in time. Similarly the efficient help and constant interactions with the editorial staffs of Springer, particularly Ms. Iris Milagros Ruiz, Developmental Editor of Springer, and Dr. Naren Aggrawal, Executive Editor, Clinical Medicine with Springer India Pvt. Ltd., are deeply appreciated. Without their continuous support and guidance, the book project could not have been completed in time.

Contents

Contributors

Premila Abraham, PhD Department of Biochemistry, Christian Medical College and Hospital, Vellore, TN, India

Dario Acuña-Castroviejo, MD, PhD Department of Physiology, Centro de Investigación Biomédica, Parque de Ciencias de la Salud, Armilla, Granada, Spain

Cecilio Álamo, MD, PhD Department of Pharmacology, Faculty of Medicine, University of Alcalá, Madrid, Spain

Nuria Álvarez-Sánchez, PhD Bioquímica Médica y Biología Molecular-Facultad de Medicina, IBiS/Hospital Universitario Virgen del Rocio/CSIC/Universidad de Sevilla, Seville, Spain

George Anderson, BSc (Hons), MPhil (Cl Psych) CRC, Glasgow, Scotland, UK

Vanessa Andrea Areco Cátedra de Bioquímica y Biología Molecular, Facultad de Ciencias Médicas, Universidad Nacional de Córdoba, Córdoba, Argentina

Maheep Bhatnagar, PhD Department of Zoology, University College of Science, MLSU, Udaipur, Rajasthan, India

Gregory M. Brown, BA, MD, PhD, FRCPC, FRSC Department of Psychiatry, Faculty of Medicine, University of Toronto, Centre for Addiction and Mental Health, Toronto, ON, Canada

Amnon Brzezinski, MD Department of Obstetrics and Gynecology, Hadassah Hebrew-University Medical Center, Jerusalem, Israel

Agata Rita Carpentieri, PhD Cátedra de Bioquímica y Biología Molecular, Facultad de Ciencias Médicas, Cátedra de Química Biológica, Facultad de Odontología, Universidad Nacional de Córdoba, Córdoba, Argentina

Antonio Carrillo-Vico, PhD Bioquímica Médica y Biología Molecular-Facultad de Medicina, IBiS/Hospital Universitario Virgen del Rocio/CSIC/Universidad de Sevilla, Seville, Spain

Marilde Cavuto, MD, BA IASM, L'Aquila, Italy

Reena Chittora, MSc Department of Zoology, University College of Science, MLSU, Udaipur, Rajasthan, India

Bruno Claustrat, PhD Hormone Laboratory, Hospices Civils de Lyon, Bron, France

INSERM, U846 Chronobiology Group, Hospices Civils de Lyon, Bron, France

Samuel Cos Corral, PhD, MD Department of Physiology and Pharmacology, and Research Institute "Marqués de Valdecilla" (IFIMAV), University of Cantabria, Santander, Spain

Gabriela Diaz de Barboza, PhD Cátedra de Bioquímica y Biología Molecular, Facultad de Ciencias Médicas, Universidad Nacional de Córdoba, Córdoba, Argentina

Domenico De Berardis, MD, PhD Department of Mental Health, Psychiatric Service of Diagnosis and Treatment, Hospital "G. Mazzini", Teramo, Italy

Nori Tolosa de Talamoni, PhD Cátedra de Bioquímica y Biología Molecular, Facultad de Ciencias Médicas, Universidad Nacional de Córdoba, Córdoba, Argentina

Massimo Di Giannantonio, MD, PhD Department of Neuroscience and Imaging, "G.D'Annunzio", University of Chieti, Chieti, Italy

Cem Ekmekcioglu, MD Department of Environmental Health, Medical University Vienna, Vienna, Austria

Vural Fidan, MD Department of Otorhinolaryngology, Yunusemre Government Hospital, Eskisehir, Turkey

Michele Fornaro, MD, PhD Department of Education Science, University of Catania, Catania, Italy

Juan M. Guerrero, PhD Bioquímica Médica y Biología Molecular-Facultad de Medicina, IBiS/Hospital Universitario Virgen del Rocio/CSIC/Universidad de Sevilla, Seville, Spain

Rüdiger Hardeland, Dr. rer. nat. Johann Friedrich Blumenbach Institute of Zoology and Anthropology, Göttingen, Lower Saxony, Germany

Asma Hayati Ahmad, MBBS, MSc Department of Physiology, School of Medical Sciences, Universiti Sains Malaysia, Kubang Kerian, Kelantan, Malaysia

Khek-Yu Ho, MBBS (Syd Hons 1), MD (NUS) Department of Gastroenterology and Hepatology, National University Hospital, Singapore, Singapore

Department of Medicine, National University of Singapore, Singapore, Singapore

Bina Isaac, MS Department of Anatomy, Christian Medical College and Hospital, Vellore, TN, India

Ayushi Jain, PhD Department of Zoology, University College of Science, MLSU, Udaipur, Rajasthan, India

Neha Jaiswal, MSc Department of Zoology, University College of Science, MLSU, Udaipur, Rajasthan, India

Onder Karaaslan, MD, FEBOPRAS Plastic, Aesthetic and Reconstructive Surgery Department, Izmir Katip Celebi University, Ataturk Training and Research Hospital, Izmir, Turkey

Hisanori Kato, PhD Organization for Interdisciplinary Research Projects, The University of Tokyo, Tokyo, Japan

Charanjit Kaur, MBBS, PhD Department of Anatomy, Yong Loo Lin School of Medicine, National University of Singapore, Singapore, Singapore

Sidney H. Kennedy, MD, FRCPC Department of Psychiatry, University Health Network, University of Toronto, Toronto, ON, Canada

Preetha Sharone Kuppuswamy, MD Department of Psychiatry and Psychology, Mayo Clinic College of Medicine, Rochester, MN, USA

Patricia J. Lardone, PhD Bioquímica Médica y Biología Molecular-Facultad de Medicina, IBiS/Hospital Universitario Virgen del Rocio/CSIC/Universidad de Sevilla, Seville, Spain

Edward C. Lauterbach, MD Department of Psychiatry and Behavioral Sciences, and the Department of Internal Medicine, Neurology Section, Mercer University School of Medicine, Macon, GA, USA

Paolo Lissoni Department of Medical Oncology, Azienda Ospedaliera San Gerardo, Monza, Italy

Amanda Lochner, MSc, DSc, PhD Division of Medical Physiology, Department of Biomedical Sciences, Faculty of Medicine and Health Sciences, University of Stellenbosch, Tygerberg, Republic of South Africa

Maria Elena Peralta Lopez, PhD Cátedra de Bioquímica y Biología Molecular, Facultad de Ciencias Médicas, Universidad Nacional de Córdoba, Córdoba, Argentina

Francisco López-Muñoz, MD, PhD Faculty of Health Sciences, Camilo José Cela University and Hospital 12 de Octubre Research Institute, Villanueva de la Cañada, Madrid, Spain

Michael Maes, MD, PhD Department of Psychiatry, Chulalongkorn University Hospital, Bangkok, Thailand

Georges Maestroni, PhD Department of Pharmacology, University of Insubria, Medical School, Varese, Italy

Giovanni Martinotti, MD, PhD Department of Neuroscience and Imaging, "G.D'Annunzio", University of Chieti, Chieti, Italy

Gianluigi Mazzoccoli, MD Division of Internal Medicine and Chronobiology Unit, Department of Medical Sciences, IRCCS Scientific Institute AND Regional General Hospital "Casa Sollievo Della Sofferenza" Opera Di Padre Pio Da Pietrelcina, S. Giovanni Rotondo, FG, Italy

Maria D. Mediavilla Aguado, PhD, MD Department of Physiology and Pharmacology, and Research Institute "Marqués de Valdecilla" (IFIMAV), University of Cantabria, Santander, Cantabria, Spain

Mahaneem Mohamed, MD, MSc, PhD Department of Physiology, School of Medical Sciences, Universiti Sains Malaysia, Kubang Kerian, Kelantan, Malaysia

Rozieyati Mohamed Saleh, DPhil School of Heath Sciences, Universiti Sains Malaysia, Kubang Kerian, Kelantan, Malaysia

Frederic Nduhirabandi, B MedSc, B (Hons) Med Bio Sc, MSc MedSc Division of Medical Physiology, Department of Biomedical Sciences, Faculty of Medicine and Health Sciences, University of Stellenbosch, Tygerberg, Republic of South Africa

Sukru Oter, MD, PhD Department of Physiology, Gulhane Military Medical Academy, Ankara, Turkey

Zahiruddin Othman, MD, MMed (Psychiatry) Department of Psychiatry, School of Medical Sciences, Hospital Universiti Sains Malaysia, Kubang Kerian, Kelantan, Malaysia

Timo Partonen, MD, PhD Department of Mental Health and Substance Abuse Services, National Institute for Health and Welfare, Helsinki, Finland

Franca M. Placenza, PhD Department of Psychiatry, University Health Network, Toronto, ON, Canada

Atul Prasad, MBBS, DM (Neurology) Department of Neurology, Dr BL Kapur Superspeciality Hospital, New Delhi, Delhi, India

Maria Angelica Rivoira, PhD Cátedra de Bioquímica y Biología Molecular, Facultad de Ciencias Médicas, Universidad Nacional de Córdoba, Córdoba, Argentina

Ana Rodríguez-Rodríguez, PhD Bioquímica Médica y Biología Molecular-Facultad de Medicina, IBiS/Hospital Universitario Virgen del Rocio/CSIC/Universidad de Sevilla, Seville, Spain

Ruth E. Rosenstein, PhD Department of Human Biochemistry, School of Medicine/CEFyBO, University of Buenos Aires/CONICET, Buenos Aires, Argentina

Emilio J. Sanchez-Barcelo, PhD, MD Department of Physiology and Pharmacology, and Research Institute "Marqués de Valdecilla" (IFIMAV), University of Cantabria, Santander, Cantabria, Spain

Francesco Saverio Moschetta, MD Department of Mental Health, Psychiatric Service of Diagnosis and Treatment, Hospital "G. Mazzini", Teramo, Italy

Nicola Serroni, MD Department of Mental Health, Psychiatric Service of Diagnosis and Treatment, Hospital "G. Mazzini", Teramo, Italy

Chhavi Sharma, MSc Department of Zoology, University College of Science, MLSU, Udaipur, Rajasthan, India

Samuel D. Shillcutt, PharmD, PhD Department of Psychiatry and Behavioral Science, Mercer University School of Medicine, Macon, GA, USA

Jarnail Singh, MBBS, Dip Av Med, MSc(OM), FAMS Department of Civil Aviation Medical Board, Civil Aviation Authority of Singapore, Singapore, Singapore

M.G. Smits, MD, PhD Department of Neurology and Sleep-Wake Disorders, Gelderse Vallei Hospital Ede, Ede, The Netherlands

Mark A. Snitselaar, MD, MSc Department of Mental Health Care, Pro Persona, Ede, The Netherlands

V. Srinivasan, MSc, PhD, MAMS Sri Sathya Sai Medical Educational and Research Foundation, An International Medical Sciences Research Study Center, Coimbatore, TN, India

National Health Service, Department of Mental Health, Psychiatric Service of Diagnosis and Treatment, Hospital "G. Mazzini", Teramo, Italy

Department of Neuroscience and Imaging, University "G.D' Annunzio", Chieti, Italy

U.S. Srinivasan, MBBS, MCh Department of Neurosurgery, Fortis Malar Hospital, Chennai, TN, India

Pooja Suhalka, PhD Department of Zoology, University College of Science, MLSU, Udaipur, Rajasthan, India

Piyu Sukhwal, PhD Department of Zoology, University College of Science, MLSU, Udaipur, Rajasthan, India

Thalhammer Theresia, PhD Department of Pathophysiology and Allergy Research (IPA), AKH, Vienna, Austria

Rahimah Zakaria, MBBS, MSc, PhD (Physiology) Department of Physiology, School of Medical Sciences, Universiti Sains Malaysia, Kubang Kerian, Kelantan, Malaysia

Darius P. Zlotos, PhD Department of Pharmaceutical Chemistry, Faculty of Pharmacy and Biotechnology, The German University in Cairo, New Cairo City, Egypt

Melatonin Receptors and Their Role in Human Diseases

1

Cem Ekmekcioglu and Theresia Thalhammer

Abstract

Melatonin acts mostly through G-protein-coupled plasma membrane receptors. MT_1 and MT_2 are the two functional melatonin membrane receptors. They are expressed in various organs of all mammals, including humans. The functional meaning of the receptors in the various organs is still not sufficiently investigated. This chapter summarizes the currently available data about MT_1 and MT_2 receptors in human tissues and human cells. Established and putative functions of melatonin after receptor activation will be described, and the clinical relevance of these findings will be discussed.

Keywords

Melatonin • Melatonin Receptors • Humans • Localization • Biological role • Diseases

Introduction

By isolating "the pineal gland factor that lightens melanocytes," Lerner et al. began the area of research on melatonin (N-acetyl-5-methoxytryptamine) in 1958 [1]. Indeed, the pineal gland is the major source of this indolamine as melatonin circulating in the body is primarily synthesized there during the night [2]. For the synthesis of melatonin in the pinealocytes, the essential amino acid L-tryptophan is provided by cerebral vessels and converted to serotonin in pineal cells. Afterward serotonin is metabolized by the rate-limiting enzyme arylalkylamine N-acetyltransferase (AA-NAT) to N-acetyl-5-hydroxytryptamine. In the last step, N-acetyl-5-HT is converted to melatonin by hydroxyindole-O-methyltransferase (HIOMT).

Regulation of circadian rhythms and seasonal responses is one major function of melatonin, but several studies further suggest that melatonin has also other functions in the body [3]. It influences the metabolism in various cell

C. Ekmekcioglu, MD (✉)
Department of Environmental Health,
Medical University Vienna, Kinderspitalgasse 15,
Vienna 1090, Austria
e-mail: cem.ekmekcioglu@meduniwien.ac.at

T. Thalhammer, PhD
Department of Pathophysiology and
Allergy Research (IPA), AKH,
Waehringer Guertel 18-20, Vienna A-1090, Austria
e-mail: theresia.thalhammer@meduniwien.ac.at

V. Srinivasan et al. (eds.), *Melatonin and Melatonergic Drugs in Clinical Practice*,
DOI 10.1007/978-81-322-0825-9_1, © Springer India 2014

types and peripheral tissues and contributes to hormonal homeostasis. Some of these functions will be presented and discussed in the chapters below.

Melatonin mediates its effects mostly through binding to G-protein-coupled plasma membrane receptors. Additionally, strong anti-oxidative effects of melatonin were demonstrated in many studies [4–8]. There is evidence that some cell- and tissue-protective functions of melatonin are mediated by an induction of anti-inflammatory genes, which are under the transcriptional regulation of redox-sensitive elements including AP-1 and NF-kappa B, and other cell redox sensors such as Nrf2/keap1 (reviewed in [9]).

Other studies showed that melatonin interacts with calmodulin or calreticulin; both are involved in intracellular signal transduction. For example, melatonin was shown to antagonize the binding of Ca^{2+} to calmodulin [10]. Thereby, it may influence tumor progression. For example, possible antiproliferative effects of melatonin on breast cancer cell proliferation may be partly mediated through this action [11].

Also, few studies suggest that melatonin could mediate its effects through nuclear transcription factors. From the nuclear receptor family, the retinoid-related orphan nuclear hormone receptor family (RZR/ROR) was suggested as melatonin target. Immunomodulatory effects and possible also part of the circadian effects may be mediated through this mechanism [12–14]. Melatonin was also shown to bind to a member of the basic helix-loop-helix transcription factors, the aryl hydrocarbon receptor (AhR), the signaling of which is also implicated in the regulation of circadian rhythms [15, 16].

This chapter discusses the plasma membrane-associated melatonin receptors and their role in humans (reviewed in [17–22]). Peripheral localization sites for the two known mammalian melatonin receptors, MT_1 and MT_2, in the human body were published by our group since 1999 [23–31]. We will summarize the data about these localization sites in human tissues and also address the biological role and clinical relevance of the melatonin receptors.

Pharmacology and Signal Transduction

Two different classes of human plasma membrane-localized melatonin receptors are known. These are designated as MT_1 (formerly Mel_{1a}, encoded by MTNR1A gene) and MT2 (Mel_{1b}, encoded by the MTNR1B gene), respectively [19, 32]. Both types of receptors were found in various organs with different expression profiles.

In general cloned melatonin receptors bind 2[125I]-melatonin at picomolar affinity. Several agonists and antagonists for melatonin receptors have been described [20, 33–36]. The best known agents are luzindole and 4-PDOT, which are especially used to demonstrate MT_2 receptor activity.

MT_1 and MT_2 receptor are coupled to similar and different signal transduction pathways. Expression of the cloned MT_1 receptors in various different cell lines, like NIH-3T3, HEK and CHO cell lines, provided evidence that these receptors are especially linked to the inhibition of cAMP via pertussis toxin-sensitive inhibitory Gi proteins. Interactions with several G proteins were described so far (reviewed in [18, 37]). MT_1 receptor activation results in a depression of forskolin-stimulated cAMP formation and inhibition of PKA activity and phosphorylation of the cAMP-responsive element-binding protein (reviewed in [20]). This signal pathway seems to lead to phase shifts of the endogenous clock [38]. Important for the prevention of cancer cell growth, via activation of MT_1 receptor, melatonin blocks the MAPK/ERK pathway in many cancer cells [39]. Additionally, it was shown to inhibit breast cancer cell proliferation, because it prevents the uptake of linoleic acid, which is metabolized to the mitogenic signaling molecule 13-hydroxyoctadecadienoic acid (13-HODE) [40].

MT_1 activation induces prostaglandin F2alpha-induced phosphoinositide turnover [41, 42] and also regulates effects of melatonin on ion channels, like calcium-activated potassium channels, which may be involved in melatonin-induced vasoconstriction of rat arteries [43]. Also activation of the inward rectifier potassium channel KIR3 was described to be induced by MT_1 activation [44].

The MT_2 receptor is also coupled to inhibition of forskolin-stimulated cAMP formation [45]. Additionally, activation of this receptor can lead to inhibition of cGMP formation [46] or, in the SCN, to an increase in PKC activity [47].

Worth to mention is the fact that both MT_1 and MT_2 can form homo- and heterodimers [48, 49]. However, the functional effects of the different receptor dimeric species are unclear.

In addition to these MT receptors, another putative MT_3 receptor was identified. It shows lower melatonin affinity in various hamster organs [50] and has a 95 % homology to the human quinone reductase 2, a cytosolic enzyme that catalyzes the reduction of quinones, such as menadione and coenzyme Q [51, 52]. Very little is known about the functions of the MT_3 receptor in different organs. It may contribute to the regulation of intraocular pressure, as shown in rabbits [53].

Finally, there also exists a melatonin-related receptor (GPR50) in mammalians, including humans. This receptor is however incapable of binding melatonin [54]. GPR50 may be involved in MT_1 (but not MT_2)-mediated signal transduction [55].

The existence of MT_1- and MT_2-deficient mice is a valuable tool for studying the function of melatonin receptors in various tissues [56, 57]. In the next sections, we briefly summarize localization sites of MT receptors in various organ systems of humans and discuss putative functional roles of melatonin.

Central Nervous System and the Eye

SCN

The master clock in the SCN controls many functions in the peripheral organs [58]. Melatonin cooperates with the SCN probably in two ways, firstly by resetting feedback signals to the SCN and secondly as an output mediator of the SCN transmitting the informations of the master clock to the periphery [59]. Here, on the cellular level, clock genes act as an integral part of the circadian system [60] influencing the expression of many genes [61]. Melatonin was shown to affect the expression of clock genes [28, 62].

Weaver and Reppert were the first to show the expression of the MT_1 receptor subtype in the SCN of humans [63]. The function of melatonin in the SCN has been described in several rodent studies. It is assumed that melatonin is an endogenous synchronizer [64] providing the SCN with the information about the night. Timed release of pineal melatonin therefore adjusts to organism the light/dark cycle. In rats it is able to stabilize circadian rhythms, reinforce them, and maintain their mutual phase relationship. Furthermore melatonin is able to entrain free-running activities in rodents [65].

Several studies in humans showed that phase shifts of major physiological parameters, such as endogenous melatonin, core temperature, and sleep timing, are present after melatonin administration. Phase delays are observed after morning administration, whereas phase advances occur after evening administration [66]. Therefore, timed intake of melatonin can facilitate the readjustment after acute phase shifts of the light–dark schedule such as in jet lag [67]. Finally, melatonin supplementation was shown to entrain free-running circadian rhythms in blind people [68].

In this context melatonin has been described to exert sleep-promoting effects, although this topic remains controversial in the scientific literature [69–71]. One reason is the short half-life of melatonin in the range of 20–40 min [69]. The MT_1 and MT_2 receptor agonist ramelteon [72] has been shown to exert sleep-promoting effects in individuals with chronic and transient insomnia (reviewed in [69]).

Furthermore, there may be an association between melatonin, melatonin receptors, and psychiatric diseases like depression. For example, a recent postmortem study showed that MT_1 receptors seemed to be highly expressed in the SCN of depressed patients. It was speculated that the number of receptors may increase with the progression of the disease [73].

Regarding depression it should be mentioned that some years ago, agomelatine, an MT_1/MT_2 agonist and 5-hydroxytryptamine 2C (5-HT2C) receptor antagonist, was introduced as a new therapeutic possibility in the treatment of depression [74, 75]. Several clinical studies showed that agomelatine improves both depressive symptoms and sleep disorders in this disease (reviewed in [74]).

Hippocampus

Both types of MT receptors are especially expressed in pyramidal neurons [76, 77], and mice studies suggested that melatonin modulates the activity of hippocampal neurons [78, 79]. Studies in Alzheimer patients showed a modulated expression of both types of melatonin receptors, with reduced levels of the MT_2 subtype and an enhanced MT_1 expression [76, 77]. The reason may be either a compensatory increase of MT_1 and/or disturbed MT_2 expression, due to Alzheimer disease-related neurodegeneration. It should also be mentioned that the antioxidative effects of melatonin can protect neurons against amyloid-β-induced neuropathology in Alzheimer disease [80].

Hippocampal MT receptors are possibly also involved in epileptic processes, and melatonin may possibly exert anticonvulsant actions. In children, for example, pharmacological doses of melatonin lead to a decrease in the severity and/or frequency of epileptiform activity [81]. Furthermore rat studies showed that pinealectomy favors epileptogenic processes that follow the long-lasting status epilepticus [82] and intra-hippocampal application of 4-PDOT, an MT_2 receptor antagonist, can exert anticonvulsant effects in rats with pilocarpine-induced seizures [83]. The putative anti-epileptic function of melatonin has been linked to a potentiation of gamma-aminobutyric acid (GABA) transmission by melatonin [59].

Central Dopaminergic System

The MT_1 receptor is expressed in the areas related to dopaminergic behavior, including the Brodmann area 10 (i.e., prefrontal cortex), putamen, substantia nigra, amygdala, and hippocampus [84]. The dopaminergic system is important for movement and psychological factors, such as reward, as well as for producing the reinforcing actions of drugs of abuse, like cocaine. For example, it was demonstrated that application of melatonin can block the development of cocaine-induced behavioral sensitizations, such as anxiety during cocaine withdrawal [85]. Furthermore, it was shown that in patients with Parkinson's disease, MT_1 and MT_2 levels are reduced in the substantia nigra and amygdala [86]. In addition, also other brain areas were shown to express melatonin receptors (reviewed in [59]).

Retina

Both types of MT receptors were identified in various cell types in the human retina [45, 87]. Additionally it is well established that melatonin is synthesized by primarily photoreceptor cells in most vertebrate species, including humans (reviewed in [88, 89]) and mainly released in the night. The function of melatonin in the retina is to regulate physiological adaptions to low light intensities. Furthermore, MT_1 and MT_2 are expressed on dopaminergic neurons in the retina where melatonin seems to exert an antagonistic action with dopamine, whose release is stimulated by light. Dopamine seems to mediate adaptions of light adaptation and circadian changes in visual sensitivity [90]. The mutual inhibition between dopamine and melatonin may be responsible for retinal adaptive processes to changes in light intensities.

Melatonin has been implicated in the modulation of intraocular pressure (IOP) [89, 91]. Therefore, melatonin or melatonin analogs are discussed to be useful in the treatment of glaucoma [92, 93]. In rabbits, topical application of melatonin or the melatonin analog 5-methoxycarbonylamino-N-acetyltryptamine (5-MCA-NAT) results in a reduction in intraocular pressure. In contrast, luzindole, an MT_1 and MT_2 receptor antagonist, abolishes the effect of both agents, which could suggest a role for MT_1

or MT_2 in the regulation of intraocular pressure [94]. In humans, oral melatonin causes some decrease in intraocular pressure in patients undergoing cataract surgery [95].

Cardiovascular System

We showed the expression of MT_1 and MT_2 receptors in left human ventricle specimens [26, 27]. The role of melatonin in human ventricular function is rather unclear. In isolated rat papillary muscle, it induces anti-adrenergic effects leading to a reduction of contractility increase [96]. Additionally, melatonin can antagonize isoproterenol-stimulated cAMP production in primary heart cell cultures [97] and also stimulate high-voltage-activated calcium currents in embryonic heart cells [98].

Evidence for melatonin receptors in vascular tissue through the use of 2-[125I] iodomelatonin binding was presented [99]. In line with these findings, we described localization of MT_1 and MT_2 receptors in human coronary arteries from pathological samples and also from healthy controls [25–27]. Furthermore we showed preliminary evidence for a circadian variation of the MT_1 receptor in coronary arteries on the protein level [26]. More studies are necessary to explore the role of melatonin in human coronary arteries. In porcine coronary arteries, melatonin mediated vasoconstriction by inhibition of NO effects and potentiation of serotonin effects [100]. Vasoconstriction could increase vasodilatatory capacities as it was shown for cerebral arteries [101]. However, relating to animal studies, it seems that melatonin can have receptor-dependent divergent effects on the vasculature [102], with vasoconstriction after MT_1 and vasorelaxation after MT_2 activation.

Our group showed that MT_1 and MT_2 are expressed in the human aorta at mRNA level [25, 27], while only MT_1 was found in the rat aorta [103].

We suggest that melatonin has vasodilatatory effects in the aorta. This was, for example, shown in aortic rings from rat and rabbits [104], an effect which is endothelium dependent and most likely mediated by NO, potentiation of acetylcholine effects, and/or inhibition of noradrenaline effects [105].

Application of melatonin during the day decreases core body temperature in humans by selective vasodilatation in distal body regions and induction of sleepiness [106, 107]. Furthermore, intravenous administration of melatonin leads to an increase in peripheral blood flow [108]. In a recent intervention trial, it was shown that melatonin differentially affects vascular blood flow in humans with a decline in renal blood flow velocity and renal vascular conductance and increase of forearm blood flow and forearm vascular conductance after per oral application of 3 mg melatonin compared with placebo [109].

Furthermore several studies provided evidence that melatonin can reduce blood pressure in humans. In healthy men [110] and postmenopausal women with hormone replacement therapy, for example [111], 1 mg melatonin orally given led to approx. Reduction in mean arterial pressure after 90 min. Furthermore norepinephrine levels were reduced.

The antihypertensive effects of melatonin may derive from a decrease in peripheral resistance through vasodilatation. Additionally, possible negative inotropic effects may be a further mechanism since cardiac ventricles also express MT receptors.

Hormone-Sensitive Organs

Prostate

MT receptors were identified in benign and malignant prostate epithelial cells [112–114]. Through especially MT_1 receptors but also partly attenuation of sex steroid-induced calcium influx, melatonin inhibits proliferation of human prostate cancer cells [115, 116]. In addition the MT_1 receptor was also identified in one patient with metastatic prostate cancer, and a timely daily treatment of the patient with 5 mg MEL stabilized PSA (prostate-specific antigen) levels for 6 weeks [117].

Female Breast

There is increasing evidence for an association between chronic light exposure in the night and the risk of cancer [118], and epidemiological studies suggest that especially night and rotating female shift workers may have an increased breast cancer risk [118–120]. A suppressed secretion of melatonin may play a role [118].

Regarding melatonin binding sites, the MT_1 receptor was identified in normal and malignant breast tissue [29, 30, 121] and in breast cancer cells (MCF-7) [122].

The pathways of the MT_1 receptor and the estrogen receptor seem to interact in breast cancer [123]. The MT_1 expression is downregulated by estradiol and melatonin as studies in MCF-7 cells showed. Additionally, the expression of the MT_1 receptor is upregulated in MDA-MB-231 cells, which are estrogen receptor-negative, and downregulated in the estrogen receptor-positive cell line MCF-7 [124].

Several papers provided convincing evidence that melatonin inhibits proliferation of estrogen-dependent human-breast-cancer cells (MCF-7) in vitro (reviewed in [11]). A significant antiproliferative effect was especially seen in MCF-7 cells transfected with the MT_1 receptor [125]. The mechanisms underlying these anticancer effects of melatonin in breast cancer may be manifold: (1) inhibition of the expression of estrogen receptor alpha (ER alpha) and/or (2) inhibition of binding of the E2-ER complex to the estrogen-responsive element on the DNA. Furthermore inhibitory effects of melatonin on calmodulin, which can phosphorylate ER alpha thus facilitating the binding of estrogen, may also apply. In a phase II study, it was, for example, shown that melatonin and tamoxifen induced visible tumor regression compared to tamoxifen alone [126].

Myometrium

The uterus shows circadian rhythms of contractility and electrical activities [127]. Also, maximal birth rates can be found during the night where secretion of melatonin is highest [128]. Both types of the melatonin receptors were found in human myocytes from nonpregnant (after hysterectomy) and pregnant women undergoing cesarean section [129]. The role of melatonin in the uterus is unclear; both inhibitory [130] and stimulatory [131, 132] effects of melatonin on the tone of the myometrium have been suggested, in animal or human studies, respectively. These differences could derive from differences in daytime/nighttime activity profiles between rats and humans.

Administration of melatonin and progesterone to women leads to a decrease in LH secretion, blockage of ovulation, and the luteal phase increase in progesterone, without influencing FSH or inhibiting estradiol synthesis [133]. Suppressive effects on LH levels were also detected in men with a negative correlation between inhibin and the LH/testosterone ratio [134]. The mechanisms may be a modulation of hypothalamic gonadotropin release [135] or may be also direct effects of melatonin on granulosa cells in the ovary [136], since both types of melatonin receptors are present in human granulosa cells [137]. Melatonin was shown to upregulate LH mRNA receptor expression [137], enhance hCG-stimulated progesterone secretion, and inhibit GnRH and GnRH receptor expression. Since LH is essential for the initiation of luteinization and GnRH is suggested to be involved in the regression of corpus luteum [138], melatonin may be involved in the maintenance of the corpus luteum during pregnancy.

Gastrointestinal and Hepatobiliary Systems

In the gastrointestinal tract, melatonin is locally produced in enterochromaffine cells [139], with considerable differences in regional distribution. The highest levels were detected in the rectum and the colon and the lowest levels in the jejunum and the ileum [140, 141].

Additionally, also the bile may contain high levels of melatonin which considerably exceed those in plasma [142]. We presented evidence for the presence of the MT_1 receptor in the epithelia of cholelithiasis and gallbladder carcinoma samples [23]. Preliminary results suggest that in gallbladder carcinoma, MT_1 receptor seemed to be less pronounced. The functional role of melatonin in the gallbladder is not really known. Melatonin can modulate gastrointestinal ion transport processes and motility [143], interfere with cholecystokinin-induced changes of ileal motility [144], and modulate nitric oxide signaling [145]. These effects could point to an effect of melatonin on gallbladder contraction.

Previously, Sjöblom et al. were able to demonstrate that melatonin influences HCO_3^- secretion from the duodenal mucosa [146, 147]. HCO_3^- is important to neutralize hydrochloric acid from the stomach. The release of HCO_3^- was inhibited by luzindole suggesting that the MT_2 receptor subtype was involved [148]. Additional studies described that melatonin stimulated the release of intracellular calcium in the enterocytes, which leads to the activation of the apical electroneutral HCO_3^-/Cl^- exchange [149]. Furthermore, melatonin was shown to increase pancreatic secretion of amylase and cholecystokinin by activation of MT_2 receptors [150]. Finally, melatonin seems to exert preventive or therapeutic effects against gastric ulcers, respectively [151–153].

Skin

Both key enzymes of melatonin synthesis, AA-NAT and HIOMT, were detected in normal and pathological skin including various skin cells, such as keratinocytes, fibroblasts, melanocytes, melanoma cell lines, and squamous cell carcinoma cells [154]. MT_1 seems to be the major melatonin receptor in the human skin [155]. The MT_2 receptor was detected in neonatal keratinocytes, one melanoma cell line, and especially normal and malignant uveal melanocytes [156]. Furthermore MT_2 receptor expression has been found in the inner root sheath, eccrine sweat gland, and blood vessel endothelium [49].

Melatonin was shown to inhibit cell proliferation in cutaneous melanoma cells. This is also true for normal and malignant uveal melanocytes [157, 158], but it has no significant effects on the proliferation of dermal fibroblasts [155]. It should also be mentioned that melatonin, through its antioxidative mechanism, exerted protective effects on UVB-induced damage in dermal fibroblasts and epidermal keratinocytes (reviewed in [159]). However, clinical studies indicated that melatonin is able to prevent sun damage only when it is administrated before UV irradiation [160].

Furthermore, few interventional trials suggest that melatonin can affect hair growth [49]. In a pilot study in women suffering from androgenic alopecia, it was shown that melatonin caused increased hair growth in patients with androgenetic alopecia. However, no effect was seen in patients with diffuse alopecia [161].

Immune System

Melatonin is important for a proper function of the immune system [162]. It is, for example, synthesized by various leukocytes and leukocyte-derived cell lines [59, 162]. In one of the first studies in this field, it was shown that pinealectomy leads to a depression in the immune system [163]. Other studies came to similar results that suppression of melatonin production was associated with compromised humoral and cellular immunological responses in mice [49].

Melatonin seems to especially modulate the synthesis and the secretion of cytokines [164, 165]. For example, melatonin increases T-helper cell activity and IL-2 production in human lymphocytes [166] and activates human monocytes by inducing cellular cytotoxic agents, such as interleukins and TNF-alpha [167]. In general, melatonin exerts its effects on the immune system through its antioxidative potential; modulation of mediators, such as endogenous opioids, cytokines, hormones, and zinc; and also receptor-mediated effects. The MT_1 receptor and also the nuclear binding sites RZR/ROR alpha were found in various immune cells of humans [168] and in the mouse immune system (MT_1, MT_2) [169]. Blockage of the receptors in human lymphocytes leads, for example, to a drop of IL-2 and IL-2 receptor production [12]. Other immunomodulatory, pro-inflammatory, but also anti-inflammatory effects of melatonin in the immune system were described in several studies (reviewed in [59, 164]).

Metabolism

Melatonin is known to affect energy expenditure and body mass regulation in mammals by, for example, modulation of the activation of fat mass or brown adipose tissue in different mammalian species [170–172]. In rats, daily oral supplementation of melatonin reduced visceral adiposity and body weight (reviewed in [173]). Also in animal models of diet-induced obesity, melatonin showed beneficial effects on body weight and metabolic parameters [174–176]. Similarly in patients with metabolic syndrome, administration of 5 mg melatonin per day reduced body mass index, systolic blood pressure (SBP), and levels of fibrinogen and thiobarbituric acid-reactive substances (TBARS) in plasma [177].

MT_1 and MT_2 receptors are expressed in the immortalized human brown adipocyte cell line, PAZ6 cells, and in white and brown adipose tissue [178]. Chronic treatment of PAZ6 adipocytes with melatonin resulted in a specific decline in GLUT4 protein levels and glucose uptake with other adipocyte marker genes (UCP1-2, PPAR-gamma, leptin, lipase) being not affected. GLUT4 mediates the uptake of glucose by insulin in fat and muscle cells with overexpression of GLUT4 leading to an increase in fat cell number and body lipids. The effects of melatonin in this adipocyte cell line were suggested to be through MT_2 receptors [46].

Both melatonin receptors are expressed in the islet of Langerhans and are involved in the modulation of insulin secretion from β-cells and in glucagon secretion from α-cells [179]. Application of melatonin decreases insulin secretion [179] possibly through downregulation of adenylate or guanylate cyclase activities, leading to reduced second messenger levels [179]. Also, long-term enteral administration of melatonin reduces plasma insulin levels. The expression of pineal insulin receptors in both healthy Wistar rats, as well as type 2 diabetic Goto-Kakizaki (GK) rats is induced [180].

Based on several experimental investigations, recent studies suggest that common genetic variations in or near the MT_2 receptor influence blood glucose and also the risk of type 2 diabetes in humans [181–183]. Furthermore, a recent meta-analysis demonstrated that the rs10830963 polymorphism on MT_2 is a risk factor for developing impaired glucose regulation and type 2 diabetes [184].

Conclusion

During the last decades, the scientific work on melatonin has increased exponentially. Many functions have been claimed for this antioxidative indolamine, including effects on circadian rhythms and sleep regulation but also, for example, on the immune system and inflammation, blood pressure, cancer, pain perception, and on blood glucose/insulin secretion and mood, which are of special clinical relevance. Many of these functions are mediated through G-protein-coupled melatonin receptors MT_1 and/or MT_2, while others are mediated via activation of different transcription factors and/or by binding to intracellular proteins. The G-protein-coupled receptors are found (almost) everywhere in the human body and open new therapeutic options with novel melatonin derivatives, e.g., agomelatine. For example, depression may be treated with this homolog [185]. Furthermore, genetic polymorphisms of MT receptors and their relation to various diseases, as, for example, for diabetes, will gain more relevance in the next years.

References

1. Lerner AB, Case JD, Takahashi Y, Lee TH, Mori W. Isolation of melatonin, a pineal factor that lightens melanocytes. J Am Chem Soc. 1958;80:2057–8.
2. Claustrat B, Brun J, Chazot G. The basic physiology and pathophysiology of melatonin. Sleep Med Rev. 2005;9(1):11–24.
3. Reiter RJ. Pineal melatonin: cell biology of its synthesis and of its physiological interactions. Endocr Rev. 1991;12(2):151–80.
4. Allegra M, Reiter RJ, Tan DX, Gentile C, Tesoriere L, Livrea MA. The chemistry of melatonin's interaction with reactive species. J Pineal Res. 2003;34(1):1–10.

5. Macchi MM, Bruce JN. Human pineal physiology and functional significance of melatonin. Front Neuroendocrinol. 2004;25(3–4):177–95.
6. Reiter RJ, Tan DX, Gitto E, Sainz RM, Mayo JC, Leon J, et al. Pharmacological utility of melatonin in reducing oxidative cellular and molecular damage. Pol J Pharmacol. 2004;56(2):159–70.
7. Rodriguez C, Mayo JC, Sainz RM, Antolin I, Herrera F, Martin V, et al. Regulation of antioxidant enzymes: a significant role for melatonin. J Pineal Res. 2004;36(1):1–9.
8. Tan DX, Manchester LC, Hardeland R, Lopez-Burillo S, Mayo JC, Sainz RM, et al. Melatonin: a hormone, a tissue factor, an autocoid, a paracoid, and an antioxidant vitamin. J Pineal Res. 2003;34(1):75–8.
9. Luchetti F, Canonico B, Betti M, Arcangeletti M, Pilolli F, Piroddi M, et al. Melatonin signaling and cell protection function. FASEB J. 2010;24(10):3603–24.
10. Benitez-King G, Anton-Tay F. Calmodulin mediates melatonin cytoskeletal effects. Experientia. 1993;49(8):635–41.
11. Sanchez-Barcelo EJ, Cos S, Mediavilla D, Martinez-Campa C, Gonzalez A, Alonso-Gonzalez C. Melatonin-estrogen interactions in breast cancer. J Pineal Res. 2005;38(4):217–22.
12. Carrillo-Vico A, Lardone PJ, Fernandez-Santos JM, Martin-Lacave I, Calvo JR, Karasek M, et al. Human lymphocyte-synthesized melatonin is involved in the regulation of the interleukin-2/interleukin-2 receptor system. J Clin Endocrinol Metab. 2005;90(2):992–1000.
13. Garcia-Maurino S, Gonzalez-Haba MG, Calvo JR, Goberna R, Guerrero JM. Involvement of nuclear binding sites for melatonin in the regulation of IL-2 and IL-6 production by human blood mononuclear cells. J Neuroimmunol. 1998;92(1–2):76–84.
14. Steinhilber D, Brungs M, Werz O, Wiesenberg I, Danielsson C, Kahlen JP, et al. The nuclear receptor for melatonin represses 5-lipoxygenase gene expression in human B lymphocytes. J Biol Chem. 1995;270(13):7037–40.
15. Abel J, Haarmann-Stemmann T. An introduction to the molecular basics of aryl hydrocarbon receptor biology. Biol Chem. 2010;391(11):1235–48.
16. Shimba S, Watabe Y. Crosstalk between the AHR signaling pathway and circadian rhythm. Biochem Pharmacol. 2009;77(4):560–5.
17. Anisimov SV, Popovic N. Genetic aspects of melatonin biology. Rev Neurosci. 2004;15(3):209–30.
18. Barrett P, Conway S, Morgan PJ. Digging deep – structure-function relationships in the melatonin receptor family. J Pineal Res. 2003;35(4):221–30.
19. Dubocovich ML, Rivera-Bermudez MA, Gerdin MJ, Masana MI. Molecular pharmacology, regulation and function of mammalian melatonin receptors. Front Biosci. 2003;8:d1093–108.
20. Masana MI, Dubocovich ML. Melatonin receptor signaling: finding the path through the dark. Sci STKE. 2001;2001(107):E39.
21. von Gall C, Stehle JH, Weaver DR. Mammalian melatonin receptors: molecular biology and signal transduction. Cell Tissue Res. 2002;309(1):151–62.
22. Witt-Enderby PA, Bennett J, Jarzynka MJ, Firestine S, Melan MA. Melatonin receptors and their regulation: biochemical and structural mechanisms. Life Sci. 2003;72(20):2183–98.
23. Aust S, Thalhammer T, Humpeler S, Jager W, Klimpfinger M, Tucek G, et al. The melatonin receptor subtype MT1 is expressed in human gallbladder epithelia. J Pineal Res. 2004;36(1):43–8.
24. Ekmekcioglu C. Melatonin receptors in humans: biological role and clinical relevance. Biomed Pharmacother. 2006;60(3):97–108.
25. Ekmekcioglu C, Haslmayer P, Philipp C, Mehrabi MR, Glogar HD, Grimm M, et al. Expression of the MT1 melatonin receptor subtype in human coronary arteries. J Recept Signal Transduct Res. 2001;21(1):85–91.
26. Ekmekcioglu C, Haslmayer P, Philipp C, Mehrabi MR, Glogar HD, Grimm M, et al. 24 h variation in the expression of the mt1 melatonin receptor subtype in coronary arteries derived from patients with coronary heart disease. Chronobiol Int. 2001;18(6):973–85.
27. Ekmekcioglu C, Thalhammer T, Humpeler S, Mehrabi MR, Glogar HD, Holzenbein T, et al. The melatonin receptor subtype MT2 is present in the human cardiovascular system. J Pineal Res. 2003;35(1):40–4.
28. Nemeth C, Humpeler S, Kallay E, Mesteri I, Svoboda M, Rogelsperger O, et al. Decreased expression of the melatonin receptor 1 in human colorectal adenocarcinomas. J Biol Regul Homeost Agents. 2011;25(4):531–42.
29. Rogelsperger O, Ekmekcioglu C, Jager W, Klimpfinger M, Konigsberg R, Krenbek D, et al. Coexpression of the melatonin receptor 1 and nestin in human breast cancer specimens. J Pineal Res. 2009;46(4):422–32.
30. Rogelsperger O, Wlcek K, Ekmekcioglu C, Humpeler S, Svoboda M, Konigsberg R, et al. Melatonin receptors, melatonin metabolizing enzymes and cyclin D1 in human breast cancer. J Recept Signal Transduct Res. 2011;31(2):180–7.
31. Toma CD, Svoboda M, Arrich F, Ekmekcioglu C, Assadian O, Thalhammer T. Expression of the melatonin receptor (MT) 1 in benign and malignant human bone tumors. J Pineal Res. 2007;43(2):206–13.
32. Dubocovich ML, Delagrange P, Krause DN, Sugden D, Cardinali DP, Olcese J. International Union of Basic and Clinical Pharmacology. LXXV. Nomenclature, classification, and pharmacology of G protein-coupled melatonin receptors. Pharmacol Rev. 2010;62(3):343–80.
33. Delagrange P, Atkinson J, Boutin JA, Casteilla L, Lesieur D, Misslin R, et al. Therapeutic perspectives for melatonin agonists and antagonists. J Neuroendocrinol. 2003;15(4):442–8.
34. Tarzia G, Diamantini G, Mor M, Spadoni G. Design and synthesis of melatonin receptors agonists and antagonists. Farmaco. 2000;55(3):184–7.

35. Witt-Enderby PA, Li PK. Melatonin receptors and ligands. Vitam Horm. 2000;58:321–54.
36. Zlotos DP. Recent advances in melatonin receptor ligands. Arch Pharm (Weinheim). 2005;338(5–6): 229–47.
37. New DC, Tsim ST, Wong YH. G protein-linked effector and second messenger systems involved in melatonin signal transduction. Neurosignals. 2003; 12(2):59–70.
38. von Gall C, Weaver DR, Kock M, Korf HW, Stehle JH. Melatonin limits transcriptional impact of phosphoCREB in the mouse SCN via the Mel1a receptor. Neuroreport. 2000;11(9):1803–7.
39. Witt-Enderby PA, MacKenzie RS, McKeon RM, Carroll EA, Bordt SL, Melan MA. Melatonin induction of filamentous structures in non-neuronal cells that is dependent on expression of the human mt1 melatonin receptor. Cell Motil Cytoskeleton. 2000;46(1):28–42.
40. Hill SM, Blask DE, Xiang S, Yuan L, Mao L, Dauchy RT, et al. Melatonin and associated signaling pathways that control normal breast epithelium and breast cancer. J Mammary Gland Biol Neoplasia. 2011;16(3):235–45.
41. Godson C, Reppert SM. The Mel1a melatonin receptor is coupled to parallel signal transduction pathways. Endocrinology. 1997;138(1):397–404.
42. Roka F, Brydon L, Waldhoer M, Strosberg AD, Freissmuth M, Jockers R, et al. Tight association of the human Mel(1a)-melatonin receptor and G(i): precoupling and constitutive activity. Mol Pharmacol. 1999;56(5):1014–24.
43. Geary GG, Duckles SP, Krause DN. Effect of melatonin in the rat tail artery: role of K+ channels and endothelial factors. Br J Pharmacol. 1998;123(8): 1533–40.
44. Jiang ZG, Nelson CS, Allen CN. Melatonin activates an outward current and inhibits Ih in rat suprachiasmatic nucleus neurons. Brain Res. 1995;687(1–2): 125–32.
45. Reppert SM, Godson C, Mahle CD, Weaver DR, Slaugenhaupt SA, Gusella JF. Molecular characterization of a second melatonin receptor expressed in human retina and brain: the Mel1b melatonin receptor. Proc Natl Acad Sci U S A. 1995;92(19): 8734–8.
46. Petit L, Lacroix I, de Coppet P, Strosberg AD, Jockers R. Differential signaling of human Mel1a and Mel1b melatonin receptors through the cyclic guanosine 3′-5′-monophosphate pathway. Biochem Pharmacol. 1999;58(4):633–9.
47. Hunt AE, Al-Ghoul WM, Gillette MU, Dubocovich ML. Activation of MT(2) melatonin receptors in rat suprachiasmatic nucleus phase advances the circadian clock. Am J Physiol Cell Physiol. 2001;280(1): C110–8.
48. Ayoub MA, Couturier C, Lucas-Meunier E, Angers S, Fossier P, Bouvier M, et al. Monitoring of ligand-independent dimerization and ligand-induced conformational changes of melatonin receptors in living cells by bioluminescence resonance energy transfer. J Biol Chem. 2002;277(24):21522–8.
49. Slominski RM, Reiter RJ, Schlabritz-Loutsevitch N, Ostrom RS, Slominski AT. Melatonin membrane receptors in peripheral tissues: distribution and functions. Mol Cell Endocrinol. 2012;351(2):152–66.
50. Paul P, Lahaye C, Delagrange P, Nicolas JP, Canet E, Boutin JA. Characterization of 2-[125I]iodomelatonin binding sites in Syrian hamster peripheral organs. J Pharmacol Exp Ther. 1999;290(1):334–40.
51. Mailliet F, Ferry G, Vella F, Thiam K, Delagrange P, Boutin JA. Organs from mice deleted for NRH:quinone oxidoreductase 2 are deprived of the melatonin binding site MT3. FEBS Lett. 2004;578(1–2):116–20.
52. Nosjean O, Ferro M, Coge F, Beauverger P, Henlin JM, Lefoulon F, et al. Identification of the melatonin-binding site MT3 as the quinone reductase 2. J Biol Chem. 2000;275(40):31311–7.
53. Pintor J, Pelaez T, Hoyle CH, Peral A. Ocular hypotensive effects of melatonin receptor agonists in the rabbit: further evidence for an MT3 receptor. Br J Pharmacol. 2003;138(5):831–6.
54. Reppert SM, Weaver DR, Ebisawa T, Mahle CD, Kolakowski Jr LF. Cloning of a melatonin-related receptor from human pituitary. FEBS Lett. 1996;386(2–3):219–24.
55. Levoye A, Dam J, Ayoub MA, Guillaume JL, Couturier C, Delagrange P, et al. The orphan GPR50 receptor specifically inhibits MT1 melatonin receptor function through heterodimerization. EMBO J. 2006;25(13):3012–23.
56. Jin X, von Gall C, Pieschl RL, Gribkoff VK, Stehle JH, Reppert SM, et al. Targeted disruption of the mouse Mel(1b) melatonin receptor. Mol Cell Biol. 2003;23(3):1054–60.
57. Liu C, Weaver DR, Jin X, Shearman LP, Pieschl RL, Gribkoff VK, et al. Molecular dissection of two distinct actions of melatonin on the suprachiasmatic circadian clock. Neuron. 1997;19(1):91–102.
58. Dibner C, Schibler U, Albrecht U. The mammalian circadian timing system: organization and coordination of central and peripheral clocks. Annu Rev Physiol. 2010;72:517–49.
59. Hardeland R, Cardinali DP, Srinivasan V, Spence DW, Brown GM, Pandi-Perumal SR. Melatonin – a pleiotropic, orchestrating regulator molecule. Prog Neurobiol. 2011;93(3):350–84.
60. Maywood ES, O'Neill J, Wong GK, Reddy AB, Hastings MH. Circadian timing in health and disease. Prog Brain Res. 2006;153:253–69.
61. Okamura H, Doi M, Fustin JM, Yamaguchi Y, Matsuo M. Mammalian circadian clock system: molecular mechanisms for pharmaceutical and medical sciences. Adv Drug Deliv Rev. 2010;62(9–10):876–84.
62. Imbesi M, Arslan AD, Yildiz S, Sharma R, Gavin D, Tun N, et al. The melatonin receptor MT1 is required for the differential regulatory actions of melatonin on neuronal 'clock' gene expression in striatal neurons in vitro. J Pineal Res. 2009;46(1):87–94.

63. Weaver DR, Reppert SM. The Mel1a melatonin receptor gene is expressed in human suprachiasmatic nuclei. Neuroreport. 1996;8(1):109–12.
64. Cajochen C, Krauchi K, Wirz-Justice A. Role of melatonin in the regulation of human circadian rhythms and sleep. J Neuroendocrinol. 2003;15(4):432–7.
65. Korf HW, Von Gall C, Stehle J. The circadian system and melatonin: lessons from rats and mice. Chronobiol Int. 2003;20(4):697–710.
66. Lewy AJ, Ahmed S, Jackson JM, Sack RL. Melatonin shifts human circadian rhythms according to a phase-response curve. Chronobiol Int. 1992;9(5):380–92.
67. Arendt J, Skene DJ, Middleton B, Lockley SW, Deacon S. Efficacy of melatonin treatment in jet lag, shift work, and blindness. J Biol Rhythms. 1997;12(6):604–17.
68. Sack RL, Brandes RW, Kendall AR, Lewy AJ. Entrainment of free-running circadian rhythms by melatonin in blind people. N Engl J Med. 2000;343(15):1070–7.
69. Spadoni G, Bedini A, Rivara S, Mor M. Melatonin receptor agonists: new options for insomnia and depression treatment. CNS Neurosci Ther. 2011;17(6):733–41.
70. van den Heuvel CJ, Ferguson SA, Macchi MM, Dawson D. Melatonin as a hypnotic: con. Sleep Med Rev. 2005;9(1):71–80.
71. Zhdanova IV. Melatonin as a hypnotic: pro. Sleep Med Rev. 2005;9(1):51–65.
72. Uchikawa O, Fukatsu K, Tokunoh R, Kawada M, Matsumoto K, Imai Y, et al. Synthesis of a novel series of tricyclic indan derivatives as melatonin receptor agonists. J Med Chem. 2002;45(19):4222–39.
73. Wu YH, Ursinus J, Zhou JN, Scheer FA, Ai-Min B, Jockers R, et al. Alterations of melatonin receptors MT1 and MT2 in the hypothalamic suprachiasmatic nucleus during depression. J Affect Disord. 2013;148(2–3):357–67.
74. Hickie IB, Rogers NL. Novel melatonin-based therapies: potential advances in the treatment of major depression. Lancet. 2011;378(9791):621–31.
75. Millan MJ, Gobert A, Lejeune F, Dekeyne A, Newman-Tancredi A, Pasteau V, et al. The novel melatonin agonist agomelatine (S20098) is an antagonist at 5-hydroxytryptamine2C receptors, blockade of which enhances the activity of frontocortical dopaminergic and adrenergic pathways. J Pharmacol Exp Ther. 2003;306(3):954–64.
76. Savaskan E, Ayoub MA, Ravid R, Angeloni D, Fraschini F, Meier F, et al. Reduced hippocampal MT2 melatonin receptor expression in Alzheimer's disease. J Pineal Res. 2005;38(1):10–6.
77. Savaskan E, Olivieri G, Meier F, Brydon L, Jockers R, Ravid R, et al. Increased melatonin 1a-receptor immunoreactivity in the hippocampus of Alzheimer's disease patients. J Pineal Res. 2002;32(1):59–62.
78. Hogan MV, El-Sherif Y, Wieraszko A. The modulation of neuronal activity by melatonin: in vitro studies on mouse hippocampal slices. J Pineal Res. 2001;30(2):87–96.
79. Musshoff U, Riewenherm D, Berger E, Fauteck JD, Speckmann EJ. Melatonin receptors in rat hippocampus: molecular and functional investigations. Hippocampus. 2002;12(2):165–73.
80. Cardinali DP, Brusco LI, Liberczuk C, Furio AM. The use of melatonin in Alzheimer's disease. Neuro Endocrinol Lett. 2002;23 Suppl 1:20–3.
81. Fauteck J, Schmidt H, Lerchl A, Kurlemann G, Wittkowski W. Melatonin in epilepsy: first results of replacement therapy and first clinical results. Biol Signals Recept. 1999;8(1–2):105–10.
82. de Lima E, Soares Jr JM, del Carmen Sanabria Garrido Y, Gomes Valente S, Priel MR, Chada Baracat E, et al. Effects of pinealectomy and the treatment with melatonin on the temporal lobe epilepsy in rats. Brain Res. 2005;1043(1–2):24–31.
83. Stewart LS, Leung LS. Hippocampal melatonin receptors modulate seizure threshold. Epilepsia. 2005;46(4):473–80.
84. Uz T, Arslan AD, Kurtuncu M, Imbesi M, Akhisaroglu M, Dwivedi Y, et al. The regional and cellular expression profile of the melatonin receptor MT1 in the central dopaminergic system. Brain Res Mol Brain Res. 2005;136(1–2):45–53.
85. Sircar R. Effect of melatonin on cocaine-induced behavioral sensitization. Brain Res. 2000;857(1–2):295–9.
86. Adi N, Mash DC, Ali Y, Singer C, Shehadeh L, Papapetropoulos S. Melatonin MT1 and MT2 receptor expression in Parkinson's disease. Med Sci Monit. 2010;16(2):BR61–7.
87. Scher J, Wankiewicz E, Brown GM, Fujieda H. MT(1) melatonin receptor in the human retina: expression and localization. Invest Ophthalmol Vis Sci. 2002;43(3):889–97.
88. Iuvone PM, Tosini G, Pozdeyev N, Haque R, Klein DC, Chaurasia SS. Circadian clocks, clock networks, arylalkylamine N-acetyltransferase, and melatonin in the retina. Prog Retin Eye Res. 2005;24(4):433–56.
89. Tosini G, Baba K, Hwang CK, Iuvone PM. Melatonin: an underappreciated player in retinal physiology and pathophysiology. Exp Eye Res. 2012;103:82–9.
90. Djamgoz MB, Wagner HJ. Localization and function of dopamine in the adult vertebrate retina. Neurochem Int. 1992;20(2):139–91.
91. Alarma-Estrany P, Crooke A, Mediero A, Pelaez T, Pintor J. Sympathetic nervous system modulates the ocular hypotensive action of MT2-melatonin receptors in normotensive rabbits. J Pineal Res. 2008;45(4):468–75.
92. Belforte NA, Moreno MC, de Zavalia N, Sande PH, Chianelli MS, Keller Sarmiento MI, et al. Melatonin: a novel neuroprotectant for the treatment of glaucoma. J Pineal Res. 2010;48(4):353–64.
93. Lundmark PO, Pandi-Perumal SR, Srinivasan V, Cardinali DP, Rosenstein RE. Melatonin in the eye: implications for glaucoma. Exp Eye Res. 2007;84(6):1021–30.

94. Pintor J, Martin L, Pelaez T, Hoyle CH, Peral A. Involvement of melatonin MT(3) receptors in the regulation of intraocular pressure in rabbits. Eur J Pharmacol. 2001;416(3):251–4.
95. Ismail SA, Mowafi HA. Melatonin provides anxiolysis, enhances analgesia, decreases intraocular pressure, and promotes better operating conditions during cataract surgery under topical anesthesia. Anesth Analg. 2009;108(4):1146–51.
96. Abete P, Bianco S, Calabrese C, Napoli C, Cacciatore F, Ferrara N, et al. Effects of melatonin in isolated rat papillary muscle. FEBS Lett. 1997;412(1):79–85.
97. Pang CS, Xi SC, Brown GM, Pang SF, Shiu SY. 2[125I]Iodomelatonin binding and interaction with beta-adrenergic signaling in chick heart/coronary artery physiology. J Pineal Res. 2002;32(4):243–52.
98. Mei YA, Lee PP, Wei H, Zhang ZH, Pang SF. Melatonin and its analogs potentiate the nifedipine-sensitive high-voltage-activated calcium current in the chick embryonic heart cells. J Pineal Res. 2001;30(1):13–21.
99. Viswanathan M, Laitinen JT, Saavedra JM. Expression of melatonin receptors in arteries involved in thermoregulation. Proc Natl Acad Sci U S A. 1990;87(16):6200–3.
100. Yang Q, Scalbert E, Delagrange P, Vanhoutte PM, O'Rourke ST. Melatonin potentiates contractile responses to serotonin in isolated porcine coronary arteries. Am J Physiol Heart Circ Physiol. 2001;280(1):H76–82.
101. Regrigny O, Delagrange P, Scalbert E, Atkinson J, Lartaud-Idjouadiene I. Melatonin improves cerebral circulation security margin in rats. Am J Physiol. 1998;275(1 Pt 2):H139–44.
102. Masana MI, Doolen S, Ersahin C, Al-Ghoul WM, Duckles SP, Dubocovich ML, et al. MT(2) melatonin receptors are present and functional in rat caudal artery. J Pharmacol Exp Ther. 2002;302(3):1295–302.
103. Schepelmann M, Molcan L, Uhrova H, Zeman M, Ellinger I. The presence and localization of melatonin receptors in the rat aorta. Cell Mol Neurobiol. 2011;31(8):1257–65.
104. Monroe KK, Watts SW. The vascular reactivity of melatonin. Gen Pharmacol. 1998;30(1):31–5.
105. Weekley LB. Pharmacologic studies on the mechanism of melatonin-induced vasorelaxation in rat aorta. J Pineal Res. 1995;19(3):133–8.
106. Krauchi K, Cajochen C, Wirz-Justice A. A relationship between heat loss and sleepiness: effects of postural change and melatonin administration. J Appl Physiol. 1997;83(1):134–9.
107. van den Heuvel CJ, Kennaway DJ, Dawson D. Thermoregulatory and soporific effects of very low dose melatonin injection. Am J Physiol. 1999;276(2 Pt 1):E249–54.
108. van der Helm-van Mil AH, van Someren EJ, van den Boom R, van Buchem MA, de Craen AJ, Blauw GJ. No influence of melatonin on cerebral blood flow in humans. J Clin Endocrinol Metab. 2003;88(12):5989–94.
109. Cook JS, Sauder CL, Ray CA. Melatonin differentially affects vascular blood flow in humans. Am J Physiol Heart Circ Physiol. 2011;300(2):H670–4.
110. Arangino S, Cagnacci A, Angiolucci M, Vacca AM, Longu G, Volpe A, et al. Effects of melatonin on vascular reactivity, catecholamine levels, and blood pressure in healthy men. Am J Cardiol. 1999;83(9):1417–9.
111. Cagnacci A, Arangino S, Angiolucci M, Melis GB, Facchinetti F, Malmusi S, et al. Effect of exogenous melatonin on vascular reactivity and nitric oxide in postmenopausal women: role of hormone replacement therapy. Clin Endocrinol (Oxf). 2001;54(2):261–6.
112. Gilad E, Laudon M, Matzkin H, Pick E, Sofer M, Braf Z, et al. Functional melatonin receptors in human prostate epithelial cells. Endocrinology. 1996;137(4):1412–7.
113. Laudon M, Gilad E, Matzkin H, Braf Z, Zisapel N. Putative melatonin receptors in benign human prostate tissue. J Clin Endocrinol Metab. 1996;81(4):1336–42.
114. Siu SW, Lau KW, Tam PC, Shiu SY. Melatonin and prostate cancer cell proliferation: interplay with castration, epidermal growth factor, and androgen sensitivity. Prostate. 2002;52(2):106–22.
115. Tam CW, Shiu SY. Functional interplay between melatonin receptor-mediated antiproliferative signaling and androgen receptor signaling in human prostate epithelial cells: potential implications for therapeutic strategies against prostate cancer. J Pineal Res. 2011;51(3):297–312.
116. Xi SC, Tam PC, Brown GM, Pang SF, Shiu SY. Potential involvement of mt1 receptor and attenuated sex steroid-induced calcium influx in the direct anti-proliferative action of melatonin on androgen-responsive LNCaP human prostate cancer cells. J Pineal Res. 2000;29(3):172–83.
117. Shiu SY, Law IC, Lau KW, Tam PC, Yip AW, Ng WT. Melatonin slowed the early biochemical progression of hormone-refractory prostate cancer in a patient whose prostate tumor tissue expressed MT1 receptor subtype. J Pineal Res. 2003;35(3):177–82.
118. Haus EL, Smolensky MH. Shift work and cancer risk: potential mechanistic roles of circadian disruption, light at night, and sleep deprivation. Sleep Med Rev. 2013;17:273–84.
119. Hansen J, Lassen CF. Nested case–control study of night shift work and breast cancer risk among women in the Danish military. Occup Environ Med. 2012;69(8):551–6.
120. Reed VA. Shift work, light at night, and the risk of breast cancer. AAOHN J. 2011;59(1):37–45; quiz 6.
121. Dillon DC, Easley SE, Asch BB, Cheney RT, Brydon L, Jockers R, et al. Differential expression of high-affinity melatonin receptors (MT1) in normal and malignant human breast tissue. Am J Clin Pathol. 2002;118(3):451–8.
122. Sanchez-Barcelo EJ, Cos S, Fernandez R, Mediavilla MD. Melatonin and mammary cancer: a short review. Endocr Relat Cancer. 2003;10(2):153–9.

123. Cos S, Gonzalez A, Martinez-Campa C, Mediavilla MD, Alonso-Gonzalez C, Sanchez-Barcelo EJ. Estrogen-signaling pathway: a link between breast cancer and melatonin oncostatic actions. Cancer Detect Prev. 2006;30(2):118–28.
124. Girgert R, Hanf V, Emons G, Grundker C. Membrane-bound melatonin receptor MT1 down-regulates estrogen responsive genes in breast cancer cells. J Pineal Res. 2009;47(1):23–31.
125. Yuan L, Collins AR, Dai J, Dubocovich ML, Hill SM. MT(1) melatonin receptor overexpression enhances the growth suppressive effect of melatonin in human breast cancer cells. Mol Cell Endocrinol. 2002;192(1–2):147–56.
126. Lissoni P, Barni S, Meregalli S, Fossati V, Cazzaniga M, Esposti D, et al. Modulation of cancer endocrine therapy by melatonin: a phase II study of tamoxifen plus melatonin in metastatic breast cancer patients progressing under tamoxifen alone. Br J Cancer. 1995;71(4):854–6.
127. Seron-Ferre M, Ducsay CA, Valenzuela GJ. Circadian rhythms during pregnancy. Endocr Rev. 1993;14(5):594–609.
128. Panduro-Baron G, Gonzalez-Moreno J, Hernandez-Figueroa E. The biorhythm of birth. Int J Gynaecol Obstet. 1994;45(3):283–4.
129. Schlabritz-Loutsevitch N, Hellner N, Middendorf R, Muller D, Olcese J. The human myometrium as a target for melatonin. J Clin Endocrinol Metab. 2003;88(2):908–13.
130. Ayar A, Kutlu S, Yilmaz B, Kelestimur H. Melatonin inhibits spontaneous and oxytocin-induced contractions of rat myometrium in vitro. Neuro Endocrinol Lett. 2001;22(3):199–207.
131. Martensson LG, Andersson RG, Berg G. Melatonin together with noradrenaline augments contractions of human myometrium. Eur J Pharmacol. 1996; 316(2–3):273–5.
132. Sharkey JT, Puttaramu R, Word RA, Olcese J. Melatonin synergizes with oxytocin to enhance contractility of human myometrial smooth muscle cells. J Clin Endocrinol Metab. 2009;94(2):421–7.
133. Voordouw BC, Euser R, Verdonk RE, Alberda BT, de Jong FH, Drogendijk AC, et al. Melatonin and melatonin-progestin combinations alter pituitary-ovarian function in women and can inhibit ovulation. J Clin Endocrinol Metab. 1992;74(1):108–17.
134. Luboshitzky R, Shen-Orr Z, Shochat T, Herer P, Lavie P. Melatonin administered in the afternoon decreases next-day luteinizing hormone levels in men: lack of antagonism by flumazenil. J Mol Neurosci. 1999;12(1):75–80.
135. Luboshitzky R, Lavie P. Melatonin and sex hormone interrelationships – a review. J Pediatr Endocrinol Metab. 1999;12(3):355–62.
136. Yie SM, Niles LP, Younglai EV. Melatonin receptors on human granulosa cell membranes. J Clin Endocrinol Metab. 1995;80(5):1747–9.
137. Woo MM, Tai CJ, Kang SK, Nathwani PS, Pang SF, Leung PC. Direct action of melatonin in human granulosa-luteal cells. J Clin Endocrinol Metab. 2001;86(10):4789–97.
138. Nathwani PS, Kang SK, Cheng KW, Choi KC, Leung PC. Regulation of gonadotropin-releasing hormone and its receptor gene expression by 17beta-estradiol in cultured human granulosa-luteal cells. Endocrinology. 2000;141(5):1754–63.
139. Raikhlin NT, Kvetnoy IM, Tolkachev VN. Melatonin may be synthesised in enterochromaffin cells. Nature. 1975;255(5506):344–5.
140. Bubenik GA. Localization of melatonin in the digestive tract of the rat. Effect of maturation, diurnal variation, melatonin treatment and pinealectomy. Horm Res. 1980;12(6):313–23.
141. Bubenik GA. Thirty four years since the discovery of gastrointestinal melatonin. J Physiol Pharmacol. 2008;59 Suppl 2:33–51.
142. Messner M, Huether G, Lorf T, Ramadori G, Schworer H. Presence of melatonin in the human hepatobiliary-gastrointestinal tract. Life Sci. 2001;69(5):543–51.
143. Bubenik GA. Gastrointestinal melatonin: localization, function, and clinical relevance. Dig Dis Sci. 2002;47(10):2336–48.
144. Bubenik GA. The effect of serotonin, N-acetylserotonin, and melatonin on spontaneous contractions of isolated rat intestine. J Pineal Res. 1986;3(1):41–54.
145. Storr M, Koppitz P, Sibaev A, Saur D, Kurjak M, Franck H, et al. Melatonin reduces non-adrenergic, non-cholinergic relaxant neurotransmission by inhibition of nitric oxide synthase activity in the gastrointestinal tract of rodents in vitro. J Pineal Res. 2002;33(2):101–8.
146. Sjoblom M, Flemstrom G. Melatonin in the duodenal lumen is a potent stimulant of mucosal bicarbonate secretion. J Pineal Res. 2003;34(4):288–93.
147. Sjoblom M, Jedstedt G, Flemstrom G. Peripheral melatonin mediates neural stimulation of duodenal mucosal bicarbonate secretion. J Clin Invest. 2001; 108(4):625–33.
148. Sjoblom M, Flemstrom G. Central nervous alpha1-adrenoceptor stimulation induces duodenal luminal release of melatonin. J Pineal Res. 2004;36(2):103–8.
149. Sjoblom M, Safsten B, Flemstrom G. Melatonin-induced calcium signaling in clusters of human and rat duodenal enterocytes. Am J Physiol Gastrointest Liver Physiol. 2003;284(6):G1034–44.
150. Jaworek J, Nawrot-Porabka K, Leja-Szpak A, Bonior J, Szklarczyk J, Kot M, et al. Melatonin as modulator of pancreatic enzyme secretion and pancreatoprotector. J Physiol Pharmacol. 2007;58 Suppl 6:65–80.
151. Brzozowska I, Ptak-Belowska A, Pawlik M, Pajdo R, Drozdowicz D, Konturek SJ, et al. Mucosal strengthening activity of central and peripheral melatonin in the mechanism of gastric defense. J Physiol Pharmacol. 2009;60 Suppl 7:47–56.
152. Celinski K, Konturek SJ, Konturek PC, Brzozowski T, Cichoz-Lach H, Slomka M, et al. Melatonin or

L-tryptophan accelerates healing of gastroduodenal ulcers in patients treated with omeprazole. J Pineal Res. 2011;50(4):389–94.
153. Ganguly K, Sharma AV, Reiter RJ, Swarnakar S. Melatonin promotes angiogenesis during protection and healing of indomethacin-induced gastric ulcer: role of matrix metaloproteinase-2. J Pineal Res. 2010;49(2):130–40.
154. Slominski A, Pisarchik A, Semak I, Sweatman T, Wortsman J, Szczesniewski A, et al. Serotoninergic and melatoninergic systems are fully expressed in human skin. FASEB J. 2002;16(8):896–8.
155. Slominski A, Pisarchik A, Zbytek B, Tobin DJ, Kauser S, Wortsman J. Functional activity of serotoninergic and melatoninergic systems expressed in the skin. J Cell Physiol. 2003;196(1):144–53.
156. Roberts JE, Wiechmann AF, Hu DN. Melatonin receptors in human uveal melanocytes and melanoma cells. J Pineal Res. 2000;28(3):165–71.
157. Hu DN, Roberts JE. Melatonin inhibits growth of cultured human uveal melanoma cells. Melanoma Res. 1997;7(1):27–31.
158. Ying SW, Niles LP, Crocker C. Human malignant melanoma cells express high-affinity receptors for melatonin: antiproliferative effects of melatonin and 6-chloromelatonin. Eur J Pharmacol. 1993; 246(2):89–96.
159. Slominski A, Wortsman J, Tobin DJ. The cutaneous serotoninergic/melatoninergic system: securing a place under the sun. FASEB J. 2005;19(2):176–94.
160. Kleszczynski K, Fischer TW. Melatonin and human skin aging. Dermatoendocrinol. 2012;4(3):245–52.
161. Fischer TW, Burmeister G, Schmidt HW, Elsner P. Melatonin increases anagen hair rate in women with androgenetic alopecia or diffuse alopecia: results of a pilot randomized controlled trial. Br J Dermatol. 2004;150(2):341–5.
162. Guerrero JM, Reiter RJ. Melatonin-immune system relationships. Curr Top Med Chem. 2002;2(2): 167–79.
163. Csaba G, Barath P. Morphological changes of thymus and the thyroid gland after postnatal extirpation of pineal body. Endocrinol Exp. 1975;9(1):59–67.
164. Carrillo-Vico A, Lardone PJ, Alvarez-Sanchez N, Rodriguez-Rodriguez A, Guerrero JM. Melatonin: buffering the immune system. Int J Mol Sci. 2013;14(4):8638–83.
165. Liu F, Ng TB, Fung MC. Pineal indoles stimulate the gene expression of immunomodulating cytokines. J Neural Transm. 2001;108(4):397–405.
166. Garcia-Maurino S, Gonzalez-Haba MG, Calvo JR, Rafii-El-Idrissi M, Sanchez-Margalet V, Goberna R, et al. Melatonin enhances IL-2, IL-6, and IFN-gamma production by human circulating CD4+ cells: a possible nuclear receptor-mediated mechanism involving T helper type 1 lymphocytes and monocytes. J Immunol. 1997;159(2):574–81.
167. Morrey KM, McLachlan JA, Serkin CD, Bakouche O. Activation of human monocytes by the pineal hormone melatonin. J Immunol. 1994;153(6):2671–80.
168. Pozo D, Garcia-Maurino S, Guerrero JM, Calvo JR. MRNA expression of nuclear receptor RZR/RORalpha, melatonin membrane receptor MT, and hydroxyindole-O-methyltransferase in different populations of human immune cells. J Pineal Res. 2004;37(1):48–54.
169. Carrillo-Vico A, Garcia-Perganeda A, Naji L, Calvo JR, Romero MP, Guerrero JM. Expression of membrane and nuclear melatonin receptor mRNA and protein in the mouse immune system. Cell Mol Life Sci. 2003;60(10):2272–8.
170. Heldmaier G, Hoffmann K. Melatonin stimulates growth of brown adipose tissue. Nature. 1974; 247(438):224–5.
171. Le Gouic S, Delagrange P, Atgie C, Nibbelink M, Hanoun N, Casteilla L, et al. Effects of both a melatonin agonist and antagonist on seasonal changes in body mass and energy intake in the garden dormouse. Int J Obes Relat Metab Disord. 1996;20(7): 661–7.
172. Viswanathan M, Hissa R, George JC. Effects of short photoperiod and melatonin treatment on thermogenesis in the Syrian hamster. J Pineal Res. 1986;3(4):311–21.
173. Tan DX, Manchester LC, Fuentes-Broto L, Paredes SD, Reiter RJ. Significance and application of melatonin in the regulation of brown adipose tissue metabolism: relation to human obesity. Obes Rev. 2011;12(3):167–88.
174. Prunet-Marcassus B, Desbazeille M, Bros A, Louche K, Delagrange P, Renard P, et al. Melatonin reduces body weight gain in Sprague Dawley rats with diet-induced obesity. Endocrinology. 2003;144(12): 5347–52.
175. Rios-Lugo MJ, Cano P, Jimenez-Ortega V, Fernandez-Mateos MP, Scacchi PA, Cardinali DP, et al. Melatonin effect on plasma adiponectin, leptin, insulin, glucose, triglycerides and cholesterol in normal and high fat-fed rats. J Pineal Res. 2010; 49(4):342–8.
176. Srinivasan V, Ohta Y, Espino J, Pariente JA, Rodriguez AB, Mohamed M, et al. Metabolic syndrome, its pathophysiology and the role of melatonin. Recent Pat Endocr Metab Immune Drug Discov. 2013;7(1):11–25.
177. Kozirog M, Poliwczak AR, Duchnowicz P, Koter-Michalak M, Sikora J, Broncel M. Melatonin treatment improves blood pressure, lipid profile, and parameters of oxidative stress in patients with metabolic syndrome. J Pineal Res. 2011;50(3):261–6.
178. Brydon L, Petit L, Delagrange P, Strosberg AD, Jockers R. Functional expression of MT2 (Mel1b) melatonin receptors in human PAZ6 adipocytes. Endocrinology. 2001;142(10):4264–71.
179. Peschke E, Bahr I, Muhlbauer E. Melatonin and pancreatic islets: interrelationships between melatonin, insulin and glucagon. Int J Mol Sci. 2013; 14(4):6981–7015.
180. Peschke E, Schucht H, Muhlbauer E. Long-term enteral administration of melatonin reduces plasma

insulin and increases expression of pineal insulin receptors in both Wistar and type 2-diabetic Goto-Kakizaki rats. J Pineal Res. 2010;49(4):373–81.

181. Bouatia-Naji N, Bonnefond A, Cavalcanti-Proenca C, Sparso T, Holmkvist J, Marchand M, et al. A variant near MTNR1B is associated with increased fasting plasma glucose levels and type 2 diabetes risk. Nat Genet. 2009;41(1):89–94.
182. Chambers JC, Zhang W, Zabaneh D, Sehmi J, Jain P, McCarthy MI, et al. Common genetic variation near melatonin receptor MTNR1B contributes to raised plasma glucose and increased risk of type 2 diabetes among Indian Asians and European Caucasians. Diabetes. 2009;58(11):2703–8.
183. Prokopenko I, Langenberg C, Florez JC, Saxena R, Soranzo N, Thorleifsson G, et al. Variants in MTNR1B influence fasting glucose levels. Nat Genet. 2009;41(1):77–81.
184. Xia Q, Chen ZX, Wang YC, Ma YS, Zhang F, Che W, et al. Association between the melatonin receptor 1B gene polymorphism on the risk of type 2 diabetes, impaired glucose regulation: a meta-analysis. PLoS One. 2012;7(11):e50107.
185. Howland RH. A benefit-risk assessment of agomelatine in the treatment of major depression. Drug Saf. 2011;34(9):709–31.

Melatonin's Antioxidant Properties: Molecular Mechanisms

2

Rüdiger Hardeland

Abstract

Melatonin acts as an antioxidant in various ways. Direct scavenging of free radicals requires elevated concentrations, which are present in some high-melatonin organisms and in melatonin-synthesizing organs and used in experimental systems designed for antagonizing oxidotoxicity. Upregulation of antioxidant enzymes occurs at physiological concentrations but is tissue and species specific. Moreover, melatonin prevents excessive radical generation by antiexcitatory and anti-inflammatory actions; by supporting mitochondrial electron flux, thereby reducing electron leakage; and, presumably, by optimizing phase relationships within the circadian multioscillator system.

Keywords

Antioxidant • Circadian • Excitotoxicity • Free radicals • Inflammation • Melatonin • Mitochondria

Introduction

Since the discovery of melatonin's superior capacity as a scavenger of the most harmful reactive oxygen species (ROS), the hydroxyl radical, by Tan et al. [1], countless publications have dealt with the antioxidant properties of this methoxyindole. However, physiological concentrations of circulating melatonin do not suffice for explaining the protective effects solely on the basis of hydroxyl radical scavenging, although physiological levels of melatonin have been shown to convey protection against the hydroxyl radical-generating oxidotoxin and carcinogen safrole [2]. Consequently, additional mechanisms have to be involved. Meanwhile, a plethora of effects is known to contribute to the reduction of oxidative damage, in numerous model systems and organisms. In addition to the elimination of free radicals already formed, melatonin can also reduce the rates of radical formation, as discussed under the term of "radical avoidance" [3]. The aim of this chapter is to outline the various relevant effects at the different levels of action that are typical for the highly pleiotropic molecule, melatonin [4].

R. Hardeland, Dr. rer. nat.
Johann Friedrich Blumenbach Institute of Zoology and Anthropology, Berliner Str. 28, Göttingen, Lower Saxony D-37073, Germany
e-mail: rhardel@gwdg.de

V. Srinivasan et al. (eds.), *Melatonin and Melatonergic Drugs in Clinical Practice*,
DOI 10.1007/978-81-322-0825-9_2, © Springer India 2014

Multiplicity of Actions

By contrast with classic antioxidants such as radical-scavenging vitamins and metabolites, or with regulator molecules that control metabolic functions by means of redox-sensitive response elements in their respective promoters, melatonin acts at multiple levels of different degrees of complexity. An overview is presented in Fig. 2.1. Scavenging of free radicals, which was first discovered and gave rise to numerous investigations on melatonin's protective functions, represents only one section within the spectrum of actions. The relevance of these effects has been controversially debated in the past. Earlier discussions as to whether the detoxification of hydroxyl radicals by melatonin are decisive appear obsolete on the background of actual knowledge. It seems rather important to distinguish between the various models and organisms. Most vertebrates do not attain physiological melatonin levels in the circulation and in the majority of organs to convey substantial protection against these devastating oxidants. Some melatonin-producing tissues may represent exceptions, not only the pineal gland but also, e.g., the Harderian gland, an organ physiologically generating free radicals at high rates because of their exceptional contents of porphyrins and their precursors, such as 5-aminolevulinic acid [5]. Whether elevated levels of the methoxyindole may be present in some brain areas has been differently judged in several studies and would urgently require clarification [6].

In most vertebrate tissues, however, the direct radical-scavenging properties of melatonin are only relevant at pharmacological concentrations. Nevertheless, this statement should not be misinterpreted in a way assuming that direct scavenging by physiological melatonin levels is generally irrelevant in nature. Numerous high-melatonin

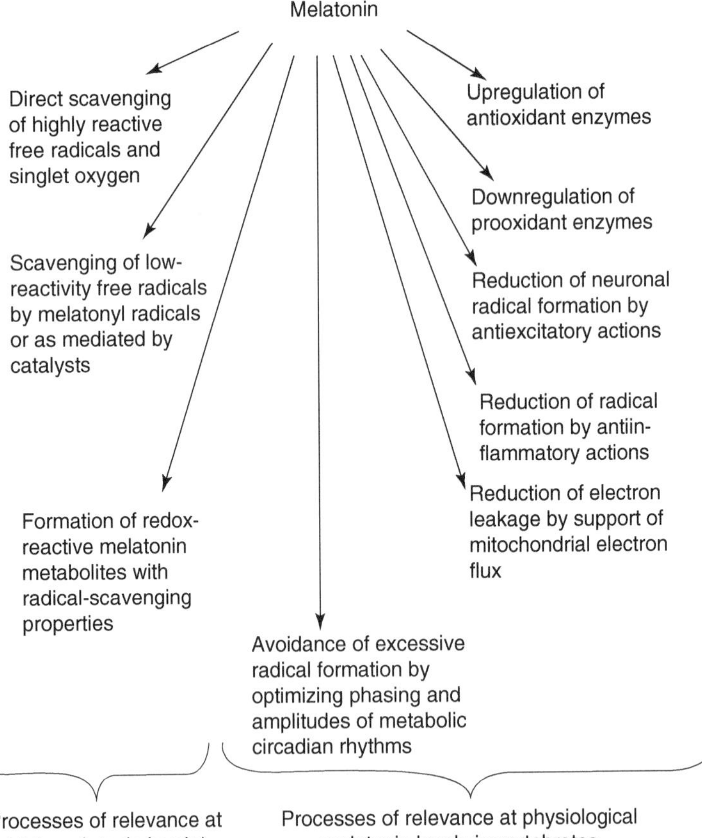

Fig. 2.1 Overview of direct and indirect antioxidant actions of melatonin. *Pharmacological or experimental concentrations applied in tissue or cell cultures and in chemical systems; natural concentrations present in some non-vertebrate high-melatonin organisms

organisms exist [7–9], in which concentrations are attained that suffice for protection by direct detoxification. This was also shown in a dinoflagellate in which antioxidant enzymes were not upregulated by melatonin [10].

Up- or downregulation of anti- or prooxidative enzymes, respectively, will be discussed below. These effects are tissue and species specific. In the absence of detailed knowledge available for the particular organ and organism, generalizations have to be avoided. Thus, the contribution of these melatonin effects can be highly variable according to the respective experimental system.

Radical avoidance is another area in which melatonin seems to play a significant role in reducing oxidative damage. This aspect has been underrated during the earlier years of research in melatonin's antioxidant effects but should be relevant under both physiological and pathological conditions. Both neuronal overexcitation and inflammatory responses represent causes of enhanced free radical formation, and their attenuation by melatonin can become an important contribution to antioxidative protection. These effects are intertwined with mitochondrial effects of prooxidant intermediates generated during excessive neuronal stimulation and inflammation, on the one hand, and reductions of damage by melatonin, on the other hand. Finally, a fourth area of radical avoidance concerns the chronobiological role of melatonin, which is involved in the coordination of phasing and maintenance of high amplitudes within the circadian multioscillator system, processes that seem to be much more important for the well functioning of an organism than previously believed [11]. In fact, disturbances of the circadian system have been shown to be a source of enhanced oxidative damage [12].

Scavenging of Free Radicals and Other Reactive Intermediates

The remarkably potent scavenging of the most devastating ROS, the hydroxyl radical (•OH) [1], has been in the focus of many studies. In experimental systems that preferentially generate •OH, melatonin interacts with two of them to give a next stable compound (Fig. 2.2). Typically, one •OH abstracts an electron or a hydrogen, whereas the other one forms an adduct. In principle, these two steps can occur at either sequence. The preferential sites at the melatonin molecule for attack by •OH have been identified [13]. Three frequently formed hydroxylated reaction products are mentioned in Fig. 2.2. 2-Hydroxymelatonin is a compound that is in a tautomeric equilibrium with a corresponding indolinone. 6-Hydroxymelatonin can be also formed by reactions with two •OH, but this nonenzymatic pathway is considerably less important compared to the hydroxylation by cytochrome P_{450} monooxygenase subforms. A structurally different hydroxylated metabolite results from •OH attack at the indolic ring atom 3. In this case, a third ring is formed to give a cyclic 3-hydroxymelatonin [14]. This compound was also identified as a urinary metabolite produced under conditions of strong oxidative stress, including ionizing radiation.

The preferential generation of •OH is rather uncommon under conditions of near-physiological oxidative stress. In this case, another free radical, the superoxide anion (O_2•$^-$), is much more abundant, so that organic free radicals formed from melatonin under the influence of electron-/hydrogen-abstracting radicals such as •OH more likely interact with O_2•$^-$ or its protonated congener, the hydroperoxyl radical (HO_2•) than with a second •OH (Fig. 2.2). This has been also observed when melatonin is oxidized by other electron- and/or hydrogen-abstracting radicals, such as the protoporphyrinyl IX cation radical or the physiologically important carbonate radical (CO_3•$^-$) [15]. While O_2•$^-$ alone has a poor affinity to melatonin, its interaction with melatonyl radicals seems to be of importance for the termination of radical reaction chains. These processes lead to pyrrole ring cleavage to give *N*^{1}-acetyl-*N*^{2}-formyl-5-methoxykynuramine (AFMK) (Fig. 2.2). AFMK has been identified as the major or, sometimes, almost exclusive product formed in numerous oxidation reactions that may involve free radicals or photochemical, pseudoenzymatic, and enzymatic mechanisms, as recently summarized [16]. AFMK is also generated by

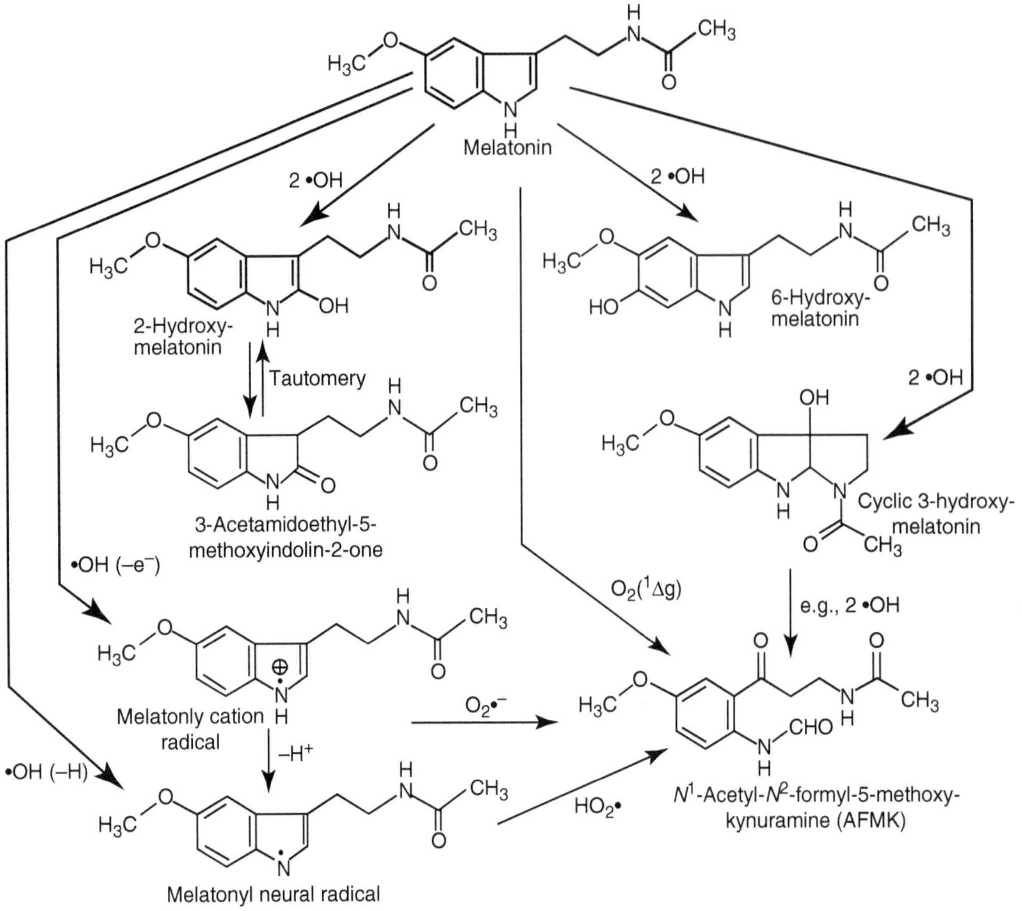

Fig. 2.2 A selection of melatonin's metabolic nonenzymatic pathways catalyzed by oxygen free radicals or singlet oxygen. Additional hydroxylation reactions exist (cf. Tan et al. [13]). Electron- or hydrogen-abstracting free radicals, in particular, several peroxyl radicals and carbonate radicals, undergo corresponding reactions with melatonin. Enzymatic reactions also lead to 6-hydroxymelatonin (major catabolic pathway) or to AFMK (e.g., by myeloperoxidase, some other peroxidases, and indoleamine 2,3-dioxygenase). Further radical reactions by AFMK and its metabolites are omitted

combining with singlet oxygen [$O_2(^1\Delta_g)$] [17] (Fig. 2.2). Interestingly, several radical reactions involving •OH or the ABTS cation radical also transform cyclic 3-hydroxymelatonin to AFMK. The sequence of steps from melatonin via cyclic 3-hydroxymelatonin to AFMK has a balance of four radicals eliminated, a finding known as a radical-scavenging cascade [18]. In a chemical system based on the ABTS cation radical, AFMK is further oxidized to previously unknown products and the cascade is extended to ten scavenged radicals [19]. Whether this extension and the novel metabolites are of biological relevance remains to be studied.

An even more potent radical scavenger than AFMK is its physiological deformylation product, *N*[1]-acetyl-5-methoxykynuramine (AMK) [16, 20]. Again, the physiological meaning remains to be demonstrated and will depend on AMK concentrations present in biological material. Considerable differences seem to exist between vertebrates and some non-vertebrate organisms, as well as between physiological and pathological, especially brain-inflammatory conditions [16]. AMK may be also of interest because of its elimination of nitrosating intermediates. All three NO congeners were shown to be efficiently scavenged by AMK, thereby forming a stable metabolite,

3-acetamidomethyl-6-methoxycinnolinone [21]. By contrast with 1-nitrosomelatonin, this compound does not easily redonate •NO.

Regulation of Pro- and Antioxidant Enzymes

The control of pro- and antioxidant enzymes represents an important contribution to melatonin's antioxidant efficacy. Some of the strongest anti-inflammatory and antiexcitatory effects of melatonin concern the downregulation and inhibition of inducible and neuronal NO synthases (iNOS and nNOS), thereby avoiding excessive radical formation [22]. Importantly, these negative regulation mechanisms do not prevent basal •NO production at physiological melatonin concentrations. Therefore, necessities of neuronal and immunological communication via •NO are not suppressed, as long as no overproduction of this reactive nitrogen species occurs. For instance, a nocturnal peak of cerebral •NO formation is observed in rats, although it approximately coincides with the melatonin maximum [23].

AMK is also an efficient blocker of iNOS and nNOS [24–26]. These findings are of interest for experimental interventions, but their physiological relevance remains to be demonstrated.

Melatonin, AFMK, and AMK downregulate cyclooxygenase-2, another proinflammatory and, thus, prooxidant enzyme [27]. However, these data have been obtained, in macrophages, at very high, unphysiological concentrations.

Two other prooxidant enzymes have been reported to be downregulated by melatonin, 5-lipoxygenase, and 12-lipoxygenase [28, 29]. While 12-lipoxygenase has been rarely investigated in this context, the effects on 5-lipoxygenase have been attributed to actions via nuclear ROR receptors [30, 31]. However, downregulation was not generally observed, and additional uncertainties exist concerning melatonin-dependent and melatonin-independent ROR signaling. In the promonocytic cell line U937, melatonin did not suppress 5-lipoxygenase expression, but rather promoted the formation of ROS [32]. The possibility remains that melatonin differently acts in cell type-specific manner. Nevertheless, these findings shed light on the problems of generalizing results on gene expression obtained in a few tissues or cell types only.

This reservation has also to be made with regard to the upregulation of antioxidant enzymes. Various studies have demonstrated their induction by melatonin in various experimental systems. This was reported for enzymes as different as glutathione peroxidase, glutathione reductase, γ-glutamylcysteine synthase, glucose-6-phosphate dehydrogenase, hemoperoxidase/catalase, Cu, Zn- and Mn-superoxide dismutases [33–35]. Especially glutathione peroxidase has been repeatedly and most consistently shown to be upregulated by melatonin, effects that have gained new relevance in the context of mitochondrial function [4, 12, 36, 37]. Glutathione reductase may mainly respond to changes in the redox equilibrium. However, the relevance of findings on other antioxidant enzymes may be easily overestimated. Especially catalase and the superoxide dismutases respond to melatonin in a highly variable manner, depending on sources and conditions [3]. Frequently, the increases were only in the lower percent range and often restricted to the mRNA level. Sometimes, no effects or even decreases were observed [4, 38]. Notably, a statistically demonstrable effect in a lower percent range may be too small for being relevant in terms of efficacious protection. Glutathione peroxidase did sometimes not respond, e.g., at the protein level in the liver of young rats [39] or at the mRNA level in the murine cerebral cortex [40]. Even when antioxidant enzymes were poorly upregulated, protection by melatonin was usually achieved. Therefore, explanations different from radical scavenging and enzyme induction have to be sought for explaining the protective potential of melatonin, especially at physiological or low pharmacological concentrations.

Radical Avoidance: Various Actions at Different Levels

The concept of radical avoidance intends to explain protective effects of melatonin primarily at the level of radical generation rather than detoxification of radicals already formed but does not exclude mechanisms of detoxification [3, 41–43]. If melatonin is capable of decreasing the processes leading to enhanced radical formation, this might already be achieved by low, physiological concentrations.

In the CNS, reduction of radical generation can be achieved by preventing neuronal overexcitation. Quite a number of antiexcitatory mechanisms have been described, some of which are effective at physiological concentrations, whereas others may require pharmacological levels of melatonin that are, however, applicable under diseased conditions. Among these, the following effects have been described: modulation of GABA and glutamate receptors, secondary effects by decreases of cytosolic Ca^{2+} via $GABA_c$ [44] or metabotropic $mGlu_3$ receptors [45], interference with neuronal NO synthase [46, 47], changes in K^+ currents [48], and potentiation of strychnine-sensitive glycine-induced currents [49]. The specific relevance of these antiexcitatory actions varies between CNS regions. The rather consistently observed attenuation of neuronal excitation by melatonin can prevent excitotoxicity and, thereby, free radical formation and neuronal apoptosis [3, 4]. Antiexcitatory activities of melatonin are largely mediated by MT_1 and/or MT_2 receptors and, thus, represent physiological responses, since corresponding effects have been observed with the synthetic MT_1-/MT_2-selective melatonergic agonist ramelteon [50].

Another important area in which oxidative damage can be attenuated results from anti-inflammatory actions of melatonin. However, the complexity of melatonin's role in inflammation should not be overlooked. It also comprises proinflammatory and prooxidant effects [4]. However, numerous other actions at different levels are involved in the suppression of overshooting inflammation. Anti-inflammatory effects of melatonin are exerted by interference with prostaglandin formation [27], inhibition of TNFα and chemokine release [51–53], and downregulation of •NO synthesis [24, 54–56]. The either pro- or anti-inflammatory behavior of melatonin is strongly conditional. Suppression of inflammatory radical formation and damage is particularly impressive in models of endotoxemia and sepsis.

To understand these properties, the main sources of free radicals have to be considered. Apart from oxidants released by leukocytes, isoforms of NAD(P)H oxidases (Nox) and mitochondria are of particular relevance. Nox isoenzymes contribute to superoxide formation in a quantitatively substantial manner [57–59]. They have been shown to be upregulated under various conditions of stress, including oxidative stress, and also during aging. Moreover, they can secondarily induce RNS formation, as demonstrated for Nox1 during microglial activation [57]. Melatonin's antagonism to both oxidative stress and excessive •NO synthesis likely attenuates these effects. Nox4 has been recently reported to be mitochondrially located as a subunit of complex IV (cytochrome oxidase) [60], another potential nexus to these organelles as a source of ROS and to beneficial actions of melatonin as a mitochondrial modulator [42, 43, 61]. Direct evidence for melatonin's beneficial actions has been obtained in a study on amyloid-β_{1-42}-exposed microglia, in which the methoxyindole inhibits the phosphorylation of the p47 Nox subunit [62].

Mitochondria as a source of superoxide anions require the consideration of sites of electron dissipation and of the crucial role of RNS, as summarized in Fig. 2.3 (for details and extensive literature, see [42, 43, 61]). Superoxide anions are mitochondrially formed by electron transfer to molecular oxygen mainly at complexes I and III. Complex IV may contribute via Nox4. The mechanisms and intrarespirasomal sites of electron leakage have been identified. Electron dissipation appears to be a normal process that results from the remarkable non-homeostatic dynamics of electron flux. Bottlenecks can lead to electron backflow and overflow at specific sites [42, 43, 61]. In addition to respirasomal single-electron dissipation, superoxide flashes have been described, which are assumed to be generated by short-term openings of the mitochondrial permeability transition pore (mtPTP) and during which relatively high amounts of $O_2^{\bullet -}$ may be released, without necessarily causing apoptosis induction [63, 64]. However, the existence of superoxide flashes has been questioned for methodological reasons [65].

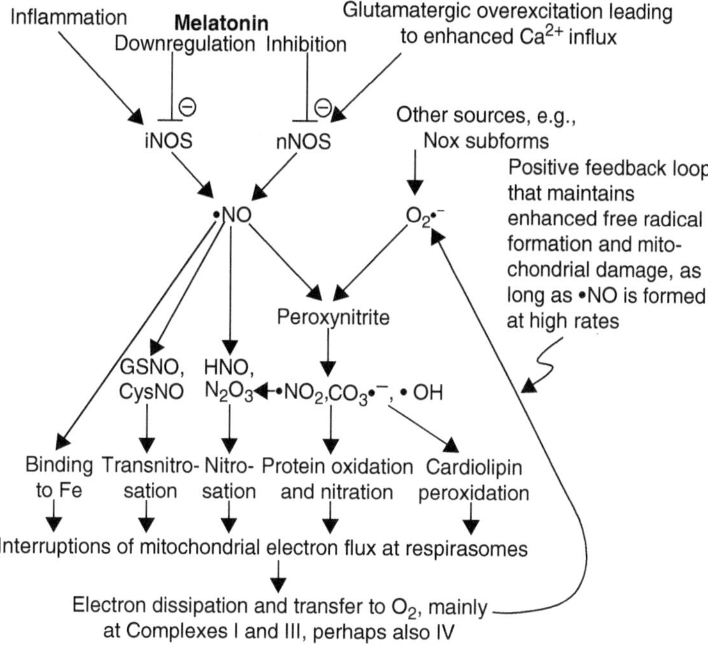

Fig. 2.3 Protective actions of melatonin concerning the reduction of oxidative damage via RNS and mitochondrial dysfunction. *Abbreviations*: *CysNO* nitrosocysteine, *Fe* iron, *GSNO* nitrosoglutathione, *iNOS* inducible *NO* synthase, *nNOS* neuronal NO synthase, *Nox* NAD(P)H oxidase

As depicted in Fig. 2.3, oxidative damage and actions of RNS are intertwined at the mitochondrial level. •NO and its derivatives are capable of partially or almost entirely blocking the electron transport chain (ETC) by binding to iron, nitrosation of SH groups, protein nitration and oxidation, and peroxidation of membrane lipids, especially cardiolipin, a compound required for correct protein conformation in complexes III and IV. A crucial •NO metabolite is peroxynitrite ($ONOO^-$), which decomposes, after protonation, to •OH and •NO_2 or, after formation of a CO_2 adduct ($ONOOCO_2^-$), to a carbonate radical (CO_3•⁻) and •NO_2 (for further details and additional reactions, see Hardeland [22]). Since the affinities of O_2•⁻ to •NO and to superoxide dismutases are similar, peroxynitrite formation is unavoidable as long as •NO synthesis is enhanced. Thus, damage to the ETC by peroxynitrite-derived radicals leads to increased electron leakage and a vicious cycle, which can, however, be interrupted by melatonin by downregulating •NO formation.

Melatonin also contributes to radical avoidance at a chronobiological level by favoring optimal phase relationships within the circadian multioscillator system [3, 11]. In fact, circadian perturbations by pharmacological means, phase shifts, or because of mutations in clock genes have been shown to cause enhanced oxidative damage or reductions in lifespan [12, 66, 67].

Conclusion

The multiple antioxidant actions of melatonin have to be seen in the context of the respective model. In high-melatonin organisms and some experimental systems, direct radical scavenging by micromolar concentrations can be decisive. In vertebrate tissues that do not synthesize melatonin, the upregulation of antioxidant enzymes may be more important, but the conditionality of these effects and their tissue specificity have to be considered. Radical avoidance can be achieved by melatonin in different ways, especially by antiexcitatory and anti-inflammatory mechanisms, by the support of mitochondrial electron flux, and also by optimizing phase relationships within the circadian multioscillator system. With regard to the multiplicity of effects, melatonin differs from all other antioxidants.

References

1. Tan D-X, Chen L-D, Poeggeler B, Manchester LC, Reiter RJ. Melatonin: a potent endogenous hydroxyl radical scavenger. Endocr J. 1993;1:57–60.
2. Tan D-X, Reiter RJ, Chen L-D, Poeggeler B, Manchester LC, Barlow-Walden LR. Both physiological and pharmacological levels of melatonin reduce DNA adduct formation induced by the carcinogen safrole. Carcinogenesis. 1994;15:615–8.
3. Hardeland R. Antioxidative protection by melatonin – multiplicity of mechanisms from radical detoxification to radical avoidance. Endocrine. 2005;27:119–30.
4. Hardeland R, Cardinali DP, Srinivasan V, Spence DW, Brown GM, Pandi-Perumal SR. Melatonin – a pleiotropic, orchestrating regulator molecule. Prog Neurobiol. 2011;93:350–84.
5. Coto-Montes A, Boga JA, Tomás-Zapico C, Rodríguez-Colunga MJ, Martínez-Fraga J, Tolivia-Cadrecha D, et al. Physiological oxidative stress model: Syrian hamster Harderian gland – sex differences in antioxidant enzymes. Free Radic Biol Med. 2001;30:785–92.
6. Hardeland R. Melatonin metabolism in the central nervous system. Curr Neuropharmacol. 2010;8:168–81.
7. Hardeland R. Melatonin and 5-methoxytryptamine in non-metazoans. Reprod Nutr Dev. 1999;39:399–408.
8. Chen G, Huo Y, Tan D-X, Liang Z, Zhang W, Zhang Y. Melatonin in Chinese medicinal herbs. Life Sci. 2003;73:19–26.
9. Hardeland R, Pandi-Perumal SR, Poeggeler B. Melatonin in plants – focus on a vertebrate night hormone with cytoprotective properties. Funct Plant Sci Biotechnol. 2007;1:32–45.
10. Antolín I, Obst B, Burkhardt S, Hardeland R. Antioxidative protection in a high-melatonin organism: the dinoflagellate *Gonyaulax polyedra* is rescued from lethal oxidative stress by strongly elevated, but physiologically possible concentrations of melatonin. J Pineal Res. 1997;23:182–90.
11. Hardeland R, Madrid JA, Tan D-X, Reiter RJ. Melatonin, the circadian multioscillator system and health: the need for detailed analyses of peripheral melatonin signaling. J Pineal Res. 2012;52:139–66.
12. Hardeland R, Coto-Montes A. New vistas on oxidative damage and aging. Open Biol J. 2010;3:39–52.
13. Tan D-X, Reiter RJ, Manchester LC, Yan MT, El-Sawi M, Sainz RM, et al. Chemical and physical properties and potential mechanisms: melatonin as a broad spectrum antioxidant and free radical scavenger. Curr Top Med Chem. 2002;2:181–97.
14. Tan D-X, Manchester LC, Reiter RJ, Plummer BF, Hardies LJ, Weintraub ST, et al. A novel melatonin metabolite, cyclic 3-hydroxymelatonin: a biomarker of in vivo hydroxyl radical generation. Biochem Biophys Res Commun. 1998;253:614–20.
15. Hardeland R, Poeggeler B, Niebergall R, Zelosko V. Oxidation of melatonin by carbonate radicals and chemiluminescence emitted during pyrrole ring cleavage. J Pineal Res. 2003;34:17–25.
16. Hardeland R, Tan D-X, Reiter RJ. Kynuramines, metabolites of melatonin and other indoles: the resurrection of an almost forgotten class of biogenic amines. J Pineal Res. 2009;47:109–26.
17. de Almeida EA, Martinez GR, Klitzke CF, de Medeiros MHG, Di Mascio P. Oxidation of melatonin by singlet molecular oxygen ($O_2(^1\Delta_g)$) produces N^1-acetyl-N^2-formyl-5-methoxykynurenine. J Pineal Res. 2003;35:131–7.
18. Tan D-X, Hardeland R, Manchester LC, Poeggeler B, Lopez-Burillo S, Mayo JC, et al. Mechanistic and comparative studies of melatonin and classic antioxidants in terms of their interactions with the ABTS cation radical. J Pineal Res. 2003;34:249–59.
19. Rosen J, Than NN, Koch D, Poeggeler B, Laatsch H, Hardeland R. Interactions of melatonin and its metabolites with the ABTS cation radical: extension of the radical scavenger cascade and formation of a novel class of oxidation products, C2-substituted 3-indolinones. J Pineal Res. 2006;41:374–81.
20. Ressmeyer A-R, Mayo JC, Zelosko V, Sáinz RM, Tan D-X, Poeggeler B, et al. Antioxidant properties of the melatonin metabolite N1-acetyl-5-methoxykynuramine (AMK): scavenging of free radicals and prevention of protein destruction. Redox Rep. 2003;8:205–13.
21. Hardeland R, Backhaus C, Fadavi A. Reactions of the NO redox forms NO+, •NO and HNO (protonated NO–) with the melatonin metabolite N1-acetyl-5-methoxykynuramine. J Pineal Res. 2007;43:382–8.
22. Hardeland R. Melatonin and its metabolites as anti-nitrosating and anti-nitrating agents. J Exp Integr Med. 2011;1:67–81.
23. Clément P, Gharib A, Cespuglio R, Sarda N. Changes in sleep-wake cycle architecture and cortical nitric oxide release during ageing in the rat. Neuroscience. 2003;116:863–70.
24. Tapias V, Escames G, López LC, López A, Camacho E, Carrión MD, et al. Melatonin and its brain metabolite N1-acetyl-5-methoxykynuramine prevent mitochondrial nitric oxide synthase induction in parkinsonian mice. J Neurosci Res. 2009;87:3002–10.
25. Entrena A, Camacho ME, Carrión MD, López-Cara LC, Velasco G, León J, et al. Kynurenamines as neural nitric oxide synthase inhibitors. J Med Chem. 2005;48:8174–81.
26. León J, Escames G, Rodríguez MI, López LC, Tapias V, Entrena A, et al. Inhibition of neuronal nitric oxide synthase activity by N1-acetyl-5-methoxykynuramine, a brain metabolite of melatonin. J Neurochem. 2006;98:2023–33.
27. Mayo JC, Sainz RM, Tan D-X, Hardeland R, Leon J, Rodriguez C, et al. Anti-inflammatory actions of melatonin and its metabolites, N1-acetyl-N2-formyl-5-methoxykynuramine (AFMK) and N1-acetyl-5-methoxykynuramine (AMK), in macrophages. J Neuroimmunol. 2005;165:139–49.
28. Manev H, Uz T, Qu T. Early upregulation of hippocampal 5-lipoxygenase following systemic administration of kainate to rats. Restor Neurol Neurosci. 1998;12:81–5.

29. Zhang H, Akbar M, Kim HY. Melatonin: an endogenous negative modulator of 12-lipoxygenation in the rat pineal gland. Biochem J. 1999;344:487–93.
30. Carlberg C, Wiesenberg I. The orphan receptor family RZR/ROR, melatonin and 5-lipoxygenase: an unexpected relationship. J Pineal Res. 1995;18:171–8.
31. Steinhilber D, Brungs M, Werz O, Wiesenberg I, Danielsson C, Kahlen JP, et al. The nuclear receptor for melatonin represses 5-lipoxygenase gene expression in human B lymphocytes. J Biol Chem. 1995;270:7037–40.
32. Radogna F, Sestili P, Martinelli C, Paolillo M, Paternoster L, Albertini MC, et al. Lipoxygenase-mediated pro-radical effect of melatonin via stimulation of arachidonic acid metabolism. Toxicol Appl Pharmacol. 2009;238:170–7.
33. Reiter RJ, Tan D-X, Mayo JC, Sainz RM, Leon J, Czarnocki Z. Melatonin as an antioxidant: biochemical mechanisms and pathophysiological implications in humans. Acta Biochim Pol. 2003;50:1129–46.
34. Pandi-Perumal SR, Srinivasan V, Maestroni GJM, Cardinali DP, Poeggeler B, Hardeland R. Melatonin: nature's most versatile biological signal? FEBS J. 2006;273:2813–38.
35. Hardeland R, Poeggeler B. Melatonin beyond its classical functions. Open Physiol J. 2008;1:1 23.
36. Acuña-Castroviejo D, Escames G, Rodríguez MI, López LC. Melatonin role in the mitochondrial function. Front Biosci. 2007;12:947–63.
37. Rodríguez MI, Escames G, López LC, López A, García JA, Ortiz F, et al. Chronic melatonin treatment reduces the age-dependent inflammatory process in senescence-accelerated mice. J Pineal Res. 2007; 42:272–9.
38. Gürdöl F, Genç S, Öner-İyidogan Y, Süzme R. Coadministration of melatonin and estradiol in rats: effects on oxidant status. Horm Metab Res. 2001; 33:608–11.
39. Mauriz JL, Molpeceres V, García-Mediavilla MV, Gonzalez P, Barrio JP, Gonzalez-Gallego J. Melatonin prevents oxidative stress and changes in antioxidant enzyme expression and activity in the liver of aging rats. J Pineal Res. 2007;42:222–30.
40. Olcese JM, Cao C, Mori T, Mamcarz MB, Maxwell A, Runfeldt MJ, et al. Protection against cognitive deficits and markers of neurodegeneration by long-term oral administration of melatonin in a transgenic model of Alzheimer disease. J Pineal Res. 2009; 47:82–96.
41. Hardeland R, Coto-Montes A, Poeggeler B. Circadian rhythms, oxidative stress, and antioxidative defense mechanisms. Chronobiol Int. 2003;20:921–62.
42. Hardeland R, Poeggeler B, Pappolla MA. Mitochondrial actions of melatonin —— an endeavor to identify their adaptive and cytoprotective mechanisms. Abh Sächs Akad Wiss Math-Nat Kl. 2009;65(Pt 3):14–31.
43. Hardeland R. Neuroprotection by radical avoidance: search for suitable agents. Molecules. 2009;14: 5054–102.
44. Prada C, Udin SB, Wiechmann AF, Zhdanova IV. Stimulation of melatonin receptors decreases calcium levels in Xenopus tectal cells by activating GABAC receptors. J Neurophysiol. 2005;94:968–78.
45. Prada C, Udin SB. Melatonin decreases calcium levels in retinotectal axons of Xenopus laevis by indirect activation of group III metabotropic glutamate receptors. Brain Res. 2005;1053:67–76.
46. León J, Vives F, Crespo E, Camacho E, Espinosa A, Gallo MA, et al. Modification of nitric oxide synthase activity and neuronal response in rat striatum by melatonin and kynurenine derivatives. J Neuroendocrinol. 1998;10:297–302.
47. León J, Macías M, Escames G, Camacho E, Khaldy H, Martín M, et al. Structure-related inhibition of calmodulin-dependent neuronal nitric-oxide synthase activity by melatonin and synthetic kynurenines. Mol Pharmacol. 2000;58:967–75.
48. Liu LY, Hoffman GE, Fei XW, Li Z, Zhang ZH, Mei YA. Delayed rectifier outward K+ current mediates the migration of rat cerebellar granule cells stimulated by melatonin. J Neurochem. 2007;102:333–44.
49. Zhang M, Cao LH, Yang XL. Melatonin modulates glycine currents of retinal ganglion cells in rat. Neuroreport. 2007;18:1675–8.
50. Fenoglio-Simeone K, Mazarati A, Sefidvash-Hockley S, Shin D, Wilke J, Milligan H, et al. Anticonvulsant effects of the selective melatonin receptor agonist ramelteon. Epilepsy Behav. 2009;16:52–7.
51. Baykal A, Iskit AB, Hamaloglu E, Guc MO, Hascelik G, Sayek I. Melatonin modulates mesenteric blood flow and TNFalpha concentrations after lipopolysaccharide challenge. Eur J Surg. 2000;166:722–7.
52. Park HJ, Kim HJ, Ra J, Hong SJ, Baik HH, Park HK, et al. Melatonin inhibits lipopolysaccharide-induced CC chemokine subfamily gene expression in human peripheral blood mononuclear cells in a microarray analysis. J Pineal Res. 2007;43:121–9.
53. Shang Y, Xu SP, Wu Y, Jiang YX, Wu ZY, Yuan SY, et al. Melatonin reduces acute lung injury in endotoxemic rats. Chin Med J (Engl). 2009;122: 1388–93.
54. Escames G, López LC, Ortíz F, Ros E, Acuña-Castroviejo D. Age-dependent lipopolysaccharide-induced iNOS expression and multiorgan failure in rats: effects of melatonin treatment. Exp Gerontol. 2006;41:1165–73.
55. Escames G, López LC, Tapias V, Utrilla P, Reiter RJ, Hitos AB, et al. Melatonin counteracts inducible mitochondrial nitric oxide synthase-dependent mitochondrial dysfunction in skeletal muscle of septic mice. J Pineal Res. 2006;40:71–8.
56. Escames G, López LC, Ortíz F, López A, García JA, Ros E, et al. Attenuation of cardiac mitochondrial dysfunction by melatonin in septic mice. FEBS J. 2007;274:2135–47.
57. Chéret C, Gervais A, Lelli A, Colin C, Amar L, Ravassard P, et al. Neurotoxic activation of microglia is promoted by a nox1-dependent NADPH oxidase. J Neurosci. 2008;28:12039–51.

58. McCann SK, Dusting GJ, Roulston CL. Early increase of Nox4 NADPH oxidase and superoxide generation following endothelin-1-induced stroke in conscious rats. J Neurosci Res. 2008;86:2524–34.
59. Chen H, Song YS, Chan PH. Inhibition of NADPH oxidase is neuroprotective after ischemia-reperfusion. J Cereb Blood Flow Metab. 2009;29:1262–72.
60. Block K, Gorin Y, Abboud HE. Subcellular localization of Nox4 and regulation in diabetes. Proc Natl Acad Sci U S A. 2009;106:14385–90.
61. Hardeland R. Melatonin, mitochondrial electron flux and leakage: recent findings and resolution of contradictory results. Adv Stud Biol. 2009;1:207–30.
62. Zhou J, Zhang S, Zhao X, Wei T. Melatonin impairs NADPH oxidase assembly and decreases superoxide anion production in microglia exposed to amyloid-β_{1-42}. J Pineal Res. 2008;45:157–65.
63. Wang W, Fang H, Groom L, Cheng A, Zhang W, Liu J, et al. Superoxide flashes in single mitochondria. Cell. 2008;134:279–90.
64. Sheu SS, Wang W, Cheng H, Dirksen RT. Superoxide flashes: illuminating new insights into cardiac ischemia/reperfusion injury. Future Cardiol. 2008;4:551–4.
65. Schwarzländer M, Logan DC, Fricke MD, Sweetlove LJ. The circularly permuted yellow fluorescent protein cpYFP that has been used as a superoxide probe is highly responsive to pH but not superoxide in mitochondria: implications for the existence of superoxide 'flashes'. Biochem J. 2011; 437:381–7.
66. Coto-Montes A, Hardeland R. Diurnal rhythm of protein carbonyl as an indicator of oxidative damage in Drosophila melanogaster: influence of clock gene alleles and deficiencies in the formation of free-radical scavengers. Biol Rhythms Res. 1999;30:383–91.
67. Coto-Montes A, Tomás-Zapico C, Rodríguez-Colunga MJ, Tolivia-Cadrecha D, Martínez-Fraga J, Hardeland R, et al. Effects of the circadian mutation 'tau' on the Harderian glands of Syrian hamsters. J Cell Biochem. 2001;83:426–34.

Past, Present, and Future of Melatonin's Clinical Uses

3

Nori Tolosa de Talamoni, Vanessa Andrea Areco, Maria Elena Peralta Lopez, Gabriela Diaz de Barboza, Maria Angelica Rivoira, and Agata Rita Carpentieri

Abstract

Melatonin (MEL) is a pleiotropic hormone which exerts its action through different mechanisms, either by binding to its receptors or by acting as an antioxidant molecule and ROS scavenger. Its mechanisms of action together with the wide distribution of MT1 and MT2 receptors have provoked an ever-increasing number of clinical trials in the last two decades. These studies have evaluated the exogenous administration of MEL in different doses and formulations to prevent or to treat many health disorders. The predominant field of research has been the treatment of insomnia and other circadian rhythm disorders due to the confirmed resynchronizing properties of this indolamine. However, in the last decade, a profound interest has arisen concerning its potential therapeutic value in different conditions such as cancer, cardiovascular diseases, gastrointestinal problems, and inflammatory states, among others. The relatively low toxicity of MEL over a wide range of doses has made the research even more promising. However, new multicenter clinical trials could shed light on different aspects of MEL's clinical uses contributing thus to clarify the conditions in which MEL might be considered as a first-line therapeutical strategy and to identify when the combination of MEL with other drugs is necessary. In this chapter, we revise the milestones in the field of MEL research from its discovery to the present time and analyze the future perspectives of its clinical uses.

N. Tolosa de Talamoni, PhD (✉)
V.A. Areco • M.E. Peralta Lopez, PhD
G. Diaz de Barboza, PhD
M.A. Rivoira, PhD
Cátedra de Bioquímica y Biología Molecular, Facultad de Ciencias Médicas, Universidad Nacional de Córdoba, Haya de la Torre S/N. Pabellón Argentina 2° Piso. Ciudad Universitaria, Córdoba 5000, Argentina
e-mail: ntolosatalamoni@yahoo.com.ar; vecaareco@hotmail.com; elenitaperalta@yahoo.com.ar; gabyediaz@yahoo.com; mariaangelicarivoira@yahoo.com.ar

A.R. Carpentieri, PhD
Cátedra de Bioquímica y Biología Molecular, Facultad de Ciencias Médicas, Cátedra de Química Biológica, Facultad de Odontología, Universidad Nacional de Córdoba, Haya de la Torre S/N. Pabellón Argentina 2° Piso. Ciudad Universitaria, Córdoba 5000, Argentina
e-mail: arcarpentieri@hotmail.com

V. Srinivasan et al. (eds.), *Melatonin and Melatonergic Drugs in Clinical Practice*, DOI 10.1007/978-81-322-0825-9_3, © Springer India 2014

Keywords
Melatonin • Agomelatine • Sleep • Neonates • Reproduction • Cancer • Antioxidant • Anti-inflammatory • Cardiovascular

Introduction

Since melatonin (MEL) isolation from bovine pineal tissue more than 50 years ago [1], the study of this hormone has raised interest in different fields such as physiology, etiopathogenesis of various disorders, and pharmacology. Evidence of this interest is the increasing number of publications (more than 17,000) approaching different aspects of MEL and its biological and biomedical applications.

During the first two decades after MEL isolation, research was mainly about its physiological properties as a light-related circadian [2]. The characterization of a functional mammalian MEL receptor [3], and the cloning of the first human MEL receptor [4] 10 years later, encouraged the study of this molecule as a potential pharmacological agent in the prevention and treatment of many diseases. Since then, the research performed in human beings has gained importance, and the clinical trials using MEL alone or in combination with other drugs have increased.

The circadian properties of the indolamine and its efficiency as a synchronizing agent have been the focus of many clinical trials in patients with primary and secondary sleep disorders and circadian dysfunctions of different kinds. These chronobiological applications have been predominant in MEL clinical research for many years. However, in the last decade, the antioxidant, antiaging, and immune regulatory properties of the molecule have deserved the attention of several groups. This has triggered an important number of clinical trials including patients suffering from a variety of diseases such as cancer, neurodegenerative disorders, gastrointestinal alterations, diabetes, and autoimmune pathologies, among others.

The different formulations of MEL as well as the synthesis of analogs, such as agomelatine, ramelteon, and tasimelteon, which function as agonists for MT receptor, are currently under investigation as potential drugs to treat many disorders. The main objectives of this chapter are an overview of the past and present MEL's clinical uses and the possible future applications of MEL in treatment and prevention of various clinical entities.

Melatonin Secretion and Human Age

MEL is secreted in a circadian manner, showing the highest levels of secretion in all species at night. The activity of the enzyme N-acetyltransferase (NAT) is increased from 30- to 70-fold at night and is rate limiting in MEL synthesis in most circumstances. The duration of darkness determines the period of MEL secretion. In humans, the onset of a circadian rhythm of MEL biosynthesis appears between 6 and 8 weeks of age [5]. A peak of MEL secretion occurs between 4 and 7 years [6], which is followed by a declination to adult levels around 15–18 years. The levels remain stable in the adulthood until old age, when a marked declination is produced, maybe as a result of a weakness of the circadian system [7].

MEL and Neonates and Children

Neonates, mainly preterm newborns, can develop oxidative stress because they are easily exposed to high oxygen concentration, have poor antioxidant defenses, and have infections or inflammation. Hence, neonates may develop pathologies named "oxygen radical diseases of neonatology" such as respiratory distress syndrome (RDS), bronchopulmonary dysplasia, periventricular leukomalacia, hypoxic-ischemic brain injury, and neonatal sepsis. The lung and brain are the two most susceptible organs. Gitto et al. [8, 9] have found in preterm newborn with RDS that MEL reduces the proinflammatory cytokines and improved the clinical outcome. Fulia et al. [10] measured serum levels of malondialdehyde (MDA) and nitrite/ nitrate in 20 asphyxiated newborns before and after MEL treatment. There were significant reductions in MDA and nitrite/nitrate levels in the asphyxiated newborns given MEL at 12 and 24 h. None of these neonates died, whereas 3 of 10 asphyxiated children not given MEL died within 72 h after birth. The beneficial MEL effects may be related to its antioxidant properties and the ability to improve the efficiency of mitochondrial electron transport. MEL treatment in septic newborns was also shown to improve the clinical outcome by decreasing serum lipid peroxidation products and parameters of inflammation such as C-reactive protein, white blood cells, and neutrophils [11]. The efficacy of MEL in ten surgical neonates has been also assayed by measuring the cytokine levels (IL-6, IL-8, TNFα) and nitrite/nitrate concentration before and after MEL treatment. The indoleamine was capable to reduce the cytokines and nitrite/nitrate levels with improvement in clinical outcome parallel to progressive reduction in parameters of inflammation [12]. Pain derived from endotracheal intubation in newborn care has been demonstrated to be diminished when MEL was added to the common sedation and analgesia used at present [13].

The efficacy of MEL on children with sleep disorders has been assayed in patients with autism, fragile X syndrome, or autism and fragile X syndrome. A reduction in the sleep-onset latency and the sleep-onset time and a longer night sleep duration have been noticed in children treated with 3 mg MEL for 2 weeks and then alternated for another 2 weeks [11]. The optimal dose of MEL for sleep disorders in children has not been established yet. Doses of 3–15 mg in children with neurodevelopmental disorders have been used. Jan et al. [14, 15] suggest starting at a lower dose (1–3 mg for infants and toddlers and 2.5–5 mg for older children) and adjusting gradually the dose according to the response.

A few clinical trials of adjunctive MEL treatment in humans have shown that MEL might improve the seizure disorders. Peled et al. [16] have shown that the combination of 3 mg of oral MEL with an antiepileptic drug improved the seizure activity in 5 of 6 children with intractable seizures. Seizure activity returned to pretreatment levels after discontinuing MEL in all patients. Gupta et al. [17] have observed that the MEL treatment associated with carbamazepine improved the quality of life of children with epilepsy. Some studies reported successful treatment of epilepsy with MEL in patients with refractory epilepsy [18]. However, a few studies have reported proconvulsant effects of MEL [19, 20]. As Banach et al. [21] suggest, it is necessary to accomplish more placebo-controlled, double-blind randomized clinical trials to establish whether MEL could be useful in the adjunctive treatment of epilepsy.

Melatonin and Sleep

Approximately one third of MEL's clinical trials in PubMed are devoted to the administration of exogenous MEL to treat different sleep disorders in various populations. This theme has received increasing attention from researchers ever since. A variety of doses and formulations have proved to produce a benefit in the treatment of primary insomnia in subjects of different ages. Van Geijlswijk et al. [22] demonstrated that 0.05 mg/kg MEL given 1–2 h before desired bedtime advanced sleep onset by approximately 1 h and decreased sleep-onset latency by 35 min in 6–12-year-old children with chronic sleep-onset insomnia. In addition, the authors found that long-term treatment (1–4 years) with the drug could have a sustained effect over sleep status without affecting pubertal and mental development [22]. Eckerberg et al. [23] observed that MEL (1 mg) given daily in the afternoon could advance sleeping time, reduce sleepiness, and increase school alertness in a group of adolescent students with sleep-onset insomnia. The drug has been also studied in middle-aged and elderly insomniacs with various results. Baskett et al. [24] demonstrated that 5 mg of fast-release MEL taken at bedtime does not improve the quality of sleep in older people with age-related sleep maintenance problems. However, positive results have been obtained among elderly population [25–27]. In a study including more than 700 patients, Wade et al. [25] reported that elderly chronic insomniacs receiving 2 mg of prolonged-release MEL (PRM), a formulation that mimics the endogenous production profile of the hormone, significantly improved sleep latency and quality. This effect was confirmed after 3 weeks of treatment and was still present after 6 months. Neither serious adverse events nor rebound insomnia nor withdrawal symptoms were reported. Similar efficacy was seen by Luthringer et al. [28], who also found a significant improvement of daytime psychomotor performance in elderly patients receiving PRM. This psychomotor preservation was also present in a trial conducted by Otmani et al. [29], in which the authors compared PRM with zolpidem (10 mg) and evaluated the coadministration of both drugs. Interestingly, PRM alone did not impair performances on any cognitive tasks while zolpidem significantly impaired early memory recall, psychomotor, and driving performances 1 and 4 h post-dosing. This effect was exacerbated when both drugs were coadministered, most probably due to a pharmacodynamic interaction. Cautious consideration on pharmacological interactions is required since elderly insomniac patients are usually subjected to polypharmacy or resort to abusive and misinformed self-medication. Organic and metabolic status should also be carefully considered when choosing a sleep promoter agent for the elderly. In this respect, MEL could be a safe sleep inducer in elderly people with cardiac risk and chronic respiratory conditions as demonstrated in several studies [30, 31]. The drug does not worsen hypoxemia and apnea/hypopnea index, as most conventional hypnotics do.

Given that insomnia is often a comorbid manifestation in the context of other conditions, MEL could play an important role in the treatment of patients with secondary sleep disorders, usually polymedicated, since it is safe and well tolerated. In this respect, several trials have been carried out among children with neurodevelopmental disabilities [32], autism [33], and attention deficit [34]. Coincidental results in most of these studies reveal that MEL in doses of 1–5 mg considerably reduces mean sleep-onset time and sleep latency and prolongs total sleep duration, slightly improving behavior and family stress. The drug was well tolerated, with only mild side effects, both in the short and long term. Larger trials including more patients as well as comparing effectiveness with other MEL formulations and MEL agonists could contribute to standardize the beneficial effects of MEL on these patients.

Sleep disorders are usual among patients suffering from depression and other mood disorders. MEL has proved to improve sleep in these patients and as a consequence to attenuate depressive symptoms [35]. Further studies evaluating the real benefit of including MEL in the treatment of depression are required, especially analyzing the potential of combining MEL with other antidepressants.

Antioxidant and Anti-inflammatory Properties of Melatonin

The beneficial properties of MEL related to its antioxidant and anti-inflammatory effects have been extensively described [36–38]. The indoleamine has direct and indirect antioxidant actions. MEL diminishes lipid peroxidation and DNA degradation due to a direct scavenging of both ROS and RNS and activation of DNA reparation enzymes. Indirectly, MEL has antioxidant actions through stimulation of SOD, CAT, and GPx activities and GSH synthesis. In acute conditions such as sepsis, asphyxia, and surgery, it has been observed a reduction in the malondialdehyde and in the nitrite/nitrate levels and in the concentration of inflammatory cytokines after MEL treatment. In chronic neuropathies as in the Alzheimer disease, Parkinson disease, and Huntington disease and amyotrophic lateral sclerosis, MEL administration has been found to inhibit the intrinsic apoptotic pathway of neurons. No adverse effects have been noted by using doses in the range of 1–300 mg/day, which encourages a long-term administration of MEL in patients with neurodegenerative diseases [15, 39, 40]. Beneficial antioxidant actions of MEL have been also detected in metabolic diseases such as type 2 diabetes mellitus (5 mg/day) and primary essential hypertension (5 mg/day). Molecular and cellular damages have been attenuated by MEL in cardiac ischemia/reperfusion and in other vascular diseases (see cardiovascular section).

With regard to the anti-inflammatory properties, MEL has been shown to block transcriptional factors that induce proinflammatory cytokines and to inhibit the activation of cyclooxygenase 2 and the inducible NO synthase, which are activated in chronic inflammatory disorders. These properties could be useful to ameliorate ulcerative colitis in combination with other drugs such as omeprazole [41, 42]. In different clinical trials in patients with irritable bowel syndrome, the use of MEL has revealed to produce symptomatic benefit, attenuation of abdominal and rectal pain, and improvement in the quality of life [43]. A reduction in the plasma levels of proinflammatory cytokines has been observed in patients with nonalcoholic steatohepatitis treated with MEL plus tryptophan [44]. Although there is an enormous amount of data about a potential hepatoprotective role of MEL, based on its antioxidant properties, there are also negative findings, which make that further data are required in order to resolve the issue of the usefulness of MEL in conditions of liver injury or liver transplantation [45]. Regarding the effects on rheumatoid arthritis, the results are controversial. A clinical trial of 75 patients with rheumatoid arthritis revealed that 10 mg MEL at night for 6 months in addition to ongoing medication did not improve the clinical assessments of patient symptoms. The authors detected increases in the concentration of some inflammatory indicators, which were not associated with any change of proinflammatory cytokine concentrations or clinical symptoms [46].

In patients with infectious diseases such as pulmonary tuberculosis [47] and human immunodeficiency virus type I (HIV-1) infection [48], MEL levels have been found to be lower in comparison with controls. MEL treatment appears to be effective in combating several bacterial and viral infections due to its antioxidant, immunomodulating, and inhibitory actions against the production of inflammatory mediators [49].

Melatonin and Cancer

The hypothesis that the diminished function of pineal gland might promote breast cancer in humans was supported by several findings: (1) pineal calcification was very common in countries with high rates of breast cancer; (2) patients taking chlorpromazine, a drug that increases serum MEL, had a lower incidence of breast cancer; (3) MEL receptor was detected in human ovary, which might influence the estrogen production; (4) impaired pineal secretion was associated with early menarche considered a risk factor for breast cancer; and (5) the demonstration that MEL might influence tumor induction in experimental animals [50]. Later, it was found that patients with estrogen receptor-positive breast cancer had decreased nocturnal plasma MEL peak [51]. Furthermore, women with estrogen or progesterone receptor-positive breast tumors showed a strong inverse correlation between the plasma MEL levels and the quantities of receptors in the primary tumor; the lower the plasma MEL levels, the greater the amount of either receptor in the tumor [52]. Similarly, an inverse correlation between plasma MEL levels and the presence of endometrial cancer has been observed. The mean plasma MEL was 6.1 pg/mL in the cancer group, while 33.2 pg/mL was observed in the control group [53].

The concomitant treatment of MEL with chemotherapy or radiation has been employed in some clinical trials in patients with different types of cancer. In this line, Lissoni et al. [54] began to evaluate the influence of MEL on interleukin-2 (IL-2) immunotherapy toxicity in metastatic renal cancer patients. The frequency of episodes of severe hypotension and depressive symptoms was lower in patients treated with IL-2 plus MEL as compared to those treated only with IL-2. In a pilot study of 14 patients with metastatic gastric cancer, a tumor regression was obtained in 3/14 (21 %) patients, and disease stabilization occurred in 6/14 (43 %) patients after a combined treatment of MEL (50 mg/day everyday starting 7 days before IL-2) and IL-2 (three million IU/day subcutaneously for 6 days/week for 4 weeks) [54].

Some clinical trials explored the use of MEL in patients with advanced cancer resistant to standard antitumor therapies. MEL intramuscular therapy (20 mg at 3:00 p.m. for 2 months followed by maintenance dose of 10 mg orally) in patients with metastatic solid tumors resistant to conventional therapies showed 1 partial response (cancer of pancreas), 2 minor responses (colon cancer and hepatocarcinoma), and 21 with stable disease. The remaining 30 patients showed disease progression within the first 2 months. The quality of life was improved in 18/54 (33 %) cases [55]. A partial response to IL-2 plus MEL was observed in patients with untreatable endocrine tumors because of disseminated disease, lack of response to other therapies, or tumors with unavailable therapy. The tumor size was reduced in 3/12 patients (25 %), and the toxicity was low in all patients [56]. A randomized study with MEL versus supportive care alone in patients with advanced non-small cell lung cancer resistant to cisplatin revealed that the percentage of both stabilization of disease and survival at 1 year was significantly higher in patients treated with MEL as compared to those receiving supportive care [57].

What are the molecular mechanisms of the antineoplastic action of MEL? There was a hypothesis that the immunomodulatory properties of MEL would alter the immune function in cancer patients through changes in the plasma cytokines. Neri et al. [58] studied 31 patients with advanced cancer resistant to conventional therapies, who were shifted to MEL therapy (10 mg/day) for 3 months. The investigators observed a significant decrease of IL-6 circulating levels and found that 39 % of patients achieved disease stabilization, with no further growth in primary or secondary tumors, and improvement in their general well-being. MEL has been also shown to increase T helper cell response by releasing IL-2, IL-10, and interferon-γ [58]. The antioxidant properties of MEL also explain, at least in part, its oncostatic function (see Section of Antioxidant properties). In breast cancer therapy, MEL is useful because of its selective estrogen receptor modulator (SERM) and selective estrogen enzyme modulator (SEEM) properties. SERM actions include modulation of cell proliferation, invasiveness, and expression of proteins and oncogenes regulated by estrogen, mediated by MT1 MEL receptors. SEEM actions consist in the inhibition of expression and activity of P450 aromatase, estrogen sulfatase, and type 1 17β-hydroxysteroid dehydrogenase and the stimulation of estrogen sulfotransferase [59]. The virtual absence of contraindications makes MEL a suitable adjuvant with the drugs used for breast cancer prevention such as antiestrogens and antiaromatases [60]. Recently, it has been demonstrated in pancreatic carcinoma cells (PANC-1 cells) a significant inhibition of cell proliferation and suppression of vascular endothelial growth factor (VEGF) expression after MEL incubation (1 mmol/L), which is an indication of the antiangiogenic properties of the indoleamine [61]. Liu et al. [62] have found that breast and colon cancer cells treated with MEL exhibit an increased DNA repair capacity by affecting several key genes involved in DNA damage-responsive pathways.

It is well known that MEL also promotes apoptosis in cancer cells, in contrast to the well-studied inhibition of apoptosis in normal cells [63, 64]. The mechanism by which the apoptotic process occurs after MEL treatment is still under investigation. Apparently, the intrinsic apoptotic pathway would be involved and so the MAPK-related pathways [65].

Epidemiological studies indicate that night workers and shift workers have slight to moderate risk to develop cancer [66]. This could be a result of increased exposure to light during nighttime provoking decreased MEL secretion. This circadian disruption seems not to affect equally people with different ethnias. Asians appear to maintain a better circadian pattern of MEL production as compared with whites, and probably Asian night and shift workers may be at reduced risk of cancer [67].

Cardiovascular System and Melatonin

Increasing interest has arisen in the last two decades concerning the use of MEL in the treatment of cardiovascular diseases, as monotherapy or in combination with other drugs. Several experiments in animals have suggested an effect of the indolamine on circulatory function via different mechanisms. The antioxidant properties of MEL seem to improve endothelial function by maintaining the availability of nitric oxide, thus exerting vasodilatation and reducing blood pressure [68]. Besides, MEL could apparently reduce adrenergic tone and increase the cholinergic tone [69]. These findings together with the identification of MT1 and MT2 MEL receptors in left human ventricle, aorta, and coronary, cerebral, and systemic peripheral arteries [70] and the occurrence of cardiovascular diseases in persons with altered circadian rhythms have supported the hypothesis of a possible pharmacological role of MEL in the treatment of cardiovascular diseases such as hypertension, myocardial ischemia, and stroke. Cagnacci et al. [71] demonstrated that MEL (1 mg) administered orally during daytime reduced systolic and diastolic pressures, pulsatility index of the internal carotid artery, and norepinephrine levels in young women and men [71, 72]. In 2004, Scheer et al. [73] evaluated the effect of a single intake of MEL and a chronic repeated oral administration of MEL 1 h before bedtime in men with untreated essential hypertension. The chronic intake of MEL (2.5 mg) improved sleep quality and reduced both systolic and diastolic sleep blood pressure. Although the reduction in blood pressure was mild, it was clinically relevant since it might contribute to counteract the cardiac risks typically present during nighttime [73]. Several studies have analyzed the use of MEL in combination with regular antihypertensive drugs. In 2000, a double-blind crossover study revealed that the coadministration of MEL (5 mg at 22 h for 4 weeks) and nifedipine (30–60 mg/day) increased blood pressure, mainly in the morning and in the afternoon [74]. This effect could be due to pharmacodynamic interaction between both drugs. However, some studies have demonstrated that MEL potentiated the effect of other antihypertensive drugs when administered in a combined treatment [75].

The chronobiological, antioxidant, and antiadrenergic properties of MEL are also involved in the cardioprotective effect of the indolamine, particularly important in myocardial infarction and ischemia/reperfusion processes. A study carried out in a murine model of acute myocardial infarction has demonstrated that certain mutations in MEL receptors are associated with higher risk of infarction [76]. Patients with coronary disease have low MEL levels and reduced 6-sulfatoxymelatonin urinary excretion [77]. There is evidence that patients with AMI have high levels of oxidized low-density lipoproteins associated with low levels of nocturnal MEL [78]. This evidence supports a potential role of MEL in the therapeutic of AMI. However, MEL did not exert a protective effect on surgical oxidative stress during the perioperative period of patients with major vascular surgery [79].

In the light of these findings, MEL could play an important role in the treatment of hypertension and myocardial infarction. By regulating the endogenous clock, MEL exerts great influence on many physiological functions, such as circulatory function. Further clinical trials including more participants and exhaustively analyzing the effects of MEL on cardiovascular function are required. Given the circadian fluctuation of the hormone, studies exploring the differential action of MEL at different times of the day would shed light on adequate pharmacological prescription.

Melatonin Secretion and Reproduction

Ovary and MEL

It has been shown that MEL has direct effects on ovary function. MEL is present in human preovulatory follicular fluid in concentrations higher than serum and there are MEL receptors in ovarian granulosa cells (GC) [80]. By its powerful antioxidant action, MEL appears to be involved in a number of reproductive events including folliculogenesis, follicular atresia, ovulation, oocyte maturation, and corpus luteum (CL) formation. Taketani et al. [81] studied the effect of MEL treatment on progesterone levels in 25 women who had luteal phase defect (serum progesterone concentrations <10 ng/mL during the mid-luteal phase). Fourteen women were given 3 mg/day MEL at 22:00 h throughout the luteal phase whereas 11 women were given no medication (controls). MEL enhanced serum progesterone concentration in 9 of 14 women (64.3 %), and only 2 of 11 women (18.1 %) had normal serum progesterone levels in the control group. Therefore, MEL may contribute to luteinization by enhancing progesterone synthesis during ovulation. Besides, MEL deficiency has been associated with endometriosis, premature ovarian failure, and polycystic ovary syndrome (PCOS) [80]. Recently, Kim et al. [82] evaluated the effect of MEL in the culture medium of granulosa cells (GC) or cumulus-oocyte complexes (COC) from patients with PCOS involved in a program of in vitro fertilization embryo transfer. The authors demonstrated that the pregnancy and implantation rates, with human chorionic gonadotrophin priming, were higher in the melatonin-supplemented group than those of the non-supplemented control. The data suggest that follicular MEL is released from luteinizing granulose cells during late folliculogenesis and plays a positive role in the maturation of oocytes. Lord et al. [83] have proven that MEL prevents post-ovulatory oocyte aging in the mouse and extends the window for optimal fertilization in vitro. Therefore, MEL could also improve oocyte quality and luteal function in infertile women.

Sperm and MEL

Earlier studies have demonstrated the presence of MEL in human seminal fluid [84] and MEL receptors in spermatozoa [85]. The effect of MEL on sperm motility is controversial. There is evidence that MEL may have inhibitory effects on sperm motility in vitro [86] or decrease not only the motility but also the sperm concentration in healthy men [87]. In contrast, Fujinoki [88] has shown hyperactivation of hamster sperm after MEL treatment. The antioxidant and antiapoptotic properties of MEL on sperm are also conflictive. Espino et al. [89] have found in 20 healthy men that ejaculated human spermatozoa exposed for a short time to MEL reversed caspase-3 and caspase-9 activation as well as PS externalization provoked by oxidants. Afterward, they have found that MEL receptor (MT1) and the survival-promoting pathway extracellular signal-regulated kinase (ERK) are likely to have a role in the protective response [90]. However, MEL did not protect testis, epididymis, and sperm in rats exposed to oxidative stress under intermittent hypobaric hypoxia [91]. Due to the fact that human spermatozoa increase ROS production through the conventional procedures used for assisted reproductive techniques, MEL supplementation could be a tool against oxidative stress and apoptosis in ejaculated spermatozoa, but more studies are needed in order to clarify molecular mechanisms triggered by MEL.

MEL and Pregnancy

MEL has protective actions on both the fetus and the mother during pregnancy. It can easily cross the placenta to enter the fetal circulation leading the photoperiodic information to the fetus [92]. At pregnancy there is a high metabolic demand for oxygen, which leads to a higher ROS production and, consequently, oxidative stress. The placenta is a major source of oxidative stress because it is rich in polyunsaturated fatty acids. Spontaneous abortion and recurrent pregnancy loss have been associated with systemic oxidative stress [93]. Due to MEL level increase during gestation in normal pregnant humans reducing the oxidative stress and abortion rate, MEL has been suggested as a potential molecule to be administered throughout compromised pregnancy such as in preeclampsia and fetal undernutrition, two entities associated with oxidative stress. In preeclampsia, lipid peroxide levels in maternal blood and placental tissue are increased and total antioxidant activities are lowered. MEL levels were found to be decreased in severe preeclampsia [94]. Some recent evidence has suggested supplements of MEL to prevent preeclampsia in humans [95].

MEL and Human Parturition

Circadian timing of parturition seems to be species specific. Rats and golden hamsters give births during daytime hours [96, 97], while human parturition occurs mainly at late nighttime and early morning hours [98]. Furthermore, both humans and nonhuman primates show nocturnally peaking uterine contractions in late pregnancy [99]. The circadian signals that drive the rapid uterine activation and strong contractions remain to be clearly understood. Sharkey et al. [100] have shown that MEL synergizes with oxytocin to increase contractility of human myometrial smooth muscle cells, recruiting similar intracellular signaling mechanisms such as activation of phospholipase C signaling, protein kinase C, and myosin light chain kinase, all of them involved in the induction or facilitation of labor. The same authors have also demonstrated a strong and parallel upregulation of the oxytocin and MEL receptors (MT2) in the myometrium of laboring pregnant humans as compared to those from myometrium of pregnant nonlaboring humans. The synergic action of MEL and oxytocin seems to be mediated by the gap junctions, which are essential in promoting synchronous myometrial contractions [101]. This novel physiological mechanism of MEL on the human uterus could explain, at least in part, the nocturnal timing of birth and may be useful to develop pharmacological strategies to handle the preterm and/or delayed parturition.

Recently, it has been reported that MEL concentration in umbilical cord blood depends on the mode of delivery. The indoleamine in the umbilical cord from the spontaneous vaginal delivery group was significantly higher both at night- and daytime than that from the cesarean section deliveries. There were no differences in the MEL levels of the umbilical cord associated with pregnancy or intrapartum complications [102].

Melatonin Agonists

The administration of MEL, alone or in combination with other drugs, may have a beneficial impact on numerous pathologies. However, the therapeutic potential of this drug is limited by some of its pharmacokinetic parameters, such as the short half-life in circulation [103]. This issue has produced an intense search for several MEL receptor agonists in the last two decades, and there are currently over 70 patients on melatoninergic agents that wait to undergo clinical assessment [104]. Some of these ligands have been recently approved or are being currently tested within clinical trials at different phases [105, 106].

Ramelteon, approved by the FDA in 2005 [107], is a hypnotic agent almost exclusively studied for the treatment of chronic primary insomnia, circadian rhythm sleep disorders, and other sleep alterations. It is a highly selective melatoninergic agonist with an affinity for MT1 and MT2 MEL receptors 3–16 times higher than the one of MEL [108]. This drug has proved to shorten the latency to persistent sleep as well as to increase total sleep duration in insomniac patients of different ages, from 18 to 83 years [109, 110]. Although the recommended dose is 8 mg, the drug has been tested in doses ranging from 4 to 160 mg [111, 112]. It is well tolerated since only mild to moderate adverse events have been detected, being the most frequent headache, dizziness, somnolence, fatigue, and nausea [106, 113].

Ramelteon has almost no affinity for MT3, opiate, dopamine, benzodiazepine, and serotonin receptors in the brain [114], which is an advantage over the other available hypnotics. This high selectivity may explain the lack of withdrawal effect, insomnia rebound, abuse, or dependence potential, property that makes ramelteon particularly beneficial for addicts [115]. The lack of depressant and sedative effect has especial interest for patients suffering from obstructive apnea, since it does not affect the control of breathing [116] and for elderly people because it does not cause significant motor or cognitive impairment [110].

Tasimelteon, similarly to ramelteon, is a selective MT1 and MT2 agonist in the suprachiasmatic nucleus. It has been through Phase III trials successfully and was shown to improve both onset and maintenance of sleep with few side effects [117].

Agomelatine is a potent synthetic MT1/MT2 receptor agonist with serotonin 5HT(2C) antagonistic properties [118]. It has been approved for the treatment of major depression in adults [119] and is now available on the market in more than 40 countries [120]. The melatoninergic modulation helps to resynchronize circadian rhythms, often disrupted in depressive disorders, thus contributing to ameliorate sleep disorders and relieving symptoms in depressed patients [121]. The serotoninergic antagonism leads to the release of norepinephrine and dopamine in the frontal cortex, partially explaining its antidepressant and anxiolytic properties [122]. Several preclinical studies have revealed that prolonged treatment with agomelatine increases dendritic neurogenesis, enhancing neuronal survival and attenuating stress-induced glutamate release [121].

Agomelatine is rapidly absorbed orally and mainly metabolized via CYP1A2 hepatic isoenzymes and has no active metabolites and an elimination half-life of 1–2 h [123]. Its atypical pharmacological profile offers important advantages over current monoaminergic antidepressants, as demonstrated by many clinical trials comparing agomelatine (25 or 50 mg/day) with venlafaxine, fluoxetine, paroxetine, and sertraline, among others [124]. One of these assets is the early onset of action-improving symptoms even in the first week of treatment [125]. This feature together with the lack of adverse effect on sexual function [126] and its relative safety with only mild adverse effects [127] result in a better adherence to treatment and low discontinuation rate [128]. Agomelatine does not exhibit discontinuation syndrome and is relatively safe in overdose [129]. Some studies have revealed agomelatine efficacy not only for the acute treatment of depression symptoms but also for the maintenance of long-term treatment showing a significant lower relapse rate [130]. However, an increase in liver transaminase activities has been observed in approximately 4 % of the patients [120], which calls for a permanent follow-up of liver function and contraindicates the drug in hepatic insufficiency. Despite the beneficial aspects of agomelatine in comparison with other antidepressants, some authors are cautious in this respect and suggest that further clinical trials should be carried out in order to define the proper niche for this innovative antidepressant in depression therapy [131]. Although the main clinical target is moderate to severe major depression, the drug has been tested with positive results in general anxiety disorder, bipolar disorder, and seasonal affective disorder [132].

A time line with the first research finding related to MEL's clinical uses according to the PubMed database is depicted in Fig. 3.1.

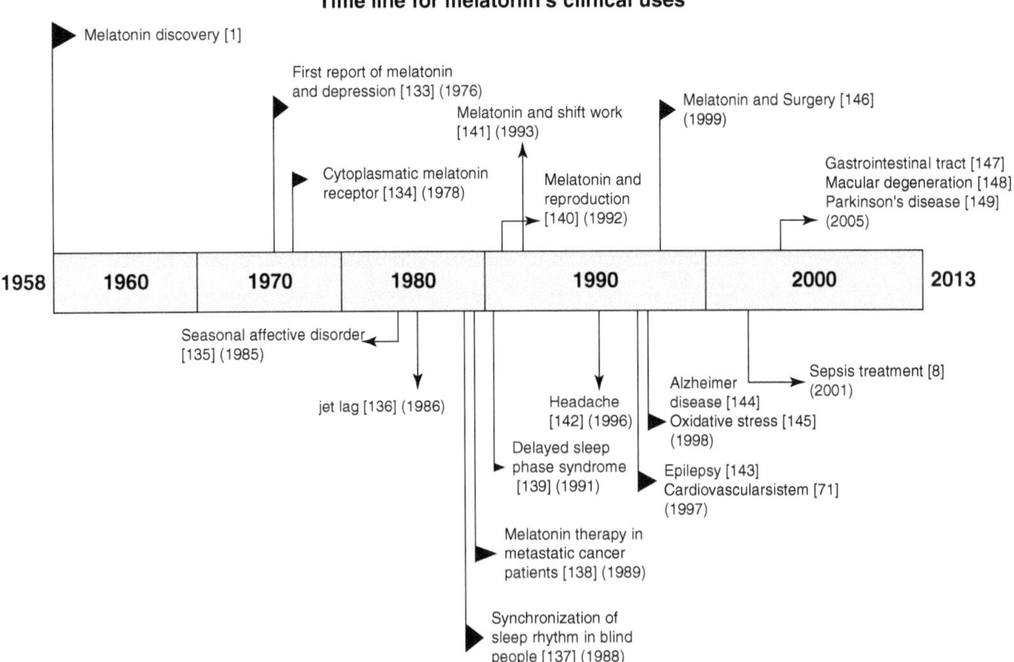

Fig. 3.1 Dates correspond to the first research findings related to MEL's clinical uses according to the PubMed database

Concluding Remarks

Many advances have been made concerning the knowledge of molecular aspects of MEL, its receptors, its physiology as a chronobiotic hormone, and its role in the pathogenesis of many diseases. The chronobiological properties of exogenous MEL, its capacity to resynchronize circadian rhythms in certain disorders such as delayed sleep-phase disorder, and its effectiveness to reduce sleep latency in primary chronic insomnia have already been proven, and, thus, MEL can be considered a first-line drug in the treatment of these conditions. The antioxidant and anti-inflammatory properties of MEL and its relative safety and good tolerability suggest that it could have a beneficial effect on the treatment and prevention of a wide spectrum of diseases such as cancer, cardiovascular and gastrointestinal diseases, reproduction disorders, neuropathies, and other pathologies. The synthesis of new MEL agonists with better pharmacokinetics has opened a novel field for the clinical uses. An increasing number of clinical trials using MEL or its agonists are ongoing and will certainly improve our understanding about the correct use of these drugs.

References

1. Lerner AB, Case JD, Heinzelman RV. Structure of melatonin. J Am Chem Soc. 1959;81:6084–5.
2. Macchi MM, Bruce JN. Human pineal physiology and functional significance of melatonin. Front Neuroendocrinol. 2004;25:177–95.
3. Dubocovich ML. Melatonin is a potent modulator of dopamine release in the retina. Nature. 1984;306: 782–4.
4. Reppert SM, Weaver DR, Godson C. Melatonin receptors step into the light: cloning and classification of subtypes. Trends Pharmacol Sci. 1996;17: 100–2.
5. Seron-Ferre M, Torres-Farfán C, Forcelledo ML, Valenzuela GJ. The development of circadian rhythms in the fetus and neonate. Semin Perinatol. 2001; 25:363–70.
6. Arendt J. Melatonin and human rhythms. Chronobiol Int. 2006;23:21–37.
7. Carlomagno G, Nordio M, Chiu TT, Unfer V. Contribution of myo-inositol and melatonin to human reproduction. Eur J Obstet Gynecol Reprod Biol. 2011;159:267–72.
8. Gitto E, Karbownik M, Reiter RJ, Tan DX, Cuzzocrea S, Chiurazzi P, et al. Effects of melatonin treatment in septic newborns. Pediatr Res. 2001;50:756–60.
9. Gitto E, Romeo C, Reiter RJ, Impellizzeri P, Pesce S, Basile M, et al. Melatonin reduces oxidative stress in surgical neonates. J Pediatr Surg. 2004;39:184–9.
10. Fulia F, Gitto E, Cuzzocrea S, Reiter RJ, Dugo L, Gitto P, et al. Increased levels of malondialdehyde and nitrite/nitrate in the blood of asphyxiated newborns: reduction by melatonin. J Pineal Res. 2001;31: 343–9.
11. Wirojanan J, Jacquemont S, Diaz R, Bacalman S, Anders TF, Hagerman RJ, et al. The efficacy of melatonin for sleep problems in children with autism, fragile X syndrome, or autism and fragile X syndrome. J Clin Sleep Med. 2009;5:145–50.
12. Jan JE, Freeman RD, Fast DK. Melatonin treatment of sleep-wake cycle disorders in children and adolescents. Dev Med Child Neurol. 1999;41:491–500.
13. Gitto E, Aversa S, Salpietro CD, Barberi I, Arrigo T, Trimarchi G, Reiter RJ, Pellegrino S. Pain in neonatal intensive care: role of melatonin as an analgesic antioxidant. J Pineal Res. 2012;52:291–5.
14. Jan JE, Freeman RD, Wasdell MB, Bomben MM. A child with severe night terrors and sleep-walking responds to melatonin therapy'. Dev Med Child Neurol. 2004;46:789.
15. Jan JE, Hamilton D, Seward N, Fast DK, Freeman RD, Laudon M. Clinical trials of controlled-release melatonin in children with sleep-wake cycle disorders. J Pineal Res. 2000;29:34–9.
16. Peled N, Shorer Z, Peled E, Pillar G. Melatonin effect on seizures in children with severe neurologic deficit disorders. Epilepsia. 2001;42:1208–10.
17. Gupta M, Aneja S, Kohli K. Add-on melatonin improves quality of life in epileptic children on valproate monotherapy: a randomized, double-blind, placebo-controlled trial. Epilepsy Behav. 2004;5: 316–21.
18. Paprocka J, Dec R, Jamroz E, Marszał E. Melatonin and childhood refractory epilepsy – a pilot study. Med Sci Monit. 2010;16:389–96.
19. Sandyk R. The pineal gland and the mode of onset of schizophrenia. Int J Neurosci. 1992;67:9–17.
20. Sheldon SH. Pro-convulsant effects of oral melatonin in neurologically disabled children. Lancet. 1998;351: 1254.
21. Banach M, Gurdziel E, Jędrych M, Borowicz KK. Melatonin in experimental seizures and epilepsy. Pharmacol Rep. 2011;63:1–11.
22. van Geijlswijk IM, Mol RH, Egberts TC, Smits MG. Evaluation of sleep, puberty and mental health in children with long-term melatonin treatment for chronic idiopathic childhood sleep onset insomnia. Psychopharmacology (Berl). 2011;216:111–20.
23. Eckerberg B, Lowden A, Nagai R, Akerstedt T. Melatonin treatment effects on adolescent students' sleep timing and sleepiness in a placebo-controlled crossover study. Chronobiol Int. 2012;29: 1239–48.
24. Baskett JJ, Broad JB, Wood PC, Duncan JR, Pledger MJ, English J, et al. Does melatonin improve sleep in

older people? A randomised crossover trial. Age Ageing. 2003;32:164–70.
25. Wade AG, Ford I, Crawford G, McMahon AD, Nir T, Laudon M, et al. Efficacy of prolonged release melatonin in insomnia patients aged 55–80 years: quality of sleep and next-day alertness outcomes. Curr Med Res Opin. 2007;23:2597–605.
26. Lemoine P, Nir T, Laudon M, Zisapel N. Prolonged-release melatonin improves sleep quality and morning alertness in insomnia patients aged 55 years and older and has no withdrawal effects. J Sleep Res. 2007; 16:372–80.
27. Peck JS, LeGoff DB, Ahmed I, Goebert D. Cognitive effects of exogenous melatonin administration in elderly persons: a pilot study. Am J Geriatr Psychiatry. 2004;12:432–6.
28. Luthringer R, Muzet M, Zisapel N, Staner L. The effect of prolonged-release melatonin on sleep measures and psychomotor performance in elderly patients with insomnia. Int Clin Psychopharmacol. 2009;24:239–49.
29. Otmani S, Demazières A, Staner C, Jacob N, Nir T, Zisapel N, et al. Effects of prolonged-release melatonin, zolpidem, and their combination on psychomotor functions, memory recall, and driving skills in healthy middle aged and elderly volunteers. Hum Psychopharmacol. 2008;23:693–705.
30. Rechciński T, Uznańska-Loch B, Trzos E, Wierzbowska-Drabik K, Krzemińska-Pakuła M, et al. Melatonin - a somniferous option which does not aggravate sleep-disordered breathing in cardiac risk patients: a Holter ECG based study. Kardiol Pol. 2012;70:24–9.
31. Nunes DM, Mota RM, Machado MO, Pereira ED, Bruin VM, Bruin PF. Effect of melatonin administration on subjective sleep quality in chronic obstructive pulmonary disease. Braz J Med Biol Res. 2008;41: 926–31.
32. De Leersnyder H, Zisapel N, Laudon M. Prolonged-release melatonin for children with neurodevelopmental disorders. Pediatr Neurol. 2011;45:23–6.
33. Malow B, Adkins KW, McGrew SG, Wang L, Goldman SE, Fawkes D, et al. Melatonin for sleep in children with autism: a controlled trial examining dose, tolerability, and outcomes. J Autism Dev Disord. 2012;42:1729–37.
34. Tjon Pian Gi CV, Broeren JP, Starreveld JS, Versteegh FG. Melatonin for treatment of sleeping disorders in children with attention deficit/hyperactivity disorder: a preliminary open label study. Eur J Pediatr. 2003;162:554–5.
35. Serfaty MA, Osborne D, Buszewicz MJ, Blizard R, Raven PW. A randomized double-blind placebo-controlled trial of treatment as usual plus exogenous slow-release melatonin (6 mg) or placebo for sleep disturbance and depressed mood. Int Clin Psychopharmacol. 2010;25:132–42.
36. Bonnefont-Rousselot D, Collin F. Melatonin: action as antioxidant and potential applications in human disease and aging. Toxicology. 2010;278:55–67.
37. Galano A, Tan DX, Reiter RJ. Melatonin as a natural ally against oxidative stress: a physicochemical examination. J Pineal Res. 2011;5:1–16.
38. Radogna F, Diederich M, Ghibelli L. Melatonin: a pleiotropic molecule regulating inflammation. Biochem Pharmacol. 2010;80:1844–52.
39. Seabra ML, Bignotto M, Pinto Jr LR, Tufik S. Randomized, double-blind clinical trial, controlled with placebo, of the toxicology of chronic melatonin treatment. J Pineal Res. 2000;29:193–200.
40. Wang X. The antiapoptotic activity of melatonin in neurodegenerative diseases. CNS Neurosci Ther. 2009;15:345–57.
41. Terry PD, Villinger F, Bubenik GA, Sitaraman SV. Melatonin and ulcerative colitis: evidence, biological mechanisms, and future research. Inflamm Bowel Dis. 2009;15:134–40.
42. Celinski K, Konturek SJ, Konturek PC, Brzozowski T, Cichoz-Lach H, Slomka M, Malgorzata P, Bielanski W, Reiter RJ. Melatonin or L-tryptophan accelerates healing of gastroduodenal ulcers in patients treated with omeprazole. J Pineal Res. 2011;50:389–94.
43. Chen CQ, Fichna J, Bashashati M, Li YY, Storr M. Distribution, function and physiological role of melatonin in the lower gut. World J Gastroenterol. 2011;17:3888–98.
44. Cichoz-Lach H, Celinski K, Konturek PC, Konturek SJ, Slomka M. The effects of L-tryptophan and melatonin on selected biochemical parameters in patients with steatohepatitis. J Physiol Pharmacol. 2010;61: 577–80.
45. Mathes AM. Hepatoprotective actions of melatonin: possible mediation by melatonin receptors. World J Gastroenterol. 2010;16:6087–97.
46. Forrest CM, Mackay GM, Stoy N, Stone TW, Darlington LG. Inflammatory status and kynurenine metabolism in rheumatoid arthritis treated with melatonin. Br J Clin Pharmacol. 2007;64:517–26.
47. Ozkan E, Yaman H, Cakir E, Deniz O, Oztosun M, Gumus S, Akgul EO, Agilli M, Cayci T, Kurt YG, Aydin I, Arslan Y, Ilhan N, Ilhan N, Erbil MK. Plasma melatonin and urinary 6-hydroxymelatonin levels in patients with pulmonary tuberculosis. Inflammation. 2012;35:1429–34.
48. Nunnari G, Nigro L, Palermo F, Leto D, Pomerantz RJ, Cacopardo B. Reduction of serum melatonin levels in HIV-1-infected individuals' parallel disease progression: correlation with serum interleukin-12 levels. Infection. 2003;31:379–82.
49. Srinivasan V, Mohamed M, Kato H. Melatonin in bacterial and viral infections with focus on sepsis: a review. Recent Pat Endocr Metab Immune Drug Discov. 2012;6:30–9.
50. Cohen M, Lippman M, Chabner B. Pineal gland and breast cancer. Lancet. 1978;2:1381–2.
51. Tamarkin L, Danforth D, Lichter A, DeMoss E, Cohen M, Chabner B, et al. Decreased nocturnal plasma melatonin peak in patients with estrogen receptor positive breast cancer. Science. 1982;216: 1003–5.

52. Danforth Jr DN, Tamarkin L, Mulvihill JJ, Bagley CS, Lippman ME. Plasma melatonin and the hormone-dependency of human breast cancer. J Clin Oncol. 1985;3:941–8.
53. Grin W, Grünberger W. A significant correlation between melatonin deficiency and endometrial cancer. Gynecol Obstet Invest. 1998;45:62–5.
54. Lissoni P, Brivio F, Ardizzoia A, Tancini G, Barni S. Subcutaneous therapy with low-dose interleukin-2 plus the neurohormone melatonin in metastatic gastric cancer patients with low performance status. Tumori. 1993;79:401–4.
55. Lissoni P, Barni S, Cattaneo G, Tancini G, Esposti G, Esposti D, et al. Clinical results with the pineal hormone melatonin in advanced cancer resistant to standard antitumor therapies. Oncology. 1991;48:448–50.
56. Lissoni P, Barni S, Tancini G, Mainini E, Piglia F, Maestroni GJ, et al. Immunoendocrine therapy with low-dose subcutaneous interleukin-2 plus melatonin of locally advanced or metastatic endocrine tumors. Oncology. 1995;52:163–6.
57. Lissoni P, Barni S, Ardizzoia A, Paolorossi F, Crispino S, Tancini G, et al. Randomized study with the pineal hormone melatonin versus supportive care alone in advanced nonsmall cell lung cancer resistant to a first-line chemotherapy containing cisplatin. Oncology. 1992;49:336–9.
58. Neri B, de Leonardis V, Gemelli MT, di Loro F, Mottola A, Ponchietti R, et al. Melatonin as biological response modifier in cancer patients. Anticancer Res. 1998;18:1329–32.
59. Sanchez-Barcelo EJ, Mediavilla MD, Alonso-Gonzalez C, Rueda N. Breast cancer therapy based on melatonin. Recent Pat Endocr Metab Immune Drug Discov. 2012;6:108–16.
60. Sanchez-Barcelo EJ, Mediavilla MD, Alonso-Gonzalez C, Reiter RJ. Melatonin uses in oncology: breast cancer prevention and reduction of the side effects of chemotherapy and radiation. Expert Opin Investig Drugs. 2012;21:819–31.
61. Lv D, Cui PL, Yao SW, Xu YQ, Yang ZX. Melatonin inhibits the expression of vascular endothelial growth factor in pancreatic cancer cells. Chin J Cancer Res. 2012,24.310–6.
62. Liu R, Fu A, Hoffman AE, Zheng T, Zhu Y. Melatonin enhances DNA repair capacity possibly by affecting genes involved in DNA damage responsive pathways. BMC Cell Biol. 2013;14:1.
63. Sainz RM, Mayo JC, Rodriguez C, Tan DX, Lopez-Burillo S, Reiter RJ. Melatonin and cell death: differential actions on apoptosis in normal and cancer cells. Cell Mol Life Sci. 2003;60:1407–26.
64. Sánchez-Hidalgo M, Guerrero JM, Villegas I, Packham G, de la Lastra CA. Melatonin, a natural programmed cell death inducer in cancer. Curr Med Chem. 2012;19:3805–21.
65. Proietti S, Cucina A, Reiter RJ, Bizzarri M. Molecular mechanisms of melatonin's inhibitory actions on breast cancers. Cell Mol Life Sci. 2013;70:2139–57.
66. Reiter RJ, Tan DX, Korkmaz A, Erren TC, Piekarski C, Tamura H, et al. Light at night, chronodisruption, melatonin suppression, and cancer risk: a review. Crit Rev Oncog. 2007;13:303–28.
67. Bhatti P, Mirick DK, Davis S. Racial differences in the association between night shift work and melatonin levels among women. Am J Epidemiol. 2013;177:388–93.
68. Simko F, Paulis L. Melatonin as a potential antihypertensive treatment. J Pineal Res. 2007;42:319–22.
69. Chuang JI, Chen SS, Lin MT. Melatonin decreases brain serotonin release, arterial pressure and heart rate in rats. Pharmacology. 1993;47:91–7.
70. Ekmekcioglu C, Thalhammer T, Humpeler S, Mehrabi MR, Glogar HD, Hölzenbein T, et al. The melatonin receptor subtype MT2 is present in the human cardiovascular system. J Pineal Res. 2003;35:40–4.
71. Cagnacci A, Arangino S, Angiolucci M, Maschio E, Melis GB. Influences of melatonin administration on the circulation of women. Am J Physiol. 1998;274:335–8.
72. Arangino S, Cagnacci A, Angiolucci M, Vacca AM, Longu G, Volpe A, Melis GB. Effects of melatonin on vascular reactivity, catecholamine levels, and blood pressure in healthy men. Am J Cardiol. 1999;83:1417–9.
73. Scheer FA, Van Montfrans GA, van Someren EJ, Mairuhu G, Buijs RM. Daily nighttime melatonin reduces blood pressure in male patients with essential hypertension. Hypertension. 2004;43:192–7.
74. Lusardi P, Piazza E, Fogari R. Cardiovascular effects of melatonin in hypertensive patients well controlled by nifedipine: a 24-hour study. Br J Clin Pharmacol. 2000;49:423–7.
75. Sánchez-Barceló EJ, Mediavilla MD, Tan DX, Reiter RJ. Clinical uses of melatonin: evaluation of human trials. Curr Med Chem. 2010;17:2070–95.
76. Sallinen P, Mänttäri S, Leskinen H, Ilves M, Vakkuri O, Ruskoaho H, et al. The effect of myocardial infarction on the synthesis, concentration and receptor expression of endogenous melatonin. J Pineal Res. 2007;42:254–60.
77. Domínguez-Rodríguez A, Pedro Abreu-González P, García MJ, Sanchez J, Marrero F, de Armas-Trujillo D. Decreased nocturnal melatonin levels during acute myocardial infarction. J Pineal Res. 2002;33:248–52.
78. Dominguez-Rodriguez A, Abreu-Gonzalez P, Garcia-Gonzalez M, Ferrer-Hita J, Vargas M, Reiter RJ. Elevated levels of oxidized low-density lipoprotein and impaired nocturnal synthesis of melatonin in patients with myocardial infarction. Atherosclerosis. 2005;180:101–5.
79. Kücükakin B, Wilhelmsen M, Lykkesfeldt J, Reiter RJ, Rosenberg J, Gögenur I. No effect of melatonin to modify surgical-stress response after major vascular surgery: a randomised placebo-controlled trial. Eur J Vasc Endovasc Surg. 2010;40:461–7.
80. Tamura H, Nakamura Y, Korkmaz A, Manchester LC, Tan DX, Sugino N, et al. Melatonin and the ovary: physiological and pathophysiological implications. Fertil Steril. 2009;92:328–43.

81. Taketani T, Tamura H, Takasaki A, Lee L, Kizuka F, Tamura I, et al. Protective role of melatonin in progesterone production by human luteal cells. J Pineal Res. 2011;51:207–13.
82. Kim MK, Park EA, Kim HJ, Choi WY, Cho JH, Lee WS, et al. Does supplementation of in-vitro culture medium with melatonin improve IVF outcome in PCOS? Reprod Biomed Online. 2013;26:22–9.
83. Lord T, Nixon B, Jones KT, Aitken RJ. Melatonin prevents postovulatory oocyte aging in the mouse and extends the window for optimal fertilization in vitro. Biol Reprod. 2013;88:67–76.
84. Bornman MS, Oosthuizen JM, Barnard HC, Schulenburg GW, Boomker D, Reif S. Melatonin and sperm motility. Andrologia. 1989;21:483–5.
85. van Vuuren RJ, Pitout MJ, van Aswegen CH, Theron JJ. Putative melatonin receptor in human spermatozoa. Clin Biochem. 1992;25:125–7.
86. Irez TO, Senol H, Alagöz M, Basmaciogullari C, Turan F, Kuru D, et al. Effects of indoleamines on sperm motility in vitro. Hum Reprod. 1992;7:987–90.
87. Luboshitzky R, Shen-Orr Z, Nave R, Lavi S, Lavie P. Melatonin administration alters semen quality in healthy men. J Androl. 2002;23:572–8.
88. Fujinoki M. Melatonin-enhanced hyperactivation of hamster sperm. Reproduction. 2008;136:533–41.
89. Espino J, Bejarano I, Ortiz A, Lozano GM, García JF, Pariente JA, et al. Melatonin as a potential tool against oxidative damage and apoptosis in ejaculated human spermatozoa. Fertil Steril. 2010;94:1915–7.
90. Espino J, Ortiz Á, Bejarano I, Lozano GM, Monllor F, García JF, et al. Melatonin protects human spermatozoa from apoptosis via melatonin receptor- and extracellular signal-regulated kinase-mediated pathways. Fertil Steril. 2011;95:2290–6.
91. Farías JG, Zepeda AB, Calaf GM. Melatonin protects the heart, lungs and kidneys from oxidative stress under intermittent hypobaric hypoxia in rats. Biol Res. 2012;45:81–5.
92. Schenker S, Yang Y, Perez A, Acuff RV, Papas AM, Henderson G, et al. Antioxidant transport by the human placenta. Clin Nutr. 1998;17:159–67.
93. Gupta S, Agarwal A, Banerjee J, Alvarez JG. The role of oxidative stress in spontaneous abortion and recurrent pregnancy loss: a systematic review. Obstet Gynecol Surv. 2007;62:335–47.
94. Nakamura Y, Tamura H, Kashida S, Takayama H, Yamagata Y, Karube A, et al. Changes of serum melatonin level and its relationship to feto-placental unit during pregnancy. J Pineal Res. 2001;30:29–33.
95. Briceño-Pérez C, Briceño-Sanabria L, Vigil-De Gracia P. Prediction and prevention of preeclampsia. Hypertens Pregnancy. 2009;28:138–55.
96. Plaut SM, Grota LJ, Ader R, Graham 3rd CW. Effects of handling and the light–dark cycle on time of parturition in the rat. Lab Anim Care. 1970; 20:447–53.
97. Siegel HI, Greenwald GS. Prepartum onset of maternal behavior in hamsters and the effects of estrogen and progesterone. Horm Behav. 1975;6:237–45.
98. Vatish M, Steer PJ, Blanks AM, Hon M, Thornton S. Diurnal variation is lost in preterm deliveries before 28 weeks of gestation. BJOG. 2010;117:765–7.
99. Olcese J. Circadian aspects of mammalian parturition: a review. Mol Cell Endocrinol. 2012;349:62–7.
100. Sharkey JT, Puttaramu R, Word RA, Olcese J. Melatonin synergizes with oxytocin to enhance contractility of human myometrial smooth muscle cells. J Clin Endocrinol Metab. 2009;94:421–7.
101. Sharkey JT, Cable C, Olcese J. Melatonin sensitizes human myometrial cells to oxytocin in a protein kinase C alpha/extracellular-signal regulated kinase-dependent manner. J Clin Endocrinol Metab. 2010;95:2902–8.
102. Bagci S, Berner AL, Reinsberg J, Gast AS, Zur B, Welzing L, et al. Melatonin concentration in umbilical cord blood depends on mode of delivery. Early Hum Dev. 2012;88:369–73.
103. Srinivasan V, Zakaria R, Othaman Z, Brzezinski A, Prasad A, Brown GM. Melatonergic drugs for therapeutic use in insomnia and sleep disturbances of mood disorders. CNS Neurol Disord Drug Targets. 2012;11:180–9.
104. Mody SM, Hu Y, Ho MK, Wong YH. In search of novel and therapeutically significant melatoninergic ligands. Recent Pat CNS Drug Discov. 2007;2: 241–5.
105. Borja NL, Daniel KL. Ramelteon for the treatment of insomnia. Clin Ther. 2006;28:1540–55.
106. Owen RT. Ramelteon: profile of a new sleep-promoting medication. Drugs Today (Barc). 2006; 42:255–63.
107. Cajochen C. TAK-375 Takeda. Curr Opin Investig Drugs. 2005;6:114–21.
108. Kato K, Hirai K, Nishiyama K, Uchikawa O, Fukatsu K, Ohkawa S, et al. Neurochemical properties of ramelteon (TAK-375), a selective MT1/MT2 receptor agonist. Neuropharmacology. 2005;48:301–10.
109. Greenblatt DJ, Harmatz JS, Karim A. Age and gender effects on the pharmacokinetics and pharmacodynamics of ramelteon, a hypnotic agent acting via melatonin receptors MT1 and MT2. J Clin Pharmacol. 2007;47:485–96.
110. Roth T, Seiden D, Wang-Weigand S, Zhang J. A 2-night, 3-period, crossover study of ramelteon's efficacy and safety in older adults with chronic insomnia. Curr Med Res Opin. 2007;23:1005–14.
111. Erman M, Seiden D, Zammit G, Sainati S, Zhang J. An efficacy, safety, and dose–response study of Ramelteon in patients with chronic primary insomnia. Sleep Med. 2006;7:17–24.
112. Johnson MW, Suess PE, Griffiths RR. Ramelteon: a novel hypnotic lacking abuse liability and sedative adverse effects. Arch Gen Psychiatry. 2006;63: 1149–57.
113. Reynoldson JN, Elliott Sr E, Nelson LA. Ramelteon: a novel approach in the treatment of insomnia. Ann Pharmacother. 2008;42:1262–71.
114. Zammit G, Schwartz H, Roth T, Wang-Weigand S, Sainati S, Zhang J. The effects of ramelteon in a

first-night model of transient insomnia. Sleep Med. 2009;10:55–9.

115. Bellon A. Searching for new options for treating insomnia: are melatonin and ramelteon beneficial? J Psychiatr Pract. 2006;12:229–43.
116. Kryger M, Wang-Weigand S, Roth T. Safety of ramelteon in individuals with mild to moderate obstructive sleep apnea. Sleep Breath. 2007;11:159–64.
117. Arendt J, Rajaratnam SM. Melatonin and its agonists: an update. Br J Psychiatry. 2008;193:267–9.
118. Levitan MN, Papelbaum M, Nardi AE. A review of preliminary observations on agomelatine in the treatment of anxiety disorders. Exp Clin Psychopharmacol. 2012;20:504–9.
119. Fornaro M. Switching from serotonin reuptake inhibitors to agomelatine in patients with refractory obsessive-compulsive disorder: a 3 month follow-up case series. Ann Gen Psychiatry. 2011;10:5.
120. Carney RM, Shelton RC. Agomelatine for the treatment of major depressive disorder. Expert Opin Pharmacother. 2011;12:2411–9.
121. Srinivasan V, Zakaria R, Othman Z, Lauterbach EC, Acuña-Castroviejo D. Agomelatine in depressive disorders: its novel mechanisms of action. J Neuropsychiatry Clin Neurosci. 2012;24:290–308.
122. Meltzer HY, Huang M. In vivo actions of atypical antipsychotic drug on serotonergic and dopaminergic systems. Prog Brain Res. 2008;172:177–97.
123. Owen RT. Agomelatine: a novel pharmacological approach to treating depression. Drugs Today (Barc). 2009;45:599–608.
124. Singh SP, Singh V, Kar N. Efficacy of agomelatine in major depressive disorder: meta-analysis and appraisal. Int J Neuropsychopharmacol. 2012;15: 417–28.
125. Di Giannantonio M, Martinotti G. Anhedonia and major depression: the role of agomelatine. Eur Neuropsychopharmacol. 2012;22 Suppl 3:S505–10.
126. Montejo AL, Prieto N, Terleira A, Matias J, Alonso S, Paniagua G, et al. Better sexual acceptability of agomelatine (25 and 50 mg) compared with paroxetine (20 mg) in healthy male volunteers. An 8-week, placebo-controlled study using the PRSEXDQ-SALSEX scale. J Psychopharmacol. 2010;24: 111–20.
127. Dolder CR, Nelson M, Snider M. Agomelatine treatment of major depressive disorder. Ann Pharmacother. 2008;42:1822–31.
128. Llorca PM. The antidepressant agomelatine improves the quality of life of depressed patients: implications for remission. J Psychopharmacol. 2010;24(2 Suppl):21–6.
129. Sansone RA, Sansone LA. Agomelatine: a novel antidepressant. Innov Clin Neurosci. 2011;8:10–4.
130. Goodwin GM, Boyer P, Emsley R, Rouillon F, de Bodinat C. Is it time to shift to better characterization of patients in trials assessing novel antidepressants? An example of two relapse prevention studies with agomelatine. Int Clin Psychopharmacol. 2013; 28:20–8.
131. Howland RH. Critical appraisal and update on the clinical utility of agomelatine, a melatonergic agonist, for the treatment of major depressive disease in adults. Neuropsychiatr Dis Treat. 2009;5:563–76.
132. da Rocha FF, Correa H. Is circadian rhythm disruption important in obsessive-compulsive disorder (OCD)? A case of successful augmentation with agomelatine for the treatment of OCD. Clin Neuropharmacol. 2011;34:139–40.
133. Carman JS, Post RM, Buswell R, Goodwin FK. Negative effects of melatonin on depression. Am J Psychiatry. 1976;133:1181–6.
134. Cohen M, Roselle D, Chabner B, Schmidt TJ, Lippman M. Evidence for a cytoplasmic melatonin receptor. Nature. 1978;274:894–5.
135. Sherer MA, Weingartner H, James SP, Rosenthal NE. Effects of melatonin on performance testing in patients with seasonal affective disorder. Neurosci Lett. 1985;58:277–82.
136. Arendt J, Aldhous M, Marks V. Alleviation of jet lag by melatonin: preliminary results of controlled double blind trial. Br Med J (Clin Res Ed). 1986;292:1170.
137. Arendt J, Aldhous M, Wright J. Synchronization of a disturbed sleep-wake cycle in a blind man by melatonin treatment. Lancet. 1988;331:772–3.
138. Lissoni P, Barni S, Crispino S, Tancini G, Fraschini F. Endocrine and immune effects of melatonin therapy in metastatic cancer patients. Eur J Cancer Clin Oncol. 1989;25:789–95.
139. Dahlitz M, Alvarez B, Vignau J, English J, Arendt J, Parkes JD. Delayed sleep phase syndrome response to melatonin. Lancet. 1991;337:1121–4.
140. Voordouw BC, Euser R, Verdonk RE, Alberda BT, de Jong FH, Drogendijk AC, et al. Melatonin and melatonin-progestin combinations alter pituitary-ovarian function in women and can inhibit ovulation. J Clin Endocrinol Metab. 1992;74:108–17.
141. Folkard S, Arendt J, Clark M. Can melatonin improve shift workers' tolerance of the night shift? Some preliminary findings. Chronobiol Int. 1993; 10:315–20.
142. Leone M, D'Amico D, Moschiano F, Fraschini F, Bussone G. Melatonin versus placebo in the prophylaxis of cluster headache: a double-blind pilot study with parallel groups. Cephalalgia. 1996;16:494–6.
143. Molina-Carballo A, Muñoz-Hoyos A, Reiter RJ, Sánchez-Forte M, Moreno-Madrid F, Rufo-Campos M, et al. Utility of high doses of melatonin as adjunctive anticonvulsant therapy in a child with severe myoclonic epilepsy: two years' experience. J Pineal Res. 1997;23:97–105.
144. Brusco LI, Márquez M, Cardinali DP. Monozygotic twins with Alzheimer's disease treated with melatonin: case report. J Pineal Res. 1998;25:260–3.
145. Dreher F, Gabard B, Schwindt DA, Maibach HI. Topical melatonin in combination with vitamins E and C protects skin from ultraviolet-induced erythema: a human study in vivo. Br J Dermatol. 1998;139:332–9.

146. Naguib M, Samarkandi AH. Premedication with melatonin: a double-blind, placebo-controlled comparison with midazolam. Br J Anaesth. 1999; 8:875–80.
147. Song GH, Leng PH, Gwee KA, Moochhala SM, Ho KY. Melatonin improves abdominal pain in irritable bowel syndrome patients who have sleep disturbances: a randomised, double blind, placebo controlled study. Gut. 2005;54:1402–7.
148. Yi C, Pan X, Yan H, Guo M, Pierpaoli W. Effects of melatonin in age-related macular degeneration. Ann N Y Acad Sci. 2005;1057:384–92.
149. Dowling GA, Mastick J, Colling E, Carter JH, Singer CM, Aminoff MJ. Melatonin for sleep disturbances in Parkinson's disease. Sleep Med. 2005; 6:459–66.

Melatonin in Human Cancer: Therapeutic Possibilities

4

Paolo Lissoni

Abstract

The recent discovery in the neuropsychoimmunology of tumors has demonstrated that human body may produce not only pro-tumoral hormones such as estrogens, androgens, and perhaps GH itself but also antitumor endocrine molecules, the most important of them represented by pineal hormones, melatonin as the most investigated of them. The antitumor activity of melatonin has been demonstrated by a great number of experimental studies, and it has been proven to be able to exert the overall potential antitumor mechanisms, commonly used by the conventional clinical oncology, including (1) antiproliferative cytotoxic action, mainly on melatonin receptor-expressing tumor cells; (2) inhibition of growth factor receptor activation; (3) inhibitory effect on tumor angiogenesis; (4) inhibition of tumor growth factor secretion; and (5) stimulation of the antitumor immunity, namely, by stimulating IL-2 secretion by T helper lymphocytes and IL-12 production by dendritic cells. In addition, melatonin could reserve interesting therapeutic results in the palliative therapy of cancer, particularly by counteracting the onset of the neoplastic cachexia by inhibiting the TNF-alpha secretion. Unfortunately, despite the great number of the experimental evidences, very few clinical studies with melatonin have been carried up to now in the treatment of human neoplasms, at least from a palliative point of view, to improve the quality of life.

Keywords

Melatonin • Cytokines • Growth factors • Antitumor immunity • Apoptosis

Introduction

The knowledge of neoplastic diseases available up to now clearly demonstrates that the prognosis of human tumors depends not only on cancer's biological characteristics, including histology, grading, and oncogene overexpression

P. Lissoni
Department of Medical Oncology,
Azienda Ospedaliera San Gerardo,
via Giovanni Battista Pergolesi 33,
Monza 20900, Italy
e-mail: p.lissoni@hsgerardo.org

V. Srinivasan et al. (eds.), *Melatonin and Melatonergic Drugs in Clinical Practice*,
DOI 10.1007/978-81-322-0825-9_4, © Springer India 2014

or mutation, but also on patient immunobiological response, which consists of the functional status of the endocrine and immune systems [1, 2]. In the same way, the impaired function of the immune system does not depend only on the activity of the immune cells but also on their physiological neuroendocrine modulation, mainly exerted by the pineal gland, brain opioid system, and brain cannabinergic system [3–5]. Most endogenous hormones exert modulatory effects on both immune responses and cell proliferation. Generally, the action of hormones tends to play a stimulatory role on cancer cell proliferation. In fact, estrogens and androgens stimulate breast cancer and prostate cancer growth, respectively [6]. PRL may also stimulate the growth of mammary and prostate tumors, while GH would exert a stimulatory activity on several tumor histotypes [7, 8]. On the contrary, somatostatin and its analogs may exert antiproliferative effects on various histotypes of cancer, namely, the endocrine tumors, by either inhibiting the growth of tumors expressing somatostatin receptors or by inhibiting the production of IGF-1 and other growth factors [9].

Moreover, a more widely extended antitumor antiproliferative action is exerted by the pineal gland through the release of several anticancer indole and peptide hormones, the most investigated of them is the indole melatonin (MLT) [10]. Despite the pineal gland's function remaining obscure until few years ago, today it is known that it would represent the most important anticancer organ in the human body. In fact, the evidence that pinealectomy stimulates tumor onset and dissemination was known before the characterization of the hormones produced by pineal gland itself [11]. MLT has appeared to inhibit cancer growth and to counteract, but not completely abolish, the stimulatory action of pinealectomy on cancer cell proliferation, by suggesting that MLT is not the only anticancer endocrine molecule produced by the pineal gland [3, 10, 12]. In fact, several studies have demonstrated that the pineal gland may produce anticancer hormones other than MLT, including the indole 5-methoxytryptamine (5-MTT) and several kinds of beta-carbolines, namely, the 6-methoxy-1,2,3,4-tetrahydro-beta-carboline, the so-called pinoline, which is also provided by psychedelic properties, and the tripeptide epithalamin [13–15]. In vitro, 5-MTT has been proven to exert an antitumor antiproliferative activity superior to that of MLT itself [13]. Then, the clinical investigation of the potential anticancer therapeutic role of MLT is only the beginning of a new approach in the treatment of human neoplasms, by using the same antitumor hormones produced by the human body; most of them are released by the pineal gland. Then, the clinical studies on the relationship between cancer growth and MLT and generally the relation between tumor progression and pineal hormones have to include not only the investigation of the therapeutic efficacy of MLT in the palliative or curative therapy of cancer but also the analysis of the pineal endocrine function in early or advanced cancer patients.

As far as the pineal function in cancer patients is concerned, more than 30 years of research studies have clearly demonstrated that cancer progression is associated with a progressive decline in MLT secretion, namely, during the night, either in animals or in humans [16–20]. Therefore, because of its anticancer activity, the progressive decline in MLT secretion with cancer development could play a role in cancer progression itself and deserves a negative prognostic significance [3, 10].

Cancer-Related Alterations of Growth Factor Activities and Antitumor Immune Responses

The recent advances in the knowledge of the mechanisms involved in tumor growth promotion, specifically those of growth factors and protein kinases acting as growth factor receptors, may disclose the possibility to arrest cancer growth by inhibiting the activation of growth factor receptors, the target therapy of cancer.

EGF receptors (EGF-R) and VEGF receptors (VEGF-R) represent the main objectives of target therapies of cancer because of their importance in the stimulation of the proliferation of several tumor histotypes and the angiogenesis processes, respectively, particularly in the treatment of lung cancer and colorectal carcinoma [21, 22]. IGF-1 and HER-2 neu receptors are also important in the growth of tumors, namely, breast cancer and gastric carcinomas. GH receptors themselves would have an important role in stimulating tumor development. Growth factors would act mainly as paracrine local factors, but their secretion would be at least partly under central regulatory control, with a stimulatory action exerted by GH itself and IGF-1 and an inhibitory one played by somatostatin system and the pineal gland through the release of MLT and other active pineal hormones [8–10]. Tumor cells may enhance their biological malignancy through two major mechanisms, consisting of mutation or overexpression of some growth factor receptors and of resistance against immune cell-mediated cytotoxicity. According to the strategy of target therapies, the treatment of human tumors is dependent on the type of tumor growth factor receptor expression, which also plays a prognostic significance. In particular, the expression of HER-2 neu would reflect a more aggressive biological malignancy in breast cancer and gastric carcinoma [23].

From an immunological point of view, presently it is known that cancer cells may be killed through both antigen-dependent and antigen-independent mechanisms, respectively, mediated by cytotoxic T lymphocytes ($CD8^+$) activated by IL-12 released from dendritic cells (DC) and by NK cells after their activation by IL-2 released from T helper 1 lymphocytes ($CD4^+$) (24). IL-2 and IL-12 production is inhibited by a subset of T lymphocytes, the $CD4^+CD25^+$, the so-called T regulatory lymphocyte (T reg) through the release of the two major immunosuppressive cytokines, consisting of IL-10 and TGF-beta [24]. In addition, T reg activation is inhibited by TH17 lymphocytes through the release of IL-17 [25]. Finally, dendritic cell maturation and differentiation is inhibited by VEGF, which would stimulate cancer growth through both angiogenic and immunosuppressive effects [26]. Until a few years ago, the failure of the immune system to destroy cancer cells was commonly considered to depend on cancer-related immunosuppressive status, primarily due to an altered neuroendocrine and immune regulation of cytokine network as well to a direct production of immunosuppressive agents by cancer cells with the progression of disease, specifically IL-10 and TGF-beta [24, 25, 27]. However, with the discovery of the importance of the interaction between Fas receptor and Fas-ligand (Fas-L) receptor in T lymphocyte and tumor cell relationship, it has been demonstrated that Fas-Fas-L interactions may induce the apoptosis of cells expressing Fas receptors on their cell surfaces [28]. Therefore, the reaction between T lymphocytes expressing Fas receptors with cancer cells expressing Fas-L receptors on their surface may allow the apoptosis of T cells themselves, with subsequent lymphocytopenia, due to lymphocyte apoptosis and cancer dissemination [28]. Therefore, lymphocytopenia occurring in the disseminated metastatic disease before the onset of chemotherapy or radiotherapy would depend on active mechanisms carried out by the tumor itself, namely, the apoptosis of T cells after their reaction with Fas-L receptor on tumor cell membrane. In fact, preliminary clinical results would suggest that tumor expression of Fas-L receptor is associated with a more aggressive disease and with a following poor prognosis and reduced survival [28, 29].

The Antitumor Mechanisms of Melatonin

MLT plays a physiological anticancer role, being responsible for the natural resistance against tumor onset, by either inhibiting cancer cell proliferation or stimulating the anticancer immunity. The biological effects of MLT may be direct or mediated by specific MLT receptors. At present, there are at least two known MLT cell surface receptors, MT1 and MT2 receptors, widely expressed by several tissue histotypes and by a nuclear receptor involved in the control of DNA transcription [30]. Luzindole is an antagonist of both MLT receptors (MT1 and MT2), whereas 4-phenyl-2-propionamido-tetralin (4P-PDOT) is a specific antagonist of only MT2 receptors. The antitumor antiproliferative action of MLT would be mainly mediated by MT1 receptor, even though other receptors and receptor-independent mechanisms are involved in the anticancer action of MLT [31]. In any case, the diminished expression of MLT receptors by tumor cells is associated with a poor prognosis and a reduced survival in cancer patients [32].

The Biological Mechanisms of the Antitumor Activity of MLT

These are listed in the following:

1. Antiproliferative cytotoxic action
   - Induction of apoptosis of cancer cells
   - Inhibition of protein kinase system activation
   - Protection against activated protein kinase-induced connexin alterations
2. Antitumor immunostimulatory activity
   - Stimulation of IL-2 production by TH1 lymphocytes
   - Stimulation of IL-12 production by dendritic cells in response to IL-2
   - Inhibition of macrophage- and T regulatory lymphocyte-mediated immunosuppressive events
   - Modulation of Fas and Fas-L expression on lymphocytes and cancer cells
3. Antiangiogenic activity
4. Neuroendocrine antitumor affects
   - Interaction with brain cannabinergic system
   - Modulation of cortisol secretion
5. Cytodifferentiating activity on tumor endocrine dependence
6. Anti-inflammatory action
7. Antioxidant activity

Additionally, the antiproliferative and antitumor immune effects of MLT, with particular regard to its relation with TGF-beta activity and with tumor expression of MLT and Fas-L receptors, are illustrated in Fig. 4.1.

The Antitumor Mechanisms of MLT in More Detail

These may be summarized as follows:

1. Antiproliferative Cytotoxic Cytostatic Activity: The antiproliferative action of MLT is due to three major mechanisms, consisting of (a) induction of the apoptosis of cancer cells through multiple pathways, including stimulation of p53 and p21 functions and activation of caspase system; (b) inhibitory modulatory control on the activation of protein kinase system at multiple levels, specifically on epidermal growth factor (EGF) receptor activation, extracellular signal-regulated protein kinase (ERK) phosphorylation, and cyclin protein activity, which is essential for the activation of cyclin-dependent protein kinases involved in the regulation of DNA transcription; and (c) protection of connexin functionless, which is responsible for the activity of gap junctional intercellular communication (GJIC) system, whose alteration may promote tumor development [33–36].
2. Antitumor Immunomodulatory Effects: MLT may induce direct immune effects by activating MLT receptors expressed on cell surfaces by most immune cells, namely, TH1 lymphocytes and dendritic cells [3]. In fact, MLT stimulates IL-2 secretion by TH1 cells and IL-12 production by dendritic cells after their activation by IL-2 [3]. In addition, MLT has been proven to counteract macrophage-mediated immunosuppressive events in response to IL-2 and the generation of T reg lymphocytes, which suppress both IL-2- and IL-12-dependent cytotoxic activities against tumor cells [3, 27, 37]. Finally, it has been demonstrated that MLT may modulate Fas-L

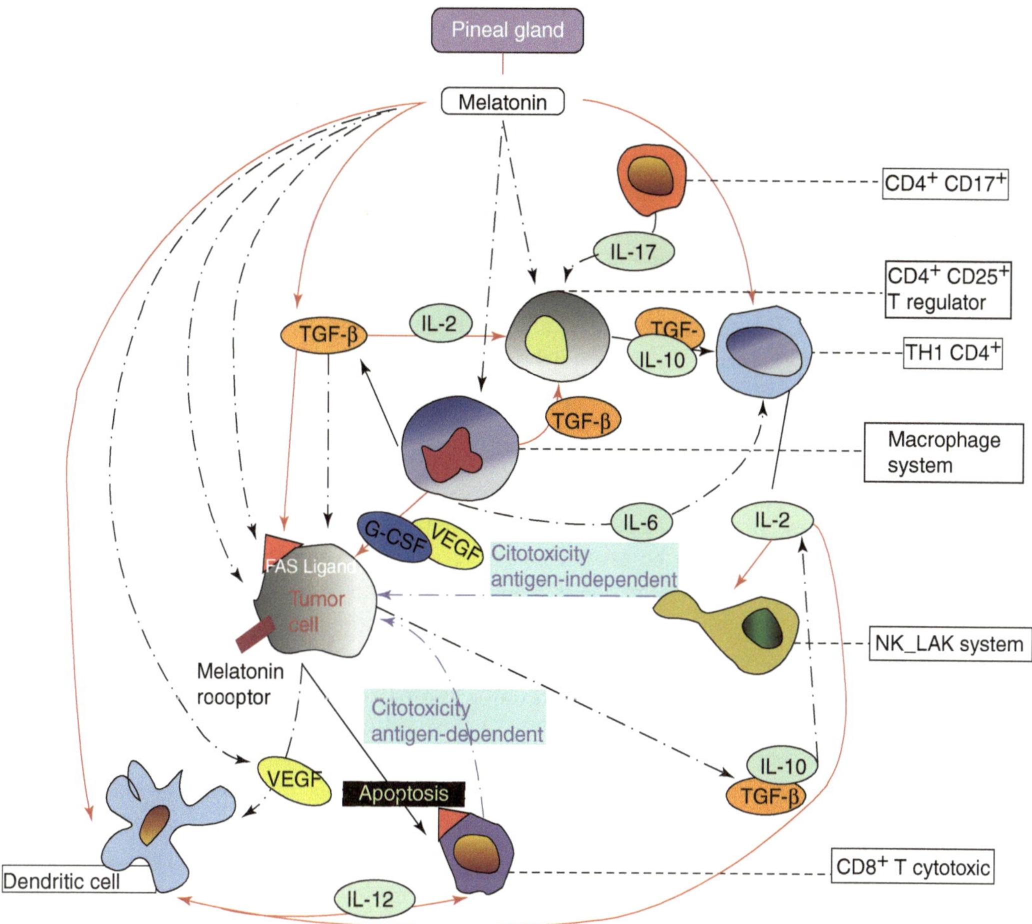

Fig. 4.1 Antitumor, antiproliferative, and immunostimulatory mechanism of melatonin. Red lines represent *stimulation*; dashed black lines represent *inhibition* effect

expression by tumor cells by reducing their biological malignancy degree [38]. Therefore, MLT would enhance the antitumor efficacy of the main antitumor cytokines, such as IL-2, IL-12, IL-7, IL-15, and IL-23, by counteracting the mechanisms involved in Fas-L expression by tumor cells, which would abolish the efficacy of the antitumor immune response by determining the apoptosis of Fas receptor-expressing T lymphocytes. In particular, the relation between MLT and TGF-beta activity needs to be better investigated and defined, since TGF-beta may exert both antitumor antiproliferative and pro-tumor immunosuppressive effects, and then it could either inhibit or stimulate cancer growth [27]. In fact, TGF-beta has been proven to be a potent growth factor inhibitor in the early phase of cancer cell transformation by acting as an antiproliferative agent and additionally to stimulate cancer progression in the advanced phases of the neoplastic disease because of its potent immunosuppressive activity on the anticancer immunity by suppressing both antigen-dependent and antigen-independent anticancer cytotoxicity, as well as by stimulating Fas-L expression by cancer cells [27, 39]. MLT, as well as other pineal indoles such as 5-MTT, has appeared to enhance the antiproliferative action of TGF-beta and to stimulate its production [40]. This finding seems to be paradoxical by taking into consideration the immunosuppressive activity of TGF-beta and the immunostimulatory one exerted by MLT on the anticancer immune reaction. These controversial evidences may be explained by suggesting that MLT may amplify the antiproliferative action of TGF-beta but counteract its immunosuppressive effect, namely, by inhibiting Fas-L expression by cancer cells, which would represent one of the main mechanisms responsible for TGF-beta-mediated immunosuppression. In fact, tumor progression has been seen to be associated with an enhanced tumor expression of Fas-L, which would make T lymphocytes as unable to attach tumor cells, and with a progressive increase in serum levels of soluble Fas-L receptor, which would further reduce the capacity of tumor cell destruction by T lymphocytes [28, 29, 38–40]. By implication, MLT may activate the anticancer immune response by stimulating T lymphocyte system and by counteracting macrophage- and T reg-mediated immunosuppressive functions and guiding the immune system to become functionless in an antitumor way [3].

3. Antiangiogenic Activity: In experimental conditions, MLT has been proven to suppress tumor angiogenesis by inhibiting the hypoxic inducible factor-1 alpha (HIF-1 alpha) [41]. Moreover, MLT has also appeared to reduce VEGF serum concentrations in advanced cancer patients [42].
4. Neuroendocrine Antitumor Effects: MLT, as well as other pineal indoles, may interact with other molecular systems also provided by anticancer activity, namely, brain endocannabinoid system and atrial natriuretic peptides. In fact, the pineal gland constitutes a functional axis, preferentially characterized by positive feedback interactions, with brain cannabinoid system, as well as with the cardiac endocrine activity, which is involved in mediating the influence of the pleasure and the spiritual sensitivity on the endocrine and cardiovascular functions in stimulating the antitumor immune reaction [3]. On the contrary, the functional axis existing between pituitary gland and brain opioid system, mainly founded on negative feedback mechanisms, is activated in stress conditions and it suppresses the anticancer immunity [3]. The cannabinoid agonists may stimulate MLT secretion from the pineal gland and directly induce the apoptosis of cancer cells and inhibit EGF-receptor activation, which is also blocked by MLT itself [5, 34]. Then, the association between MLT and cannabinoid agonists could further enhance their single antiproliferative activity. Natriuretic peptides may also exert an antitumor action through both antiproliferative and immunostimulatory effects, consisting of the stimulation of T lymphocyte differentiation and activation [43, 44].
5. Cytodifferentiating Activity: MLT has appeared to modulate tumor gene expression and counteract the biological malignancy of cancer cells by stimulating endocrine receptor expression in both breast and prostate carcinomas, with a following enhancement of tumor endocrine dependency and a possible reversal of hormone resistance [10].
6. Anti-inflammatory Activity: It has been known that the inflammatory status is associated with a suppression of the antitumor immunity through the action of inflammatory cytokines mainly released from macrophages, such as IL-6, which may counteract LAK cell generation from NK cells in response to IL-2 [27]. Then, since MLT may exert an anti-inflammatory action by reducing IL-6 secretion and PgE2 production, MLT-induced inhibition of the inflammatory response may also contribute to explain the antitumor immunostimulatory role of MLT itself [1, 3, 10].
7. Antioxidant Activity: MLT is one of the most potent natural antioxidant agents [10]. Obviously, the antioxidant activity is not synonymous than the anticancer one, which is depending on specific antiproliferative or

apoptotic mechanisms. However, since free radicals may enhance the biological malignancy of tumor cells by determining a progressive DNA damage, the antioxidant activity may play also a role within a natural biological strategy to control cancer growth.

Melatonin Secretion in Cancer Patients

MLT decline would represent the main cancer progression-related endocrine deficiency [10, 17–19]. In fact, several experimental studies have shown that cancer progression is constantly associated with a progressive decline in the pineal endocrine function, with a diminished secretion of MLT during the night and the following disappearance of the physiological circadian light/dark rhythm in the production of the pineal hormone [10]. The preliminary studies in cancer patients have confirmed that the clinical course of the neoplastic disease is also characterized by a progressive MLT deficiency [18, 19]. Then, because of the importance of MLT in the regulation of the overall biological rhythms, including endocrine secretions, immune response, and cardiovascular function, the alteration in the pineal endocrine activity occurring during the clinical course of the neoplastic disease may allow a more general systemic alteration of the overall biological rhythms, namely, cortisol circadian secretion [10, 20]. The evidence of alterations in cortisol secretion and rhythm in cancer patients would play also a negative prognostic significance [20].

Melatonin Application in the Medical Oncology

According to the experimental studies in animals, MLT may in vivo exert antitumor activity only when it is administered at pharmacological doses and during the dark phase of the day, since light inhibits MLT receptor expression [45]. The minimal dosage required to achieve an in vivo antitumor efficacy of MLT has to be of at least 0.3 mg/kg b.w./day. Therefore, an adequate schedule of MLT therapy in medical oncology has to be at least 20 mg/day orally in late evening, every day. At present, however, no defined MLT dose–response clinical study has been performed, but preliminary results would suggest that the anticancer activity of MLT is a dose-dependent phenomenon. In fact, cancer patients progressing on MLT therapy at a dose of 5 mg/day have been observed to achieve a further stabilization of their disease by increasing MLT dosage at 20 mg/day [46]. In the same way, cancer patients progressing on MLT at 20 mg/day would seem to achieve a further disease control at higher doses of MLT, such as 100 mg/day (Porro et al., unpublished data). However, according to the clinical results available up to now, it seems that all tumor histotypes may obtain some benefits from MLT therapy in terms of both disease control and treatment of cancer related symptoms, even though non-small cell lung cancer (NSCLC), pancreatic adenocarcinoma, gastric cancer, prostate carcinoma, and malignant melanoma would represent the neoplasms most responsive and most suitable to obtain some benefit from MLT therapy [3, 10, 47–50]. Moreover, experimental studies have suggested that tumors expressing MLT receptors, namely, the MT1 receptor, are more sensitive to the antiproliferative action of MLT [31]. At present, however, it has to be established whether tumor positivity for MLT receptor expression may be essential or not for the clinical antitumor efficacy of MLT itself. Preliminary experimental data seem to suggest that the lack of MLT receptor expression by cancer cells would not exclude the efficacy of MLT treatment in human neoplasms, since the antiproliferative action of MLT, which is mediated by a stimulation of MLT receptor, is not the only mechanism responsible for the anticancer activity of MLT that depends also on an activation of IL-2- and IL-12- dependent anticancer immunity as well as on an inhibition of tumor angiogenesis through complex interactions with brain cannabinoid system [3, 5]. In any case, it has to be taken into consideration that MLT therapy of cancer may also deserve the significance of an endocrine substitutive treatment to replace and correct the progressive cancer-related MLT deficiency during the clinical history of the neoplastic disease [17–19]. The dosage of MLT required to replace its physiological daily production is corresponding to 1 mg/day only, but higher pharmacological doses of MLT are necessary to in vivo achieve a clinically evident anticancer efficacy, at least from a palliative point of view [47–50]. In a novel clinical investigation, at present more than thousand advanced cancer patients have been treated with MLT for several months; most of them were suffering from an untreatable disseminated disease [3, 10, 42, 50]. Most studies have been carried out with MLT at a dose of at least 20 mg/day in a single oral administration during the dark phase of the day, every day without interruption, according to the following eligibility criteria: histologically proven metastatic cancer, measurable lesions, no availability of conventional therapies because of poor clinical status and/or lack of response to previous chemotherapies, and an expected survival time less than 1 year. The meta-analysis of the main clinical studies has shown that MLT therapy of cancer may significantly reduce the risk of death at 1 year, irrespective of the histotype of tumor [50]. In more detail, the treatment with MLT alone at a dose of at least 20 mg/day in the late evening may allow 1-year survival in about 25 % of patients with untreatable metastatic solid neoplasms, with a stable disease (SD) and life expectancy lower than 1 year [47–50]. It is extremely rare (<5 %) to observe objective tumor regression under treatment with MLT alone. The most evident clinical benefit of MLT cancer therapy is consisting of the prevention of the neoplastic cachexia, which is due to an inhibition of TNF-alpha secretion, which plays a fundamental role in the pathogenesis of the neoplastic cachexia [3, 10, 42]. In addition, MLT therapy has been proven to normalize platelet count in cancer patients affected by thrombocytopenia due to different reasons, including previous chemotherapies, bone marrow neoplastic infiltration, and liver failure [3, 47–50]. The mechanisms responsible for the thrombopoietic activity of MLT need to be better investigated, but they would depend at least in part on a direct stimulation of megakaryocyte fragmentation, as well as on interactions with the main thrombopoietic cytokines, consisting of IL-3, IL-11, and thrombopoietin.

In a second group of clinical studies, MLT therapy has been evaluated in association with the conventional anticancer therapies, including chemotherapy, immunotherapy with cytokines, endocrine therapy, and radiotherapy. MLT was given in association of chemotherapy, as a chemoneuroendocrine combination in an attempt to achieve a possible control of chemotherapy-related toxicities and an increase in chemotherapy efficacy. The mechanisms responsible for the possible potentiation of chemotherapy-induced cancer cell destruction by MLT are dependent on the fact that the antioxidant agents have been proven to enhance the cytotoxic potency of cancer chemotherapies [51]. Therefore, since MLT is one of the most potent antioxidant agents available in the nature, it is not exaggerated to expect an increased efficacy of chemotherapy in cancer patients under chronic therapy of MLT, which may also promote the apoptosis of tumor cells [10, 33]. In fact, preliminary clinical studies have shown that a chronic concomitant administration of MLT may enhance the cytotoxic efficacy of the most commonly used chemotherapeutic drugs, including cisplatin and its analogs, 5-fluorouracil, and anthracyclines, in terms of both tumor regression rate and survival time, which is constantly associated with an acceptable quality of life, and this benefit is particularly evident in cancer patients with poor clinical status [10, 52–54]. In fact, MLT chronic administration in patients under chemotherapy would act as a maintenance treatment after chemotherapy-induced tumor regression or stabilization of disease on the basis of its oncostatic properties, since chemotherapeutic drugs cannot be administered without interruption because of their cumulative toxicity. At present, the most recent oncological strategies tend to propose a maintenance therapy after the planned chemotherapeutic cycles, but this strategy is generally realized by the administration of some particular chemotherapeutic drugs, such as pemetrexed in

NSCLC patients, or monoclonal antibodies against growth factor receptors or angiogenic factors. Therefore, MLT chronic administration could constitute another simple strategy of maintenance therapy of cancer. Then, the maintenance therapy of cancer by MLT would represent a first historical example showing that the complementary medicine may be a potential source of new therapeutic strategies of cancer. On the other hand, as far as the influence of MLT on chemotherapy-induced side effects is concerned, the pineal hormone has been proven to reduce some chemotherapy-related toxicities, namely, cardiotoxicity, neuropathy, renal damage, thrombocytopenia, lymphocytopenia and lymphocyte functional immune damage, asthenia, and anticipatory vomiting, whereas neutropenia, anemia, alopecia, and vomiting are not substantially improved by MLT alone [3, 10, 52–54]. Another new therapeutic strategy of cancer of MLT is consisting of cancer neuroimmunotherapy (NIT) with MLT in association with subcutaneous (SC) low-dose IL-2, which is the main antitumor cytokine in humans [24, 25, 27]. It is known that IL-2 alone is substantially effective in the only treatment of renal cell carcinoma and melanoma, whereas in association with a chronic therapy with MLT, IL-2 becomes potentially effective in most solid tumor histotypes at least from an immunobiological point of view, since the pineal hormone may promote the generation of an effective anticancer reaction in response to IL-2 [55]. The neuroendocrine combination with MLT in association with the standard endocrine therapy of cancer is a potential new therapeutic approach elaborated in an attempt to counteract and to reverse the hormonal resistance of cancer cells. In fact, MLT has been shown to reverse the endocrine resistance in hormone-dependent neoplasms, even though the low number of patients does not allow us to define conclusions on the relation between MLT and tumor endocrine dependency [56, 57].

Finally, MLT may be successfully associated with the radiotherapy as a radioneuroendocrine combination on the basis of either its anticancer activity or its well experimentally demonstrated radioprotective action against radiation-induced lymphocyte and neuronal damages, even though the radioprotective activity of MLT would seem to require very high pharmacological doses [55]. Preliminary clinical studies have also suggested that a concomitant chronic administration of MLT may enhance the efficacy of radiotherapy in the treatment of both brain tumors and brain metastases due to solid neoplasms [58, 59]. Obviously, the efficacy of MLT in combination with the standard therapies of cancer, including chemotherapy, radiotherapy, endocrine therapy, and immunotherapy with cytokines, is constantly significantly superior to that achieved by MLT alone [52–59]. On the other hand, when MLT is administered as a palliative therapy of cancer in patients for whom no other standard treatment is available, its oncostatic efficacy in terms of both tumor regression rate and survival time may be biologically enhanced through a concomitant association with other natural anticancer agents, provided by a well scientifically documented antitumor activity at least in experimental conditions, primarily consisting of the other antiproliferative pineal indole hormones, mainly the pineal hormone 5-MTT, which could deserve a reputation as having anticancer activity superior to that of MLT itself [13]. According to the recent advances in the investigation of the psychoneuroendocrine mechanisms involved in the control of the immune system, the anticancer activity of MLT could be further amplified by a psychoneurochemical strategy consisting of the concomitant administration of the opioid antagonist naltrexone (NTX) as a poly-neuroendocrine therapy of cancer because of the involvement of brain opioid system in stress-induced predisposition to cancer development [1–5, 60]. However, at present the results concerning the anticancer efficacy of MLT-NTX combination are too preliminary and controversial [3].

Finally, within the group of plants provided by anticancer activity due to the content of well-known molecules with experimentally proven antitumor action, the most effective or at least the most investigated anticancer plants are represented by Aloe arborescens, which would be more active than Aloe vera, myrrh, curcuma, and Cannabis indica [5, 61–63]. These are the results obtained up to now with MLT in the treatment palliative or curative of solid tumors. On the other hand, as far as the possible application of MLT in the treatment of the hematological neoplasms is concerned, preliminary results have shown that MLT may counteract the leukemic evolution of the myelodysplastic syndromes secondary to cancer chemotherapy [64]. Moreover, other preliminary results have demonstrated the potential efficacy of a neuroimmunotherapeutic regimen consisting of MLT in association with SC low-dose IL-2 in the treatment of hematological malignancies progressing on the standard antitumor therapies, with particular benefits in multiple myeloma and chronic myeloid leukemia [65]. No biological toxicity has been reported during MLT therapy, also in the case of a long duration of treatment for several years [46–51]. The only described subjective side effects would consist of headache, excitation, and paradoxical insomnia, in a percentage, however, less than 1 % [42, 50]. On the contrary, most patients referred an improvement in well-being and mood, relief of asthenia, and amelioration in the quality of sleep under MLT chronic therapy. Then, in addition to its potential anticancer curative activity either alone or in combination with the classical antitumor therapies, MLT may play a fundamental role in the palliative therapy of cancer patients, being active in the treatment of symptoms, for whom no effective standard therapy is available, including neoplastic cachexia, cancer-related asthenia, mood disturbances, sleep disorders, and thrombocytopenia [42]. Moreover, MLT could be usefully associated with opioids in the treatment of cancer pain because of its capacity of counteracting opioid-induced suppression of the anticancer immunity, and of inhibiting the glutamate receptor NMDA, which is involved in determining the opioid dependence, with a following potential reduction of the opioid dosage required to control cancer pain [66].

Future Perspectives of Melatonin in Cancer Therapy

A further improvement in the therapeutic benefits of MLT in the treatment of human tumors would require to better define the dose–response rate in the antiproliferative efficacy of the pineal indole, to identify the more responsive tumor histotypes to MLT, and to establish the real importance of MLT receptor expression by tumor cells to predict the oncostatic effects of the pineal hormone.

Future perspectives could include the use of MLT as an adjuvant therapy after the radical removal of tumor and as a possible primary chemoprevention of cancer development. As far as the adjuvant therapy is concerned, preliminary results have shown that MLT may enhance the progression-free period in node-positive melanoma patients after resection of the primary tumor [67]. Obviously, the adjuvant therapy with MLT has an opposite significance with respect to the other commonly adjuvant endocrine therapies, such as the antiestrogen treatment for estrogen receptor positive-breast cancer and the antiandrogen therapy in prostate cancer. In fact, whereas the stimulation of estrogen receptor in breast cancer and androgen receptor in prostate cancer may promote cancer cell proliferation, MLT-induced stimulation of tumor MLT receptor would allow an inhibition of tumor growth. Finally, as far as the possible use of MLT as a primary chemoprevention of tumors, this hypothesis is justified by the evidence of an age-dependent progressive decline in MLT secretion, which has been proven to be responsible at least in part for the enhanced frequency of tumors with age because of its fundamental role in the natural resistance against tumor development [10]. In fact, in experimental conditions it has been demonstrated that MLT administration may prevent both spontaneous and carcinogen-induced tumor development [3, 10]. However, since there is a great variety in age-dependent MLT decline, an eventual primary chemoprevention with MLT would have to be performed on the basis of a general screening in the aged population to evaluate the pineal function by determining the urinary excretion during the day and the night of the main MLT metabolite, 6-sulphatoxy-melatonin (6-MTS), in an attempt to identify a real decline in the endogenous production of MLT and with a successive MLT administration only in the presence of a well-documented initial MLT deficiency [10].

Conclusion

According to the data already available in the treatment of cancer patients, it is possible to affirm that simple application of MLT therapy in the clinical management of the neoplastic diseases as either palliative or curative treatment of human tumors would be sufficient to profoundly modify the medical oncology in terms of humanization. Then, in agreement with the great number of both experimental and clinical data confirming the antitumor properties of MLT, it is not scientifically exaggerated to conclude that at present it is not ethical to further exclude MLT from the drugs commonly used in the medical treatments of cancer, at least as a palliative therapy of tumor-related symptoms in addition to the other most known palliative drugs, such as steroids, opioids, and progestative agents. In fact, by considering that there are up to now five essential medical strategies in the treatment of human neoplasms, consisting of cytotoxic chemotherapy, endocrine therapy, immunotherapy, antiangiogenic treatment, and target therapies against tumor growth factors or their receptors, it appears that MLT is the only drug capable of exerting the overall five fundamental medical approaches elaborated by oncologists in the treatment of tumors because of its antiproliferative, immunostimulatory, antiangiogenic, cytodifferentiating, and antigrowth factor receptor properties without any biological toxicity and at a very low social cost. Therefore, MLT would provide a preponderance of possible medical therapeutic strategies for treating cancer. Without concomitant chronic administration of MLT, the quality of life of cancer patients is clearly worse, and the conventional anticancer therapies are often more toxic and less effective with respect to the results observed in cancer patients under chronic treatment with MLT [42, 52–59]. Presently, the more recent medical strategies in cancer therapy are founded on the identification of specific tumor molecules involved in malignant cell proliferation and dissemination, and on the consequent inhibition of their activities through several mechanisms, including monoclonal antibodies against angiogenic or tumor growth factors and tyrosine kinase inhibitors (TKI), by constituting the so-called target therapies of cancer. Then, the type of cancer therapy will depend on the type of molecule, whose activity has to be inhibited.

The recent advances in the knowledgements of both tumor biology and the immunobiological status of cancer patients have identified the importance of two new tumor markers, not yet considered by the conventional medical oncology, consisting of expression of MLT receptors and Fas-L on tumor cell surface, which could represent, respectively, the most prognostically positive and negative tumor biological markers irrespective of tumor histotype, since MLT receptor-expressing cancer cells would be more sensitive to the antiproliferative action of MLT, whereas the expression of Fas-L would make cancer cells as completely resistant to the cytotoxic action of T lymphocytes and capable of determining cell death of Fas-expressing T lymphocytes, with a consequent lymphocytopenia [28–30]. Then, the prognostic significance of tumor expression of MLT receptors and Fas-L could be superior with respect to that of the other most commonly considered tumor biological parameters, including growth factor receptor and VEGF receptor expression. In addition, since prognostic factor may be identified within both tumor and patient biological variables, the future therapies of human neoplasms would have to be elaborated to influence the mechanisms responsible for the interactions between tumor biological characteristics and neuroimmune status of cancer patients, rather than to act separately on tumor variables and on patient biological response, since the degree of tumor malignancy is negatively correlated with the efficiency of patient antitumor immunobiological reactivity. In this project of the future medical oncology, the pineal hormone MLT would play a fundamental role [3, 10].

In fact, if we define the target therapy of cancer as a treatment carried out against a single tumor parameter, only MLT may be already considered within itself a multi-target therapy, because of its capacity of acting at different levels and on different tumor targets and on the different molecules involved in promoting tumor cell proliferation and dissemination.

References

1. Foon KA. Biological response modifiers: the new immunotherapy. Cancer Res. 1989;49:1621–7.
2. Rubinow DR. Brain, behaviour and immunity: an interactive system. J Natl Cancer Inst Monogr. 1994;10:79–82.
3. Maestroni GJM. The immunoneuroendocrine role of melatonin. J Pineal Res. 1993;14:1–10.
4. Plotnikoff NP, Miller GC. Enkephalins as immunomodulators. Int J Immunopharmacol. 1983;5:437–42.
5. Grotenhermen F. Pharmacology of cannabinoids. Neuro Endocrinol Lett. 2004;25:14–22.
6. Roberts AB, Sporn AB. Growth factors and transformation. Cancer Surv. 1986;5:405–11.
7. Welsch C, Nagasawa H. Prolactin and murine tumorigenesis: a review. Cancer Res. 1977;37:951–63.
8. Ben-Shlomo A, Melmed S. Growth hormone excess and cancer. J Antiag Med. 2001;4:301–9.
9. Benlot C, Lévy L, Fontanaud P, Roche A, Rouannet P, Joubert D. Somatostatin and growth hormone-releasing hormone in normal and tumoral breast tissue: endogenous content, in vitro pulsatile release, and regulation. J Clin Endocrinol Metab. 1997;82:690–6.
10. Brzezinski A. Melatonin in humans. N Engl J Med. 1997;336:186–95.
11. Buswell RS. The pineal and neoplasia. Lancet. 1975;1:34–5.
12. El-Domeiri AAH, Das Gupta TK. Reversal by melatonin of the effect of pinealectomy on tumor growth. Cancer Res. 1973;33:2830–3.
13. Sze SF, Ng TB, Liu WK. Antiproliferative effect of pineal indoles on cultured tumor cell lines. J Pineal Res. 1993;14:27–33.
14. Tsuchiya H, Shimizu H, Inuma M. Beta-carboline alkaloids in crude drugs. Chem Pharm Bull. 1999;47:440–3.
15. Anisomov VN, Arutjunyan V, Khavinson VK. Effects of pineal peptide preparation epithalamin on free-radical processes in humans and animals. Neuro Endocrinol Lett. 2001;22:9–18.
16. Lapin V. Pineal gland and malignancy. Oster Z Onkol. 1976;3:51–60.
17. Bartsch C, Bartsch H, Lippert TH. The pineal gland and cancer: facts, hypotheses and perspectives. Cancer J. 1992;5:194–9.
18. Maestroni JGM, Conti A, Pierpaoli W. Pineal melatonin, its fundamental immunoregulatory role in aging and cancer. Ann N Y Acad Sci. 1988;521:140–8.
19. Mazzocchi G, Carughi S, De Cata A, La Viola M, Vendemmiale G. Melatonin and cortisol serum levels in lung cancer patients at different stages of disease. Med Sci Monit. 2005;11:284–8.
20. Hajdu SI, Porro RS, Lieberman PH, Foote Jr FW. Degeneration of the pineal gland of patients with cancer. Cancer. 1972;29:706–9.
21. Huang Y, .Chang Y, Wang X, Jiang J, Frank SJ. Growth hormone alters epidermal growth factor receptor binding affinity via activation of extracellular signal-regulated kinases in 3T3-F442A cells. Endocrinology. 2004;145:3297–306.
22. Siejka A, Awinicka H, Komorowski J, Schally AV, Stpie T, Krupi R, Stpie H. GH-RH antagonist (MZ-4-71) inhibits VEGF secretion and proliferation of murine endothelial cells. Life Sci. 2003;72: 2473–9.
23. Taverna D, Groner B, Hynes NE. Epidermal growth factor receptor, platelet-derived growth factor receptor and c-erb B-2 receptor activation all promote growth but have distinctive effects upon mouse mammary epithelial cell differentiation. Cell Growth Differ. 1991;2:145–54.
24. Zou W. Regulatory T, cells, tumour immunity and immunotherapy. Nat Rev Immunol. 2006;6:295–307.
25. Battelli E, Oukka M, Kuchroo VK. TH-17 cells in the circle of immunity and autoimmunity. Nat Immunol. 2007;8:345–50.
26. Gabrilovich DL, Chen HL, Girgis KR, Cunningham HT, Meny GM, Nadaf S, Kavanaugh D, Carbone DP. Production of vascular endothelial growth factor by human tumor inhibits the functional maturation of dendritic cells. Nat Med. 1996;2:1096–103.
27. Reiss M. TGF-beta and cancer. Microbes Infect. 1999;1:1327–47.
28. Kim R, Emi M, Tanabe K, Uchida Y, Toge T. The role of Fas ligand and transforming growth factor-beta in tumor progression: molecular mechanisms of immune privilege via Fas-mediated apoptosis and potential target for cancer therapy. Cancer. 2004;100:2281–91.
29. Lerma E, Romero M, Callardo A, Pons C, Munoz J, Fuentes J, Llovera B, Catasus L, Prati J. Prognostic significance of the Fas receptor/Fas-ligand system in cervical squamous cell carcinoma. Virchows Arch. 2008;452:65–74.
30. Danielczyk K, Dzjegiel P. MT 1 melatonin receptors and their role in the oncostatic action of melatonin. Postepy Hig Med Dosw. 2009;63:425–34.
31. Winczyk K, Fuss-Chmielewska K, Lawnika H, Pawlilkowski M, Karasek M. Luzindol but not 4P-PDOT diminishes the inhibitory effect of melatonin on murine colon cancer growth in vitro. Neuro Endocrinol Lett. 2009;30:657–62.
32. Named C, Humpeler S, Kallay E, Msteri I, Sloboda M, Rogelsperger O, Klammert N, Thalhammer T, Ekmekaoglu C. Decreased expression of the melatonin receptor 1 in human colorectal carcinomas. J Biol Regul Homeost Agents. 2011;25:531–42.
33. Hill SM, Erasch T, Xiang S, Yuan L, Duplessis T, Mao L. Molecular mechanisms of melatonin anticancer effects. Integr Cancer Ther. 2009;8:337–46.
34. Reiter RJ, Tan DX, Fuentes-Broto L. Melatonin. A multitasking molecule. Prog Brain Res. 2010;181:127–51.
35. Cos S, Fernandez R. Melatonin effects on intercellular junctional communication in MCF-7 human breast cancer cells. J Pineal Res. 2000;29:166–71.
36. Trosko JE, Ruch RJ. Cell-cell communication in carcinogenesis. Front Biosci. 2004;3:1171–86.

37. Lissoni P, Messina G, Brivio F, Fumagalli L, Vigoré L, Rovelli F, Maruelli L, Miceli M, Marchiori P, Porro G, Held M, Di Fede G, Uchiyamada T. Modulation of the anticancer immunity by natural agents: inhibition of T regulatory lymphocyte generation by arabinoxylan in patients with locally limited or metastatic solid tumors. Cancer Ther. 2008;6:1007–12.
38. Casado-Apico S, Martin V, Garcia-Santos G, Rodriguez-Bianco J, Sanchez-Sanchez AM, Luno E, Suarez G, Garcia-Pedrera JM, Menendez ST, Antolin I, Rodriguez C. Regulation of the expression of death receptors and their ligands by melatonin in haematological cancer cell lines and in leukaemia cell from patients. J Pineal Res. 2011;50:345–55.
39. Hagimoto N, Kuwand K, Inashima I, Yashimi M, Nakamura N, Fujita M, Moeyama T, Hara N. TGF-beta-1 as an enhancer of Fas-mediated apoptosis of lung epithelial cells. J Immunol. 2002;168:6470–8.
40. Liu F, Ng TB, Fung ML. Pineal indoles stimulate the gene expression of immunomodulating cytokines. J Neural Transm. 2001;108:397–405.
41. Park SY, Yang WJ, Yi EY, Jang JY, Jung Y, Leong JW, Kim YJ. Melatonin suppresses tumor angiogenesis by inhibiting HIF- 1 alpha stabilization under hypoxia. J Pineal Res. 2010;48:178–84.
42. Lissoni P. Is there a role for melatonin in supportive care? Support Care Cancer. 2000;10:110–6.
43. Kong X, Wang X, Xu W, Behera S, Hellermann G, Kumar A, Lockey RF, Mohapatra S, Mohapatra SS. Natriuretic peptide receptor as a novel anticancer target. Cancer Res. 2008;68:249–56.
44. Lissoni P, Pittalis S, Vigoré L, Rovelli F, Vezzo R, Bramati S, Menin E, Rescaldani R, Fondrini G, Pelizzoni F, Grugni G, Morabito F. The heart as an immunomodulator organ: in vitro immune effects of the cardiac hormone atrial natriuretic peptide-alpha and their possible relevance in cardiac failure and aging. Cardiol Eld. 1993;1:227–31.
45. Bartsch H, Bartsch C. Effect of melatonin on experimental tumors under different photoperiods and times of administration. J Neural Transm. 1981;52:269–79.
46. Lissoni P, Tisi E, Brivio F, Ardizzoia A, Crispino S, Barni S, Tancini G, Conti A, Maestroni GJM. Modulation of interleukin-2-induced macrophage activation in cancer patients by the pineal hormone melatonin. J Biol Regul Homeost Agents. 1991;5:154–6.
47. Starr KW. Growth and new growth: environmental carcinogens in the process of human ontogeny. Prog Clin Cancer. 1970;4:1–13.
48. Lissoni P, Barni S, Crispino S, Tancini G, Fraschini F. Endocrine and immune effects of melatonin therapy in metastatic cancer patients. Eur J Cancer. 1989;25:789–95.
49. Gonzales R, Sanchez A, Ferguson JA, Palmer C, Daniel C, Cohn A, Robinson WA. Melatonin therapy of advanced human malignant melanoma. Melanoma Res. 1991;1:237–43.
50. Millis E, Wu P, Seely D, Guyatt G. Melatonin in the treatment of cancer: a systemic review of randomized controlled trials and meta-analysis. J Pineal Res. 2005;39:360–6.
51. Chinery R, Brockman JA, Peeler MO, Shyr Y, Beauchamps RD, Coffey RJ. Antioxidants enhance the cytotoxicity of chemotherapeutic agents in colorectal cancer: a p53-independent induction of p21 via F1/CIP1 via c/EBP-beta. Nat Med. 1997;3:1233–8.
52. Conti A, Maestroni GJM. The clinical neuroimmunotherapeutic role of melatonin in oncology. J Pineal Res. 1995;19:103–10.
53. Lissoni P, Paolorossi F, Ardizzoia A, Barni S, Chilelli M, Tancini G, Conti A, Maestroni GJM. A randomized study of chemotherapy with cisplatin plus etoposide versus chemoendocrine therapy with cisplatin, etoposide and the pineal hormone melatonin as a first- line treatment of advanced non-small cell lung cancer patients in poor clinical state. J Pineal Res. 1997;23:15–9.
54. Lissoni P, Barni S, Mandala M, Ardizzoia A, Paolorossi F, Vaghi M, Longarini R, Malugani F, Tancini G. Decreased toxicity and increased efficacy of cancer chemotherapy using the pineal hormone melatonin in metastatic solid tumor patients with poor clinical status. Eur J Cancer. 1999;35:1688–92.
55. Lissoni P, Barni S, Tancini G, Ardizzoia A, Ricci G, Aldeghi R, Brivio F, Tisi E, Rovelli F, Rescaldani R, Quadro G, Maestroni GJM. A randomised study with subcutaneous low-dose interleukin-2 alone vs interleukin-2 plus the pineal neurohormone melatonin in advanced solid neoplasms other than renal cancer and melanoma. Br J Cancer. 1994;69:196–9.
56. Siu SW, Lau TK, Tam PC, Shiu SY. Melatonin and prostate cancer cell proliferation: interplay with castration, epidermal growth factor, and androgen sensitivity. Prostate. 2002;52:106–22.
57. Lissoni P, Ardizzoia A, Barni S, Paolorossi F, Tancini G, Meregalli S, Esposti D, Zubelewicz B, Braczowski R. A randomized study of tamoxifen alone versus tamoxifen plus melatonin in estrogen receptor-negative heavily pretreated metastatic breast cancer patients. Oncol Rep. 1995;2:871–3.
58. Lissoni P, Barni S, Ardizzoia A, Tancini G, Conti A, Maestroni GJM. A randomized study with the pineal hormone melatonin versus supportive care alone in patients with brain metastases due to solid neoplasms. Cancer. 1994;73:699–701.
59. Lissoni P, Meregalli S, Nasetto L, Barni S, Tancini G, Fossati V, Maestroni G. Increased survival time in brain glioblastoma by a radioneuroendocrine strategy with radiotherapy plus melatonin compared to radiotherapy alone. Oncology. 1996;53:43–6.
60. Lewis JW, Shavit Y, Terman GW. Apparent involvement of opioid peptides in stress-induced enhancement of tumor growth. Peptides. 1983;4:635–8.
61. Lissoni P, Giani L, Zerbini S, Trabattoni P, Rovelli F. Biotherapy with the pineal immunomodulating hormone

melatonin plus Aloe vera in untreatable advanced solid neoplasms. Nat Immun. 1998;16:27–33.
62. Shishodia S, Harikumar KB, Dass S, Ramawat KG, Aggarwal BB. The guggul for chronic diseases: ancient medicine, modern targets. Anticancer Res. 2008;28:3647–64.
63. Somparn P, Phisalaphong C, Nakornchal S, Unchern S, Morales NP. Comparative antioxidant activities of curcumin and its demethoxy and hydrogenated derivatives. Biol Pharm Bull. 2007;30:74–8.
64. Viviani S, Negretti E, Orazi A, Sozzi G, Santoro A, Lissoni P, Esposti G, Fraschini F. Preliminary studies on melatonin in the treatment of myelodysplastic syndromes following cancer chemotherapy. J Pineal Res. 1990;8:347–51.
65. Lissoni P, Mandalà M, Rossini F, Fumagalli L, Barni S. Thrombopoietic property of the pineal hormone melatonin. Hematology. 1999;4:335–43.
66. Lissoni P, Mandalà M, Brivio F. Abrogation of the negative influence of opioids on IL-2 immunotherapy of renal cell cancer by melatonin. Eur Urol. 2000;38:115–8.
67. Lissoni P, Brivio O, Brivio F, Barni S, Tancini G, Crippa D, Meregalli S. Adjuvant therapy with the pineal hormone melatonin in patients with lymph node relapse due to malignant melanoma. J Pineal Res. 1996;21:239–42.

5 Melatonin: Its Microbicidal Properties and Clinical Applications

V. Srinivasan, Mahaneem Mohamed, and Hisanori Kato

Abstract

Melatonin is a versatile molecule, synthesized mainly by the pineal gland and in small amounts by other organs like retina, gastrointestinal tract, thymus, bone marrow, and lymphocytes. Other than its important role in various body functions like sleep and circadian rhythm regulation, antioxidant functions, and control of reproductive functions, melatonin has been found to be effective in combating infections by various bacteria including chlamydia and *Mycobacterium tuberculosis*, as well as by viruses. Molecular mechanisms of antimicrobial actions of melatonin have been proposed to be due to its effects on free radical formation, direct regulation of bacterial duplication, and depletion of intracellular substrates like iron. It also has protective effect against sepsis as shown in various animal models of septic shock. This protective effect is suggested to be due to its antioxidant, immunomodulating, and inhibitory actions against the production and activation of pro-inflammatory mediators. Clinical studies have shown the potential beneficial use of melatonin in treating septic shock with severe respiratory distress syndrome and associated multiorgan failure in addition to its antimicrobial and antiviral actions.

V. Srinivasan, MSc, PhD, MAMS (✉)
Sri Sathya Sai Medical Educational and Research Foundation, An International Medical Sciences Research Study Center, Prasanthi Nilayam, 40-Kovai Thirunagar Extn, Goldwins, Coimbatore, TN 641014, India

National Health Service, Department of Mental Health, Psychiatric Service of Diagnosis and Treatment, Hospital "G. Mazzini", ASL 4, Teramo, Italy

Department of Neuroscience and Imaging, University "G.D' Annunzio", Chieti 66013, Italy
e-mail: sainivasan@yahoo.com; venkataramanujamsrinivasan6@gmail.com

M. Mohamed, MD, MSc, PhD
Department of Physiology, School of Medical Sciences, Universiti Sains Malaysia, Kubang Kerian, Kelantan 16150, Malaysia
e-mail: mahaneem@kck.usm.my

H. Kato, PhD
Organization for Interdisciplinary Research Projects, The University of Tokyo, 1-1-1 Yayoi, Bunkyo-ku, Tokyo 113-8657, Japan
e-mail: akatoq@mail.ecc.u-tokyo.ac.jp

V. Srinivasan et al. (eds.), *Melatonin and Melatonergic Drugs in Clinical Practice*, DOI 10.1007/978-81-322-0825-9_5, © Springer India 2014

Keywords
Anti-inflammatory • Antimicrobial • Melatonin • Sepsis

Abbreviations

4HDA	4-hydroxyalkenals
cAMP	Cyclic adenosine monophosphate
CLP	Cecal ligation and puncture
cNOS	Constitutive nitric oxide synthase
GSH	Reduced glutathione
GSSG	Oxidized glutathione
H_2O_2	Hydrogen peroxide
HEp-2	Human epithelial type 2
IFN	Interferon
IL	Interleukin
iNOS	Inducible nitric oxide synthase
LPS	Lipopolysaccharide
MDA	Malondialdehyde
MIC	Minimum inhibitory concentrations
MODS	Multiorgan dysfunction syndrome
MOF	Multiorgan failure
MPO	Myeloperoxidase
mtNOS	Mitochondrial nitric oxide synthase
MTP	Mitochondrial transition pore
NO	Nitric oxide
NOS	Nitric oxide synthase
$O_2^{\bullet-}$	Superoxide anion radical
$ONOO^-$	Peroxynitrite
RNS	Reactive nitrogen species
ROS	Reactive oxygen species
TNF	Tumor necrosis factors
VEE	Venezuelan equine encephalomyelitis

Introduction

There is a growing problem of antibiotic-resistant bacteria that has to be eradicated seriously for the effective control and management of infectious diseases. The management and control of infectious diseases is an important public health issue as there are seasonal outbreaks of many infectious diseases with their predictable occurrence [1, 2]. Annual variations in the incidence of many infectious diseases link to changes in the light/dark cycle which in turn link to the temporal secretion of melatonin (5-methoxy-N-acetyltryptamine), the major hormone produced by the pineal gland of all mammals [3].

Melatonin is also synthesized by other organs such as retina, gastrointestinal tract, bone marrow, thymus, skin, platelets, and lymphocytes [4, 5]. Melatonin has recently been shown to protect against both bacterial and viral infections by a number of mechanisms like its pro-oxidant properties [6–8]. Protective effect of melatonin against the symptoms of severe septic shock has been reported in both animals and humans, suggesting its beneficial role in the treatment of septic shock [9, 10]. This review paper will discuss on the detailed mechanisms of melatonin action in combating bacterial and viral infections, inflammation, and septic shock as well as its potential therapeutic value.

Receptors for Melatonin

The physiological and pharmacological actions of melatonin are mediated by membrane-bound melatonin receptors, namely, MT_1 and MT_2 or nuclear receptors, although some of its actions are also receptor independent. MT_1 and MT_2 belong to the superfamily of G-protein-coupled receptors that contain seven transmembrane domains [11, 12]. Activated MT_1 and MT_2 cause a decrease in cyclic adenosine monophosphate (cAMP) concentration and stimulation of inositol phosphate [13]. Another melatonin receptor, namely, MT_3, has also been identified that is characterized as the enzyme quinone reductase [14]. Melatonin receptors are found distributed in several peripheral tissues as well in the central nervous system of both humans and animals [15]. The genomic action of melatonin has also been identified which occurs through RZR/ROR receptors [16]. The RZR/ROR receptors are widely expressed in normal tissues [17] and belong to a novel class of orphan nuclear receptors with several isoforms (RORα, RORβ—formerly known as RZR). These orphan receptors' affinity to melatonin is lower as compared to MT_1. Melatonin receptors exhibit circadian variations in their expression and mediate a plethora of intracellular effects depending upon the cellular milieu. Changes in melatonin receptor concentrations have been reported in circadian rhythm sleep disorders, depressive disorders, Alzheimer's disease, breast and prostate cancer, hepatoma, melanoma, and other pathological conditions [18, 19].

Role of Melatonin as an Antioxidant in Bacterial Infections

In various in vitro and in vivo models, melatonin has been shown as a potent free radical scavenger and antioxidant in which it reduces lipid peroxidation and scavenges hydroxyl and peroxyl radicals [20–26]. Tan et al. [20] first discovered melatonin as a remarkable potent scavenger of reactive and highly destructive hydroxyl radicals [27]. Under numerous experimental conditions, supraphysiological concentration for melatonin is required to exert its effective antioxidant effect. Therefore, the role of melatonin as an antioxidant at physiological concentrations has become a matter for debate [19]. In chemical system, a single melatonin molecule generates products in a scavenger cascade that collectively eliminates up to ten free radicals [28], and this finding may not be fully applicable to physiological systems [19]. However, melatonin has been shown to act as an antioxidant whereby it protects the cells and tissues from oxidotoxicity both in vitro and in vivo models [20]. Melatonin also upregulates several antioxidant enzymes such as glutathione peroxidase, glutathione reductase, γ-glutamylcysteine synthetase, glucose-6-phosphate dehydrogenase, and catalase [18, 29]. On the other hand, melatonin also functions as pro-oxidant whereby it stimulates the formation of reactive oxygen species (ROS) by monocytes [30] and in the promonocytic cell line U937 [31].

Role of Melatonin in Microbicidal and Antiviral Actions

Melatonin also demonstrates pro-oxidant activity which is essential for its microbicidal actions [6, 7]. In a study conducted on normal mice infected with Semliki Forest virus, subcutaneous administration of melatonin daily from 3 days before through 10 days after virus inoculation significantly reduces viremia and postpones the onset of disease and death by 7–10 days. Melatonin also reduces the mortality of Semliki Forest virus-inoculated mice from 100 to 44 %. In high doses melatonin postpones the death and reduces the mortality by 20 %. The mechanism of its protection against infection is attributed to the pro-oxidative properties of melatonin [6, 7]. The protective action of melatonin against bacterial infections has been evaluated in a cultured medium containing *Mycobacterium (M.) tuberculosis* (H37Rv strain) enriched with albumin dextrose catalase. The antibacterial action of melatonin is assessed with isoniazid, a frontline drug used in the treatment of tuberculosis. Isoniazid concentrations of 0.005–0.01 μg/ml and melatonin concentrations between 0.26 nM to 0.1 mM slightly inhibit the growth of H37Rv growth. However, at isoniazid concentration of 0.005 μg/ml, and at the melatonin concentration of 0.01 mM, the bacterial growth is inhibited 3- to 4-fold more than the sum of the inhibition obtained when either of these compounds is used alone [8]. In this study, intracellular bacterial growth is also studied in monocyte-derived macrophages, which are infected with *M. tuberculosis* H37Rv. Addition of either isoniazid or melatonin alone (16 h later) does not have any effect on macrophage mortality or viability. The growth rate of *M. tuberculosis* is also studied for 5 days in both control and drug-treated human macrophages. Addition of 1.6 mM melatonin or 0.08 μg/ml isoniazid alone shows no significant effect on mycobacterial growth. However, their combination has resulted in a marked reduction in bacterial load showing the potentiation of isoniazid killing of the mycobacteria by melatonin in macrophages. It is suggested that the microbicidal action of melatonin is attributed to its action of forming stable radicals that either could modify the isoniazid action or could be due to its binding with mycobacterial cell wall resulting in destabilization of the cell wall which causes enhanced permeability to isoniazid molecules. One of the suggested possible mechanisms for the bactericidal activity of isoniazid and melatonin combination is the formation of free radicals [8].

The microbicidal action of melatonin has also been evaluated in chlamydial infections. The Chlamydiae cause a variety of diseases in animals and humans [27]. Persistent infections with *Chlamydophila pneumoniae* cause acute and chronic respiratory diseases including asthma [32] while infection with *C. trachomatis* might lead to infertility [33]. The main mechanism for chlamydial infection is through its effect on tryptophan synthesis [34–36]. The main defense mechanism against chlamydial infection is the synthesis of interferon (IFN)-γ, which induces indoleamine 2,3-dioxygenase resulting in the depletion of tryptophan from human cell [35–38]. Melatonin increases the levels of IFN-γ during viral infection in a mouse model [39]. The effect of melatonin and tryptophan on chlamydial infection has been studied on human epithelial type 2 (HEp-2) cells (ATCC CCL-23) infected with *C. pneumoniae* to assess its mechanism of microbicidal activity. Both serotonin and melatonin reduce the chlamydial infection by about 50 % compared with controls. They exhibit a dose-dependent inhibition of *C. pneumoniae*, and their concentration at 100 μM shows the optimum effect [40]. The relationship of melatonin and IFN-γ has also been evaluated to understand the mechanism of melatonin's microbicidal activity. In this study, addition of tryptophan reverses the chlamydial infection caused by IFN-γ inhibition. However, addition of tryptophan does not reverse melatonin-mediated inhibition suggesting that the inhibitory mechanism of melatonin is independent of IFN-γ.

Pretreatment of HEp-2 cells with melatonin or serotonin reduces the chlamydial infection while pretreatment with chlamydial cells does not produce any effect. Melatonin-mediated reduction in chlamydial infection in HEp-2 cells is abolished by treatment with 20 ng/ml of pertussis toxin suggesting the involvement of G-protein-coupled melatonin receptors [40]. Melatonin receptor (either MT_1 or MT_2) activation causes increased intracellular Ca^{2+} concentration, regulation of adenyl cyclase activity, and consequent increased cAMP. Chlamydial infection has been shown to be inhibited by high concentrations of extracellular cAMP or cGMP [41]. Therefore, it is suggested that melatonin inhibits chlamydial infection by modulating intracellular Ca^{2+} and/or cAMP levels which in turn result in increased phagolysosomal activity of host cells that is responsible for inhibiting chlamydial infection [40].

The antimicrobial action of melatonin is also confirmed on microorganisms up to 48 h of incubation. Melatonin at concentrations of 31.25–125 μg/ml (0.13–0.53 mM) inhibits microbial growth of microorganisms such as *Staphylococcus aureus*, *Acinetobacter baumannii*, and *Pseudomonas aeruginosa* at both 24 and 48 h incubation [42]. The minimum inhibitory concentrations (MIC) of melatonin required for inhibiting the growth of microorganisms are also evaluated in this study (growth <0.05, evaluated with absorbance measurement at 625 nm). At 24 h, the MIC of melatonin is 250 μg/ml (1.07 mM) for gram-positive microorganisms and 125 μg/ml for gram-negative microorganisms (0.53 mM). After 48 h incubation, the MIC of melatonin is decreased to 125 μg/ml (0.53 mM) for gram-positive microorganisms and 31.25 μg/ml (0.13 mM) for gram-negative microorganisms. As melatonin is known to reduce the lipid levels in microorganisms [43] and has high metal-binding capacity [9], it is possible to suggest that melatonin shows microbicidal activity by reducing the intracellular substrates in these microorganisms [42].

Melatonin and Myeloperoxidase

The main component of neutrophil azurophilic granules is myeloperoxidase (MPO) [44]. Myeloperoxidase catalyzes hydrogen peroxide (H_2O_2)-dependent peroxidation of halides and pseudohalides to produce hypohalous acid, an antimicrobial agent [45]. It also has been associated in the pathogenesis of various diseases like atherosclerosis, asthma, arthritis, and pulmonary and heart diseases [46–50]. To date, effective inhibitors for this enzyme have not been identified. Recently, few studies have been carried out to investigate melatonin and have tried to find out whether it acts as a potent inhibitor of MPO. Indeed it was found that melatonin was able to

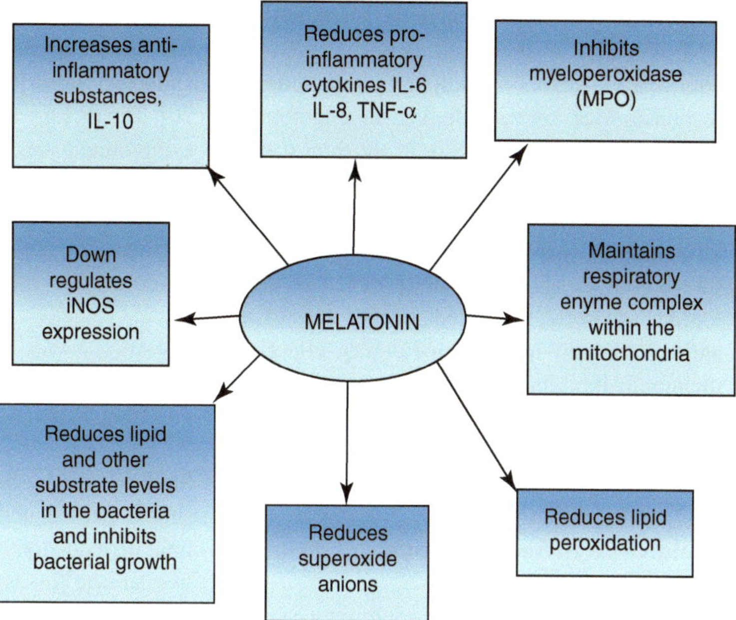

Fig. 5.1 Schematic diagram showing beneficial effects of melatonin in bacterial infections and sepsis

inhibit the catalytic activity of MPO by multiple pathways. Melatonin causes allosteric binding to the entrance of the heme pocket which in turn accelerates formation and decay of MPO compound II. Then the MPO catalytic activity switches from peroxidation to catalase-like activity. Chloride ion binding to the halide-binding site enhances the allosteric binding to the MPO-heme pocket which therefore prevents the access of H_2O_2 to the catalytic site of the enzyme. Under physiological conditions, the affinity of MPO for melatonin is very high, and inhibition of MPO activity by melatonin will be beneficial for combating increased inflammation and infectious diseases [50]. A schematic diagram depicting the beneficial effects of melatonin in bacterial infections is presented in Fig. 5.1.

Melatonin, Immune Modulation, and Viral Infections

In 1995, re-emergence of Venezuelan equine encephalomyelitis (VEE) virus, a mosquito-borne virus that caused deaths of thousands of people, horses, and donkeys from 1920 to 1970, caused mortality of affected people [51, 52]. Administration of melatonin at 250, 500, and 1,000 μg/kg to mice infected with the VEE virus reduces the mortality to 45, 40, and 16 %, respectively, compared to 100 % mortality in control-infected mice [53]. Pretreatment of melatonin also increases the survival rate to 73 % compared to 60 % obtained with standard 3 days of pre-treatment. The virus levels also reduce significantly in the blood and brain of mice treated with melatonin as compared with non-treated infected mice. Melatonin reduces the VEE virus levels in the brains of immunocompetent mice but not in the brains of immunodepressed mice. This finding may suggest that melatonin needs the integrity of immune system for its antiviral activity [54]. As melatonin has stimulatory effect on endogenous production of IFN-γ, interleukin (IL)-1β, and tumor necrosis factor (TNF)-α, it is suggested that melatonin and IFN-γ create an immunoregulatory circuit for the antiviral and antiproliferative actions of IFN-γ [55]. However, there is 100 % mortality of VEE virus-infected mice treated with melatonin when IL-1β is blocked with anti-murine IL-1β antibodies. This finding may suggest that IL-1β induced by melatonin treatment is the main target for immune-enhanced state for rapid viral clearance [40].

VEE virus infection increases the brain levels of TNF-α, which is suggested as one of the main contributory factors for producing inflammatory responses due to their leukocyte chemotactic properties. Reduced TNF-α in the brain when melatonin is administrated to VEE virus-infected mice could be responsible for reducing the inflammatory responses occurring in VEE virus-infected mice [56]. The antiviral action of melatonin has been suggested to be due to its antioxidant and immunomodulatory effects as melatonin inhibits nitric oxide synthase (NOS) activity and scavenges nitric oxide radicals (•NO) [57].

Melatonin in Septic Shock

As sepsis often results in multiorgan failure (MOF), sepsis causes high mortality rate seen in intensive care units [58, 59]. It is an infection which is associated with systemic inflammation caused by either bacterial pathogens, viruses, parasites, or fungal attack [60, 61]. Lipopolysaccharide (LPS), a component of the cell walls of gram-negative bacteria, has been suggested as the major agent responsible for the initiation of sepsis [62]. LPS is responsible for activation of intracellular signaling pathways such as nuclear factor κB, which triggers rapid gene induction and expression of inflammatory mediators like cytokines, chemokines, iNOS, and heat shock proteins [63, 64]. During sepsis, normal equilibrium between pro-inflammatory and anti-inflammatory mediators is disrupted causing the release of different inflammatory mediators [65].

TNF-α and IL-1, the important soluble mediators of inflammation, are released during early sepsis. After binding with the receptors, TNF-α causes cell activation through translation of nuclear factor κB. IL-1 is responsible for generation of ROS and stimulation of proteases production [66]. Increased release of other pro-inflammatory mediators such as IL-8, IL-12, IL-4, IL-13, and interferon is also involved in the pathogenesis of sepsis [66, 67]. Pro-inflammatory mediators causing increased production of inducible nitric oxide synthase (iNOS) are suggested to be responsible for cellular damage in sepsis [68]. Mitochondrial dysfunction during sepsis has been attributed to overexpression of mitochondrial nitric oxide synthase (mtNOS) [69, 70]. The therapy for septic shock remains largely symptomatic despite major advances in understanding the pathophysiology of sepsis. During septic shock, high doses of corticosteroids and nonsteroidal anti-inflammatory drugs are used for controlling inflammatory responses [60, 71].

Melatonin in Septic Shock: Animal Studies

Studies done by Sewerynek and coworkers have shown that melatonin is able to reduce membrane lipid peroxidation in bacterial LPS-induced oxidative damage [24] as evidenced by decreased hepatic malondialdehyde (MDA) and 4-hydroxyalkenals (4HDA). Melatonin also prevents LPS-induced endotoxemia as revealed by the reduction of TNF-α, superoxide ($O_2\bullet^-$) production in the aorta, and suppression of iNOS in the liver [72].

An animal study has been done to evaluate the possible protective effects of melatonin administration in the Swiss mouse model of lethal endotoxemia caused by i.p. injection of LPS [73]. LPS at the dose of 0.75 mg/animal was injected (i.p.) between 17:00 and 18:00 h to optimize the melatonin action. Melatonin (10 mg/kg body weight) was injected (i.p.) twice, i.e., 30 min before LPS and 60 min after LPS. Nitric oxide (NO), MDA, and 4HDA were measured in brain and liver samples of control, LPS-injected, and LPS+ melatonin-injected mice. Cytokines such as IL-1, IL-6, IL-12, IFN-γ, IL-10, and TNF-α were also measured in peritoneal fluids and serum of animals. After 72 h of LPS injection, the survival rate of LPS-injected mice was 20 %, whereas the survival rate of LPS+ melatonin-injected mice was 90 %. A significant decrease of pro-inflammatory cytokines TNF-α, IL-12, and IFN-γ was observed in the peritoneal fluid (at the site of LPS injection), but no significant effects on pro-inflammatory cytokine levels were observed in the serum of melatonin-treated mice. Melatonin stimulated the production of anti-inflammatory cytokine IL-10 in the peritoneal fluid and serum. Nitric oxide level was significantly reduced in the liver and brain samples of LPS-treated mice. The effects of melatonin in counteracting the increase of nitrite/nitrate in the brain and liver samples might suggest that the inflammation induced in sepsis by pro-inflammatory mediators is prevented by melatonin [73]. The decrease of programmed cell death in spleen found in this study might suggest the anti-apoptotic effect of melatonin via its stimulatory effects on IL-10 levels. It is concluded that melatonin protected the mice from the lethal effects of LPS-induced sepsis via its multifactorial nature such as modulation of immune function and antioxidant and anti-apoptotic actions [73].

Antioxidant effect of melatonin in cecal ligation and puncture (CLP) method induced septic shock associated with multiorgan dysfunction syndrome (MODS) has been done in 10–12-week-old male Wistar rats. Septic shock was induced by CLP. Melatonin was administered 3 mg/kg i.v. at 3, 6, and 12 h after CLP. The blood levels of pH, PaO_2, $PaCO_2$, and lactate dehydrogenase were analyzed to evaluate the extent of organ injury. Nitric oxide and IL-1β levels in the plasma as well as $O_2\bullet^-$ production in lungs, thoracic aorta, and liver were assayed. It was found that the treatment of septic animals with melatonin protected the animals against circulatory failure and organ injury resulting from the CLP model [74]. The pathogenesis of systemic inflammatory response syndrome and organ failure has been suggested to be due to the release of inflammatory mediators and oxidants from the gut [75]. Free radicals cause inflammatory reactions by mediating immune cell activation in sepsis. The release of multiple ROS and RNS (reactive nitrogen species) constitutes a part of cytokine inflammatory cascade and is also essential for bacterial killing [74]. Antioxidant therapy has been found beneficial in the clinical setting of sepsis-induced MODS [76]. Melatonin has been suggested to have beneficial effects in sepsis through its ability to (i) reduce plasma IL-1β and NO concentrations, (ii) suppress $O_2\bullet^-$ level, and (iii) decrease polymorph leukocyte infiltrations in the lungs and liver [74].

The role of ROS in the pathogenesis of LPS-induced gastrointestinal disturbances such as ileus and mucosal barrier dysfunctions was evaluated. Ileus is suggested to play an important role in the development of sepsis and MOF by promoting bacterial stasis, bacterial overgrowth, and bacterial translocation [77]. In a study conducted on male Swiss mice, melatonin (10 mg/kg) was administered at 16:00 h to all mice which were then divided in two groups, namely, control and LPS groups. Control groups received saline while LPS groups received *Escherichia coli* 20 mg/kg. Melatonin was again (10 mg/kg) administered to these mice 6 h after saline or LPS injection. LPS activates NO-mediated oxidative pathways which in turn causes disturbances in the intestinal motility [78]. These motility disturbances were reversed by melatonin. Reduction in lipid peroxidation as shown by decreased MDA levels was noted in LPS mice treated with melatonin, but with its vehicle, p38 expression, the active form of p38 MAP kinase was markedly increased by LPS. Melatonin but not its vehicle reversed the LPS-induced increase in p38 levels. It also reversed the LPS-induced increase of iNOS mRNA and protein expression. The antioxidative effects of melatonin and its beneficial effects on LPS-induced intestinal motility disturbances are due to downregulation of iNOS expression. These findings might suggest that switching off the pro-oxidant pathways induced by endotoxins is the major mechanism of the beneficial effect of melatonin in systemic inflammation during sepsis [78].

Melatonin, Mitochondrial Dysfunction, and Sepsis

The source of excessive intra-mitochondrial NO levels has suggested to increase expression and activity of mtNOS in sepsis [70]. Sepsis is often associated with ventilatory failure mainly due to reduction in contractility of the skeletal muscles such as diaphragm and intercostal muscles [79]. In a study conducted on both wild-type and ($iNOS^{+/+}$) iNOS knockout ($iNOS^{-/-}$) mice with the CLP sepsis model, glutathione (GSH) and nitrite levels as well as respiratory complexes activities (complex 1; NADH:CoQ oxidoreductase) were measured in skeletal muscle mitochondrial samples [10]. In iNOS$^{+/+}$ mice, sepsis induced a significant increase in mitochondrial iNOS activity whereas cNOS (constitutive NOS) remained unchanged. Knockout (iNOS$^{-/-}$) mice expressed only mitochondrial cNOS activity which was unaffected by sepsis. Melatonin administration counteracted sepsis-induced iNOS in iNOS$^{+/+}$ mice, and it did not affect cNOS activity in either mouse strain. In septic iNOS$^{+/+}$ mice, mitochondrial nitrite levels also increased significantly, but melatonin treatment significantly reduced nitrite levels to control values. Nitrite concentration did not change in septic iNOS$^{-/-}$mice. Sepsis reduced mitochondrial content of total and reduced GSH in iNOS$^{+/+}$ mice. Significant increases of oxidized glutathione (GSSG) level and GSSG/GSH ratio were also observed in septic iNOS$^{+/+}$ mice. During sepsis melatonin administration counteracted all these changes in mitochondrial GSH pool [10]. Mitochondria express cNOS and iNOS under physiological conditions suggesting that both enzymes produce NO for regulatory purposes [80]. The induction of mitochondrial iNOS in sepsis has been suggested to release excess of NO which could affect mitochondria through several mechanisms. Increased concentrations of NO that inhibits respiratory complexes I, II, III, and IV in mitochondria have been reported. The inhibition of respiratory complexes generates more free radicals such as $O_2^{\bullet-}$ which in turn reacts with NO forming peroxynitrite ($ONOO^-$) [81]. Under normal circumstances, the excess of free radicals generated within mitochondria is neutralized by its antioxidant defense system such as superoxide dismutase and glutathione redox cycling system. However, in sepsis there is an increase in GSSG/GSH ratio showing the failure of glutathione redox cycling system to protect mitochondria. This has been supported by the findings of Escames et al. [70] in which increased oxidative stress caused by excess NO produced in LPO-induced sepsis caused electron transport chain failure. Under oxidative stress, melatonin has been shown to be an excellent antioxidant that restores GSH homeostasis and mitochondrial function in organelles. Melatonin treatment has been shown to increase mitochondrial respiratory complex activities I and IV of liver and brain samples in a time-dependent manner [82]. It also stimulates the activity of enzymes glutathione peroxidase and glutathione reductase which are involved in GSH/GSSG balance in mitochondria [83]. The antioxidant and free radical scavenging activity of melatonin protects proteins of the electron transport chain and mtDNA from oxidative damage by ROS/RNS [84]. Melatonin also directly interacts with mitochondrial membrane and inhibits the opening of the mitochondrial transition pore (MTP) and blocks the MTP-dependent cytochrome release, the downstream activation of caspase 3, and cell death by apoptosis [85]. Melatonin maintains the mitochondrial homeostasis by all these actions, free radical scavenging and antioxidant actions, stimulation of respiratory complexes activities, and its direct interaction with MTPs [86]. Melatonin has a potential therapeutic value in treating septic conditions based on its ability in mediating mitochondrial bioenergetics and in limiting inflammatory response and oxidative damage [87, 88].

Melatonin in Septic Disease: Clinical Studies

Sepsis-induced MODS is a common cause of death in 30–100 % of critically ill patients depending upon the number of organs involved [89]. There are several studies measuring melatonin levels in critically ill patients to determine the correlation between melatonin and intensity of septic shock. Sixteen of 17 septic patients had a high urinary excretion of 6-sulfatoxymelatonin with disturbance in its circadian rhythm while non-septic patients had normal urinary 6-sulfatoxymelatonin [90]. Increased stress associated with increased sympathetic activity as well as increased norepinephrine and cortisol secretions were suggested as possible causes [91]. In another study, 7 out of 8 septic patients showed disturbed melatonin rhythm [92]. Twelve out of 16 intensive care unit patients also showed disturbed melatonin rhythm and reduced urinary 6-sulfatoxymelatonin levels [93]. However, a negative correlation between disease severity and melatonin levels was detected in another study conducted on 302 patients admitted in medical Intensive Care Unit of the University Hospital in Lübeck, Germany. This observation is important in view of the accumulating evidence "that melatonin supports the body defense against septic disease" [94].

Melatonin: A Potential Therapeutic Agent for Severe Sepsis

In ten septic newborns, melatonin treatment (2×10 mg oral doses 1 h apart) significantly reduced white cell counts and C-reactive proteins and increased platelet levels when compared with controls [95]. In ten asphyxiated newborns administered with a total of 80 mg of melatonin (eight doses of 10 mg each separated by 2 h intervals) orally, there were significant reduction in MDA and nitrite/nitrate levels at both 12 and 24 h. Three of the other ten asphyxiated newborns who did not receive melatonin died suggesting that melatonin is beneficial in newborn infants with asphyxia. The protective action of melatonin was attributed to its ability to increase the efficiency of mitochondrial electron transport and antioxidant property [96]. Clinical improvement was also observed as assessed by daily sepsis score [97]. Pro-inflammatory mediators such as IL-1β, TNF-α, and IL-8 were higher in bronchoalveolar lavage fluid obtained from babies with chronic lung disease. Treatment with ten doses of melatonin (10 mg/kg per dose) greatly limited the serum rise of IL-6, IL-8, and TNF-α when compared to non-melatonin-treated infants with respiratory distress syndrome. Nitrite/nitrate values were also lowered in these infants with chronic lung disease treated with melatonin. Therefore, it was concluded that melatonin is beneficial in improving the clinical outcome of newborns with respiratory distress syndrome by preventing its progression to chronic lung disease [9]. One of the suggested early indicators for infants to develop bronchopulmonary dysplasia is increase of pro-inflammatory indicators. In a study, measurement of pro-inflammatory cytokines such as IL-6, IL-8, and TNF-α in 103 premature newborns with respiratory distress syndrome of III and IV degree was undertaken whereby 55 infants received 10 intravenous injections of melatonin (10 mg/kg each). The first four doses were separated by 2 h intervals while the fifth and sixth were separated by 4 h intervals. Melatonin caused significant modifications in several parameters at 24 h, 72 h, and 7 days of treatment. The levels of pro-inflammatory cytokines such as IL-6, IL-8, and TNF-α in tracheobronchial aspirate were significantly reduced in melatonin-treated infants. These beneficial actions of melatonin were attributed to its antioxidative actions [97]. Melatonin reduces oxidative stress by reducing nitrite/nitrate levels and modifying serum inflammatory mediators in surgical neonates with sepsis [98]. Melatonin also has been tried in critically ill patients placed in mechanical ventilation to study the alterations of the sleep-wake parameters and augmented oxidative/nitrosative stress [91]. In a randomized, double-blind placebo-controlled study undertaken on 24 patients with tracheotomy, melatonin or placebo was administered (10 mg/day orally) at 21:00 h for four nights. Melatonin improved the sleep quality in these patients compared to placebo [99]. Although a lower dose of melatonin (1–2 mg) is able to improve the sleep, a higher dose of melatonin (10 mg/day) was administered to reduce ischemia/reperfusion injury, prevent MOF, and treat the sepsis. The therapeutic use of melatonin in different clinical conditions is summarized in Table 5.1.

Table 5.1 Melatonin for therapeutic use in different clinical conditions

Melatonin dose	Number of patients	Effects observed in newborn infants or adults	Nature of response	References
2×10 mg	20	Reduction in white blood cell and C-reactive protein	Beneficial	Gitto et al. [95]
8×10 mg	10	Reduction of MDA and nitrite/nitrate	Beneficial	Gitto et al. [96]
10×10 mg/kg	110 (chronic lung disease)	Reduced the serum IL-6, IL-8, and TNF-α	Beneficial	Gitto et al. [9]
10 mg/day	24 adults	Reduced ischemic reperfusion injury	Beneficial	Bourne et al. [99]

Conclusions

Melatonin has been found to be effective in fighting bacterial infections in various animal studies. It potentiates the effects of isoniazid in killing *M. tuberculosis* by the formation of free radicals or binding with the membranes of mycobacteria. It also inhibits chlamydial infections by activating G-protein-coupled melatonin receptors and subsequently by increasing adenyl cyclase and intracellular cAMP in host cells. Melatonin administration protects mice infected with the VEE virus by increasing the production of IL-1β. Melatonin has a potential therapeutic value in the treatment of septic shock in various animal models as well as in critically ill patients. Beside its antimicrobial and antiviral actions, the protective action of melatonin against septic shock has been attributed to its remarkable properties of cytokine modulating, antioxidant, and anti-apoptotic actions.

References

1. Srinivasan V, Spence DW, Pandi-Perumal SR, Cardinali DP, Maestroni GJ. Immunomodulation by melatonin: its significance for seasonally occurring diseases. Neuroimmunomodulation. 2008;15:93–101.
2. Baysallar M, Kilic A, Aydogan H, Cilli F, Doganci L. Linezolid and quinupristin resistance in vancomycin-resistant enterococci and methicillin-resistant *staphylococcus aureus* prior to clinical use in Turkey. Int J Antimicrob Agents. 2004;23:510–2.
3. Srinivasan V. The pineal gland: its physiological and pharmacological role. Indian J Physiol Pharmacol. 1989;33:263–72.
4. Pandi-Perumal SR, Srinivasan V, Maestroni GJ, Cardinali DP, Poeggeler B, Hardeland R. Melatonin. Nature's most versatile signal? FEBS J. 2006;273: 2813–38.
5. Claustrat B, Brun J, Chazot G. The basic physiology and pathophysiology of melatonin. Sleep Med Rev. 2005;9:11–24.
6. Ben-Nathan D, Maestroni GJ, Lustig S, Conti A. Protective effects of melatonin in mice infected with encephalitis viruses. Arch Virol. 1995;140:223–30.
7. Ben-Nathan D, Maestroni GJM, Conti A. The protective effect of melatonin in viral and bacterial infections. In: Maestroni GJM, Conti A, Reiter RJ, editors. Therapeutic potential of melatonin. Basel: Karger; 1997. p. 71–80.
8. Wiid I, Hoal-van Helden E, Hon D, Lombard C, van Helder P. Potentiation of isoniazid activity against Mycobacterium tuberculosis by melatonin. Antimicrob Agents Chemother. 1999;43:975–7.
9. Gitto E, Reiter RJ, Amodio A, Romeo C, Cuzzocrea E, Sabatino G, et al. Early indicators of chronic lung disease in preterm infants with respiratory distress syndrome and their inhibition by melatonin. J Pineal Res. 2004;36:250–5.
10. Escames G, Lopez LC, Tapias V, Utrilla P, Reiter RJ, Hitos AB, et al. Melatonin counteracts inducible mitochondrial nitric oxide synthase-dependent mitochondrial dysfunction in skeletal muscle of septic mice. J Pineal Res. 2006;40:71–8.
11. Reppert SM, Weaver DR, Ebisawa T. Cloning and characterization of a mammalian melatonin receptor that mediates reproductive and circadian responses. Neuron. 1994;13:1177–85.
12. Reppert SM, Godson C, Mahle CD, Weaver DR, Slaugenhaupt SA, Gusella JF. Molecular characterization of a second melatonin receptor expressed in human retina and brain: the Mel_{1b} melatonin receptor. Proc Natl Acad Sci U S A. 1995;92:8734–8.
13. Godson C, Reppert SM. The Mel1a melatonin receptor is coupled to parallel signal transduction pathways. Endocrinology. 1997;138:397–404.
14. Nosjean O, Ferro M, Coge F, Beauverger P, Henlin JM, Lefoulon F, et al. Identification of the melatonin binding site MT_3 as the quinone reductase 2. J Biol Chem. 2001;275:31311–7.
15. Ekmekcioglu C. Melatonin receptors in humans. Biological role and clinical relevance. Biomed Pharmacother. 2006;60:97–101.
16. Becker-Andre M, Wiesenberg I, Schaeren-Wiemer N, Andre E, Missbach M, Saurat JH, et al. Pineal gland hormone melatonin binds and activates an orphan of the nuclear receptor superfamily. J Biol Chem. 1994;269:28531–4.
17. Giguere V. Orphan nuclear receptors: from gene to function. Endocr Rev. 1999;20:689–725.
18. Pandi-Perumal SR, Trakht I, Srinivasan V, Spence DW, Maestroni GJM, Zisapel N, et al. Physiological effects of melatonin: role of melatonin receptors and signal transduction pathways. Prog Neurobiol. 2008; 85:335–53.
19. Hardeland R, Cardinali DP, Srinivasan V, Spence DW, Brown GM, Pandi-Perumal SR. Melatonin A pleiotropic orchestrating molecule. Prog Neurobiol. 2011;93: 350–84.
20. Tan DX, Chen LD, Poeggeler B, Manchester LD, Reiter RJ. Melatonin: a potent, endogenous hydroxyl radical scavenger. Endocr J. 1993;1:57–60.
21. Tan DX, Poeggeler B, Reiter RJ. The pineal hormone melatonin inhibits DNA adduct formation induced by the chemical carcinogen safrole in vivo. Cancer Lett. 1993;70:65–71.
22. Pieri C, Marra M, Moroni F, Recchioni R, Marcheselli F. Melatonin: a peroxyl radical scavenger more effective than vitamin E. Life Sci. 1994;55:L271–6.

23. Sewerynek E, Melchiorri D, Ortiz GG, Poeggeler B, Reiter RJ. Melatonin reduces H_2O_2 induced lipid peroxidation in homogenates of different rat brain regions. J Pineal Res. 1995;19:51–6.
24. Sewerynek E, Melchiorri D, Reiter RJ, Ortiz GG, Lewinski A. Lipopolysaccharide-induced hepatotoxicity is inhibited by the antioxidant melatonin. Eur J Pharmacol. 1995;293:327–34.
25. Gilad E, Cuzzocrea S, Zingarelli B, Salzman AL, Szabo C. Melatonin is a scavenger of peroxynitrite. Life Sci. 1997;60:169–74.
26. Reiter RJ, Tan DX, Manchester LC, Qi W. Biochemical reactivity of melatonin with reactive oxygen and nitrogen species. Cell Biochem Biophys. 2001;34:237–54.
27. Rottenberg ME, Gigliotti-Rothfuchs A, Wigzell H. The role of IFN-gamma in the outcome of chlamydial infection. Curr Opin Immunol. 2001;14:444–51.
28. Rosen J, Than NN, Koch D, Poeggeler B, Laatsch H, Hardeland R. Interactions of melatonin and its metabolites with ABTS cation radical: extension of radical scavenger cascade and formation of a novel class of oxidation products, C2-substituted 3-indolinones. J Pineal Res. 2006;41:374–81.
29. Reiter RJ. Interactions of the pineal hormone melatonin with oxygen centered free radicals: a brief review. Braz J Med Biol Res. 1993;26:1141–55.
30. Morrey KM, McLachlan JA, Serkin CD, Bakouche O. Activation of monocytes by the pineal hormone melatonin. J Immunol. 1994;153(267):1–80.
31. Cristafanon S, Uguccioni F, Cerella C, Radogna F, Dicato M, Ghibelli L, et al. Intracellular prooxidant activity of melatonin induces a survival pathway involving NF-κB activation. Ann N Y Acad Sci. 2009;1171:472–8.
32. Hahn DL, Dodge RW, Golubjatnikov R. Association of Chlamydia pneumoniae (strain TWAR) infection with wheezing, asthma, bronchitis and adult-onset asthma. JAMA. 1991;266:225–30.
33. Schachter J. Chlamydial infections (first of three parts). N Engl J Med. 1978;298:428–35.
34. Kalman SMW, Marathe R, Lammel C, Fan J, Hyman RW, Olinger L, et al. Comparative genomes of Chlamydia pneumoniae and C. trachomatis. Nat Genet. 1999;21:385–9.
35. Pantoja LG, Miller RD, Ramirez JA, Molestina RE, Summersgill JT. Inhibition of Chlamydia pneumoniae replication in human aortic smooth muscle cells by gamma interferon-induced indoleamine 2,3-dioxygenase activity. Infect Immun. 2000;68:6478–81.
36. Xie GBC, Bonner CA, Jensen RA. Dynamic diversity of the tryptophan pathway in chlamydiae: reductive evolution and a novel operon for tryptophan metabolism recapture. Genome Biol. 2002;51:1–17.
37. Mehta SJ, Miller RD, Ramirez JA, Summersgill JT. Inhibition of Chlamydia pneumonia replication in HEp-2 cells by interferon-gamma: role of tryptophan catabolism. J Infect Dis. 1998;177:1326–31.
38. Moffett JR, Namboodiri MA. Tryptophan and the immune response. Immunol Cell Biol. 2003;81:247–65.
39. Valero N, Bonilla E, Pons H, Chacin-Bonilla L, Anez F, Espina LM, et al. Melatonin induces changes to serum cytokines in mice infected with the Venezuelan equine encephalomyelitis virus. Trans R Soc Trop Med Hyg. 2002;96:348–51.
40. Rahman MA, Azuma Y, Fukunaga H, Murakami T, Sugi K, Fukushi K, et al. Serotonin and melatonin, neurohormones for homeostasis, as novel inhibitors of infections by the intracellular parasite Chlamydia. J Antimicrob Chemother. 2005;56:861–8.
41. Ward ME, Salari H. Control mechanisms governing the infectivity of Chlamydia trachomatis for hela cells: modulation by cyclic nucleotides, prostaglandins and calcium. J Gen Microbiol. 1982;128:639–50.
42. Tekbas OF, Ogur R, Korkmaz A, Killic A, Reiter RJ. Melatonin as an antibiotic: new insights into the actions of this ubiquitous molecule. J Pineal Res. 2008;44:222–6.
43. Konar V, Yilmaz O, Ozturk AI, Kirbag S, Arslan M. Antimicrobial and biological effects of bomphos and phomphos on bacterial and yeast cells. Bioorg Chem. 2000;28:214–25.
44. Nauseef WM, Malech HL. Analysis of the peptide subunits of human neutrophil myeloperoxidase. Blood. 1986;67:1504–7.
45. Klebanoff SJ, Waltersdorph AM, Rosen H. Antimicrobial activity of myeloperoxidase. Methods Enzymol. 1984;105:399–403.
46. Podrez EA, Abu-Soud HM, Hazen SL. Myeloperoxidase-generated oxidants and atherosclerosis. Free Radic Biol Med. 2000;28:1717–25.
47. Nicholls SJ, Hazen SL. Myeloperoxidase and cardiovascular disease. Arterioscler Thromb Vasc Biol. 2005;25:1102–11.
48. Xu W, Zheng S, Dweik RA, Erzurum SC. Role of epithelial nitric oxide in airway viral infections. Free Radic Biol Med. 2006;41:19–28.
49. Pattison DI, Davies MJ. Reactions of myeloperoxidase -derived oxidants with biological substrates: gaining chemical insight into human inflammatory diseases. Curr Med Chem. 2006;13:3271–90.
50. Glijasevic S, Abdulhamid I, Husam M, Abu-Sood HM. Melatonin is a potent inhibitor for myeloperoxidase. Biochemistry. 2008;47:2668–77.
51. Bowen GS, Calisher CH. Virological and serological studies of Venezuelan equine encephalomyelitis in humans. J Clin Microbiol. 1976;4:22–7.
52. Weaver SC, Salas R, Rico-Hesse R, Ludwig GV, Oberste MS, Boshell J, et al. Reemergence of epidemic Venezuelan equine encephalomyelitis virus in South America. Lancet. 1996;358:436–40.
53. Bonilla E, Valero N, Pons H, Chacin-Bonilla L. Melatonin protects mice infected with Venezuelan equine encephalomyelitis virus. Cell Mol Life Sci. 1997;53:430–4.

54. Bonilla E, Rodon C, Valero N, Pons H, Chacin-Bonilla L, Garcia Tamayo J, et al. Melatonin prolongs survival of immunodepressed mice infected with the Venezuelan equine encephalomyelitis virus. Trans R Soc Trop Med Hyg. 2001;95:207–10.
55. Finocchiaro LM, Artz ES, Fernandez S, Crisculo M, Finkielman S, Nahmod VE. Serotonin and melatonin synthesis in peripheral blood mononuclear cells stimulation by interferon -gamma as part of the immunomodulatory pathway. J Interferon Res. 1988;8:705–16.
56. Bonilla E, Valero N, Chacin-Bonilla L, Pons H, Larreal Y, Medina-Leendert S, et al. Melatonin increases interleukin-1β and decreases tumor necrosis factor alpha in the brain of mice infected with the Venezuelan equine encephalomyelitis virus. Neurochem Res. 2003;28:687–92.
57. Bonilla E, Valero N, Chacin-Bonilla L, Medina-Leendertz S. Melatonin and viral infections. J Pineal Res. 2004;36:73–9.
58. Baker CC, Huynh T. Sepsis in the critically ill patients. Curr Probl Surg. 1995;32:1013–92.
59. Cohen J. The immunopathogenesis of sepsis. Nature. 2002;420:885–91.
60. Annane D, Bellissant E, Cavallion JM. Septic shock. Lancet. 2005;365:63–78.
61. Calandra T, Cohen J. The international sepsis forum consensus conference on definitions of infection in the intensive care unit. Crit Care Med. 2005;33: 1538–48.
62. Sriskandan S, Cohen J. The pathogenesis of septic shock. J Infect. 1995;30:201–6.
63. Victor VM, Rocha M, De La Fuente M. Immune cells: free radicals and antioxidants in sepsis. Int Immunopharmacol. 2004;4:327–47.
64. Tsiotoo AG, Sakorafas GH, Anagnostopoolos G, Bramis J. Septic shock: current pathogenetic concepts from a clinical perspective. Med Sci Monit. 2005;11: RA76–85.
65. Pinsky MR. Sepsis, a pro and anti-inflammatory disequilibrium. Contrib Nephrol. 2001;132:354–66.
66. Baggiolini M, Dewald B, Moser B. Interleukin-8 and related chemotactic cytokines. Adv Immunol. 1994;55:97–179.
67. Kumar A, Thota V, Dee L, Olson J, Uretz E, Parrillo JE. Tumor necrosis factor α and interleukin 1 beta are responsible for *in vitro* myocardial cell depression induced by human septic shock. J Exp Med. 1996;183: 949–58.
68. Carreras MC, Franco MC, Peralta JG, Poderoso JJ. Nitric oxide, complex I, and the modulation of mitochondrial reactive species in biology and disease. Mol Aspects Med. 2004;25:125–39.
69. Boveris DJ, Alvarez S, Navarro A. The role of mitochondrial nitric oxide synthase in inflammation and septic shock. Free Radic Biol Med. 2002;33:1186–93.
70. Escames G, León J, Macías M, Khaldy H, Acuña-Castroviejo D. Melatonin counteracts lipopolysaccharide-induced expression and activity of mitochondrial nitric oxide synthase in rats. FASEB J. 2003;17:932–4.
71. Annane D, Bellisant E, Bollaert P, Brigel J, Keh D, Kupfer Y. Corticosteroids for severe sepsis and septic shock: a systematic review and meta-analysis. Br Med J. 2004;329:480.
72. Wu CC, Chiao CW, Hsiao G, Chen A, Yen MH. Melatonin prevents endotoxin-induced circulatory failure in rats. J Pineal Res. 2001;30:147–56.
73. Carrillo-Vico A, Lardone PJ, Naji L, Fernandez-Santos JM, Martin-Lacave I, Guerrero JM, et al. Beneficial pleiotropic actions of melatonin in an experimental model of septic shock in mice: regulation of pro-/anti-inflammatory cytokine network, protection against oxidative damage and anti-apoptotic effects. J Pineal Res. 2005;39:400–8.
74. Wu J-Y, Tsou MY, Chen TH, Chen SJ, Tsao CM, Wu CC. Therapeutic effects of melatonin on peritonitis-induced septic shock with multiple organ dysfunction syndrome in rats. J Pineal Res. 2008;45:106–16.
75. Adams JM, Hauser CJ, Adams Jr CA, Xu DZ, Livingston DH, Deitch EA. Entry of gut lymph into the circulation primes rat neutrophil respiratory burst in hemorrhagic shock. Crit Care Med. 2001;29: 2194–8.
76. Heller AR, Groth G, Heller SC, Breitkreutz R, Nebe T, Quintel M, et al. N-acetylcysteine reduces respiratory burst but augments neutrophil phagocytosis in intensive care unit patients. Crit Care Med. 2001;29:272–6.
77. De Filipps D, Iuvone T, Esposito G, Sterdo L, Arnold GH, Paul AP, et al. Melatonin reverses lipopolysaccharide-induced gastro-intestinal motility disturbances through the inhibition of oxidative stress. J Pineal Res. 2008;44:45–51.
78. De Winter BY, van Nassaow L, de Man JG, De Jonge F, Bredenoord AJ, Seerden TC, et al. Role of the oxidative stress in the pathogenesis of septic ileus in mice. Neurogastroenterol Motil. 2005;17:251–61.
79. Hussain SN. Respiratory muscle dysfunction in sepsis. Mol Cell Biochem. 1998;179:125–34.
80. Ghafourifar P, Cadenas E. Mitochondrial nitric oxide synthase. Trends Pharmacol Sci. 2005;26:190–5.
81. Poderoso JJ, Carreras MC, Lisdero C. Nitric oxide inhibits electron transfer and increases O_2^- radical production in rat heart mitochondria and submitochondrial particles. Arch Biochem Biophys. 1996;308: 89–95.
82. Martin M, Macias M, Escames G, Reiter RJ, Agapito MT, Ortiz GG, et al. Melatonin induced increased activity of the respiratory chain complexes I and IV can prevent mitochondrial damage induced by ruthenium red in vivo. J Pineal Res. 2000;28:242–8.
83. Martin M, Macias M, Escames G, Leon J, Acuna-Castroviejo D. Melatonin but not vitamin C and E maintains glutathione homeostasis in t-butyl hydroperoxide-induced mitochondrial oxidative stress. FASEB J. 2000;14:1677–9.
84. Karbownik M, Tan D, Manchester LC, Reiter RJ. Renal toxicity of the carcinogen delta-aminolevulinic acid: antioxidant effects of melatonin. Cancer Lett. 2000;161:1–7.

85. Park JW, Youn YC, Kwon OS, Jang YY, Han ES, Lee CS. Protective effect of serotonin on 6-hydroxydopamine and dopamine induced oxidative damage of brain mitochondria and synaptosomes and PC12 cells. Neurochem Int. 2002;40:223–33.
86. Leon J, Acuna-Castroviejo D, Escames G, Tan DX, Reiter RJ. Melatonin mitigates mitochondrial malfunction. J Pineal Res. 2005;38:1–9.
87. Srinivasan V, Pandi-Perumal SR, Spence DW, Kato H, Cardinali DP. Melatonin septic shock. J Crit Care. 2010;25:656.e1–6.
88. Srinivasan V, Spence DW, Pandi-Perumal SR, Brown GM, Cardinali DP. Melatonin in mitochondrial dysfunction and related disorders. Int J Alzheimers Dis. 2011;2011:326320.
89. Kirton OC, Civetta JM. Ischemia-reperfusion injury in the critically ill: a progenitor of multiple organ failure. New Horiz. 1999;7:87–95.
90. Mundigler G, Delle-Karth G, Koreny M, Zehetgruber M, Steindl-Munda P, Marktl W, et al. Impaired circadian rhythm of melatonin secretion in sedated critically ill patients with severe sepsis. Crit Care Med. 2002;30:536–40.
91. Bourne RS, Mills GH. Melatonin: possible implications for the postoperative and critically ill patient. Intensive Care Med. 2006;32:371–9.
92. Olofsson K, Alling C, Lundberg D, Malmros C. Abolished circadian rhythm of melatonin secretion in sedated and artificially ventilated intensive care patients. Acta Anaesthesiol Scand. 2004;48:679–84.
93. Frisk U, Olsson J, Nylen P, Hahn RG. Low melatonin excretion during mechanical ventilation in the intensive care unit. Clin Sci. 2004;107:47–53.
94. Perras B, Kurowski V, Dodt C. Nocturnal melatonin concentration is correlated with illness severity in patients with septic disease. Intensive Care Med. 2006;32:624–5.
95. Gitto E, Karbownik M, Reiter RJ, Tan DX, Cuzzocrea S, Chiurazzi S, et al. Effects of melatonin treatment in septic newborns. Pediatr Res. 2001;50:756–60.
96. Fulia F, Gitto E, Cuzzocrea S, Reiter RJ, Dugo L, Gitto P, et al. Increased levels of malondialdehyde and nitrite/nitrate in the blood of asphyxiated newborns: reduction by melatonin. J Pineal Res. 2001;31:343–9.
97. Gitto E, Reiter RJ, Sabatino G, Buonocore G, Romeo C, Gitto P, et al. Correlation among cytokines, bronchopulmonary dysplasia and modality of ventilation in preterm newborns: improvement with melatonin treatment. J Pineal Res. 2005;39:287–93.
98. Gitto E, Pellegrino S, Gitto P, Barberi I, Reiter RJ. Oxidative stress of the new born in the pre- and postnatal period and the clinical utility of melatonin. J Pineal Res. 2009;46:128–39.
99. Bourne RS, Mills GH, Minelli C. Melatonin therapy to improve nocturnal sleep in critically ill patients: encouraging results from a small randomized controlled trial. Crit Care. 2008;12:R52.

6 Melatonin and the Metabolic Syndrome

Frederic Nduhirabandi and Amanda Lochner

Abstract

The ongoing worldwide obesity epidemic is paralleled by an elevated incidence of the metabolic syndrome, a disorder referred to as a clustering of metabolic abnormalities that increase the risk for cardiovascular disease and type 2 diabetes. Considered as a multifunctional molecule, the pineal gland hormone melatonin is also involved in body fat mass and energy metabolism regulation. A large body of evidence supports the beneficial effects of melatonin on the cardiovascular function in normal and pathophysiological conditions. However, melatonin's role in cardiovascular risk factors such as obesity and other related disorders including the metabolic syndrome needs further investigations, particularly in humans. This chapter will address the effects of melatonin on the metabolic syndrome focusing on obesity and insulin-resistant conditions. Since cardiovascular disease is the primary outcome of the metabolic syndrome, the effects of melatonin on cardiovascular function will be also described focusing on normal and pathological conditions. In view of the current knowledge, we aim to reveal the potential clinical relevance of melatonin or melatonin receptor agonists in the setting of obesity-induced metabolic syndrome.

Keywords

Cardiovascular disease • Insulin resistance • Melatonin • Melatonin agonist • Metabolic syndrome • Obesity disorders

Introduction

Excessive food intake and reduced physical activity associated with modern lifestyle have led to the dramatic increase in the prevalence of obesity [1–3] which is paralleled by an elevated incidence of other metabolic disorders including, among others, the metabolic syndrome (MetS), type 2 diabetes (T2D), cardiovascular diseases

F. Nduhirabandi, B MedSc, B (Hons) Med Bio Sc, MSc MedSc (✉) • A. Lochner, MSc, DSc, PhD
Division of Medical Physiology,
Department of Biomedical Science,
Faculty of Medicine and Health Sciences,
University of Stellenbosch,
19063, Tygerberg 7505, Republic of South Africa
e-mail: nduhirabandi@sun.ac.za; alo@sun.ac.za

V. Srinivasan et al. (eds.), *Melatonin and Melatonergic Drugs in Clinical Practice*,
DOI 10.1007/978-81-322-0825-9_6, © Springer India 2014

(CVD), and some cancers [4–7]. The concept of MetS refers to the clustering of common metabolic alterations that increase the risk for CVD and T2D [8]. The most widely recognized MetS components include abdominal obesity, insulin resistance, raised blood pressure, atherogenic dyslipidemia, glucose intolerance, and a proinflammatory state [8]. Apart from an increased risk for CVD and T2D, additional numerous comorbidities have been observed in MetS including nonalcoholic fatty liver disease [9], reproductive disorders [10], obstructive sleep apnea syndrome [11], chronic kidney disease [12], osteoarthritis [13], periodontal diseases [14], some cancers [7], sleep/wake disturbances, as well as other circadian alterations [15, 16]. Furthermore, patients with MetS were recently indicated to be at high risk for neurological disorders such as depression and Alzheimer's disease [17].

Epidemiological studies have shown that the prevalence of MetS continues to rise in most developed and developing countries, comprising 20–30 % of the adult population. Although not all obese people have the syndrome, the major driving force behind MetS prevalence is the actual obesity epidemic [4]. In 2008, more than 1.46 billion of the global adult population were overweight or obese [body mass index (BMI) ≥25 kg/m^2] with more than 500 million among them being identified as obese (BMI ≥30 kg/m^2) [1, 3], and it is predicted that by 2030 up to 58 % of the worldwide adult population (3.3 billion) could be either overweight or obese [18]. This alarming prevalence is not only a concern among adults, overweight and obesity prevalence is also dramatically increasing in children. In 2010, 43 million children (35 million in developing countries) were estimated to be overweight and obese, while 92 million were at risk of overweight [2]. Therefore, obesity and related metabolic abnormalities present serious socioeconomic challenges for both government and society [19].

Clinical approaches to treat or prevent obesity-induced MetS are still a challenging task. The pathophysiological mechanisms involved in the progression of obesity to MetS and other associated comorbidities are complex and not well understood. It is well established that genetic background, lifestyle behaviors, age, and gender contribute significantly in the development of obesity as well as MetS [20]. Several pathophysiological mechanisms associated with increased fat accumulation and insulin resistance have been proposed: adipose tissue dysfunction, generation of lipid metabolites, inflammation, and cellular stress (oxidative and endoplasmic reticulum stress) [21–23]. In this regard, the significance of elevated oxidative stress in obesity and its potential role in the development of insulin resistance and MetS have largely been studied by many workers [24–28].

Patients with MetS were reported to have a low serum antioxidant status with a concomitant increased levels of inflammatory markers compared with those without MetS [29, 30]. Interestingly, a higher dietary antioxidant intake has been shown to be beneficial in patients with MetS by preventing the body weight and abdominal fat gain during a 3-year follow-up [31]. Therefore, although the overall clinical relevance of conventional antioxidants (e.g., vitamins C and E, beta-carotene, zinc, and selenium) in metabolic diseases is still challenging [32], it appears that along with other substantial interventions (e.g., sustained lifestyle modification, calorie restriction, physical activity), the potential use of nonclassical antioxidants for an effective therapy to reduce or prevent obesity-related metabolic disorders is attracting many investigators.

In this chapter we consider the potential therapeutic role of melatonin in MetS. Besides its powerful antioxidant activities [33], melatonin has been shown to play an important role in metabolic regulation [34, 35]. Membrane melatonin receptors (MT1 and MT2) have been identified in the central and peripheral organs/tissues involved in the regulation of energy metabolism (e.g., hypothalamus, adipose tissue, pancreas, liver, skeletal muscle, heart, vessels, kidney) [36, 37]. It is well known that MetS features (e.g., obesity, insulin resistance, dyslipidemia, and hypertension) are more prevalent in the elderly [38, 39] where melatonin production levels decrease [40]. In addition to this, a positive association between melatonin suppression, sleep deprivation, and circadian rhythms system alteration has recently been described in obesity and MetS [15]. As consequence, the potential clinical use of either melatonin or its analogs in several pathological conditions appears exciting, and it is being used in aging and several metabolic diseases [41, 42].

We aim to review the current literature on the effects of melatonin and other melatonergic drugs in obesity and insulin-resistant conditions and the potential mechanisms underlying these effects. To better understand the overall activities of melatonin, the recent view of melatonin as a multifunctional molecule is summarized. Since CVD are the primary clinical outcome of the MetS, the effects of melatonin on cardiovascular function are also addressed. Because of space limitations, the description of obesity-associated oxidative stress, inflammation, and eventual antioxidant interventions as well as the role of melatonin in other features of MetS such as nonalcoholic fatty liver disease is not included.

Melatonin: A Multifunctional Molecule

Melatonin or 5-methoxy-N-acetyltryptamine is the neurohormone mainly produced by the pineal gland upon the activation of the suprachiasmatic nucleus (SNC) of the hypothalamus during the night (for details on biosynthesis and metabolism of melatonin, see [43]). It is a highly conserved indolamine found in almost all organisms including bacteria, algae, plants, fungi, insects, nematodes, and vertebrates including mammals [44]. In humans, the normal circulating melatonin levels vary between 1–10 pM and 43–400 pM, during the day and the night, respectively [45, 46]. The use of high doses of melatonin as frequently found in in vitro (1 μM–100 mM) or in vivo (1–300 mg/day) studies has been supported as a requirement to obtain therapeutic effects in some conditions [45, 47, 48].

Viewed as multifunctional molecule [49], melatonin is a small compound able to cross all morphological barriers and acts within every subcellular compartment due to its highly lipophilic and hydrophilic properties [47]. Since its isolation by Lerner et al. [50], apart from its classical role as a chronobiotic or endogenous synchronizer participating in the regulation of seasonal as well as circadian rhythm along with its sleep-inducing effects [43], melatonin has been shown to play a role in all most physiological functions in animals and humans [41, 49]. Indeed, melatonin has anti-excitatory, antioxidant, immunomodulatory, anti-inflammatory, oncostatic, and vasomotor properties [49, 51, 52]. However, besides its universal availability and, presumably, its presence in our daily food consumption [53], its potential beneficial effects and their underlying mechanisms are still vast and not fully explored [54].

Melatonin has powerful antioxidant properties with strong cytoprotective activities [33, 55]. It has been proved to be more effective than other classical antioxidants [56, 57] due to its multiple free radical scavenger cascades and its ability to stimulate the natural antioxidant capacity [58]. In addition to this, its metabolites have also free radical scavenging activities, and, moreover, melatonin does not have a pro-oxidant action [33, 59]. Recently, the efficacy of melatonin to improve oxidative stress-mediated metabolic disorders via its gene regulation has been shown to be linked to epigenetic mechanisms [60].

Besides its pineal production, melatonin is also secreted by wide variety of tissues including retina, thymus, spleen, heart, muscle, liver, stomach, intestine, placenta, testis, cerebral cortex, and striatum [47, 61–63]. Melatonin content in these tissues varies and decreases with age to a similar extent as the pineal melatonin production [61, 63]. Commonly, nocturnal melatonin production as shown by its circulating levels as well as its primary urinary metabolite, 6-sulfatoxymelatonin (aMT6s), is lowered in various pathologies characterized by increased oxidative stress such as neurological disorders, CVD, and T2D as well as obstructive sleep apnea syndrome [41, 64]. Importantly, circulating melatonin levels can be influenced by the diet [65, 66]. Melatonin was recently identified in common ingredients of the traditional Mediterranean diet [67] which has been reported to be efficient in improving MetS features such as waist circumference, the levels of triglycerides (TGs), high-density lipoprotein (HDL)-cholesterol (HDL-c), and blood pressure (BP) as well as glucose metabolism [68]. Interestingly, along with resveratrol, the minute amounts of melatonin present in red wine protect the heart against myocardial ischemia/reperfusion damage [69], indicating its therapeutic potential in CVD.

Melatonin and Cardiovascular Function

The Link Between Cardiovascular Function and Melatonin

The link between cardiovascular function and melatonin as well as the influence of endogenous melatonin on the cardiovascular function is well established [70]. Diurnal variations can be seen in BP, heart rate, cardiac output, and endothelial dilatory capacity of peripheral and coronary arteries, sympathetic activity, cardiac electrical stability, and platelet aggregation [70, 71]. In pathological conditions, adverse cardiovascular events including myocardial infarction [72], sudden cardiac death [73], and arrhythmias [74] have also been linked to the circadian rhythm in humans, having a higher incidence in the early morning hours, where circulating melatonin levels are considerably low [75].

The most important evidence linking melatonin to the cardiovascular function was the identification of membrane MT1 and MT2 receptors along with other intracellular binding sites such as the cytosolic quinone reductase 2 enzyme [also called the putative melatonin receptor 3 (QR2/MT3) and melatonin nuclear receptors (e.g., retinoic acid subfamily of orphan receptors (RORx)] in the heart and the arteries [76–78]. These receptors offer possibilities for melatonin signaling to interact with the cardiovascular function. Melatonin may indirectly affect cardiovascular function via MT receptors in the SCN which is known to modulate the cardiovascular function via multisynaptic autonomic neurons [79]. Melatonin may also influence the cardiovascular physiology via its direct actions on the peripheral intrinsic circadian clocks identified in both cardiomyocytes [78, 80] and vessels [81]. More surprisingly, melatonin has been shown to be also secreted within the heart [61, 63]. However, the exact role for this cardiac melatonin remains unknown.

Effects of Melatonin on the Heart

Animal studies showed that prolonged melatonin consumption under normal conditions affects cardiac metabolism, reduces the absolute and relative heart weights [82, 83], and increases its glycogen content [84] with no effects on heart function in vivo [85] and ex vivo [82]. Similarly, in healthy male volunteers, administration of 3 mg of melatonin had no effect on their heart rate [86].

Although raising circulating melatonin concentration by administration of exogenous melatonin does not appear to be harmful to the heart, the presence of very low circulating concentrations (as occurring during daytime) is essential and pinealectomy has profound effects on the heart. Surgical removal of pineal gland followed by 2 months of stabilization caused increase in serum cholesterol and cardiac malondialdehyde (MDA) levels as well as the heart weight. Other morphological changes such as increased myocardial fibrosis, myxomatous degeneration of the valves, and thickening of left atrial endocardium were also observed in the hearts isolated from these pinealectomized rats [87]. Importantly, despite failure to improve morphological alterations (presumably due to the short treatment time), melatonin administration (4 mg/kg/day) for 2 days reversed the changes in circulating cholesterol and cardiac MDA levels [87].

In pathological conditions, patients with coronary heart disease have impaired nocturnal melatonin secretion [75, 88] and subjects with myocardial infarction were reported to have reduced circulating melatonin levels [72]. Concordantly, a significant association between single nucleotide polymorphisms (SNPs) (rs28383653) of melatonin receptor type 1A (MT1A) and coronary artery disease has been demonstrated in a recent case–control study [89].

In a cohort of survivors of acute myocardial infarction, reduction of circulating melatonin was also associated with greater adverse remodeling [90]. As a consequence, reduced serum melatonin concentrations measured at admission were considered as an independent predictor of left ventricular remodeling [90]. Importantly, in a double-blind randomized clinical trial, melatonin supplementation (3 mg/day for 2 months) was able to improve left ventricular ejection fraction in patients with heart failure [91].

Melatonin and Experimental Myocardial Infarction

In view of the above, it is expected that melatonin treatment could play a clinically relevant role in the pharmacotherapy of ischemic heart disease. The role of oxidative stress and excessive free radical production in the pathogenesis of myocardial infarction as well as experimental ischemia/reperfusion damage is well established [92]. The ability of melatonin to attenuate ischemia/reperfusion damage in rodent hearts has been demonstrated in isolated hearts (in vitro) [69, 93–96], isolated cardiomyocytes [97], as well as in situ heart (in vivo) [98–100]. These beneficial actions were undiscovered by the observations that hearts from pinealectomized animals exhibited a bigger post-ischemic myocardial infarction compared to those from non-pinealectomized rats [101]. Melatonin was able to attenuate ventricular fibrillation and reduce infarct size and mortality rate of the pinealectomized rats [101]. Additional investigations in our own laboratory have shown that long-term effects of melatonin evaluated 1 day after melatonin administration (2.5 or 5.0 mg/kg, i.p.) or after oral administration for 7 days (20 or 40 μg/ml) were also cardioprotective, and this cardioprotection persisted for 2–4 days after withdrawal of treatment [102]. Finally, melatonin at either physiological or pharmacological doses, given before or after ischemia period, was able to protect the heart against myocardial ischemia/reperfusion damage (for review, see [103]).

Mechanism of Melatonin-Induced Cardioprotection

The mechanism underlying the beneficial effects of melatonin on the ischemic heart is complex and not yet fully explored. Several investigations agreed that melatonin protects the heart against ischemia/reperfusion injury directly via its antioxidant properties and indirectly via its free radical scavenging actions and stimulatory effects on antioxidant capacity activities, respectively [85, 104]. Other melatonin's effects such as anti-adrenergic, anti-inflammatory, and anti-excitatory [85, 105, 106] as well as the MT receptors may also be involved [102, 106, 107].

Although it was reported that patients with myocardial infarction have reduced circulating melatonin levels [72], experimental myocardial infarction was shown to increase circulating melatonin levels, followed by enhancement of MT receptors expression [107]. The observation that luzindole, a melatonin receptor antagonist, was able to suppress the cardioprotection induced by melatonin [102] stressed the importance of these receptors in cardioprotection. These events may affect the probability of the opening of mitochondrial permeability transition pore (MPTP): Petrosillo and co-workers [108] reported that melatonin protected the hearts against reperfusion injury by inhibiting the opening of the MPTP probably via prevention of cardiolipin peroxidation. Downstream signaling events include activation of the reperfusion injury salvage kinase (RISK) pathway (PI-3K, PKB/AKT, ERK1/2) and the protective survivor activating factor enhancement (SAFE) pathway (JAK/STAT-3) [103].

Additional studies have documented the beneficial effects of exogenous melatonin on the heart in physiological conditions such as aging [109] and in other pathophysiological conditions such as hyperthyroidism [110], cadmium-induced oxidative damage [111], and myocardial hypertrophy [112]. However, more investigations using melatonin agonists are warranted. To the best of our knowledge, only one study investigated a melatonin agonist on myocardial ischemia/reperfusion injury in mice: the melatonin receptor agonist 8-methoxy-2-propionamidotetralin which has no antioxidant activity was not found to be cardioprotective [113].

Melatonin and the Blood Vessels

Melatonin and Blood Pressure

Hypertension is more frequent in overweight or obese than in lean subjects [114, 115]. Melatonin's ability to modulate and regulate BP and its potential therapeutic use in patients with hypertension have been a subject of interest for many investigators for several years [104, 116–119]. Early animal studies showed that pinealectomy caused a gradual and sustained elevation in arterial BP [120, 121], while chronic melatonin administration was able to reverse hypertension in the pinealectomized animals [122]. Additional animal investigations using spontaneously hypertensive rats confirmed this BP reduction following melatonin supplementation [104, 119]. Furthermore, the BP lowering effect of melatonin was demonstrated in healthy [119] as well as in hypertensive individuals [123]. A double-blind controlled clinical trial found that the bedtime melatonin (5 mg/day) ingestion for 4 weeks effectively reduced the BP in normotensive young subjects [124]. Acute oral melatonin (1–3 mg) was able to reduce BP of healthy male volunteers [86, 125] with a concomitant reduction of the aortic pulse wave velocity (PWV) which is considered as an important indicator of total cardiovascular risk estimation [125]. The PWV negatively correlated with diurnal levels of melatonin in young healthy men and women [126]. Importantly, low nocturnal melatonin production was suggested to be an independent pathophysiologic risk factor in the development of hypertension among young women [127]. A decrease in nocturnal melatonin levels indicating impairment of pineal melatonin secretion has consistently been observed in non-dipper hypertensive patients [128, 129].

In view of the above observations, melatonin supplementation is currently considered as a potential pharmacological agent in non-dippers or individuals with nocturnal hypertension and hypertensive heart disease [104]. Melatonin could also be administered in the elderly in order to attenuate the development of hypertension [130]. A recent meta-analysis of randomized controlled trials by Grossman et al. [117] indicated that melatonin administration (at 2–3 mg, controlled-release preparation, but not 5 mg, fast release) was effective to reduce nocturnal systolic and diastolic BP in patients with nocturnal hypertension. However, in patients with coronary artery disease, caution must be taken to monitor the circadian BP profile, before and during melatonin treatment, because of the danger of induction of arterial hypertension during daytime, hereby indicating a contraindication for melatonin in patients with "high normal" BP values [118]. The role of melatonin in the pathogenesis of hypertension has recently been demonstrated in MetS subjects [48, 131–133]. This is described in the section of obesity.

Mechanisms of BP Regulation by Melatonin

Unfortunately, early studies aimed at determining the effects of melatonin on vascular reactivity yielded controversial results [119]. In addition, involvement of intracellular signaling pathways further complicated matters. Melatonin causes a receptor-mediated reduction in cAMP and phosphatidylinositol-4,5-biphosphate (PIP2) hydrolysis, leading to vasoconstriction [134, 135]. However, improved nitric oxide (NO) signaling via enhancement of NOS activity and cGMP levels also appears to play an important role in melatonin-induced vasodilation [136, 137].

Other factors independent of NO pathway are also involved: for a 6-week treatment, only melatonin (10 mg/kg/day) but not antioxidant N-acetylcysteine (1.5 g/kg/day) was able to reduce the blood pressure of adult spontaneously hypertensive rats [138]. These results demonstrated thereby a possible involvement of additional mechanisms. This was later confirmed in renovascular hypertensive rats where hypertension caused a significant decrease in tissue antioxidant capacity and Na^+, K^+-ATPase activities, while MDA levels and myeloperoxidase (MPO) activity were increased [139]. In these rats, early or late administration of melatonin (10 mg/kg/day/i.p. for 9 or 6 weeks) not only lowered blood pressure but also improved the left ventricular function as well as the hypertensive profile by alleviating oxidative injury and increasing antioxidant capacity [139]. From these findings, it appears that melatonin might exhibit these effects presumably via both its direct antioxidant and receptor-mediated activities.

The overall regulation and modulation of BP is a complex mechanism with multifactorial aspects involving sympathetic neural mechanisms and central and peripheral nonneural factors including vasoactive substances and hormones. In this regard, while the role of endogenous melatonin on the BP is being recognized, the implication of neural vasomotor and alteration in renin-angiotensin-aldosterone system (RAAS) in the effects of melatonin reversing pinealectomy-induced hypertension is still hypothetic [140]. The potential antagonistic activities of angiotensin and melatonin in cardiovascular and metabolic diseases have been recently supported [141].

Furthermore, exogenous melatonin has been shown to differently affect the blood flow in humans depending on the vascular bed type or region [116]. For example, in healthy men and women, melatonin administration (3 mg) caused a reduction in renal blood flow and an increase in forearm blood flow with no effect on the cerebral blood flow [116, 142]. Consistently, this lack of effect on hemodynamic parameters (arterial and cerebral blood flows) was also reported in healthy men after acute melatonin premedication (0.2 mg/kg), suggesting that melatonin premedication may be safe under clinical conditions, such as postural changes, hemorrhage, and other operative stimuli in which arterial pressure decreases temporally [143].

Studies have also shown that these vascular effects could also differ depending on the type of experimental conditions. For example, in vitro melatonin caused vasoconstriction in porcine isolated coronary arteries [144], while in vivo intracoronary infusion of melatonin (70 pg/ml/min of coronary blood flow) in anesthetized pigs increased coronary blood flow and cardiac function through the beta-adrenoreceptors and NO pathways [137]. Similarly, intravenous infusion of melatonin (0.5 μg/kg/min) caused vasodilation in the umbilical vascular bed in pregnant sheep [145]. These controversial observations could be due to differences between the expression of MT1 and MT2 receptors in some vascular regions with eventual vasoconstriction for MT1 [144], vasodilation for MT2 [137], and involvement of the autonomic nervous system in in vivo experiments [137].

Although few clinical investigations on small number of patients have been done so far [123] and despite the controversies reported in experimental data, melatonin appears to be a suitable candidate for effective treatment for CVD and hypertension, in particular. It is well known that obesity increases the risk for the development of cardiovascular disorders [114]. These have been linked to derangement of melatonin's circadian rhythm [70–75, 140]. As a consequence, the eventual role of melatonin in obesity and other cardiovascular risk factors is currently receiving much attention.

Melatonin and Obesity

Obesity, Circadian Rhythm, and Melatonin

Convincing evidence supports a link between the development of obesity (increased body fat accumulation) and a disrupted circadian system [15, 16, 146, 147]. Epidemiological and experimental studies have shown that the alteration of the circadian rhythm in obesity as shown by the decrease of the amplitude of daily pineal melatonin rhythm in shift workers [148], T2D patients [149], as well as in rats fed with a high-fat diet [150] is accompanied by alterations of other circulating metabolic factors including, among others, glucose, insulin, leptin, corticosterone, thyroid-stimulating hormone, prolactin, luteinizing hormone, and testosterone [148, 150]. Although the causal relationship between chronodisruption and obesity can be somehow considered as bidirectional [146], the supplementation of melatonin as well as melatonin agonists has been beneficial in resetting the circadian rhythm [43] and improving the obesity-related abnormalities [41, 151–153]. In addition to this, obesity was found to be associated with various comorbidities including sleep disorders, and melatonin or melatonergic drugs have been proved to be effective in treating sleep disorders [151].

Animal Studies

Body Weight and Fat Mass Regulation

Melatonin may play an important role in body weight regulation and energy metabolism. The involvement of melatonin in the regulation of body fat mass and energy metabolism was first observed in seasonal animals [154] and attributed to its role as regulator of seasonal and circadian rhythms [155]. In these seasonal animals, any increase in circulating melatonin levels due to photoperiodic changes or exogenous melatonin administration, depending on the animal species, was eventually associated with a reduction or an increase in body fat mass [154, 156]. Interestingly, nonseasonal animals like the obese Zucker rats exposed to long photoperiod conditions (characterized by a low nocturnal melatonin production) had an increased body mass gain compared to those exposed to short photoperiods [157]. In line with this, surgical removal of the pineal gland caused a reduction in circulating melatonin levels and an increase in body weight after 3 weeks in obese but not in normal rats [158]. When the postoperative period was extended to 2 months, the normal rats had also increased their body and heart weight [159]. These pinealectomy-induced changes could be prevented by melatonin (30 mg/kg/day, i.p. at 1 h before lights-out) for 3 weeks [158]. The same workers also showed that melatonin administered in the same manner was able to reduce high-fat-diet-induced body weight gain without affecting the total food intake [158]. In young normal rats a decrease in body weight and visceral fat mass was also noticed following 3 or 6 months of prolonged melatonin consumption in drinking water (4 μg/ml) [84, 160]. Similar effects have also been reported in normal middle-aged rats [161, 162] without altering food consumption [163]. These metabolic effects were independent of gonadal function [164].

Several animal investigations have consistently demonstrated the efficacy for melatonin to prevent the development of obesity or reduce obesity-related metabolic features [46, 82, 152, 158, 165–168] (see Fig. 6.1a), and the potential therapeutic value of melatonin treatment in obesity and MetS has recently been summarized

Fig. 6.1 (**a**) Obesity-induced metabolic abnormalities without melatonin treatment and (**b**) potential metabolic effects of melatonin in obesity and insulin resistance. Obesity induces systemic metabolic abnormalities associated with adipose tissue dysfunction and insulin resistance. Melatonin treatment reduces body weight and visceral fat gain of obese subjects. The overall melatonin's effect in obesity is a combination of direct effects in peripheral organs involved in metabolism and indirect effects via systemic regulation. Melatonin reduces dyslipidemia, hyperglycemia, hyperinsulinemia, hyperleptinemia, oxidative stress, and inflammatory markers and increases adiponectinemia and antioxidants status. It increases insulin sensitivity in peripheral organs including liver, skeletal muscle, heart, vessels, and adipose tissue. Melatonin may affect indirectly the cardiovascular function (heart and vessels) via its effects on central nervous system reducing sympathetic activities. Melatonin may also affect indirectly the adipose tissue function and plasticity via sympathetic effects. The adipose tissue in turn may influence other peripheral organs via its secreted hormones (adipokines) such as adiponectin which has cardiovascular protective activities behind its insulin sensitizing properties. The overall effects will lead to body weight reduction and insulin sensitivity in peripheral organs and the improvement of cardiovascular functions. ?, no available data in obesity/MetS; ↓ or ↑, decrease or increase; solid lines (*arrow*), indirect systemic effects (from adipose tissue and other secretory organs, e.g., liver, pancreas); square dots (*arrow*), indirect sympathetic effects; *BW* body weight, *MEL* melatonin, *IR* insulin resistance, *FFA* free fatty acids, *FA* fatty acids, *TG* triglycerides, *LDL-c* low-density lipoprotein cholesterol, *HDL-c* high-density lipoprotein cholesterol, *VLDL* very low-density lipoprotein, *TNF-α* tumor necrosis factor alpha, *IL-6* interleukin-6, *NO* nitric oxide, *MI* myocardial infarction, *CHD* coronary heart disease, *ApoA-I,A-II* apolipoprotein A-I and A-II, *CRP* C-reactive protein, *HbA1c* hemoglobin A1c, *LPO* lipid peroxidation, *TBARS* thiobarbituric acid reactive substances

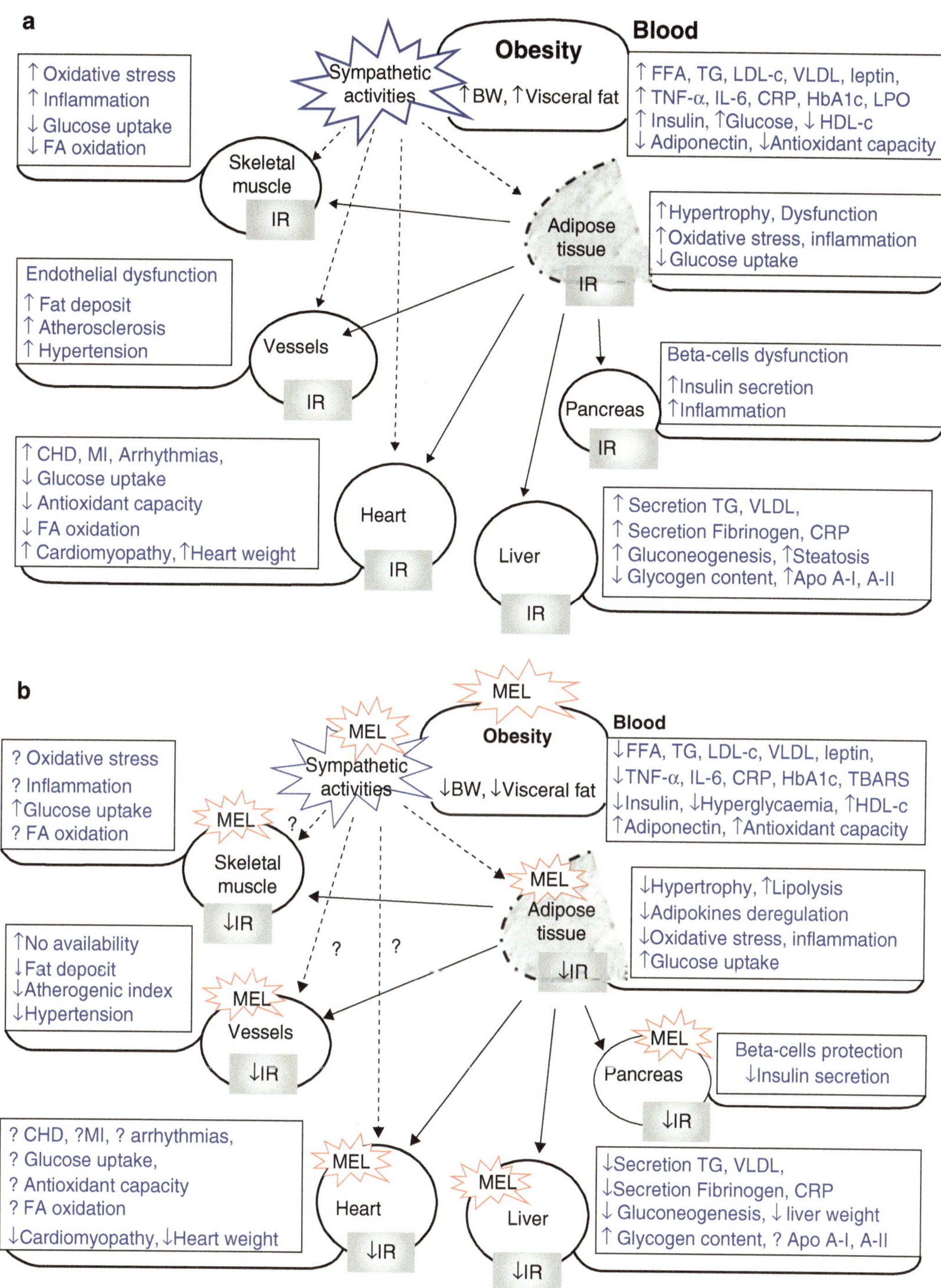
a
Obesity
↑BW, ↑Visceral fat
Blood
↑ FFA, TG, LDL-c, VLDL, leptin,
↑ TNF-α, IL-6, CRP, HbA1c, LPO
↑ Insulin, ↑Glucose, ↓ HDL-c
↓ Adiponectin, ↓Antioxidant capacity
Sympathetic activities
↑ Oxidative stress
↑ Inflammation
↓ Glucose uptake
↓ FA oxidation
Skeletal muscle
IR
Adipose tissue
IR
↑Hypertrophy, Dysfunction
↑Oxidative stress, inflammation
↓Glucose uptake
Endothelial dysfunction
↑ Fat deposit
↑ Atherosclerosis
↑ Hypertension
Vessels
IR
Pancreas
IR
Beta-cells dysfunction
↑Insulin secretion
↑Inflammation
↑ CHD, MI, Arrhythmias,
↓ Glucose uptake
↓ Antioxidant capacity
↓ FA oxidation
↑ Cardiomyopathy, ↑Heart weight
Heart
IR
Liver
IR
↑ Secretion TG, VLDL,
↑ Secretion Fibrinogen, CRP
↑ Gluconeogenesis, ↑Steatosis
↓ Glycogen content, ↑Apo A-I, A-II
b
MEL
Obesity
↓BW, ↓Visceral fat
Blood
↓FFA, TG, LDL-c, VLDL, leptin,
↓TNF-α, IL-6, CRP, HbA1c, TBARS
↓Insulin, ↓Hyperglycaemia, ↑HDL-c
↑Adiponectin, ↑Antioxidant capacity
MEL
Sympathetic activities
? Oxidative stress
? Inflammation
↑Glucose uptake
? FA oxidation
MEL
Skeletal muscle
↓IR
?
MEL
Adipose tissue
↓IR
↓Hypertrophy, ↑Lipolysis
↓Adipokines deregulation
↓Oxidative stress, inflammation
↑Glucose uptake
↑No availability
↓Fat depocit
↓Atherogenic index
↓Hypertension
MEL
Vessels
↓IR
? ?
MEL
Pancreas
↓IR
Beta-cells protection
↓Insulin secretion
? CHD, ?MI, ? arrhythmias,
? Glucose uptake,
? Antioxidant capacity
? FA oxidation
↓Cardiomyopathy, ↓Heart weight
MEL
Heart
↓IR
MEL
Liver
↓IR
↓Secretion TG, VLDL,
↓Secretion Fibrinogen, CRP
↓ Gluconeogenesis, ↓ liver weight
↑ Glycogen content, ? Apo A-I, A-II

[169]. It was shown that long-term melatonin administration significantly reduced body weight and visceral fat mass as well as circulating glucose, insulin, leptin, TG, free fatty acid (FFA), and total cholesterol levels in young Zucker diabetic fatty (ZDF) rats [165, 170], in middle-aged rats fed with a high-fat diet [166, 171], in young rats with high-fat/high-sucrose diet [152], as well as rats drinking 10 % fructose solution [48]. In these studies, daily melatonin was administered in drinking water at 0.2–4 μg/ml [172] and 25 μg/ml [48, 166] or via intraperitoneal injection at 4 mg/kg [152] for a period of 8–12 weeks and did not affect the total food intake. A study in rabbits fed with a high-fat diet has however reported a reduction in food intake after 4 weeks of melatonin treatment (1 mg/kg/day subcutaneously at 2–3 h before lights-off) [167]. This weight-loss-inducing effect of melatonin was also confirmed in other animal models of obesity, for example, a rat model of ovariectomized-induced obesity [172, 173] and female rats treated with olanzapine [174].

Obesity-Induced Dyslipidemia

Melatonin has been shown to improve obesity-induced dyslipidemia. This was first documented in nonobese hypercholesterolemic rats [175, 176] and thereafter confirmed in various rat models of obesity [82, 158, 165, 169, 177]. For example, oral melatonin (4–10 mg/kg/day for 6–12 weeks) raised the HDL-c in both obese and lean Zucker rats [165] or in high-fat-/high-sucrose-diet-induced obese rats [152]. This has also been confirmed in obese rabbits [167], associated with a concomitant reduction in circulating TGs, FFA, and low-density lipoprotein cholesterol (LDL-c) with [152, 167] or without [165, 166] effect on total cholesterol levels. Similar results were recently confirmed in ApoE knockout C57BL/6 J male mice fed with a high-fat diet [177] and in rats fed with a high-fructose diet for 4 weeks [178]. Although the latter model did not gain weight, 2 weeks of coadministration of oral melatonin (10 mg/kg/day) reduced the intra-abdominal fat mass and circulating FFA levels as well as hepatic TG and cholesterol contents [178]. These studies strongly support the suggestion that melatonin supplement may ameliorate overweight and lipid metabolism in humans.

Obesity-Induced Low Antioxidant Status

Obesity is associated with elevated oxidative stress and low antioxidant status [179, 180]. The antioxidant as well as anti-inflammatory activities of melatonin have been well established [33, 60]. Daily melatonin administration to obese rabbits (1 mg/kg subcutaneously for 4 weeks) [167] or rats (4 mg/kg i.p. for 8 weeks) [152] increased the HDL-c levels, glutathione peroxidase (GSH-Px), and superoxide dismutase (SOD) activities and reduced oxidative stress as indicated by low plasma MDA levels. Furthermore, in young obese ZDF rats, chronic oral melatonin administration (10 mg/kg/day) for 6 weeks attenuated circulating biomarkers of systemic oxidative stress (basal plasma lipid peroxidation and Fe2+/H_2O_2-induced lipid oxidation) and low-grade inflammation [plasma interleukin 6 (IL-6), tumor necrosis factor-α (TNF-α), and C-reactive protein (CRP) values] without affecting their profile in non-obese animals [181]. It is well established that low-grade chronic inflammation contributes to the pathogenesis of insulin resistance and diabetes as well as cardiovascular complications [182]. The antioxidant properties of melatonin have been reported along with the improvement of metabolic profile in diabetes [165, 181, 183] and diet-induced obesity [152, 167]. However, whether the improvement of insulin resistance by melatonin precedes or follows its suppressive effects on oxidative stress and inflammation is still not yet known.

Cardiovascular Effects of Melatonin in Obesity

Melatonin supplementation was able to improve cardiovascular function in obesity. A decrease in melatonin secretion was associated with hypertension in fructose-fed rats [131]. Administration of melatonin to these fructose-induced MetS rats reduced the BP rise and other metabolic abnormalities [48, 131]. Similarly, in animals receiving a high-fat diet, intake of melatonin was associated with a lowering of BP, heart rate, and sciatic nerve activity [167]. Melatonin prevented the appearance of fatty streaks produced by a mass of foam cells covered by the endothelium and a thin layer of mononucleated cells in the carotid artery intima of hypercholesterolemic rats [184]. It was also able to prevent deposition of fat in the liver and subintimal lipid in the blood vessels, kidney, and heart [167], indicating melatonin's potential anti-atherosclerotic activities. In spontaneously hypertensive Wistar-Kyoto male rats, chronic (but not acute) administration of the selective melatonin receptor agonist, ramelteon, in drinking water (8 mg/kg/day, from 4 to 12 weeks of age) attenuated the age-associated increase of systolic BP by 45 % [153].

We recently showed that long-term oral melatonin consumption (4 mg/kg/day for 16 weeks) starting before the establishment of obesity prevented the increase in the heart weight and protected the hearts against obesity-induced increased susceptibility to myocardial ischemia/reperfusion damage [82]. We also found that melatonin treatment prevented the development of obesity-induced metabolic alterations (elevated visceral fat, serum insulin, leptin, and TG and reduced HDL-c) [82]. This finding was of particular significance since to date there is no effective cardioprotective strategy available in obesity, diabetes, as well as aging conditions [185–187]. However, how melatonin protected the heart in obesity remains unknown. We hypothesized that the direct effects of melatonin to the heart via its receptor-mediated effects may be involved, but this requires further investigation.

The melatonin-induced improvement of the cardiovascular function in MetS could also be linked to the body weight loss and improvement of dyslipidemia with eventual reduction of oxidative stress, inflammation, insulin resistance, and hyperglycemia [48, 82, 153, 167]. These two latter states are reviewed in the section of insulin resistance.

Human Studies

The overall circulating melatonin levels in obese humans are not consistent. For example, the mean nocturnal serum melatonin levels were reported to be reduced in patients with severe obesity [188] as well as with T2D [149], autonomic neuropathy [189], retinopathy [190], and coronary heart disease [191] as well as obese craniopharyngioma [192]. Surprisingly, despite a lack of difference in BMI or waist circumference between the obese nondiabetic and T2D subjects, nocturnal plasma melatonin levels were significantly higher in obese nondiabetic subjects compared to weight-matched T2D subjects [193] who failed to produce any detectable melatonin [193]. However, in young male and female obese MetS patients [194, 195] and in obese girls [196], circulating melatonin or urinary 6-sulfatoxymelatonin levels were not different from controls subjects, confirming the early observation that obesity had no effect on melatonin secretion and excretion [197]. Furthermore, it has been noticed that in MetS patients, the levels of melatonin per se are not as important as the melatonin/insulin ratio which correlates negatively with the lipid profile [194].

The reasons for these inconsistencies in melatonin secretion in obese subjects remain complex and not well understood. It is possible that the increased sympathetic tone in obesity and a consecutive alteration in sympathetic innervation of the pineal gland increased melatonin concentration in obese nondiabetic subjects [193]. Furthermore, low circulating melatonin levels have been linked to many factors including elevated oxidative stress and inflammation [198], but not by low testosterone levels in young men with MetS [195]. It appears therefore that melatonin circulating levels could vary depending on age of patients and severity of obesity [188].

Few clinical investigations on melatonin or melatonergic drugs have considered body weight change and adiposity mass in their aims. However, as discussed above, these parameters are affected by the long-term melatonin treatment [82]. A pilot study investigating the role of melatonin in obese craniopharyngioma survivors reported that low nocturnal and early morning melatonin levels were associated with increased daytime sleepiness and BMI, suggesting potential involvement of hypothalamic lesions [199]. Melatonin substitution (6 mg/day) in these subjects increased circulating melatonin and improved the sleep rhythms with no clear effect on BMI due probably to small sample size [199]. Interestingly, melatonin treatment (5 mg/day, 2 h before bedtime) in MetS patients significantly reduced their BMI, systolic BP, and plasma fibrinogen as well as lipid peroxidation levels after 1 month [132]. After 2 months, these patients had a further amelioration of BP and improved antioxidative capacity (e.g., catalase activity) and lipid profile (reduced LDL-c) [132].

Mechanism of Actions of Melatonin in Obesity

The mechanism of action of melatonin in obesity is complex and not well understood. As mentioned above, melatonin is a small pleiotropic molecule able to cross each membrane layer and enter each cellular compartment to exert its various activities with and/or without receptor-mediated pathways [47, 49]. Melatonin receptors as well as adipose tissue function and plasticity may be involved.

Melatonin Receptors

Involvement of the melatonin receptors in body fat mass regulation has been known for many years [200]. Administration of a melatonin receptor agonist or antagonist to seasonal animals (before night) affected the body weight and adiposity mass regulation as well as the onset of seasonal obesity: a melatonin agonist and the short day (6 h light/18 h dark) had a same effect, whereas an antagonist and the long day (18 h light/6 h dark) had also similar effects [200]. This involvement of MT receptors in the body weight and fat mass regulation was recently demonstrated in spontaneously hypertensive rats, using ramelteon, a potent selective MT1/MT2 receptors agonist [153], and in obese rats, using the melatonin agonist NEU-P11 [152].

MT receptors have been identified in the major organs involved in metabolism regulation: liver, pancreas, and skeletal muscle [201] as well as adipose tissue [202]. They have been involved in the regulation of insulin secretion and may play an active role in the glucose regulation [201]. Recently, it was reported that variation in MTNR1B, the gene encoding for MT2, was associated with increased risk of T2D, increased fasting plasma glucose, and impaired insulin secretion in populations of European ancestry [203, 204]. Similar observations were also made in Chinese [205] as well as in Japanese [206] populations. Thus, the overall effects of melatonin in obesity appear to be partly mediated through these receptors in addition to activation of the sympathetic nervous system via hypothalamic receptors and subsequent effects on lipolysis and adipose tissue plasticity [156, 207].

Adipose Tissue

The exact mechanisms whereby melatonin reduces body fat mass and the role of adipose tissue are complex and not clear. In vivo melatonin treatment prevents the increase in circulating TG and eventually body fat accumulation and weight gain in overweight and obese subjects [82, 170]. In vitro melatonin treatment of adipocytes inhibits its differentiation and limits adipose tissue hypertrophy [208] by inhibiting fatty acid-induced TG accumulation in cells exposed to physiological levels of oleic acid [209]. The reduction in body weight gain might be due to a significant decrease in fat content as opposed to lean body mass [163] and could be related to melatonin-induced improvements in the compromised insulin and leptin signaling associated with obesity [210] accompanied by modulation of plasma levels of insulin, glucose, TG, cholesterol, and leptin [166] (see following section on "Leptin Resistance").

The involvement of brown adipose tissue has also been suggested [35]. While white adipose tissue is specialized for energy storage, brown adipose tissue has a high concentration of mitochondria and uniquely expresses uncoupling protein 1(UCP-1), enabling it to be specialized for energy expenditure and thermogenesis [211]. Brown adipose tissue has been suggested to be the factor whereby animals lose weight in response to melatonin administration (and gain weight when there is a deficiency of melatonin) independently of food intake [35]. The exploitation of the functional role of brown adipose tissue could be of great interest in obesity management. Clearly, more research is required to elucidate the role of melatonin in weight loss.

Leptin Resistance

Leptin is one of adipose tissue-secreted hormones that plays a central role in modulation of food intake, body weight, and energy expenditure [212]. Leptin resistance is an essential feature of human obesity and refers to the inability of elevated circulating leptin levels to reduce common obesity [213]. It is associated with insulin resistance and an increased proinflammatory state [214]. Pinealectomy increases circulating leptin [215], while exogenous melatonin decreases serum leptin levels in both pinealectomized [216] and intact rat models of diet-induced obesity [163] before decreasing plasma insulin levels [171]. These observations suggest a secondary modulatory effect of leptin on insulin in body weight reduction [217]. However, increased leptin levels have also been observed following melatonin administration to normal and pinealectomized rats (3 mg/kg/day i.p. for 6 months) [218] and male C57BL/6 adult mice (10 μg/ml in drinking water for 1 month) [219]. In this regard, surprisingly, Baltaci and Mogulkoc [218] reported that pinealectomy decreased body weight gain and leptin levels. To further complicate matters, it has also been observed that melatonin had no effect on leptin levels in ovariectomized rats [172], obese horse [220], and menopausal women [221]. However, as expected, in a rat model of high-fructose-diet-induced MetS [178] and in young ZDF rats [165], melatonin administration reduced serum leptin levels. Apart from differences in experimental protocols and animal models, the causes of these controversial results remain unclear.

At a molecular level, the mechanism of leptin resistance and impaired leptin signaling has been associated with increased activity of suppressor of cytokine signaling 3 (SOCS3) [222, 223], which is a member of a family of proteins which inhibits the JAK/STAT signaling cascade [224]. It has been found that melatonin, leptin, and insulin activated the same intracellular signaling pathways, namely, PI-3K and STAT-3 [225–227]. Therefore, melatonin may attenuate or reverse the insulin resistance in obesity by mimicking the actions of insulin and leptin signaling via cross talk between these pathways. In this regard, insulin has been shown to modulate leptin-induced STAT3 activation in rat hypothalamus [225]. Thus, melatonin may act initially on hypothalamic insulin and leptin receptor sensitivity (as these hormones do under normal conditions) and eventually relay information about peripheral fat stores to central effectors in the hypothalamus to modify food intake and energy expenditure [207, 212]. It appears that an intricate relationship exists between leptin, melatonin, and insulin, synchronized in circadian fashion with profound effects on metabolism. However, this has not yet been studied in diet-induced obesity setting.

Melatonin and Insulin Resistance

Insulin resistance is the most important pathophysiological feature in the development of the MetS as well as T2D [228] and is referred to as a decrease or inhibition of cellular sensitivity to the effect of normal circulating insulin on glucose uptake, metabolism, and storage in peripheral tissues [21, 228]. Insulin resistance results in increased postprandial and fasting circulating insulin levels in order to normalize glycemia in prediabetic subjects and is closely associated with dyslipidemia and other metabolic abnormalities [228, 229]. It has recently been shown to be the best predictor of the metabolic syndrome in subjects with a first-degree relative with T2D [230]. Although not all forms of obesity result in insulin resistance [231], obesity (particularly abdominal obesity) is currently accepted as the major factor in the incidence and etiology of insulin resistance [21, 232], a condition which is generally considered as the common links between obesity and its vascular complications [229].

Effects of Melatonin on Insulin Resistance

Melatonin has been shown to play a role in the regulation of insulin secretion and glucose/lipid metabolism [183, 233, 234]. Studies have shown that in normal rats, pinealectomy-induced insulin resistance and glucose intolerance [235, 236] and increased serum cholesterol [87]. To demonstrate the role of endogenous melatonin on insulin secretion, the study done by Nishida et al. [237] using T2D rats found that after 21 weeks of pinealectomy, there was a significant increase in plasma insulin and accumulation of TG. The same study found also that when the post-pinealectomy period was extended to 35 weeks, circulating insulin levels were significantly decreased. This decrease is a clear indicator of impairment of insulin release from pancreatic β-cells as seen in patients at an advanced stage of T2D [238]. Additionally, it was found that pineal gland melatonin synthesis is decreased in T2D Goto-Kakizaki (GK) rats [239].

Since insulin resistance precedes the establishment of T2D, the possibility that melatonin replacement could reverse insulin resistance has been a subject of numerous investigators in the field of obesity and diabetes as well as MetS. In this regard, it was found that long-term melatonin consumption (2.5 mg/kg/day for 9 weeks) increased plasma melatonin levels with a concomitant reduction in insulin levels in T2D GK rats [240]. In mice fed with a high-fat diet, 8-week oral melatonin (100 mg/kg/day) markedly improved insulin sensitivity and glucose tolerance [210]. Using the same model, 2 weeks of melatonin administration (10 mg/kg/day i.p), attenuated insulin resistance, and glucose intolerance associated with an increase in hepatic glycogen and improvement in liver steatosis [168]. Furthermore, in high-fat-/high-sucrose-fed rats, 8-week treatment with melatonin or its agonist NEU-P11 increased insulin sensitivity [152]. In rats with T2D, 30 weeks of melatonin treatment (1.1 mg/kg/day, subcutaneously via implanted melatonin-releasing pellets) reduced circulating insulin, leptin, and TG levels [241]. These findings were also confirmed by additional studies in young ZDF rats [165, 170] and fructose-fed rats [48, 178]. In the latter model, administration of melatonin (1 or 10 mg/kg/day for 2 weeks) improved the abnormal serum insulin response curve in oral glucose tolerance test [178], indicating potential insulin sensitizing effects of melatonin.

Mechanism of Actions of Melatonin in Insulin Resistance

The mechanism of actions of melatonin on obesity-induced insulin-resistant state is complex and not fully explored. The reduction of circulating insulin levels in these obese animals may be linked to a reduced body weight and improved lipid metabolism as it was recently demonstrated in young ZDF rats [165] or rats drinking 10 % fructose solution [48]. In these rat models, the amelioration of insulin resistance was also characterized by improvement in glucose tolerance [48, 170]. In addition, in young ZDF rats melatonin treatment reduced fasting blood glucose, plasma insulin, hemoglobin A1c (HbA1c), HOMA-IR, and FFA levels and increased index of beta-cell function [170].

The improvement in lipid and glucose regulation could be also linked to amelioration of the proinflammatory state and oxidative stress [181]. It is well established that oxidative stress and proinflammatory states are important pathological features that underlie the development of insulin resistance, MetS, diabetes, and CVD. Therefore, in insulin-resistant condition, the reduction of oxidative stress and proinflammatory state may lead to the avoidance of lipid peroxidation resulting from free radical generation due to the continuous hyperglycemia and hyperlipidemia. As expected, melatonin administration for 2 or 6 weeks (1 or 10 mg/kg/day) attenuated the levels of circulating IL-6 and TNF-α [178, 181] accompanied by a reduction in serum and hepatic lipid peroxidation concentrations and increase in hepatic GSH concentration [178]. Interestingly, melatonin treatment was associated with increase in serum adiponectin levels and reduction in leptin levels with [170] or without

[178] effects on body weight. Adiponectin (which is reduced in MetS subjects) has been shown to have insulin sensitizing actions in the liver and peripheral tissues and other beneficial properties associated with cardiovascular protection (anti-apoptotic, anti-inflammatory, and antiatherogenic properties) [242]. Therefore, increased circulating adiponectin levels may play important role in melatonin's effects.

On a molecular level, insulin resistance is associated with abnormal or compromised intracellular insulin signaling cascade in peripheral tissues/organs that are more involved in the glucose metabolism regulation (skeletal muscle, liver, and adipose tissue). This cascade principally includes binding of insulin to insulin receptor (IR), tyrosine phosphorylation of insulin receptor substrate (IRS) proteins, and activation of phosphotidylinositol-3-kinase (PI-3K), protein kinase B (PKB/Akt), and protein kinase C (PKC) isoforms (for details see [228]). Melatonin (1nM) treatment has been shown to stimulate glucose transport in skeletal muscle via the phosphorylation and activation of IRS-1 and PI-3K, respectively [243]. It was further demonstrated that melatonin improves glucose homeostasis by restoring the vascular actions of insulin which were characterized by increased phosphorylation of Akt and endothelial nitric oxide synthase (eNOS) in aortic tissue [210]. In addition to the phosphorylation of Akt and PKC-ζ, melatonin (1 nM) stimulated glycogen synthesis and increased the phosphorylation of glycogen synthase kinase 3 β (GSK3-β) in hepatic cells [168]. More interestingly, these effects of melatonin could be blocked by using the nonselective MT1/MT2 antagonist, luzindole, or the MT2 selective antagonist, 4-phenyl-2-propionamidotetralin (4P-PDOT) [168, 243], suggesting possible MT receptor involvement. However, it is not clear how activation of the high affinity MT receptors which are G-protein linked leads to stimulation of the IRS-1/PI-3K pathway and the role of PKC-ζ in this regard. In addition, the role of PKB/Akt is not clear in view of the different results that have been reported showing its activation in skeletal muscle cells [243] as opposed to its inactivation in hepatic cells [168].

Melatonin treatment (100 ng/ml and 500 pg/ml) enhanced the insulin-stimulated glucose uptake of adipocytes obtained from female fruit bat (*Cynopterus sphinx*) [244]. There was however no correlation between glucose uptake and the protein expression of glucose transporter 4 (GLUT-4) in these cells [244]. In this regard, investigation of GLUT4-translocation could give more insight in the results obtained. Pinealectomy was shown to reduce the expression of GLUT-4 protein translocation in adipose tissue [235, 236]. Although a decrease in GLUT-4 gene expression was reported following melatonin treatment (1 μM for 14 days) in human brown adipocyte cell lines (PAZ6) [202], Zanquetta et al. [235] found that 30 days of calorie restriction or melatonin replacement (50 μg/100 g/day i.p.) to pinealectomized rats was accompanied by improvement of insulin resistance and increased plasma membrane GLUT-4 protein content in white adipose tissue. Importantly, in the hyperthyroid rat heart, melatonin administration was able to protect the heart against oxidative damage and restored expression of GLUT-4 gene, establishing the ability of antioxidants to reverse oxidative stress-mediated metabolic alterations [110]. However, whether melatonin affects glucose regulation in the normal or obese heart is still not yet explored.

Melatonin receptors may play an important role in regulation of glucose metabolism. An important support for the role of melatonin in the regulation of energy metabolism came from the finding that removal of the MT1 receptor significantly impairs the ability of mice to metabolize glucose and probably induces insulin resistance in these animals [245]. Epidemiological studies have also revealed that variants near/in the MTNR1B (or MT2) receptor are associated with impaired pancreatic beta-cell function as shown by impaired early insulin secretion and concomitant elevated plasma fasting glucose levels [246, 247]. Indeed, MT1/MT2 receptors are expressed in pancreatic islets [248] and as insulin levels exhibit a nocturnal drop, its production has been suggested to be controlled, at least in part, by melatonin [249]. Melatonin reduced the fasting insulin levels [152, 171] probably via its inhibitory effects on insulin secretion in rat pancreatic islets [233, 250]. Catecholamines have been indicated as a key feature to understand the biological relevance of insulin-melatonin antagonisms in type 1 and T2D [251]. It was found that catecholamines (noradrenaline and adrenaline) and melatonin levels were reduced in T2D GK rats (characterized by high insulin levels) and elevated in T1D rats (associated with reduced insulin levels) [251], assuming that elevated catecholamines decrease insulin secretion via stimulation of melatonin synthesis [251].

Clinical Implications

The exploitation of melatonin's inhibitory effect on insulin secretion by phototherapy as a potential therapy to increase insulin secretion has been effective in treating an insulin-dependent diabetes mellitus (IDDM) patient [252]. However, in the case of T2D, the exploitation of melatonin-insulin interaction as a potential therapy to reduce hyperinsulinemia is not currently suggested [234] before further large clinical studies.

Conclusions

The effects of melatonin in obesity and the MetS have been largely studied in experimental animals, particularly in rodents. Few clinical studies have considered the role of melatonin in obesity and MetS. However, available data show that melatonin treatment may influence and improve all metabolic abnormalities found in MetS patients (Fig. 6.1b). Similar effects have also been found following administration of melatonin agonists (ramelteon, NEU-P1). Behind its antioxidant properties, the overall metabolic action of melatonin is a combined result from its various pleiotropic activities associated with multiple signaling in areas of the central nervous system and in peripheral organs [49]. The current findings suggested melatonin treatment as a suitable candidate for effective therapy of CVD at both preventive and curative levels especially when circulating melatonin levels are decreased. In this regard, a randomized controlled trial of melatonin supplementation in men and women with the MetS has been recently designed to determine the feasibility, efficacy, and safety of melatonin supplementation in humans [253]. The use of high doses of melatonin compared to the physiological concentration has been explained as a requirement to obtain therapeutic effects in some conditions [45, 47, 48]. Melatonin is an affordable molecule having exceptional beneficial effects without toxicity [45].

References

1. Swinburn BA, Sacks G, Hall KD, McPherson K, Finegood DT, Moodie ML, Gortmaker SL. The global obesity pandemic: shaped by global drivers and local environments. Lancet. 2011;378:804–14.
2. de Onis M, Blössner M, Borghi E. Global prevalence and trends of overweight and obesity among preschool children. Am J Clin Nutr. 2010;92:1257–64.
3. Finucane MM, Stevens GA, Cowan MJ, Danaei G, Lin JK, Paciorek CJ, Singh GM, Gutierrez HR, Lu Y, Bahalim AN, Farzadfar F, Riley LM, Ezzati M. National, regional, and global trends in body-mass index since 1980: systematic analysis of health examination surveys and epidemiological studies with 960 country-years and 9·1 million participants. Lancet. 2011;377:557–67.
4. Grundy SM. Metabolic syndrome pandemic. Arterioscler Thromb Vasc Biol. 2008;28:629–36.
5. Danaei G, Finucane MM, Lu Y, Singh GM, Cowan MJ, Paciorek CJ, Lin JK, Farzadfar F, Khang Y, Stevens GA, Rao M, Ali MK, Riley LM, Robinson CA, Ezzati M. National, regional, and global trends in fasting plasma glucose and diabetes prevalence since 1980: systematic analysis of health examination surveys and epidemiological studies with 370 country-years and 2·7 million participants. Lancet. 2011;378:31–40.
6. Murphy NF, MacIntyre K, Stewart S, Hart CL, Hole D, McMurray JJV. Long-term cardiovascular consequences of obesity: 20-year follow-up of more than 15000 middle-aged men and women (the Renfrew–Paisley study). Eur Heart J. 2006;27:96–106.
7. Pothiwala P, Jain SK, Yaturu S. Metabolic syndrome and cancer. Metab Syndr Relat Disord. 2009;7:279–88.
8. Alberti KGMM, Eckel RH, Grundy SM, Zimmet PZ, Cleeman JI, Donato KA, Fruchart J, James WPT, Loria CM, Smith SC. Harmonizing the metabolic syndrome. Circulation. 2009;120:1640–5.
9. Uchil D, Pipalia D, Chawla M, Patel R, Maniar S, Narayani, Juneja A. Non-alcoholic fatty liver disease (NAFLD)–the hepatic component of metabolic syndrome. J Assoc Physicians India. 2009;57:201–4.

10. Michalakis K, Mintziori G, Kaprara A, Tarlatzis BC, Goulis DG. The complex interaction between obesity, metabolic syndrome and reproductive axis: A narrative review. Metabolism. 2013;62:457–78.
11. Wolk R, Somers VK. Sleep and the metabolic syndrome. Exp Physiol. 2007;92:67–78.
12. Ruan X, Guan Y. Metabolic syndrome and chronic kidney disease. J Diabetes. 2009;1:236–45.
13. Katz JD, Agrawal S, Velasquez M. Getting to the heart of the matter: osteoarthritis takes its place as part of the metabolic syndrome. Curr Opin Rheumatol. 2010;22:512–9.
14. Pietropaoli D, Monaco A, Del Pinto R, Cifone MG, Marzo G, Giannoni M. Advanced glycation end products: possible link between metabolic syndrome and periodontal diseases. Int J Immunopathol Pharmacol. 2012;25:9–17.
15. Reiter RJ, Tan D, Korkmaz A, Ma S. Obesity and metabolic syndrome: association with chronodisruption, sleep deprivation, and melatonin suppression. Ann Med. 2012;44:564–77.
16. Gomez-Abellan P, Madrid JA, Ordovas JM, Garaulet M. Chronobiological aspects of obesity and metabolic syndrome. Endocrinol Nutr. 2012;59:50–61.
17. Farooqui AA, Farooqui T, Panza F, Frisardi V. Metabolic syndrome as a risk factor for neurological disorders. Cell Mol Life Sci. 2012;69:741–62.
18. Kelly T, Yang W, Chen CS, Reynolds K, He J. Global burden of obesity in 2005 and projections to 2030. Int J Obes (Lond). 2008;32:1431–7.
19. Wang YC, McPherson K, Marsh T, Gortmaker SL, Brown M. Health and economic burden of the projected obesity trends in the USA and the UK. Lancet. 2011;378:815–25.
20. Naukkarinen J, Rissanen A, Kaprio J, Pietiläinen KH. Causes and consequences of obesity: the contribution of recent twin studies. Int J Obes. 2012;36:1017–24.
21. Boden G. Obesity, insulin resistance and free fatty acids. Curr Opin Endocrinol Diabetes Obes. 2011;18:139–43.
22. Rizvi AA. Cytokine biomarkers, endothelial inflammation, and atherosclerosis in the metabolic syndrome: emerging concepts. Am J Med Sci. 2009;338:310–8.
23. de Ferranti S, Mozaffarian D. The perfect storm: obesity, adipocyte dysfunction, and metabolic consequences. Clin Chem. 2008;54:945–55.
24. Otani H. Oxidative stress as pathogenesis of cardiovascular risk associated with metabolic syndrome. Antioxid Redox Signal. 2011;15:1911–26.
25. Ozgen IT, Tascilar ME, Bilir P, Boyraz M, Guncikan MN, Akay C, Dundaroz R. Oxidative stress in obese children and its relation with insulin resistance. J Pediatr Endocrinol Metab. 2012;25:261–6.
26. Ando K, Fujita T. Metabolic syndrome and oxidative stress. Free Radic Biol Med. 2009;47:213–8.
27. Grattagliano I, Palmieri VO, Portincasa P, Moschetta A, Palasciano G. Oxidative stress-induced risk factors associated with the metabolic syndrome: a unifying hypothesis. J Nutr Biochem. 2008;19:491–504.
28. Furukawa S, Fujita T, Shimabukuro M, Iwaki M, Yamada Y, Nakajima Y, Nakayama O, Makishima M, Matsuda M, Shimomura I. Increased oxidative stress in obesity and its impact on metabolic syndrome. J Clin Invest. 2004;114:1752–61.
29. Beydoun MA, Shroff MR, Chen X, Beydoun HA, Wang Y, Zonderman AB. Serum antioxidant status is associated with metabolic syndrome among U.S. adults in recent national surveys. J Nutr. 2011;141:903–13.
30. Beydoun MA, Canas JA, Beydoun HA, Chen X, Shroff MR, Zonderman AB. Serum antioxidant concentrations and metabolic syndrome are associated among U.S. adolescents in recent national surveys. J Nutr. 2012;142:1693–704.
31. Bahadoran Z, Golzarand M, Mirmiran P, Shiva N, Azizi F. Dietary total antioxidant capacity and the occurrence of metabolic syndrome and its components after a 3-year follow-up in adults: Tehran Lipid and Glucose Study. Nutr Metab. 2012;9:70.
32. Tiganis T. Reactive oxygen species and insulin resistance: the good, the bad and the ugly. Trends Pharmacol Sci. 2011;32:82–9.
33. Korkmaz A, Reiter RJ, Topal T, Manchester LC, Oter S, Tan DX. Melatonin: an established antioxidant worthy of use in clinical trials. Mol Med. 2009;15:43–50.
34. Korkmaz A, Topal T, Tan DX, Reiter RJ. Role of melatonin in metabolic regulation. Rev Endocr Metab Disord. 2009;10:261–70.
35. Tan DX, Manchester LC, FuentesBroto L, Paredes SD, Reiter RJ. Significance and application of melatonin in the regulation of brown adipose tissue metabolism: relation to human obesity. Obes Rev. 2011;12:167–88.
36. Dubocovich ML, Markowska M. Functional MT1 and MT2 melatonin receptors in mammals. Endocrine. 2005;27:101–10.
37. Slominski RM, Reiter RJ, Schlabritz-Loutsevitch N, Ostrom RS, Slominski AT. Melatonin membrane receptors in peripheral tissues: distribution and functions. Mol Cell Endocrinol. 2012;351:152–66.
38. Carr MC. The emergence of the metabolic syndrome with menopause. J Clin Endocrinol Metab. 2003;88:2404–11.
39. Mendes KG, Theodoro H, Rodrigues AD, Olinto MT. Prevalence of metabolic syndrome and its components in the menopausal transition: a systematic review. Cad Saude Publica. 2012;28:1423–37.
40. Reiter RJ. The ageing pineal gland and its physiological consequences. Bioessays. 1992;14:169–75.
41. Hardeland R. Melatonin in aging and disease – multiple consequences of reduced secretion, options and limits of treatment. Aging Dis. 2012;3:194–225.
42. Shatilo VB, Bondarenko EV, Antoniuk-Shcheglova IA. Metabolic disorders in elderly patients with hypertension and their correction with melatonin. Adv Gerontol. 2012;25:84–9.

43. Zawilska JB, Skene DJ, Arendt J. Physiology and pharmacology of melatonin in relation to biological rhythms. Pharmacol Rep. 2009;61:383–410.
44. Hardeland R, Fuhrberg B. Ubiquitous melatonin—presence and effects in unicells, plants and animals. Trends Comp Biochem Physiol. 1996;2:25–45.
45. Bonnefont-Rousselot D, Collin F. Melatonin: action as antioxidant and potential applications in human disease and aging. Toxicology. 2010;278:55–67.
46. Barrenetxe J, Delagrange P, Martinez JA. Physiological and metabolic functions of melatonin. J Physiol Biochem. 2004;60:61–72.
47. Venegas C, Garcia JA, Escames G, Ortiz F, Lopez A, Doerrier C, GarciaCorzo L, Lopez LC, Reiter RJ, AcunaCastroviejo D. Extrapineal melatonin: analysis of its subcellular distribution and daily fluctuations. J Pineal Res. 2012;52:217–27.
48. Cardinali DP, Bernasconi PA, Reynoso R, Toso CF, Scacchi P. Melatonin may curtail the metabolic syndrome: studies on initial and fully established fructose-induced metabolic syndrome in rats. Int J Mol Sci. 2013;14:2502–14.
49. Hardeland R, Cardinali DP, Srinivasan V, Spence DW, Brown GM, Pandi-Perumal SR. Melatonin–a pleiotropic, orchestrating regulator molecule. Prog Neurobiol. 2011;93:350–84.
50. Lerner AB, Case JD, Takahashi Y, Lee TH, Mori W. Isolation of melatonin, the pineal gland factor that lightens melanocytes. J Am Chem Soc. 1958;80:2587.
51. Hardeland R, Pandi-Perumal SR, Cardinali DP. Melatonin. Int J Biochem Cell Biol. 2006;38:313–6.
52. Pandi-Perumal SR, Srinivasan V, Maestroni GJ, Cardinali DP, Poeggeler B, Hardeland R. Melatonin: nature's most versatile biological signal? FEBS J. 2006;273:2813–38.
53. Tan D, Hardeland R, Manchester LC, Korkmaz A, Ma S, RosalesCorral S, Reiter RJ. Functional roles of melatonin in plants, and perspectives in nutritional and agricultural science. J Exp Bot. 2012;63:577–97.
54. Hardeland R, Madrid JA, Tan DX, Reiter RJ. Melatonin, the circadian multioscillator system and health: the need for detailed analyses of peripheral melatonin signaling. J Pineal Res. 2012;52:139–66.
55. Reiter RJ, Tan DX, Jou MJ, Korkmaz A, Manchester LC, Paredes SD. Biogenic amines in the reduction of oxidative stress: melatonin and its metabolites. Neuro Endocrinol Lett. 2008;29:391–8.
56. Sener G, Sehirli AÖ, Ayanoğlu-Dülger G. Protective effects of melatonin, vitamin E and N-acetylcysteine against acetaminophen toxicity in mice: a comparative study. J Pineal Res. 2003;35:61–8.
57. Montilla-Lopez P, Munoz-Agueda MC, Feijoo Lopez M, Munoz-Castaneda JR, Bujalance-Arenas I, Tunez-Finana I. Comparison of melatonin versus vitamin C on oxidative stress and antioxidant enzyme activity in Alzheimer's disease induced by okadaic acid in neuroblastoma cells. Eur J Pharmacol. 2002;451:237–43.
58. Tan DX, Manchester LC, Terron MP, Flores LJ, Reiter RJ. One molecule, many derivatives: a never-ending interaction of melatonin with reactive oxygen and nitrogen species? J Pineal Res. 2007; 42:28–42.
59. Tan DX, Manchester LC, Terron MP, Flores LJ, Tamura H, Reiter RJ. Melatonin as a naturally occurring co-substrate of quinone reductase-2, the putative MT3 melatonin membrane receptor: hypothesis and significance. J Pineal Res. 2007;43:317–20.
60. Korkmaz A, Rosales-Corral S, Reiter RJ. Gene regulation by melatonin linked to epigenetic phenomena. Gene. 2012;503:1–11.
61. Sanchez-Hidalgo M, Montavez JMG, Carrascosa Salmoral MP, Gutierrez MCN, Lardone PJ, Lardone PJ, de la Lastra Romero CA. Decreased MT1 and MT2 melatonin receptor expression in extrapineal tissues of the rat during physiological aging. J Pineal Res. 2009;46:29–35.
62. Stefulj J, Hörtner M, Ghosh M, Schauenstein K, Rinner I, Wölfler A, Semmler J, Liebmann PM. Gene expression of the key enzymes of melatonin synthesis in extrapineal tissues of the rat. J Pineal Res. 2001;30:243–7.
63. Sanchez-Hidalgo M, de la Lastra CA, Carrascosa-Salmoral MP, Naranjo MC, Gomez-Corvera A, Caballero B, Guerrero JM. Age-related changes in melatonin synthesis in rat extrapineal tissues. Exp Gerontol. 2009;44:328–34.
64. Hernandez C, Abreu J, Abreu P, Castro A, Jimenez A. Nocturnal melatonin plasma levels in patients with OSAS: the effect of CPAP. Eur Respir J. 2007;30:496–500.
65. Sae-Teaw M, Johns J, Johns NP, Subongkot S. Serum melatonin levels and antioxidant capacities after consumption of pineapple, orange, or banana by healthy male volunteers. J Pineal Res. 2013;55:58–64.
66. Johns NP, Johns J, Porasuphatana S, Plaimee P, Sae-Teaw M. Dietary intake of melatonin from tropical fruit altered urinary excretion of 6-sulfatoxymelatonin in healthy volunteers. J Agric Food Chem. 2013;61:913–9.
67. Iriti M, Varoni EM, Vitalini S. Melatonin in traditional Mediterranean diets. J Pineal Res. 2010;49:101–5.
68. Kastorini CM, Milionis HJ, Esposito K, Giugliano D, Goudevenos JA, Panagiotakos DB. The effect of Mediterranean diet on metabolic syndrome and its components: a meta-analysis of 50 studies and 534,906 individuals. J Am Coll Cardiol. 2011;57:1299–313.
69. Lamont KT, Somers S, Lacerda L, Opie LH, Lecour S. Is red wine a SAFE sip away from cardioprotection? Mechanisms involved in resveratrol- and melatonin-induced cardioprotection. J Pineal Res. 2011;50:374–80.
70. Dominguez-Rodriguez A, Abreu-Gonzalez P, Sanchez-Sanchez JJ, Kaski JC, Reiter RJ. Melatonin and circadian biology in human cardiovascular disease. J Pineal Res. 2010;49:14–22.
71. Takeda N, Maemura K. Circadian clock and cardiovascular disease. J Cardiol. 2011;57:249–56.
72. Dominguez-Rodriguez A, Abreu-Gonzalez P, Garcia MJ, Sanchez J, Marrero F, de Armas-Trujillo D.

Decreased nocturnal melatonin levels during acute myocardial infarction. J Pineal Res. 2002;33:248–52.
73. Muller JE, Ludmer PL, Willich SN, Tofler GH, Aylmer G, Klangos I, Stone PH. Circadian variation in the frequency of sudden cardiac death. Circulation. 1987;75:131–8.
74. Siegel D, Black DM, Seeley DG, Hulley SB. Circadian variation in ventricular arrhythmias in hypertensive men. Am J Cardiol. 1992;69:344–7.
75. Altun A, Yaprak M, Aktoz M, Vardar A, Betul UA, Ozbay G. Impaired nocturnal synthesis of melatonin in patients with cardiac syndrome X. Neurosci Lett. 2002;327:143–5.
76. Schepelmann M, Molcan L, Uhrova H, Zeman M, Ellinger I. The presence and localization of melatonin receptors in the rat aorta. Cell Mol Neurobiol. 2011;31:1257–65.
77. Ekmekcioglu C, Thalhammer T, Humpeler S, Mehrabi MR, Glogar HD, Holzenbein T, Markovic O, Leibetseder VJ, Strauss-Blasche G, Marktl W. The melatonin receptor subtype MT2 is present in the human cardiovascular system. J Pineal Res. 2003;35:40–4.
78. Peliciari-Garcia RA, Zanquetta MM, Andrade-Silva J, Gomes DA, Barreto-Chaves ML, Cipolla-Neto J. Expression of circadian clock and melatonin receptors within cultured rat cardiomyocytes. Chronobiol Int. 2011;28:21–30.
79. Scheer FA, Kalsbeek A, Buijs RM. Cardiovascular control by the suprachiasmatic nucleus: neural and neuroendocrine mechanisms in human and rat. Biol Chem. 2003;384:697–709.
80. Durgan DJ, Young ME. The cardiomyocyte circadian clock. Circ Res. 2010;106:647–58.
81. Reilly DF, Westgate EJ, FitzGerald GA. Peripheral circadian clocks in the vasculature. Arterioscler Thromb Vasc Biol. 2007;27:1694–705.
82. Nduhirabandi F, Du Toit EF, Blackhurst D, Marais D, Lochner A. Chronic melatonin consumption prevents obesity-related metabolic abnormalities and protects the heart against myocardial ischemia and reperfusion injury in a prediabetic model of diet-induced obesity. J Pineal Res. 2011;50:171–82.
83. Bojkova B, Orendas P, Friedmanova L, Kassayova M, Datelinka I, Ahlersova E, Ahlers I. Prolonged melatonin administration in 6-month-old Sprague–Dawley rats: metabolic alterations. Acta Physiol Hung. 2008;95:65–76.
84. Kassayova M, Markova M, Bojkova B, Adamekova E, Kubatka P, Ahlersova E, Ahlers I. Influence of long-term melatonin administration on basic physiological and metabolic variables of young Wistar:Han rats. Biologia. 2006;61:313–20.
85. Patel V, Upaganlawar A, Zalawadia R, Balaraman R. Cardioprotective effect of melatonin against isoproterenol induced myocardial infarction in rats: a biochemical, electrocardiographic and histoarchitectural evaluation. Eur J Pharmacol. 2010;644:160–8.
86. Kitajima T, Kanbayashi T, Saitoh Y, Ogawa Y, Sugiyama T, Kaneko Y, Sasaki Y, Aizawa R, Shimisu T. The effects of oral melatonin on the autonomic function in healthy subjects. Psychiatry Clin Neurosci. 2001;55:299–300.
87. Mizrak B, Parlakpinar H, Acet A, Turkoz Y. Effects of pinealectomy and exogenous melatonin on rat hearts. Acta Histochem. 2004;106:29–36.
88. Brugger P, Marktl W, Herold M. Impaired nocturnal secretion of melatonin in coronary heart disease. Lancet. 1995;345:1408.
89. SamimiFard S, AbreuGonzalez P, DominguezRodriguez A, JimenezSosa A. A case–control study of melatonin receptor type 1A polymorphism and acute myocardial infarction in a Spanish population. J Pineal Res. 2011;51:400–4.
90. Dominguez-Rodriguez A, Abreu-Gonzalez P, Arroyo-Ucar E, Reiter RJ. Decreased level of melatonin in serum predicts left ventricular remodelling after acute myocardial infarction. J Pineal Res. 2012;53:319–23.
91. Garakyaraghi M, Siavash M, Alizadeh MK. Effects of melatonin on left ventricular ejection fraction and functional class of heart failure patients: a randomized, double-blind, placebo-controlled trial. J Res Med Sci. 2012;17:S13–6.
92. Opie LH. Heart physiology from cell to circulation. Philadelphia: Williams & Wilkens; 2004.
93. Kaneko S, Okumura K, Numaguchi Y, Matsui H, Murase K, Mokuno S, Morishima I, Hira K, Toki Y, Ito T, Hayakawa T. Melatonin scavenges hydroxyl radical and protects isolated rat hearts from ischemic reperfusion injury. Life Sci. 2000;67:101–12.
94. Lagneux C, Joyeux M, Demenge P, Ribuot C, Godin-Ribuot D. Protective effects of melatonin against ischemia-reperfusion injury in the isolated rat heart. Life Sci. 2000;66:503–9.
95. Szarszoi O, Asemu G, Vanecek J, Ost'adal B, Kolar F. Effects of melatonin on ischemia and reperfusion injury of the rat heart. Cardiovasc Drugs Ther. 2001;15:251–7.
96. Tan DX, Manchester LC, Reiter RJ, Qi W, Kim SJ, El-Sokkary GH. Ischemia/reperfusion-induced arrhythmias in the isolated rat heart: prevention by melatonin. J Pineal Res. 1998;25:184–91.
97. Salie R, Harper I, Cillie C, Genade S, Huisamen B, Moolman J, Lochner A. Melatonin protects against ischaemic-reperfusion myocardial damage. J Mol Cell Cardiol. 2001;33:343–57.
98. Lee YM, Chen HR, Hsiao G, Sheu JR, Wang JJ, Yen MH. Protective effects of melatonin on myocardial ischemia/reperfusion injury in vivo. J Pineal Res. 2002;33:72–80.
99. Sahna E, Acet A, Ozer MK, Olmez E. Myocardial ischemia-reperfusion in rats: reduction of infarct size by either supplemental physiological or pharmacological doses of melatonin. J Pineal Res. 2002;33:234–8.
100. Sahna E, Parlakpinar H, Turkoz Y, Acet A. Protective effects of melatonin on myocardial ischemia/reperfusion induced infarct size and oxidative changes. Physiol Res. 2005;54:491–5.
101. Sahna E, Olmez E, Acet A. Effects of physiological and pharmacological concentrations of melatonin on

ischemia-reperfusion arrhythmias in rats: can the incidence of sudden cardiac death be reduced? J Pineal Res. 2002;32:194–8.

102. Lochner A, Genade S, Davids A, Ytrehus K, Moolman JA. Short- and long-term effects of melatonin on myocardial post-ischemic recovery. J Pineal Res. 2006;40:56–63.

103. Lochner A, Huisamen B, Nduhirabandi F. Cardioprotective effect of melatonin against ischaemia/reperfusion damage. Front Biosci (Elite Ed). 2013;5:305–15.

104. Reiter RJ, Tan DX, Paredes SD, Fuentes-Broto L. Beneficial effects of melatonin in cardiovascular disease. Ann Med. 2010;42:276–85.

105. Dominguez-Rodriguez A, Abreu-Gonzalez P, Reiter RJ. Clinical aspects of melatonin in the acute coronary syndrome. Curr Vasc Pharmacol. 2009;7:367–73.

106. Genade S, Genis A, Ytrehus K, Huisamen B, Lochner A. Melatonin receptor-mediated protection against myocardial ischaemia/reperfusion injury: role of its anti-adrenergic actions. J Pineal Res. 2008;45:449–58.

107. Sallinen P, Manttari S, Leskinen H, Ilves M, Vakkuri O, Ruskoaho H, Saarela S. The effect of myocardial infarction on the synthesis, concentration and receptor expression of endogenous melatonin. J Pineal Res. 2007;42:254–60.

108. Petrosillo G, Colantuono G, Moro N, Ruggiero FM, Tiravanti E, Di Venosa N, Fiore T, Paradies G. Melatonin protects against heart ischemia-reperfusion injury by inhibiting mitochondrial permeability transition pore opening. Am J Physiol Heart Circ Physiol. 2009;297:H1487–93.

109. Petrosillo G, Moro N, Paradies V, Ruggiero FM, Paradies G. Increased susceptibility to Ca(2+)-induced permeability transition and to cytochrome c release in rat heart mitochondria with aging: effect of melatonin. J Pineal Res. 2010;48:340–6.

110. Ghosh G, De K, Maity S, Bandyopadhyay D, Bhattacharya S, Reiter RJ, Bandyopadhyay A. Melatonin protects against oxidative damage and restores expression of GLUT4 gene in the hyperthyroid rat heart. J Pineal Res. 2007;42:71–82.

111. Mukherjee R, Banerjee S, Joshi N, Singh PK, Baxi D, Ramachandran AV. A combination of melatonin and alpha lipoic acid has greater cardioprotective effect than either of them singly against cadmium-induced oxidative damage. Cardiovasc Toxicol. 2011;11:78–88.

112. Reiter RJ, Manchester LC, FuentesBroto L, Tan D. Cardiac hypertrophy and remodelling: pathophysiological consequences and protective effects of melatonin. J Hypertens. 2010;28:S7–12.

113. Chen Z, Chua CC, Gao J, Hamdy RC, Chua BH. Protective effect of melatonin on myocardial infarction. Am J Physiol Heart Circ Physiol. 2003;284:H1618–24.

114. Poirier P, Giles TD, Bray GA, Hong Y, Stern JS, Pi-Sunyer FX, Eckel RH. American Heart Association, Obesity Committee of the Council on Nutrition, Physical Activity, and Metabolism. Obesity and cardiovascular disease: pathophysiology, evaluation, and effect of weight loss: an update of the 1997 American Heart Association Scientific Statement on Obesity and Heart Disease from the Obesity Committee of the Council on Nutrition, Physical Activity, and Metabolism. Circulation. 2006;113:898–918.

115. Qin X, Zhang Y, Cai Y, He M, Sun L, Fu J, Li J, Wang B, Xing H, Tang G, Wang X, Xu X, Xu X, Huo Y. Prevalence of obesity, abdominal obesity and associated factors in hypertensive adults aged 45–75 years. Clin Nutr. 2013;32(3):361–7.

116. Cook JS, Sauder CL, Ray CA. Melatonin differentially affects vascular blood flow in humans. Am J Physiol Heart Circ Physiol. 2011;300:H670–4.

117. Grossman E, Laudon M, Zisapel N. Effect of melatonin on nocturnal blood pressure: meta-analysis of randomized controlled trials. Vasc Health Risk Manag. 2011;7:577–84.

118. Rechcinski T, Trzos E, Wierzbowska-Drabik K, Krzeminska-Pakula M, Kurpesa M. Melatonin for nondippers with coronary artery disease: assessment of blood pressure profile and heart rate variability. Hypertens Res. 2010;33:56–61.

119. Paulis L, Simko F. Blood pressure modulation and cardiovascular protection by melatonin: potential mechanisms behind. Physiol Res. 2007;56:671–84.

120. Karppanen H, Lahovaara S, Mannisto P, Vapaatalo H. Plasma renin activity and in vitro synthesis of aldosterone by the adrenal glands of rats with spontaneous, renal, or pinealectomy-induced hypertension. Acta Physiol Scand. 1975;94:184–8.

121. Zanoboni A, Zanoboni-Muciaccia W. Experimental hypertension in pinealectomized rats. Life Sci. 1967;6:2327–31.

122. Holmes SW, Sugden D. Proceedings: the effect of melatonin on pinealectomy-induced hypertension in the rat. Br J Pharmacol. 1976;56:360P–1.

123. Katsi V, Karagiorgi I, Makris T, Papavasileiou M, Androulakis AE, Tsioufis C, Tousoulis D, Stefanadis C, Kallikazaros IE. The role of melatonin in hypertension: a brief review. Cardiovasc Endocrinol. 2012;1:13–8.

124. Lusardi P, Preti P, Savino S, Piazza E, Zoppi A, Fogari R. Effect of bedtime melatonin ingestion on blood pressure of normotensive subjects. Blood Press Monit. 1997;2:99–103.

125. Yildiz M, Sahin B, Sahin A. Acute effects of oral melatonin administration on arterial distensibility, as determined by carotid-femoral pulse wave velocity, in healthy young men. Exp Clin Cardiol. 2006;11:311–3.

126. Yildiz M, Akdemir O. Assessment of the effects of physiological release of melatonin on arterial distensibility and blood pressure. Cardiol Young. 2009;19:198–203.

127. Forman JP, Curhan GC, Schernhammer ES. Urinary melatonin and risk of incident hypertension among young women. J Hypertens. 2010;28:446–51.

128. Zeman M, Dulková K, Bada V, Herichová I. Plasma melatonin concentrations in hypertensive patients with the dipping and non-dipping blood pressure profile. Life Sci. 2005;76:1795–803.
129. Jonas M, Garfinkel D, Zisapel N, Laudon M, Grossman E. Impaired nocturnal melatonin secretion in non-dipper hypertensive patients. Blood Press. 2003;12:19–24.
130. Simko F. Chronobiology of blood pressure: emerging implications of melatonin. Eur J Clin Invest. 2012;42:1252–4.
131. Leibowitz A, Peleg E, Sharabi Y, Shabtai Z, Shamiss A, Grossman E. The role of melatonin in the pathogenesis of hypertension in rats with metabolic syndrome. Am J Hypertens. 2008;21:348–51.
132. Kozirog M, Poliwczak AR, Duchnowicz P, KoterMichalak M, Sikora J, Broncel M. Melatonin treatment improves blood pressure, lipid profile, and parameters of oxidative stress in patients with metabolic syndrome. J Pineal Res. 2011;50:261–6.
133. Pechanova O, Parohova J, Vrankova S, Barta A, Kovacsova M, Janega P. 604 Effect of melatonin on blood pressure and fibrosis enlargement in the heart and aorta in experimental metabolic syndrome. J Hypertens. 2012;30:e177.
134. Witt-Enderby PA, Dubocovich ML. Characterization and regulation of the human ML1A melatonin receptor stably expressed in Chinese hamster ovary cells. Mol Pharmacol. 1996;50:166–74.
135. Dubocovich ML. Melatonin receptors: are there multiple subtypes? Trends Pharmacol Sci. 1995;16:50–6.
136. Anwar MM, Meki AR, Rahma HH. Inhibitory effects of melatonin on vascular reactivity: possible role of vasoactive mediators. Comp Biochem Physiol C Toxicol Pharmacol. 2001;130:357–67.
137. Grossini E, Molinari C, Uberti F, Mary DA, Vacca G, Caimmi PP. Intracoronary melatonin increases coronary blood flow and cardiac function through beta-adrenoreceptors, MT1/MT2 receptors, and nitric oxide in anesthetized pigs. J Pineal Res. 2011;51:246–57.
138. Pechanova O, Zicha J, Paulis L, Zenebe W, Dobesova Z, Kojsova S, Jendekova L, Sladkova M, Dovinova I, Simko F, Kunes J. The effect of N-acetylcysteine and melatonin in adult spontaneously hypertensive rats with established hypertension. Eur J Pharmacol. 2007;561:129–36.
139. Ersahin M, Sehirli O, Toklu HZ, Suleymanoglu S, EmekliAlturfan E, Yarat A, Tatldede E, Yegen BC, Sener G. Melatonin improves cardiovascular function and ameliorates renal, cardiac and cerebral damage in rats with renovascular hypertension. J Pineal Res. 2009;47:97–106.
140. Reiter RJ, Tan D, Korkmaz A. The circadian melatonin rhythm and its modulation: possible impact on hypertension. J Hypertens. 2009;27:S17–20.
141. Campos LA, Cipolla-Neto J, Amaral FG, Michelini LC, Bader M, Baltatu OC. The Angiotensin-melatonin axis. Int J Hypertens. 2013;2013:521783.
142. van der Helm-van Mil Annette HM, van Someren EJW, van den Boom R, van Buchem MA, de Craen AJM, Blauw GJ. No influence of melatonin on cerebral blood flow in humans. J Clin Endocrinol Metab. 2003;88:5989–94.
143. Bang J, Park YS, Jeong S, Song J, Kim Y, Hwang G. Melatonin does not attenuate dynamic cardiovascular and cerebrovascular reflex responses to acute hypotension in healthy men. Korean J Anesthesiol. 2012;63:245–52.
144. Tunstall RR, Shukla P, Grazul-Bilska A, Sun C, O'Rourke ST. MT2 receptors mediate the inhibitory effects of melatonin on nitric oxide-induced relaxation of porcine isolated coronary arteries. J Pharmacol Exp Ther. 2011;336:127–33.
145. Thakor AS, Herrera EA, SeronFerre M, Giussani DA. Melatonin and vitamin C increase umbilical blood flow via nitric oxide-dependent mechanisms. J Pineal Res. 2010;49:399–406.
146. Bray MS, Young ME. Chronobiological effects on obesity. Curr Obes Rep. 2012;1:9–15.
147. Boer-Martins L, Figueiredo VN, Demacq C, Martins LC, Consolin-Colombo F, Figueiredo MJ, Cannavan FP, Moreno Jr H. Relationship of autonomic imbalance and circadian disruption with obesity and type 2 diabetes in resistant hypertensive patients. Cardiovasc Diabetol. 2011;10:24.
148. Lund J, Arendt J, Hampton SM, English J, Morgan LM. Postprandial hormone and metabolic responses amongst shift workers in Antarctica. J Endocrinol. 2001;171:557–64.
149. Peschke E, Frese T, Chankiewitz E, Peschke D, Preiss U, Schneyer U, Spessert R, Muhlbauer E. Diabetic Goto Kakizaki rats as well as type 2 diabetic patients show a decreased diurnal serum melatonin level and an increased pancreatic melatonin-receptor status. J Pineal Res. 2006;40:135–43.
150. Cano P, Jimenez-Ortega V, Larrad A, Reyes Toso CF, Cardinali DP, Esquifino AI. Effect of a high-fat diet on 24-h pattern of circulating levels of prolactin, luteinizing hormone, testosterone, corticosterone, thyroid-stimulating hormone and glucose, and pineal melatonin content, in rats. Endocrine. 2008;33:118–25.
151. Cardinali DP, Pagano ES, Scacchi Bernasconi PA, Reynoso R, Scacchi P. Disrupted chronobiology of sleep and cytoprotection in obesity: possible therapeutic value of melatonin. Neuro Endocrinol Lett. 2011;32:588–606.
152. She M, Deng X, Guo Z, Laudon M, Hu Z, Liao D, Hu X, Luo Y, Shen Q, Su Z, Yin W. NEU-P11, a novel melatonin agonist, inhibits weight gain and improves insulin sensitivity in high-fat/high-sucrose-fed rats. Pharmacol Res. 2009;59:248–53.
153. Oxenkrug GF, Summergrad P. Ramelteon attenuates age-associated hypertension and weight gain in spontaneously hypertensive rats. Ann N Y Acad Sci. 2010;1199:114–20.
154. Bartness TJ, Wade GN. Body weight, food intake and energy regulation in exercising and melatonin-treated siberian hamsters. Physiol Behav. 1985;35:805–8.

155. Arendt J. Melatonin and human rhythms. Chronobiol Int. 2006;23:21–37.
156. Bartness TJ, Demas GE, Song CK. Seasonal changes in adiposity: the roles of the photoperiod, melatonin and other hormones, and sympathetic nervous system. Exp Biol Med (Maywood). 2002;227:363–76.
157. Larkin LM, Moore BJ, Stern JS, Horwitz BA. Effect of photoperiod on body weight and food intake of obese and lean Zucker rats. Life Sci. 1991;49: 735–45.
158. Prunet-Marcassus B, Desbazeille M, Bros A, Louche K, Delagrange P, Renard P, Casteilla L, Penicaud L. Melatonin reduces body weight gain in Sprague Dawley rats with diet-induced obesity. Endocrinology. 2003;144:5347–52.
159. Kurcer Z, Sahna E, Olmez E. Vascular reactivity to various vasoconstrictor agents and endothelium-dependent relaxations of rat thoracic aorta in the long-term period of pinealectomy. J Pharmacol Sci. 2006;101:329–34.
160. Bojkova B, Markova M, Ahlersova E, Ahlers I, Adamekova E, Kubatka P, Kassayova M. Metabolic effects of prolonged melatonin administration and short-term fasting in laboratory rats. Acta Vet Brno. 2006;75:21–32.
161. Rasmussen DD, Boldt BM, Wilkinson CW, Yellon SM, Matsumoto AM. Daily melatonin administration at middle age suppresses male rat visceral fat, plasma leptin, and plasma insulin to youthful levels. Endocrinology. 1999;140:1009–12.
162. Rasmussen DD, Mitton DR, Larsen SA, Yellon SM. Aging-dependent changes in the effect of daily melatonin supplementation on rat metabolic and behavioral responses. J Pineal Res. 2001;31:89–94.
163. Wolden-Hanson T, Mitton DR, McCants RL, Yellon SM, Wilkinson CW, Matsumoto AM, Rasmussen DD. Daily melatonin administration to middle-aged male rats suppresses body weight, intraabdominal adiposity, and plasma leptin and insulin independent of food intake and total body fat. Endocrinology. 2000;141:487–97.
164. Puchalski SS, Green JN, Rasmussen DD. Melatonin effects on metabolism independent of gonad function. Endocrine. 2003;21:169–73.
165. Agil A, Navarro-Alarcon M, Ruiz R, Abuhamadah S, El-Mir MY, Vazquez GF. Beneficial effects of melatonin on obesity and lipid profile in young Zucker diabetic fatty rats. J Pineal Res. 2011;50:207–12.
166. Ríos-Lugo MJ, Cano P, Jiménez-Ortega V, Fernández-Mateos MP, Scacchi PA, Cardinali DP, Esquifino AI. Melatonin effect on plasma adiponectin, leptin, insulin, glucose, triglycerides and cholesterol in normal and high fat? Fed rats. J Pineal Res. 2010;49:342–8.
167. Hussein MR, Ahmed OG, Hassan AF, Ahmed MA. Intake of melatonin is associated with amelioration of physiological changes, both metabolic and morphological pathologies associated with obesity: an animal model. Int J Exp Pathol. 2007;88:19–29.
168. Shieh JM, Wu HT, Cheng KC, Cheng JT. Melatonin ameliorates high fat diet-induced diabetes and stimulates glycogen synthesis via a PKCzeta-Akt-GSK3beta pathway in hepatic cells. J Pineal Res. 2009;47:339–44.
169. Nduhirabandi F, du Toit EF, Lochner A. Melatonin and the metabolic syndrome: a tool for effective therapy in obesity-associated abnormalities? Acta Physiol (Oxf). 2012;205:209–23.
170. Agil A, Rosado I, Ruiz R, Figueroa A, Zen N, Fernandez-Vazquez G. Melatonin improves glucose homeostasis in young Zucker diabetic fatty rats. J Pineal Res. 2012;52:203–10.
171. Puchalski SS, Green JN, Rasmussen DD. Melatonin effect on rat body weight regulation in response to high-fat diet at middle age. Endocrine. 2003;21:163–7.
172. Sanchez-Mateos S, Alonso-Gonzalez C, Gonzalez A, Martinez-Campa CM, Mediavilla MD, Cos S, Sanchez-Barcelo EJ. Melatonin and estradiol effects on food intake, body weight, and leptin in ovariectomized rats. Maturitas. 2007;58:91–101.
173. Baxi D, Singh PK, Vachhrajani K, Ramachandran AV. Melatonin supplementation therapy as a potent alternative to ERT in ovariectomized rats. Climacteric. 2012;15:382–92.
174. Raskind MA, Burke BL, Crites NJ, Tapp AM, Rasmussen DD. Olanzapine-induced weight gain and increased visceral adiposity is blocked by melatonin replacement therapy in rats. Neuropsychopharmacology. 2007;32:284–8.
175. Hoyos M, Guerrero JM, Perez-Cano R, Olivan J, Fabiani F, Garcia-Perganeda A, Osuna C. Serum cholesterol and lipid peroxidation are decreased by melatonin in diet-induced hypercholesterolemic rats. J Pineal Res. 2000;28:150–5.
176. Hussain SA. Effect of melatonin on cholesterol absorption in rats. J Pineal Res. 2007;42:267–71.
177. Zhang K, Lv Z, Jia X, Huang D. Melatonin prevents testicular damage in hyperlipidaemic mice. Andrologia. 2012;44:230–6.
178. Kitagawa A, Ohta Y, Ohashi K. Melatonin improves metabolic syndrome induced by high fructose intake in rats. J Pineal Res. 2012;52:403–13.
179. D'Archivio M, Annuzzi G, Vari R, Filesi C, Giacco R, Scazzocchio B, Santangelo C, Giovannini C, Rivellese AA, Masella R. Predominant role of obesity/insulin resistance in oxidative stress development. Eur J Clin Invest. 2012;42:70–78.
180. Vincent HK, Taylor AG. Biomarkers and potential mechanisms of obesity-induced oxidant stress In humans. Int J Obes (Lond). 2006;30:400–18.
181. Agil A, Reiter RJ, Jimenez-Aranda A, Iban-Arias R, Navarro-Alarcon M, Marchal JA, Adem A, Fernandez-Vazquez G. Melatonin ameliorates low-grade inflammation and oxidative stress in young zucker diabetic fatty rats. J Pineal Res. 2013;54:381–88.
182. de Rooij SR, Nijpels G, Nilsson PM, Nolan JJ, Gabriel R, Bobbioni-Harsch E, Mingrone G, Dekker

JM, Relationship Between Insulin Sensitivity and Cardiovascular Disease (RISC) Investigators. Low-grade chronic inflammation in the relationship between insulin sensitivity and cardiovascular disease (RISC) population: associations with insulin resistance and cardiometabolic risk profile. Diabetes Care. 2009;32:1295–301.
183. Nishida S. Metabolic effects of melatonin on oxidative stress and diabetes mellitus. Endocrine. 2005;27:131–6.
184. Pita ML, Hoyos M, Martin-Lacave I, Osuna C, Fernández-Santos JM, Guerrero JM. Long-term melatonin administration increases polyunsaturated fatty acid percentage in plasma lipids of hypercholesterolemic rats. J Pineal Res. 2002;32: 179–86.
185. Boengler K, Schulz R, Heusch G. Loss of cardioprotection with ageing. Cardiovasc Res. 2009;83: 247–61.
186. Kloner RA, Schwartz LL. State of the science of cardioprotection: challenges and opportunities – proceedings of the 2010 NHLBI Workshop on Cardioprotection. J Cardiovasc Pharmacol Ther. 2011;16:223–32.
187. Downey JM, Cohen MV. Why do we still not have cardioprotective drugs? Circ J. 2009;73:1171–7.
188. Shafii M, MacMillan DR, Key MP, Kaufman N, Nahinsky ID. Case study: melatonin in severe obesity. J Am Acad Child Adolesc Psychiatry. 1997;36:412–6.
189. Tutuncu NB, Batur MK, Yildirir A, Tutuncu T, Deger A, Koray Z, Erbas B, Kabakci G, Aksoyek S, Erbas T. Melatonin levels decrease in type 2 diabetic patients with cardiac autonomic neuropathy. J Pineal Res. 2005;39:43–9.
190. Hikichi T, Tateda N, Miura T. Alteration of melatonin secretion in patients with type 2 diabetes and proliferative diabetic retinopathy. Clin Ophthalmol. 2011;5:655–60.
191. Cardinali DP, Cano P, Jimenez-Ortega V, Esquifino AI. Melatonin and the metabolic syndrome: physiopathologic and therapeutical implications. Neuroendocrinology. 2011;93:133–42.
192. Lipton J, Megerian JT, Kothare SV, Cho YJ, Shanahan T, Chart H, Ferber R, Adler-Golden L, Cohen LE, Czeisler CA, Pomeroy SL. Melatonin deficiency and disrupted circadian rhythms in pediatric survivors of craniopharyngioma. Neurology. 2009;73:323–5.
193. Mantele S, Otway DT, Middleton B, Bretschneider S, Wright J, Robertson MD, Skene DJ, Johnston JD. Daily rhythms of plasma melatonin, but not plasma leptin or leptin mRNA, vary between lean, obese and type 2 diabetic men. PLoS One. 2012;7:e37123.
194. Robeva R, Kirilov G, Tomova A, Kumanov P. Melatonin-insulin interactions in patients with metabolic syndrome. J Pineal Res. 2008;44:52–6.
195. Robeva R, Kirilov G, Tomova A, Kumanov P. Low testosterone levels and unimpaired melatonin secretion in young males with metabolic syndrome. Andrologia. 2006;38:216–20.
196. Lee J, Yoon J, Lee JA, Lee SY, Shin CH, Yang SW. Urinary 6-sulfatoxymelatonin level in girls and its relationship with obesity. Korean J Pediatr. 2012;55:344–9.
197. Rojdmark S, Berg A, Rossner S, Wetterberg L. Nocturnal melatonin secretion in thyroid disease and in obesity. Clin Endocrinol (Oxf). 1991;35:61–5.
198. Ozguner F, Koyu A, Cesur G. Active smoking causes oxidative stress and decreases blood melatonin levels. Toxicol Ind Health. 2005;21:21–6.
199. Muller HL, Handwerker G, Gebhardt U, Faldum A, Emser A, Kolb R, Sorensen N. Melatonin treatment in obese patients with childhood craniopharyngioma and increased daytime sleepiness. Cancer Causes Control. 2006;17:583–9.
200. LeGouic S, Delagrange P, Atgie C, Nibbelink M, Hanoun N, Casteilla L, Renard P, Lesieur D, GuardiolaLemaitre B, Ambid L. Effects of both a melatonin agonist and antagonist on seasonal changes in body mass and energy intake in the garden dormouse. Int J Obes. 1996;20:661–7.
201. Muhlbauer E, Gross E, Labucay K, Wolgast S, Peschke E. Loss of melatonin signalling and its impact on circadian rhythms in mouse organs regulating blood glucose. Eur J Pharmacol. 2009;606:61–71.
202. Brydon L, Petit L, Delagrange P, Strosberg AD, Jockers R. Functional expression of MT2 (Mel1b) melatonin receptors in human PAZ6 adipocytes. Endocrinology. 2001;142:4264–71.
203. Prokopenko I, Langenberg C, Florez JC, Saxena R, Soranzo N, Thorleifsson G, Loos RJ, Manning AK, Jackson AU, Aulchenko Y, Potter SC, Erdos MR, Sanna S, Hottenga JJ, Wheeler E, Kaakinen M, Lyssenko V, Chen WM, Ahmadi K, Beckmann JS, et al. Variants in MTNR1B influence fasting glucose levels. Nat Genet. 2009;41:77–81.
204. Bouatia-Naji N, Bonnefond A, Cavalcanti-Proenca C, Sparso T, Holmkvist J, Marchand M, Delplanque J, Lobbens S, Rocheleau G, Durand E, De Graeve F, Chevre JC, Borch-Johnsen K, Hartikainen AL, Ruokonen A, Tichet J, Marre M, et al. A variant near MTNR1B is associated with increased fasting plasma glucose levels and type 2 diabetes risk. Nat Genet. 2009;41:89–94.
205. Ling Y, Li X, Gu Q, Chen H, Lu D, Gao X. A common polymorphism rs3781637 in MTNR1B is associated with type 2 diabetes and lipids levels in Han Chinese individuals. Cardiovasc Diabetol. 2011;10:27.
206. Tabara Y, Osawa H, Kawamoto R, Onuma H, Shimizu I, Makino H, Kohara K, Miki T. Genotype risk score of common susceptible variants for prediction of type 2 diabetes mellitus in Japanese: the Shimanami Health Promoting Program (J-SHIPP study). Development of type 2 diabetes mellitus and genotype risk score. Metabolism. 2011;60:1634–40.
207. Song CK, Bartness TJ. CNS sympathetic outflow neurons to white fat that express MEL receptors may

mediate seasonal adiposity. Am J Physiol Regul Integr Comp Physiol. 2001;281:R666–72.
208. Alonso-Vale MI, Peres SB, Vernochet C, Farmer SR, Lima FB. Adipocyte differentiation is inhibited by melatonin through the regulation of C/EBPbeta transcriptional activity. J Pineal Res. 2009;47:221–7.
209. Sanchez-Hidalgo M, Lu Z, Tan DX, Maldonado MD, Reiter RJ, Gregerman RI. Melatonin inhibits fatty acid-induced triglyceride accumulation in ROS17/2.8 cells: implications for osteoblast differentiation and osteoporosis. Am J Physiol Regul Integr Comp Physiol. 2007;292:R2208–15.
210. Sartori C, Dessen P, Mathieu C, Monney A, Bloch J, Nicod P, Scherrer U, Duplain H. Melatonin improves glucose homeostasis and endothelial vascular function in high-fat diet-fed insulin-resistant mice. Endocrinology. 2009;150:5311–7.
211. Townsend K, Tseng Y. Brown adipose tissue: recent insights into development, metabolic function and therapeutic potential. Adipocyte. 2012;1:13–24.
212. Benoit SC, Clegg DJ, Seeley RJ, Woods SC. Insulin and leptin as adiposity signals. Recent Prog Horm Res. 2004;59:267–85.
213. Scarpace PJ, Zhang Y. Leptin resistance: a predisposing factor for diet-induced obesity. Am J Physiol Regul Integr Comp Physiol. 2009;296:R493–500.
214. Lago R, Gomez R, Lago F, Gomez-Reino J, Gualillo O. Leptin beyond body weight regulation–current concepts concerning its role in immune function and inflammation. Cell Immunol. 2008;252:139–45.
215. Baydas G, Gursu F, Canpolat S, Konar V, Yasar A, Canatan H, Kelestimur H. Effects of pinealectomy on the circadian release pattern of leptin in male rat. Neuro Endocrinol Lett. 2001;22:449–52.
216. Canpolat S, Sandal S, Yilmaz B, Yasar A, Kutlu S, Baydas G, Kelestimur H. Effects of pinealectomy and exogenous melatonin on serum leptin levels in male rat. Eur J Pharmacol. 2001;428:145–8.
217. Morrison CD, Huypens P, Stewart LK, Gettys TW. Implications of crosstalk between leptin and insulin signaling during the development of diet-induced obesity. Biochim Biophys Acta. 2009;1792:409–16.
218. Baltaci AK, Mogulkoc R. Pinealectomy and melatonin administration in rats: their effects on plasma leptin levels and relationship with zinc. Acta Biol Hung. 2007;58:335–43.
219. Song YM, Chen MD. Effects of melatonin administration on plasma leptin concentration and adipose tissue leptin secretion in mice. Acta Biol Hung. 2009;60:399–407.
220. Buff PR, Morrison CD, Ganjam VK, Keisler DH. Effects of short-term feed deprivation and melatonin implants on circadian patterns of leptin in the horse. J Anim Sci. 2005;83:1023–32.
221. Cagnacci A, Malmusi S, Zanni A, Arangino S, Cagnacci P, Volpe A. Acute modifications in the levels of daytime melatonin do not influence leptin in postmenopausal women. J Pineal Res. 2002;33:57–60.
222. Bjorbaek C, El-Haschimi K, Frantz JD, Flier JS. The role of SOCS-3 in leptin signaling and leptin resistance. J Biol Chem. 1999;274:30059–65.
223. Emilsson V, Arch JR, de Groot RP, Lister CA, Cawthorne MA. Leptin treatment increases suppressors of cytokine signaling in central and peripheral tissues. FEBS Lett. 1999;455:170–4.
224. Myers MG, Cowley MA, Munzberg H. Mechanisms of leptin action and leptin resistance. Annu Rev Physiol. 2008;70:537–56.
225. Carvalheira JB, Siloto RM, Ignacchitti I, Brenelli SL, Carvalho CR, Leite A, Velloso LA, Gontijo JA, Saad MJ. Insulin modulates leptin-induced STAT3 activation in rat hypothalamus. FEBS Lett. 2001;500:119–24.
226. Anhe GF, Caperuto LC, Pereira-Da-Silva M, Souza LC, Hirata AE, Velloso LA, Cipolla-Neto J, Carvalho CR. In vivo activation of insulin receptor tyrosine kinase by melatonin in the rat hypothalamus. J Neurochem. 2004;90:559–66.
227. Picinato MC, Hirata AE, Cipolla-Neto J, Curi R, Carvalho CR, Anhe GF, Carpinelli AR. Activation of insulin and IGF-1 signaling pathways by melatonin through MT1 receptor in isolated rat pancreatic islets. J Pineal Res. 2008;44:88–94.
228. Benito M. Tissue specificity on insulin action and resistance: past to recent mechanisms. Acta Physiol (Oxf). 2011;201:297–312.
229. Tesauro M, Cardillo C. Obesity, blood vessels and metabolic syndrome. Acta Physiol (Oxf). 2011;203:279–86.
230. Utzschneider KM, Van de Lagemaat A, Faulenbach MV, Goedecke JH, Carr DB, Boyko EJ, Fujimoto WY, Kahn SE. Insulin resistance is the best predictor of the metabolic syndrome in subjects with a first-degree relative with type 2 diabetes. Obesity (Silver Spring). 2010;18:1781–7.
231. McLaughlin T, Allison G, Abbasi F, Lamendola C, Reaven G. Prevalence of insulin resistance and associated cardiovascular disease risk factors among normal weight, overweight, and obese individuals. Metabolism. 2004;53:495–9.
232. Hardy OT, Czech MP, Corvera S. What causes the insulin resistance underlying obesity? Curr Opin Endocrinol Diabetes Obes. 2012;19:81–7.
233. Peschke E. Melatonin, endocrine pancreas and diabetes. J Pineal Res. 2008;44:26–40.
234. Peschke E, Muhlbauer E. New evidence for a role of melatonin in glucose regulation. Best Pract Res Clin Endocrinol Metab. 2010;24:829–41.
235. Zanquetta MM, Seraphim PM, Sumida DH, Cipolla-Neto J, Machado UF. Calorie restriction reduces pinealectomy-induced insulin resistance by improving GLUT4 gene expression and its translocation to the plasma membrane. J Pineal Res. 2003;35:141–8.
236. Lima FB, Machado UF, Bartol I, Seraphim PM, Sumida DH, Moraes SM, Hell NS, Okamoto MM, Saad MJ, Carvalho CR, Cipolla-Neto J. Pinealectomy causes glucose intolerance and decreases adipose cell responsiveness to insulin in rats. Am J Physiol. 1998;275:E934–41.
237. Nishida S, Sato R, Murai I, Nakagawa S. Effect of pinealectomy on plasma levels of insulin and leptin

and on hepatic lipids in type 2 diabetic rats. J Pineal Res. 2003;35:251–6.

238. Kuzuya T, Nakagawa S, Satoh J, Kanazawa Y, Iwamoto Y, Kobayashi M, Nanjo K, Sasaki A, Seino Y, Ito C, Shima K, Nonaka K, Kadowaki T, Committee of the Japan Diabetes Society on the diagnostic criteria of diabetes mellitus. Report of the Committee on the classification and diagnostic criteria of diabetes mellitus. Diabetes Res Clin Pract. 2002;55:65–85.
239. Frese T, Bach AG, Muhlbauer E, Ponicke K, Bromme HJ, Welp A, Peschke E. Pineal melatonin synthesis is decreased in type 2 diabetic Goto-Kakizaki rats. Life Sci. 2009;85:526–33.
240. Peschke E, Schucht H, Muhlbauer E. Long-term enteral administration of melatonin reduces plasma insulin and increases expression of pineal insulin receptors in both Wistar and type 2-diabetic Goto-Kakizaki rats. J Pineal Res. 2010;49:373–81.
241. Nishida S, Segawa T, Murai I, Nakagawa S. Long-term melatonin administration reduces hyperinsulinemia and improves the altered fatty-acid compositions in type 2 diabetic rats via the restoration of Delta-5 desaturase activity. J Pineal Res. 2002;32:26–33.
242. Hui X, Lam KS, Vanhoutte PM, Xu A. Adiponectin and cardiovascular health: an update. Br J Pharmacol. 2012;165:574–90.
243. Ha E, Yim SV, Chung JH, Yoon KS, Kang I, Cho YH, Baik HH. Melatonin stimulates glucose transport via insulin receptor substrate-1/phosphatidylinositol 3-kinase pathway in C2C12 murine skeletal muscle cells. J Pineal Res. 2006;41:67–72.
244. Banerjee A, Udin S, Krishna A. Regulation of leptin synthesis in white adipose tissue of the female fruit bat, Cynopterus sphinx: role of melatonin with or without insulin. Exp Physiol. 2011;96:216–25.
245. Contreras-Alcantara S, Baba K, Tosini G. Removal of melatonin receptor type 1 induces insulin resistance in the mouse. Obesity (Silver Spring). 2010;18(9):1861–3.
246. Kan MY, Zhou DZ, Zhang D, Zhang Z, Chen Z, Yang YF, Guo XZ, Xu H, He L, Liu Y. Two susceptible diabetogenic variants near/in MTNR1B are associated with fasting plasma glucose in a Han Chinese cohort. Diabet Med. 2010;27: 598–602.
247. Tam CH, Ho JS, Wang Y, Lee HM, Lam VK, Germer S, Martin M, So WY, Ma RC, Chan JC, Ng MC. Common polymorphisms in MTNR1B, G6PC2 and GCK are associated with increased fasting plasma glucose and impaired beta cell function in Chinese subjects. PLoS One. 2010;5: e11428.
248. Peschke E, Fauteck JD, Musshoff U, Schmidt F, Beckmann A, Peschke D. Evidence for a melatonin receptor within pancreatic islets of neonate rats: functional, autoradiographic, and molecular investigations. J Pineal Res. 2000;28:156–64.
249. Mulder H, Nagorny CL, Lyssenko V, Groop L. Melatonin receptors in pancreatic islets: good morning to a novel type 2 diabetes gene. Diabetologia. 2009;52:1240–9.
250. Picinato MC, Haber EP, Carpinelli AR, Cipolla-Neto J. Daily rhythm of glucose-induced insulin secretion by isolated islets from intact and pinealectomized rat. J Pineal Res. 2002;33:172–7.
251. Peschke E, Hofmann K, Ponicke K, Wedekind D, Muhlbauer E. Catecholamines are the key for explaining the biological relevance of insulin-melatonin antagonisms in type 1 and type 2 diabetes. J Pineal Res. 2012;52:389–96.
252. Nieuwenhuis RF, Spooren PF, Tilanus JJ. Less need for insulin, a surprising effect of phototherapy in insulin-dependent diabetes mellitus. Tijdschr Psychiatr. 2009;51:693–7.
253. Terry PD, Goyal A, Phillips LS, Superak HM, Kutner MH. Design and rationale of a randomized controlled trial of melatonin supplementation in men and women with the metabolic syndrome. Open Access J Clin Trials. 2013;5:51–9.

Development of Agonists and Antagonists for Melatonin Receptors

7

Darius P. Zlotos

Abstract

Numerous physiological actions of melatonin are mediated by two G-protein-coupled MT_1 and MT_2 receptors. The melatonergic drugs on the market, ramelteon and agomelatine, as well as the most advanced melatonergic ligands under clinical evaluation, tasimelteon and TIK-301, are high-affinity nonselective MT_1 and MT_2 agonists. However, exploring the exact physiological role of the MT_1 and MT_2 melatonin receptors requires subtype-selective MT_1 and MT_2 ligands. This chapter summarizes the progress in the development of melatonergic agonists and antagonists focusing on high-affinity and subtype-selective agents.

Keywords

Melatonin • Melatonin receptor agonists • Melatonin receptor antagonists Melatonin receptor partial agonists • MT_1 receptors • MT_2 receptors • Selective ligands

Introduction

Many physiological effects of melatonin are mediated through activation of the high-affinity G-protein-coupled receptors named MT_1 and MT_2. Both receptor subtypes have been found in mammals, including humans, and were cloned in the mid-1990s [1]. Melatonin displays high affinity toward both MT_1 and MT_2 receptors ($K_i \sim 0.5$ nM) as determined in binding experiments using the standard radioligand 2-[^{125}I]-iodomelatonin. Additionally, a low-affinity melatonin binding site *MT_3* has been characterized as a melatonin-sensitive form of the human enzyme quinone reductase 2 [2]. MT_1 and MT_2 receptors are expressed both centrally (suprachiasmatic nucleus, cortex, *pars tuberalis*, etc.) and peripherally (kidney, adipocytes, retina, blood vessels, etc.) [3]. However, their exact physiological roles are not well defined. While MT_1 receptors seem to be involved in the sleep-promoting effects of melatonin [4, 5] and in mediating vasoconstriction [6], MT_2 receptors appear to play a major role in the resynchronizing activity of MLT [3, 7, 8] and in mediating vasodilation.

D.P. Zlotos, PhD
Department of Pharmaceutical Chemistry,
Faculty of Pharmacy and Biotechnology,
The German University in Cairo,
Al Tagamoa Al Khames,
New Cairo City, 11835, Egypt
e-mail: darius.zlotos@guc.edu.eg

V. Srinivasan et al. (eds.), *Melatonin and Melatonergic Drugs in Clinical Practice*,
DOI 10.1007/978-81-322-0825-9_7, © Springer India 2014

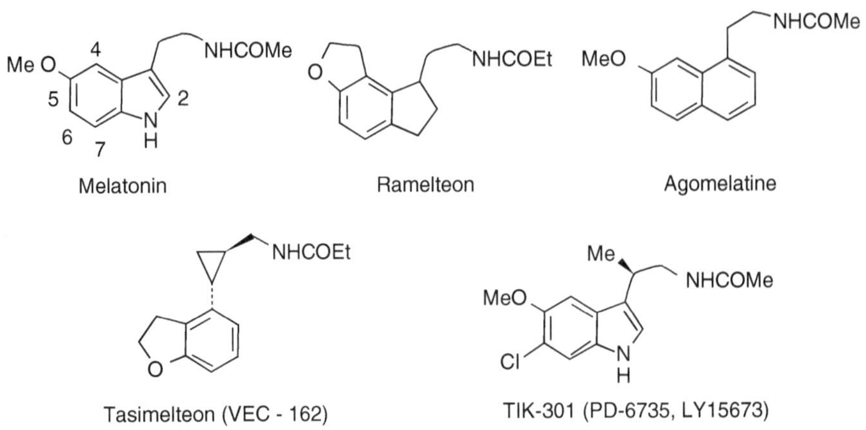

Fig. 7.1 Melatonin and melatonergic agonists on the market (ramelteon, agomelatine) and in clinical studies (tasimelteon, TIK-301)

Melatonergic Ligands in Clinical and Preclinical Practice

Melatonin is classified as a dietary supplement in the USA and other countries and is often used to alleviate the symptoms of jet lag and as a sleep-promoting agent. It shows an unfavorable pharmacokinetic profile, such as high first-pass metabolism and rapid elimination (half-life 20–30 min) limiting its efficacy for many possible treatment purposes. To overcome this obstacle, a prolonged-released formulation of melatonin, Circadin® (Neurim), has been developed and approved in Europe for the treatment of insomnia in elderly patients [9]. An alternative approach is the development of metabolically stable long-acting melatonergic agonists. The first synthetic melatonergic agent on the market introduced in the USA in 2005 is ramelteon (Rozerem™, Takeda Pharmaceuticals Inc.) [10, 11]. Ramelteon is a nonselective high-affinity MT_1/MT_2 agonist approved for the treatment of insomnia. It is characterized by a half-life of 0.83–1.93 h that is, indeed, longer than that of melatonin [12]. Another nonselective MT_1/MT_2 agonist agomelatine (Valdoxan®, Servier) has been approved in Europe for the treatment of major depression in 2009. The antidepressive effect of agomelatine is caused by its antagonist behavior at 5-HT_{2C} serotonin receptors, a pharmacological action which is not attributed to melatonin [13]. Tasimelteon (VEC-162) [14] and TIK-301 (PD-6735, LY-156735) [15], both nonselective MT_1/MT_2 agonists, are the most advanced drug candidates undergoing clinical trials for the treatment of sleep disorders. Interestingly, TIK-301 (β-methyl-6-chloromelatonin) has been recently reported to act as an antagonist at the serotonin receptor subtypes 5-HT_{2C} and 5-HT_{2B} opening new perspectives for its possible antidepressive action [16] (Fig. 7.1).

Numerous patents claiming the use of melatonergic agonists, mostly for the treatment of sleep disorders, have been filed in the last decade. Advances in the field have been summarized in several recently published review articles [17–19]. Melatonin receptor antagonists have been only evaluated in preclinical studies, for instance, luzindole for its antidepressant-like effects [20], S22153 in circadian rhythm entrainment experiments [21], and ML-23 in the treatment of Parkinson's disease [22]. Recently, a MT_2-selective partial agonist UCM765 has been shown to promote non-rapid eye movement sleep in rats and mice [23] (Fig. 7.2).

Structure-Activity Relationships of Melatonin at Native Tissues Containing Melatonin Receptors

Numerous melatonin receptor ligands belonging to different structural classes and their affinities toward melatonin receptors were reported in the

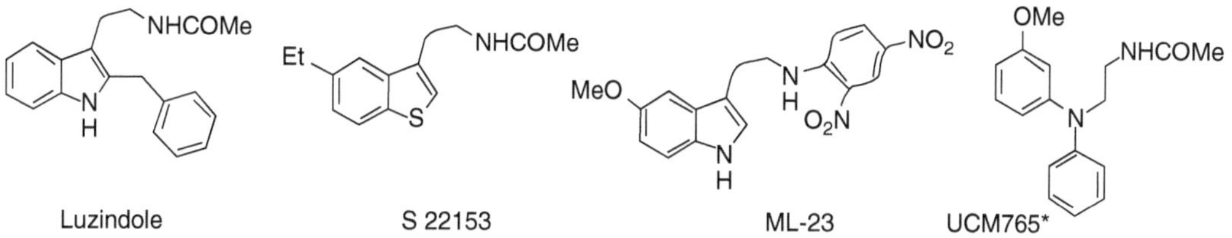

Fig. 7.2 Melatonergic antagonists evaluated in preclinical studies (*MT_2-selective partial agonist)

1980s and early 1990s. Although different native tissue preparations, such as chicken brain and retina, hamster brain, rabbit retina, ovine pars tuberalis, and *Xenopus melanophore*, each containing not clearly defined receptor subtypes, were used by different research groups, the SARs for different series of compounds were similar [24, 25]. The presence of both the methoxy and the amide group in an appropriate spatial arrangement is essential for high receptor affinity and mostly intrinsic activity. Removal of the methoxy group leading to *N*-acetyltryptamine results in over a 1,000-fold lower affinity for the receptors in chicken brain (K_i=730 nM) compared to melatonin (K_i=0.24 nM). 5-Methoxytryptamine, which lacks the *N*-acetyl group in the amide side chain moiety exhibits no affinity for melatonin receptors. Relocation of the methoxy group from C5 to C4, C6, or C7 leads to a dramatic loss of affinity. Replacement of the 5-methoxy substituent by H, OH, halogen, or bulkier alkoxy groups reduces receptor binding. Increasing the length of the alkyl substituent attached to the amide carbonyl group from CH_3 to C_3H_7 enhances affinity, but any increase in the size larger than C_3H_7 or branching is detrimental for binding. Conversion of the ethylamide side chain to an ethyl ester reduces binding. Substitutions at the 2-position of melatonin with a halogen, a methyl, or a phenyl group generate compounds with increased binding. Substitutions at the 6-position are also well tolerated. For instance, 6-chloromelatonin demonstrates comparable affinity to melatonin for the receptor in chicken brain. On the other hand, substitution at the indole nitrogen or the 7-position of melatonin reduces affinity. The structure of the aromatic ring is not crucial for binding to melatonin receptors as the exchange of indole in melatonin by various aromatic scaffolds, such as naphthalene, benzofuran, benzothiophene, indane, tetralin, and quinoline, maintains high binding. On the contrary, substitution of the melatonin indole scaffold with benzimidazole, i.e., the formal replacement of C3 with N, dramatically reduced binding affinity.

Melatonergic Ligands Characterized at Human MT_1 and MT_2 Receptors

The determination of the exact physiological functions of the melatonin receptors MT_1 and MT_2 will only be possible using subtype-selective ligands as pharmacological tools. Cloning of the human MT_1 and MT_2 receptors and the development of recombinant receptor cellular models expressing homogenous populations of a defined melatonin receptor subtype facilitated the development of subtype-selective melatonin receptor ligands in the 1990s. Indeed, during the last two decades, medicinal chemistry in the field focused on the development of subtype-selective agonists and antagonists as pharmacological tools and potential therapeutic agents [24, 25]. However, while selectivity toward MT_2 can be easily achieved and many series of MT_2-selective agents have been reported, most of them acting as competitive antagonists or partial agonists, pronounced MT_1 selectivity is still a challenge with only few examples of selective ligands reported so far.

Nonselective MT_1/MT_2 Ligands

According to the guidelines of the International Union of Basic and Clinical Pharmacology, a selective ligand should display at least 50–100

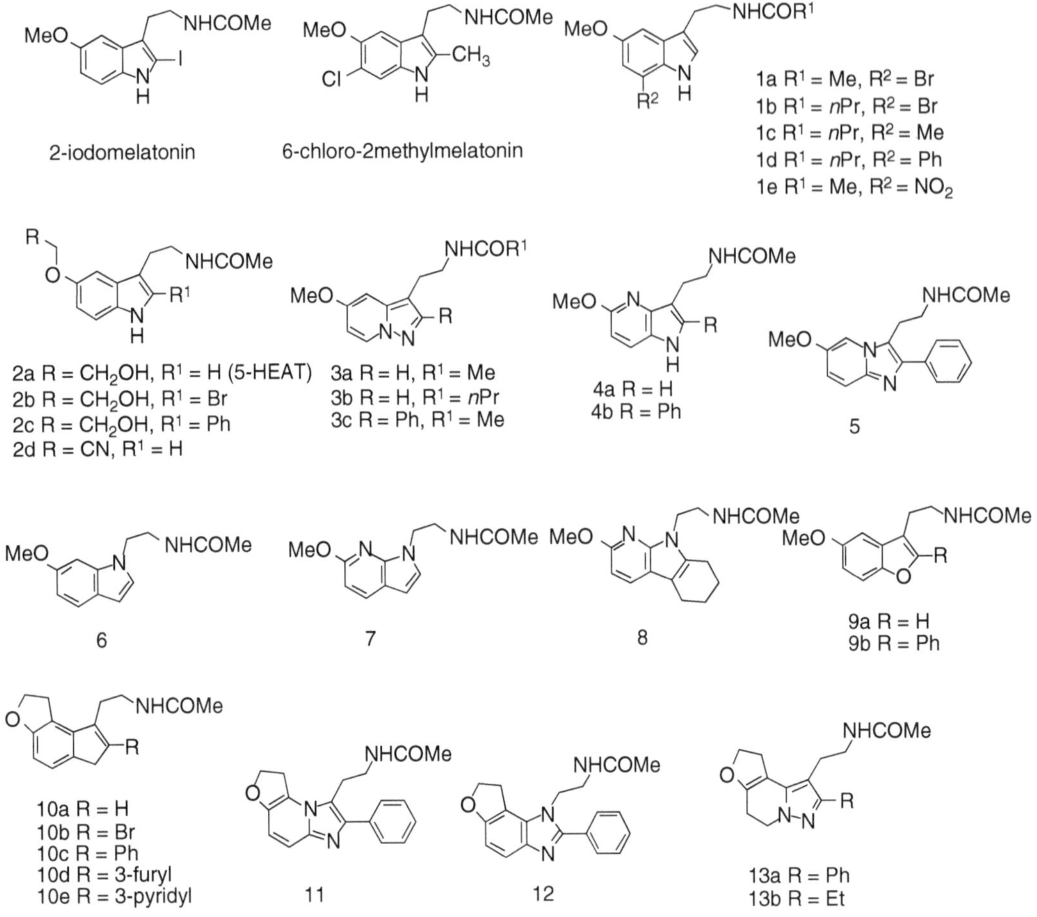

Fig. 7.3 Nonselective MT_1/MT_2 ligands

times higher binding affinity and/or potency for one receptor subtype relative to the other [26]. Applying these criteria, compounds with moderate, approximately 10–50-fold selectivity and agents showing just two to tenfold preference for one of the melatonin receptor subtypes are considered to be nonselective (Fig. 7.3).

Most high-affinity nonselective MT_1/MT_2 ligands were designed based on the SARs from previous studies carried out on native tissue preparations summarized previously in this chapter. Their structures range from bioisosteric melatonin analogs obtained by exchange of the indole nucleus with others, mostly heteroaromatic rings, to ring-opened derivatives and conformationally constrained compounds with the amide side chain incorporated into an additional ring. Moreover, substitution in a position equivalent to C2 of melatonin with methyl, phenyl, or halogen often resulted in an increased MT_1 and MT_2 affinity. The structures of the representative nonselective MT_1/MT_2 ligands are compiled in Figs. 7.3 and 7.4.

Melatonin, the natural agonist at both MT_1 and MT_2 receptors, displays equal subnanomolar affinity toward both MT_1 and MT_2. The binding constants K_i determined in either 2-[^{125}I]-iodomelatonin or [3H]melatonin displacement assays range between 0.15 and 1.00 nM depending on the cell lines used for receptor expression and on the research laboratory. Introduction of iodine into C2 of melatonin leads to an increase in affinity toward both MT_1 ($K_i = 0.068$ nM) and MT_2 ($K_i = 0.22$ nM) receptors as determined in receptors expressed in COS-7

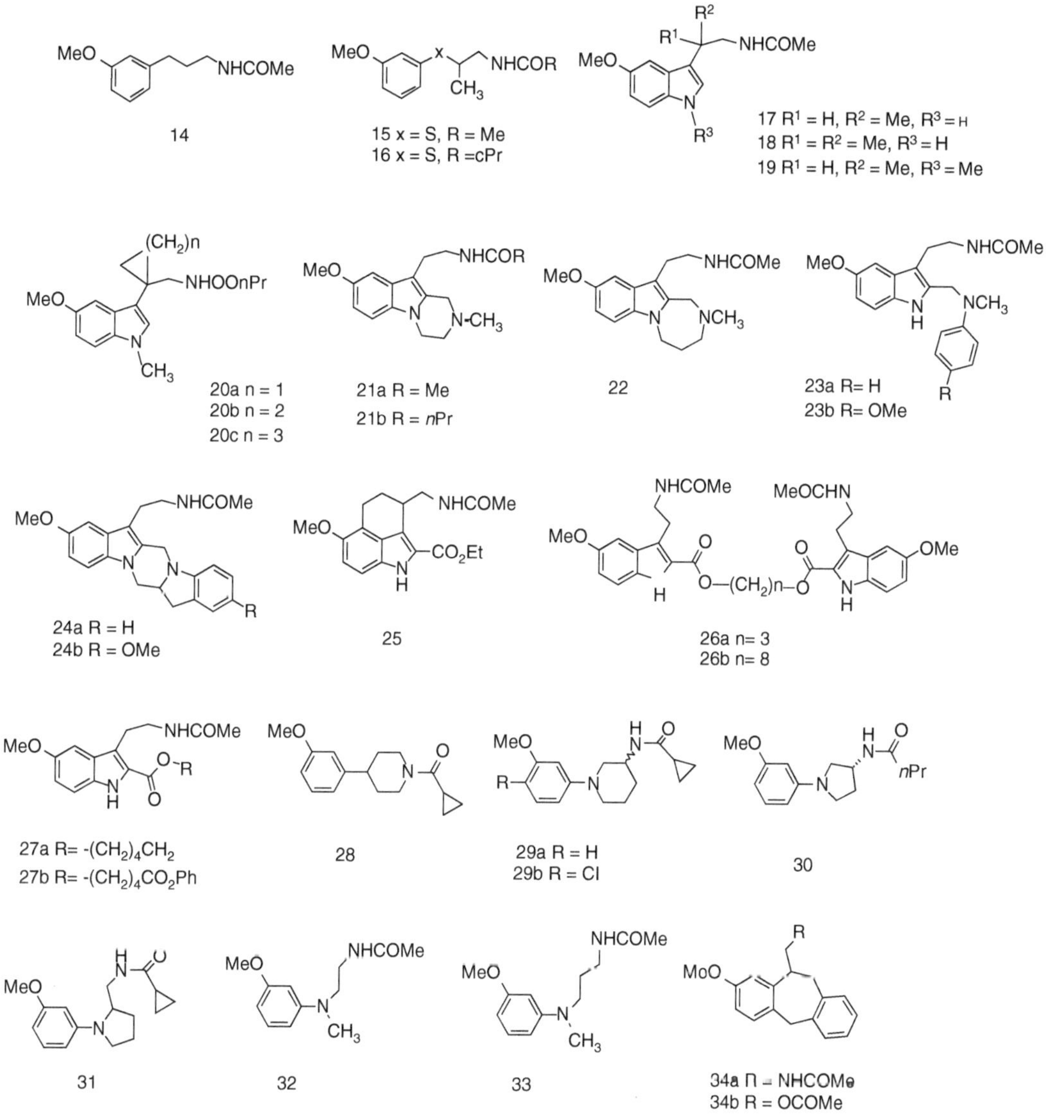

Fig. 7.4 Nonselective MT_1/MT_2 ligands (continued)

cells [27]. A simultaneous substitution with chlorine at C6 and with methyl at C2 is well tolerated at both subtypes. The resulting 6-chloro-2-methylmelatonin displays equal affinity for MT_1 (K_i=1.34 nM) and MT_2 (K_i=2.2 nM) in receptors expressed in COS-7 cells [27]. Interestingly, 6-chloromelatonin is a high-affinity MT_2 ligand (MT_2: K_i=0.22 nM, COS-7 cells) showing a 57-fold selectivity for MT_2 (MT_1: K_i=11.4 nM, COS-7 cells) [27]. Monosubstitution in position 7 of melatonin with bromine or methyl is also better tolerated at MT_2 than at MT_1 receptors. For example, the 7-bromomelatonin **1a** (MT_1: K_i=3.5 nM; MT_2: K_i=0.68 nM) and the corresponding butyramide **1b** (MT_1: K_i=5.1 nM; MT_2: K_i=0.35 nM) are high-affinity MT_2 ligands showing significantly reduced MT_1 binding at receptors expressed in NIH3T3 cells [28]. Both ligands, **1a** and **1b**, are 40 times less potent agonists than melatonin as determined in the pigment aggregation assay using *Xenopus laevis* melanophore cells. Replacement of the bromine substituent by a methyl group in the butyramide ligand **1b** to give ligand **1c** has just a marginal effect on receptor binding reducing four times intrinsic activity. On the contrary, the 7-phenyl substituted analog **1d** displays strongly reduced binding at both MT_1 and MT_2 receptors (MT_1: K_i=0.95 μM; MT_2: K_i=0.87 μM) and agonist potency. The 7-nitromelatonin ligand, **1e**, displays also only moderate affinities for both receptors expressed in HEK 293 cells (MT_1: K_i=49 nM; MT_2: K_i=29 nM) [29].

5-Hydroxyethoxy-*N*-acetyltryptamine **2a** (5-HEAT) is a full agonist at MT_1 and an antagonist/partial agonist at the MT_2 receptors binding with relatively low affinities to MT_1 (K_i=17 nM) and MT_2 (K_i=76 nM) receptors [30]. In order to enhance binding, substituents, such as C2-phenyl and C2-bromine, having an affinity increasing effect on melatonin have been introduced to ligand **2a** [31]. C2-bromination of **2a** to give **2b** generates a substantial increase in MT_1 (K_i=1.4 nM) and MT_2 (K_i=20 nM) affinity at receptors expressed in NIH3T3 cells, while the intrinsic activity profile in the GTPγS assay is virtually unchanged. In contrast, the C2-phenyl analog **2c** acts as agonist at both MT_1 and MT_2 exhibiting considerably higher affinities for MT_1 (K_i=0.3 nM) and MT_2 (K_i=1.1 nM) than analogs **2a**,**b**. Replacement of the 2-hydroxyethyl moiety of 5-HEAT with a cyanomethyl group to give ligand **2d** generates enhanced MT_1 (K_i=3.8 nM) and MT_2 (K_i=2.6 nM) binding and switches the antagonist behavior at MT_2 receptors to full agonist action.

Melatonergic ligands, **3a** [32] and **4a** [33], have been designed by exchange of one carbon atom at different positions of the indole ring in melatonin by nitrogen. 7a-Azamelatonin, **3a**, displays K_i (MT_1)=12.3 nM and K_i (MT_2)=4.0 nM at receptors expressed in NIH3T3 cells behaving as a considerably less potent agonist (EC_{50}=10.2 nM) than melatonin (EC_{50}=0.02 nM) in *Xenopus laevis* melanophore assay. The corresponding butyramide analog **3b** displays K_i (MT_1)=7.61 nM and K_i (MT_2)=0.52 nM. As expected, 2-phenyl substitution of ligand **3a** to give compound **3c** (MT_1: K_i=0.58 nM; MT_2: K_i=0.40 nM) caused an increase in MT_1 and MT_2 affinity as well as in intrinsic activity (EC_{50}=0.09 nM). 4-Azamelatonin, **4a**, shows identical MT_1 (K_i=0.24 nM) and MT_2 (K_i=0.36 nM) binding affinities as melatonin for receptors expressed in HEK-293 cells indicating that 4-azaindole is an equipotent bioisostere of indole. Introduction of a phenyl substituent in position 2 to give ligand **4b** (MT_1: *Ki*=0.04 nM; MT_2: K_i=0.20 nM) leads to a 6-fold and less pronounced 1.7-fold increase in MT_1 and MT_2 binding, respectively. In contrast, the 2-phenyl-3*a*-azamelatonin analog **5** is characterized by 700-fold and 40-fold reduced affinity for MT_1 (K_i=28 nM) and MT_2 (K_i=8 nM), respectively.

The structure of compound **6** is designed from that of melatonin by relocation of the methoxy group to position 6 and of the amide side chain to *N1*. Ligand **6** was reported to display fivefold higher binding affinity for quail optic tecta membranes than melatonin [34]. Compound **7**, which is the 7-aza analog of **6**, exhibits K_i (MT_1)=1.4 nM and K_i (MT_2)=0.6 nM at receptors expressed in HEK-293 cells acting as MT_1 and MT_2 agonist in GTPγS test performed on receptors expressed in CHO cells [35]. While C3-substitution of compound **7** with tertiary methylamino groups of different size leads to strongly reduced affinity at both receptors, the C2–C3 cyclohexane annulated tricyclic compound **8** is a high-affinity MT_2 ligand (K_i=0.68 nM) exhibiting 13-fold preference for MT_2 and agonist activity at both receptor subtypes [35].

Another high-affinity nonselective melatonergic ligand **9a** was obtained by a bioisosteric exchange of the indole ring of melatonin with a benzofuran scaffold [36]. While ligand **9a** displays almost identical binding constants to those of melatonin (MT_1: K_i=0.15 nM; MT_2: K_i=0.34 nM, HEK cells), the 2-phenyl analog **9b** shows 15 times higher affinities at MT_1 (0.01 nM) and MT_2 (0.02 nM) acting as MT_1/MT_2 full agonist in GTPγS assay performed on receptors expressed in CHO cells. The findings confirm the presence of an additional lipophilic binding site surrounding the C2 position in both MT_1 and MT_2 receptor subtypes. Interestingly, introduction of bulkier substituents, such as benzyl groups, in position 2 reduces affinity toward

MT_1, while MT_2 binding remains high generating pronounced MT_2 selectivity.

The thiophene analog of melatonin **S22153** (Fig. 7.2) has been reported to display equal binding affinities at MT_1 and MT_2 receptors (K_i=8 nM, HEK cells) acting as antagonist at MT_2 and partial agonist at MT_1 [37]. Its moderate affinity and antagonistic behavior are caused by the absence of the methoxy group which is essential for both strong binding and agonistic action. The bioisosteric exchange of the indole ring in melatonin by a naphthalene scaffold to give agomelatine also retains high MT_1 and MT_2 binding (K_i=0.1 nM at both receptor subtypes in CHO cells and agonist activity [37]).

Compound **10a** is another bioisostere of melatonin obtained by replacement of the indole nucleus with indene scaffold and simultaneous incorporation of the ether oxygen into furan ring [38]. The latter structural motif is also present in ramelteon (MT_1: K_i=0.014 nM; MT_2: K_i=0.112 nM, CHO cells) being responsible for increased binding. Compound **10a** shows indeed five to ten times higher affinities at both subtypes than melatonin in receptors expressed in CHO cells. Introduction of a bromine or a phenyl group in position 7 of the parent compound **10a** enhances binding, generating highest-affinity ligands **10b** (MT_1: K_i=0.0087 nM; MT_2: K_i=0.014 nM) and **10c** (MT_1: K_i=0.0082 nM; MT_2: K_i=0.0065 nM), respectively. While the 3-furyl derivative **10d** (MT_1: K_i=0.0065 nM; MT_2: K_i=0.0096 nM) is an extremely high-affinity ligand equipotent to the phenyl derivative **10c**, the corresponding 3-pyridyl-substituted analog **10e** exhibits similar MT_1 and MT_2 binding to the unsubstituted parent ligand **10a**. As frequently reported for other series of melatonergic agents, introduction of more bulky substituents in position 7 of analog **10a**, such as benzyl, generates pronounced MT_2 selectivity. These ligands are discussed in detail in the following section.

The further structure modification of the tricyclic ligands **10a–10e** is an example of an ADME-guided ligand optimization in the early stage of drug development. Three diaza analogs of **10c** obtained by replacing two carbon atoms at different positions of the indene ring with nitrogens have been explored [39]. The resulting ligands **11**, **12**, and **13a** possess lower lipophilicity and, consequently, are expected to exhibit a more favorable ADME profile and in vivo activity than **10c**. The parent compound **10c** and the diaza analogs have been compared in terms of not only binding affinity but also lipophilicity (log*D* values measured at pH 7.4), ligand-lipophilicity efficiency (LLE) (defined as $pK_i - \log D$, LLE is a parameter estimating the potential of the binding interaction without the contribution of lipophilicity [40]), and metabolic stability. Compounds **11**, **12**, and **13a** show considerably lower lipophilicity (log*D*=1.66, 1.39, and 2.04, respectively) than the parent compound **10c** (log*D*=3.49). The less lipophilic agents **11** and **12** are more stable against oxidative metabolism showing a much slower metabolic clearance than compounds **13a** and **10c** in rat hepatic microsomes. Unfortunately, compounds **11** (MT_1: K_i>100 nM; MT_2: K_i=6.1 nM) and **12** (MT_1: K_i=20 nM; MT_2: K_i=4.5 nM) display much lower binding affinities than compound **13a** (MT_1: K_i=0.082 nM; MT_2: K_i=0.085 nM). Moreover, the LLE values of compounds **11** (MT_1: LLE<5.3; MT_2: LLE=6) and **12** (MT_1: LLE=6.3; MT_2: LLE=7) are much lower than those of compound **10c** (MT_1: LLE=7.6; MT_2: LLE=7.7), suggesting that other factors than lipophilicity contribute to their reduced binding. On the contrary, compound **13a** is characterized by LLE=8.0 at both receptor subtypes equally high as LLE for compound **10c** which makes this compound the best choice for the development of less lipophilic melatonergic ligands. To improve the metabolic clearance of compound **10c**, the phenyl group has been replaced by less lipophilic substituents, such as methyl, ethyl, cyclopropyl, and trifluoromethyl substituents. The binding affinities of the new analogs are in a subnanomolar concentration range both for MT_1 and MT_2. Interestingly, the LLE values of these compounds are comparable to those of the lead compound **13a**, and their pK_i values correlate with the log*D* values suggesting the presence of hydrophobic pockets in the C2 region of melatonin in the MT_1 and MT_2 receptors. The ethyl derivative **13b** (MT_1: K_i=0.062 nM; MT_2: K_i=0.420 nM) has been chosen for further evaluation because of its highest metabolic stability. It is a full agonist in the cAMP assay equipotent to melatonin. Compound **13b** significantly decreases the percentage of wakefulness and increases the percentage of slow wave sleep in freely moving cats, making it a promising candidate for further clinical evaluation (Fig. 7.3).

The phenylalkyl amide derivative, compound **14**, is a ring-opened analog of melatonin representing the minimal structure required for the ligand recognition by melatonin receptors [41]. In a series of phenoxyalkyl and phenylthioalkyl amides formally obtained from compound **14** by an isosteric exchange of the benzylic methylene group with oxygen and sulfur and branching the side chain by introduction of one or two methyl groups, the (*S*) enantiomers behave as eutomers at both receptor subtypes [42]. The highest stereoselectivity was observed for the thio analogs. For example, the acetamide, compound **15**, shows a K_i eutomer (5.75 nM)/K_i distomer (2,754 nM) *ratio* of 480 for MT_1 receptors. The (*S*) enantiomer of the *N*-cyclopropyl-substituted phenoxyalkyl derivative (*S*)-**16** displays the highest affinity of the whole series for melatonin receptors expressed in NIH3T3 cells with K_i=0.72 nM for MT_2 and K_i=4.4 nM for MT_1 behaving as full agonist in [^{35}S]GTPγS binding assay.

Melatonin analogs substituted at the β-position by one or two methyl groups or by a three-, four-, or five-membered ring have also been investigated [43]. Racemic β-methylmelatonin, compound **17** (MT_1: K_i=1.67 nM; MT_2: K_i=2.94 nM) and β,β-dimethylmelatonin, compound **18** (MT_1: K_i=1.12 nM; MT_2: K_i=2.75 nM) show decreased binding at MT_1 and MT_2 receptors expressed in NIH3T3 cells when compared to melatonin (MT_1: K_i=0.39 nM; MT_2: K_i=0.35 nM). Interestingly, both compounds **17** and **18** are more potent agonists than melatonin in the *Xenopus laevis* melanophore assay. An additional methyl group at the indole nitrogen of compound **17** to give racemic compound **19** led to a drop in MT_1 binding affinity (K_i=5.48 nM) and increased MT_2 binding (K_i=0.41 nM). The enantiomers of compound **19** have been separated revealing compound (−)-**19** to be responsible for MT_2 preference. Compound (−)-**19** displays an excellent affinity (K_i=0.27 nM) and 28-fold selectivity for MT_2 receptors. The absolute configuration of the enantiomers of compound **19** is still to be determined.

Among the melatonin analogs with a cyclopropane, cyclobutane, or cyclopentane ring attached to the β-position of the side chain and a methyl group at *N*1, the cyclopropane butyramide, compound **20a**, shows 28-fold binding preference for the MT_2 receptors (MT_1: K_i=212 nM; MT_2: K_i=7.5 nM). The homologous cyclobutane analog **20b** shows increased affinity to both receptor subtypes, K_i (MT_1)=10.6 nM and K_i (MT_2)=0.86 nM, and MT_1/MT_2 affinity ratio reduced to 12. A further ring extension resulting in the cyclopentane analog **20c** led to dramatic reduction of affinity at both receptors (MT_1: K_i=589 nM; MT_2: K_i=85.1 nM). In the forskolin-stimulated cAMP release assays, analogs **20b** and **20c** behave as antagonists at MT_1 receptors. Interestingly, at the MT_2 receptors, analog **20b** is an agonist equipotent to melatonin, whereas analog **20c** showed no action representing one of the first examples of a functionally MT_1-selective antagonist (Fig. 7.4).

In order to explore the sterical tolerance of melatonin receptors for substituents around the positions *N*1 and C2 of melatonin, a series of tetrahydropyrazino[1,2]indoles and 2-[(phenylmethylamino)-methyl]-indoles have been prepared [44]. The tricyclic acetamide, compound **21a** (MT_1: K_i=11.7 nM; MT_2: K_i=7.8 nM) and butyramide, compound **21b** (MT_1: K_i=6.6 nM; MT_2: K_i=6.9 nM) show moderate affinities at both receptor subtypes with compound **21b** acting as a partial agonist at MT_1 and antagonist at MT_2. Expansion of the six-membered piperazine ring of compound **21a** to the seven-membered 1,4-diazepane analog **22** produced a dramatical drop in binding affinity at both receptors. In the series of 2-[(phenylmethylamino)-methyl]-indole analogs, compound **23a** is characterized by the highest MT_2 binding (K_i=2.3 nM) and preference for the MT_2 receptors (K_i MT_1/MT_2 ratio=7). In the cAMP release assay, compound **23a** acts as MT_1 agonist and MT_2 antagonist. Substitution of the benzene ring of ligand **23a** with *para*-Cl and *para*-CF_3 and replacement by a longer benzyl group substantially reduced MT_1 and MT_2 binding. In contrast, the *para*-OCH_3-substituted analog **23b** maintains moderate affinity for both MT_1 (K_i = 8 nM) and MT_2 (K_i = 9 nM).

The pentacyclic ligands **24a,b** represent bulkier analogs of the tricyclic compound **21a** formally obtained by attaching an indoline moiety to *N*1 and C2 of melatonin via methylene linkers [45, 46]. Increasing the size of the *N*1-C2-linked moiety of ligand **21a** by adding a benzene ring resulted in substantially decreased MT_1 and MT_2 affinity. The resulting ligands **24a** (MT_1: K_i = 319 nM; MT_2: K_i = 65 nM) and **24b** (MT_1: K_i = 1.8 μM; MT_2: K_i = 410 nM) show fivefold preference toward MT_2 receptors. Interestingly, the conformationally more flexible analog **49a** obtained by opening of the central piperazine ring in ligand **24a** is a high-affinity MT_2-selective antagonist described in the following chapter.

In order to estimate the bioactive conformation of the acetylaminoethyl side chain of melatonin, the racemic mixture of the constrained agonist (+/−)-**25** was resolved, and the structure of the levorotatory enantiomer was determined by X-ray analysis assigning its absolute configuration as *R* [47]. The (+)-(*S*) enantiomer is the eutomer displaying ~500 times higher affinity for both receptors expressed in NIH3T3 cells (MT_1: K_i = 0.18 nM; MT_2: K_i = 0.29 nM) and acting as a full MT_1 and MT_2 agonist. The intrinsic activity of (−)-**25** is 2.5 and 3.5 times lower at MT_1 and MT_2, respectively, as determined in the [^{35}S] GTPγS assay.

Applying the bivalent ligand approach, two melatonin units were connected by polymethylene spacers of variable length ranging from C_3 to C_{12} via an ester linkage at C2 [48]. No clear correlation between spacer length and affinity, intrinsic activity, and/or subtype selectivity has been observed. The highest-affinity ligands **26a,b** are characterized by $(CH_2)_3$ and $(CH_2)_8$ spacers and display K_i = 9.5 nM and 7.9 nM at MT_1 and K_i = 14.3 nM and 7.9 nM at MT_2, respectively, on receptors expressed in NIH3T3 cells behaving as full agonists in the GTPγS test. To assess the influence of the alkyl spacer itself, the monovalent ligands **27a,b** bearing pentyl and (benzyloxy)nonyl chains, respectively, have been pharmacologically evaluated. The MT_2 affinities of the monomeric ligands **27a** (MT_1: K_i = 70 nM; MT_2: K_i = 4.8 nM) and **27b** (MT_1: K_i = 83 nM; MT_2: K_i = 20 nM) are similar to those of the dimeric ligands **26a,b** indicating that the presence of the second pharmacophoric unit does not greatly influence binding at MT_2 receptors, even if intrinsic activity of the monomeric agents at MT_2 is three to four times lower. As for the MT_1 receptors, the second pharmacophore seem to contribute more significantly to higher binding and to higher agonistic potency of these bivalent ligands.

An extensive series of arylpiperidine derivatives has been evaluated for affinity and functional activity in a FLIPR assay for rat MT_1 and MT_2 receptors [49]. The cyclopropane carboxamide compound **28** (MT_1: K_i = 40 nM; MT_2: K_i = 10 nM) displays 40- and 20-fold lower MT_1 and MT_2 affinity than melatonin. Moreover, compound **28** is a 100-fold and 10-fold weaker agonist than melatonin at MT_1 and MT_2, respectively. In a series of structurally related *N*-arylpiperidine-3-yl-cyclopropane carboxamide, the enantiomers of compound **29a** display different activities. The (*S*) enantiomer (MT_1: K_i = 9.9 nM; MT_2: K_i = 2.7 nM) is a potent nonselective partial to full agonist with binding affinities similar to those of the previously reported (*S*)-aminopyrrolidine amide **30** (MT_1: K_i = 3.7 nM; MT_2: K_i = 2.6 nM) [50]. In contrast, the mirror image (*R*)-**29a** (MT_1: K_i = 1 μM; MT_2: K_i = 95 nM) is a low-affinity ligand acting as MT_2 antagonist and weak partial MT_1 agonist. Similar to melatonin, introduction of chlorine at the position adjacent to the methoxy-substituted carbon of compound (*S*)-**29a** is well tolerated. The resulting highest-affinity ligand in this series, (*S*)-**29b** (MT_1: K_i = 1.2 nM; MT_2: K_i = 2.1 nM), behaves as a potent MT_1/MT_2 partial agonist. The *R* enantiomer of **29b** displays considerably lower binding (MT_1: K_i = 130 nM; MT_2: K_i = 31 nM) and acts as MT_1/MT_2 full antagonist. Whereas replacing the piperidine ring in compound **29a** by other heterocycles, such as pyridine and tetrahydroisoquinoline, is detrimental for binding at MT_1 and MT_2 receptors, reducing its size by one carbon is well tolerated. The resulting pyrrolidine analog **31** (racemate) is a MT_1/MT_2 full agonist with sixfold preference for the MT_2 subtype (MT_1: K_i=21 nM; MT_2: K_i=3.3 nM).

The (anilinoethyl)amide **32** is an opened-ring analog of **31** with increased conformational flexibility of the side chain. It displays substantially enhanced affinity for MT_1 (K_i=0.81 nM) and MT_2 (K_i=0.65 nM) at receptors expressed in NIH3T3 cells acting as full MT_1/MT_2 agonist in GTPγS assay [51]. Chain elongation by one carbon to give compound **33** is tolerated at MT_1 (K_i=0.83 nM), whereas it causes reduced MT_2 binding (K_i=20.0 nM) generating 24-fold preference for MT_1. Compound **33** behaves as full MT_1/MT_2 agonist. Replacement of the *N*-methyl group in compound **32** by phenyl or naphthyl generates MT_2-selective ligands discussed in the following chapter.

Rigid tricyclic dibenzocycloheptene ligands exemplified by compounds **34a,b** have been reported to display binding preference toward MT_2 receptors [52]. Compound **34a** shows K_i (MT_1)=27 nM and K_i (MT_2)=1.3 nM at receptors expressed in NIH3T3 cells acting as antagonist at both subtypes in GTPγS assay. The enantiomers of **34a** have been separated showing binding affinities and intrinsic activities almost identical to those of the racemate. Surprisingly, the ester analog **34b** (MT_1: K_i=141 nM; MT_2: K_i=11 nM) retains remarkable binding, even if the corresponding esters derived from melatonin or agomelatine were reported to show ~1,000 times lower affinity relative to their parent amides at receptors expressed in native tissues. This discrepancy may be caused by the fact that while melatonin and agomelatine are agonists, compound **34a** is an antagonist at both receptor subtypes.

MT_2-Selective Ligands

Most melatonergic ligands are not able to distinguish between MT_1 and MT_2 receptors or they show just a preference, e.g., maximally 50-fold selectivity, in binding affinity for one of the subtypes.

Selectivity toward MT_2 is much easier to be accomplished than for MT_1, and many series of MT_2-selective ligands have been reported. MT_2 receptors possess an additional hydrophobic pocket in an area corresponding to the *N*1-C2 binding region of melatonin which is not present at the MT_1 subtype. This lipophilic pocket is positioned out of plane of the indole nucleus of melatonin, and, when occupied, the corresponding ligands show reduced intrinsic activity behaving as MT_2-selective antagonists or partial agonists. Accordingly, all MT_2-selective antagonists reported to date include a flexible bulky hydrophobic substituent surrounding the position topologically equivalent to *N*1 or C2 of melatonin. The importance of this structural element has been confirmed by 3D-QSAR and by docking within the putative receptor models [53].

Modest MT_2 selectivity can also be generated by introduction of Cl and OCH_3 in position 6 of melatonin. The resulting 6-chloromelatonin **35a** (MT_1: K_i=11.4 nM; MT_2: K_i=0.20 nM, COS-7 cells) and 6-methoxymelatonin **35b** (MT_1: K_i=207 nM; MT_2: K_i=3.5 nM, COS-7 cells) have been reported to display 60-fold selectivity toward MT_2, both behaving as MT_1/MT_2 agonists [27] (Fig. 7.5).

The first melatonin receptor antagonist that has been used to distinguish the functions of MT_1 and MT_2 receptors in melatonin-mediated effects is luzindole, **36a** [27]. While luzindole shows just a modest affinity and 15-fold preference for the MT_2 subtype (MT_1: K_i=158 nM; MT_2: K_i=10.2 nM, COS-7 cells), the respective 5-methoxy analog, **36b**, is 130 times more selective for MT_2 than for MT_1 receptors (MT_1: K_i=32.7 nM; MT_2: K_i=0.25 nM, COS-7 cells) acting as partial agonist in mediating inhibition of the calcium-dependent release of dopamine in an assay using rabbit retinas [27]. Another MT_2-selective ligand behaving as antagonist in the same assay is the simple derivative of melatonin GR128107, compound **37**, with the acetamide side chain incorporated into a piperidine ring (MT_1: K_i=90.4 nM; MT_2: K_i=9.1 nM, COS-7 cells) [27].

4-P-PDOT (4-phenyl-2-propionamidotetralin) is a standard highly MT_2-selective antagonist displaying 330 times higher affinity for the MT_2 (K_i=1.5 nM) than for the MT_1 (K_i=501 nM) in receptors expressed in COS-7 cells [27]. Because

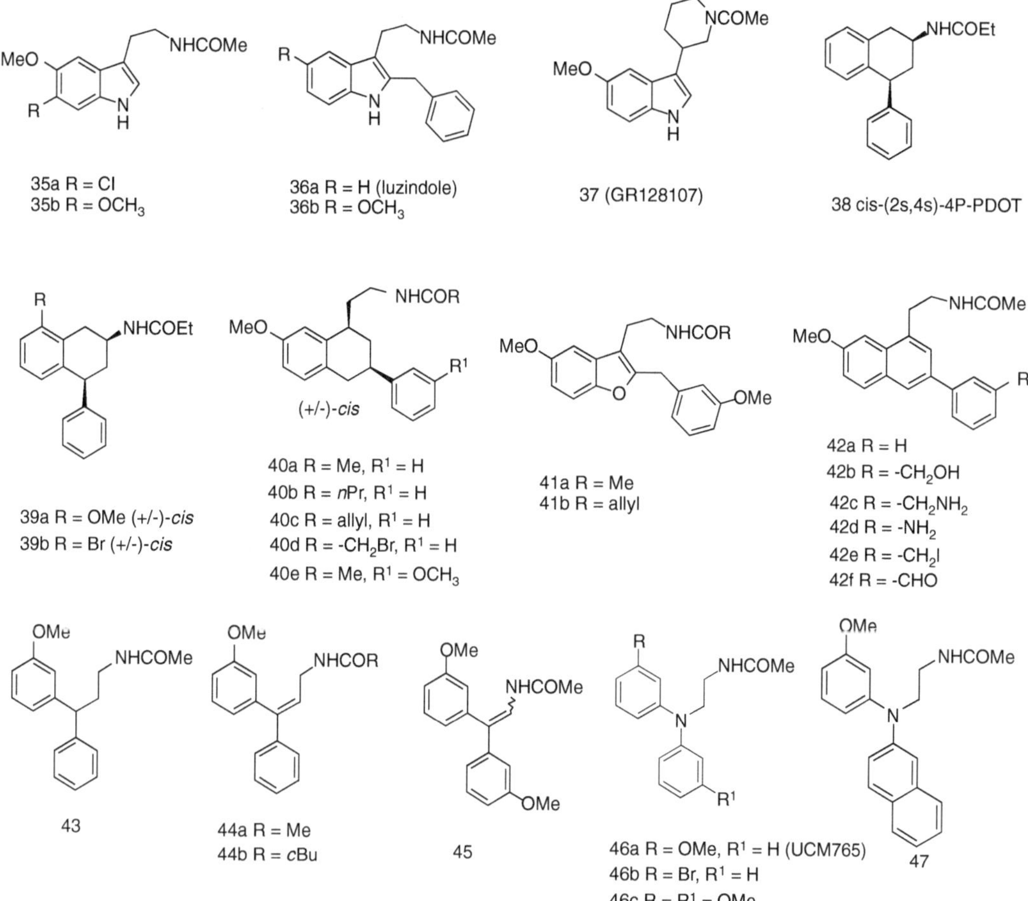

Fig. 7.5 MT_2-selective ligands

of the presence of two stereogenic centers, four stereoisomers of 4-P-PDOT exist, a pair of *cis* and a pair of *trans* enantiomers. Most older reports on 4-P-PDOT did not specify the stereochemistry of the mixtures employed. Recently, all four single stereoisomers of 4-P-PDOT have been separated [54] and pharmacologically evaluated at receptors expressed in NIH3T3 cells in terms of their binding affinities and intrinsic activities (GTPγS assay) [55]. The racemic mixtures (+/−)-*cis* and (+/−)-*trans* 4-P-PDOT have been also included in the study. The eutomer for (+/−)-*cis*-4-P-PDOT (MT_1: K_i=76 nM; MT_2: K_i=0.69 nM) is the (+)-(2*S*,4*S*) enantiomer **38** displaying ~170-fold higher affinity for MT_2 (K_i=0.55 nM) than for MT_1 receptors (K_i=95nM) and 15 and 45 % intrinsic activity at MT_1 and MT_2 relative to melatonin. The (−)-(2*R*,4*R*) mirror image shows MT_1 (K_i=257 nM) and MT_2 (K_i=98 nM) exhibiting ~3 times lower agonist potency than compound **38**. For the less MT_2-selective (+/−)-*trans*-4-P-PDOT (MT_1: K_i=223 nM; MT_2: K_i=8.7 nM), the eutomer is the (+)-(2*R*,4*S*) stereoisomer exhibiting just a 13-fold MT_2 binding preference (MT_1: K_i=129 nM; MT_2: K_i=9.5 nM). Introduction of a methoxy group in position 8 of the racemic mixtures of 4P-PDOT generates enhanced MT_1 and MT_2 affinity. The *cis* analog **39a** (MT_1: K_i=14.8 nM; MT_2: K_i=0.06 nM) is characterized by ~250-fold MT_2 selectivity and shows 6-fold higher affinity for the MT_2 receptors than melatonin displaying 20 and 40 % intrinsic activity relative to melatonin at MT_1 and MT_2 receptors, respectively. Replacement of the methoxy group in analog **39a** by bromine to give analog **39b** maintains the high MT_1 (K_i=1.0 nM) and MT_2 (K_i=0.014 nM) affinity reducing the MT_2 selectivity to 70-fold. Compound **39b** possesses 49 and 65 % intrinsic activity at MT_1 and MT_2 relative to melatonin. These pharmacological data have been used to build a new superposition model for MT_2-selective antagonists postulating that MT_1/MT_2 agonists and MT_2 antagonists can share similar spatial orientation of their pharmacophoric elements [55].

2-Phenyltetraline analogs exemplified by compounds **40a–40e** are highly MT_2-selective melatonergic ligands showing selectivity ratios between 10 and 426 [56]. All reported compounds are (+/−)-*cis* racemates. The butyramide analog **40b** displays the highest MT_2 affinity (K_i=0.1 nM) and 350-fold MT_2 selectivity (MT_1: K_i=35 nM) in receptors expressed in HEK 293 or CHO cells (not specified) behaving as MT_1 agonist and MT_2 partial agonist. Introduction of a double bond into the amide side chain of ligand **40b** to give the allyl analog **40c** (MT_1: K_i=127 nM; MT_2: K_i=0.66 nM) causes a slight reduction of MT_1 and MT_2 binding retaining high 192-fold MT_2 selectivity. The bromomethyl derivative **40d** displays considerably reduced MT_1 binding (K_i=809 nM), while its MT_2 affinity (K_i=1.9 nM) is only slightly reduced when compared to the acetamide, **40a** (MT_1: K_i=20.5 nM; MT_2: K_i=0.31 nM), resulting in the highest, 426-fold MT_2 selectivity. In the previously published series of benzofuran derivatives, the *meta*-OMe benzyl-substituted analogs, **41a** (MT_1: K_i=40.6 nM; MT_2: K_i=0.33 nM) and **41b** (MT_1: K_i=21.6 nM; MT_2: K_i=0.11 nM), were characterized by the highest MT_2 selectivity [36]. Introduction of the *m*-OMe group at the phenyl ring of analog **40a** leads indeed to a fourfold increase of MT_2 selectivity caused by a strong reduction of MT_1 binding. The resulting compound **40e** (MT_1: K_i=247 nM; MT_2: K_i=0.89 nM) exhibits 278-fold MT_2 selectivity.

A series of differently substituted 3-phenyl analogs of the nonselective agonist agomelatine (MT_1: K_i=0.06 nM; MT_2: K_i=0.27 nM) exemplified by compounds **42a–42f** has been evaluated on melatonin receptors expressed in CHO or HEK 293 cells [57]. Introduction of a phenyl ring at C3 of agomelatine to give compound **42a** retains high binding for MT_2 (K_i=0.37 nM), whereas the MT_1 affinity (K_i=53 nM) is 140 times reduced leading to 132-fold MT_2 selectivity. The high MT_2 selectivity is unexpected because the C3-phenyl ring is coplanar with the naphthalene ring, and consequently, the structure of compound **42a** is not in accordance with the pharmacophore model for MT_2 antagonist requiring a bulky lipophilic substituent arranged out of plane of the core ring. On the other hand compound **42a** is not an antagonist but a partial agonist at MT_2 receptors exhibiting 56 % activity of melatonin in the GTPγS assay. Introduction of a hydroxymethyl substituent at *meta* position generates the most favorable ligand in this series, **42b**, displaying MT_2 affinity (K_i=0.36 nM) similar to that of melatonin and 763-fold selectivity toward MT_2 (MT_1: K_i=275 nM) and behaving as a MT_2 antagonist. Bioisosteric replacement of the hydroxyl group in compound **42b** by an amino moiety to give compound **42c** leads to similar reductions in MT_1 (K_i=1,390 nM) and MT_2 (K_i=3.4 nM) binding maintaining the high MT_2 selectivity (409-fold). The corresponding primary aromatic amine, compound **42d**, exhibits ~15 times higher affinities for both receptors (MT_1: K_i=82 nM; MT_2: K_i=0.27 nM) than compound **42c** maintaining high MT_2 selectivity (304-fold) and behaving also as MT_2 antagonist [37]. The iodomethyl analog, **42e** exhibits slightly changed MT_1 (126 nM) and MT_2 (0.71 nM) affinities when compared to the hydroxymethyl derivative **42b** resulting in MT_1/MT_2 ratio of 178. Interestingly, replacement of the hydroxymethyl group in compound **42b** by an aldehyde function to give compound **42f** has no effect on MT_1 (0.42 nM) and slightly enhances MT_2 binding (137 nM) maintaining high MT_2 selectivity (326-fold).

Ligands obtained by opening of the tetralin ring and removal of the upper methylene group of methoxy-4P-PDOT **39a** have been evaluated on melatonin receptors expressed in NIH3T3 cells [58]. The acetamide, compound **43** (MT_1: K_i=2,187 nM; MT_2: K_i=5.4 nM), shows the highest MT_2 selectivity (405-fold) acting as MT_1

partial agonist and MT_2 antagonist. Introduction of a double bond into the side chain of compound **43** leads to increased binding at both receptor subtypes. While the (*E*) isomer (MT_1: K_i=2.7 nM; MT_2: K_i=0.22 nM) displays only 12-fold preference for MT_2 and high MT_2 affinity comparable to that of melatonin, the corresponding (*Z*) analog **44a** is characterized by considerably lower MT_1 (229 nM) and MT_2 (2.5 nM) affinity and 90-fold selectivity for MT_2. The (*Z*) cyclobutane carboxamide **44b** (MT_1: K_i=257 nM; MT_2: K_i=1.5 nM) exhibits ~170-fold MT_2 selectivity. Introduction of an OMe group in the *meta* position of the second benzene ring of compound **44a** to give analog **45** (stereochemistry not indicated) increased MT_2 selectivity. **45** is a high-affinity MT_2 ligand (0.28 nM) exhibiting 210-fold MT_2 selectivity.

Exchange of the central carbon atom in analog **43** by nitrogen retains high binding and selectivity toward MT_2 receptors [51]. The resulting ligand **46a** displays very high affinity (K_i=0.066 nM) and 64-fold selectivity for the MT_2 receptors behaving as MT_1/MT_2 partial agonist. Replacement of the methoxy group in ligand **46a** with bromine is well tolerated. The resulting ligand **46b** exhibits only slightly reduced binding affinities (MT_1: K_i=17.0 nM; MT_2: K_i=0.20 nM) and intrinsic activities. As already known for other ligand series, the introduction of a methoxy group at the second phenyl ring is expected to increase MT_2 selectivity. The corresponding ligand **46c** is characterized by very high MT_2 binding (0.036 nM) and MT_2 selectivity (527-fold) behaving as MT_1 partial agonist. Replacement of the phenyl group in **46a** by a bulkier 2-naphthyl moiety to give ligand **47** greatly reduces MT_1 binding and MT_2 intrinsic activity. Compound **47** (MT_1: K_i=132 nM; MT_2: K_i=0.11 nM) exhibits the highest, 1,200-fold MT_2 selectivity in whole series acting as MT_1 partial agonist and MT_2 antagonist.

The moderately MT_2-selective (64-fold) high-affinity partial agonist **46a** (UCM765) has been recently reported to promote non-rapid eye movement sleep (NREMS) in rats and mice [23]. This effect is nullified by the pharmacological blockage or genetic deletion of MT_2 receptors. Remarkably, the effects of ligand **46a** on sleep are different from those of nonselective MT_1/MT_2 agonists. For example, the structurally related MT_1/MT_2 agonists UCM793 slightly decrease sleep onset without effect on NREMS maintenance, similar to ramelteon, indicating that dual MT_1/MT_2 agonistic activity accounts for the effect on sleep onset, whereas selectivity for MT_2 receptors has an additional effect on NREMS maintenance. Because of the selective promotion of NREMS, MT_2 receptors could become an interesting future target for the treatment of sleep disorders.

Benzyloxy substituted 3-(3-methoxyphenyl) propylamides, **48a–48c**, have been reported to exhibit extraordinarily high affinity for MT_2 receptors in pM to sub-pM range and MT_2 selectivities up to ~1,000,000-fold in a binding assay on melatonin receptors expressed in CHO cells using [^{3}H]melatonin as radioligand [59]. In this assay, melatonin displays K_i (MT_1)=0.296 nM and K_i (MT_2)=0.429 nm, which are very similar values compared to the binding constants obtained using 2-[^{125}I]-iodomelatonin. The propionamide, **48b**, exhibits the highest MT_2 affinity (K_i=0.55 pM) and 473,000-fold MT_2 selectivity. The butyramide, ligand **48c**, is the most MT_2-selective (1,140,000-fold) compound displaying K_i (MT_1)=1,172 nM and K_i (MT_2)=1.03 pM. Shortening of the amido alkyl side chain from ethyl (ligand **48b**) to methyl (ligand **48a**) leads to a ~100-fold reduction of MT_2 affinity (47 pM) which decreases the MT_2 selectivity to 18,700-fold. Introduction of a methoxy group in the *meta* position of the benzyl substituent in ligand **48b** leads to increased MT_2 selectivity. The resulting ligand **48d** is 1,021,739 times more selective for MT_2 (K_i=0.69 pM) than for MT_1 (K_i=705 nM) receptors. Compound **48d** has been recently used by another group as a reference MT_2-selective ligand in a 2-[^{125}I]-iodomelatonin binding assay displaying similar affinity for the MT_1 receptors (K_i=1,350 nM) but dramatically decreased MT_2 binding (K_i=1.7 nM) resulting in a reduced MT_1/MT_2 ratio of 790 [60]. Surprisingly, instead of the expected antagonistic/partial agonistic action, ligands **48a–48d** are full MT_2 agonists in Ca^{2+} FLIPR and cAMP assays [61].

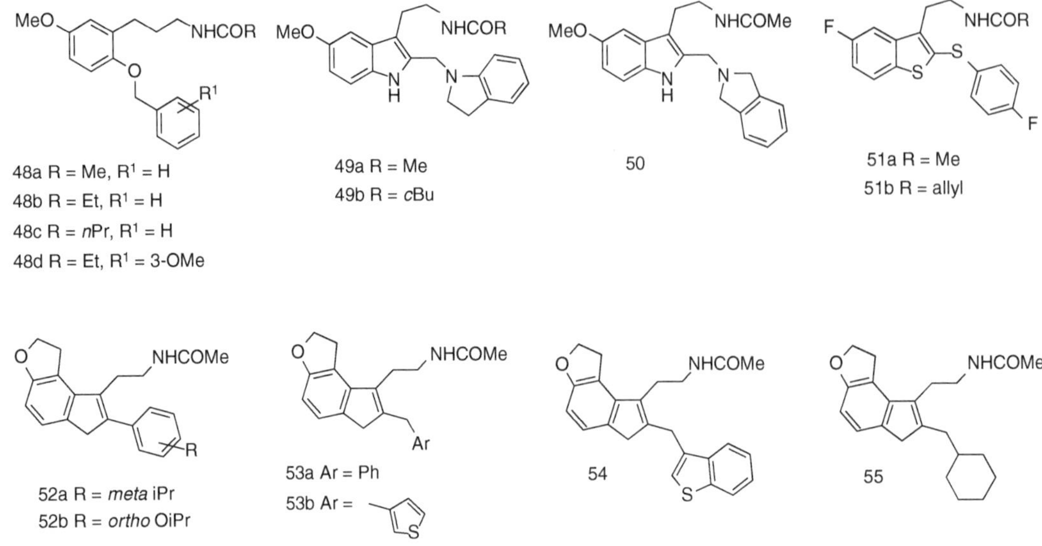

Fig. 7.6 MT_2-selective ligands (continued)

In order to achieve selectivity toward MT_2 receptors, the open chain approach has been applied to the nonselective pentacyclic ligands **24a,b** [62]. In the conformationally restricted compounds **24a,b**, the indoline moiety is a part of a relatively plane pentacyclic ring system being approximately coplanar with the indole ring. In contrast, the methylindoline group in the novel ligands **49a,b** is conformationally flexible and, therefore, able to occupy the postulated lipophilic binding pocket located in the MT_2 receptors out of plane of the ligand's core nucleus. The acetamide **49a** displays K_i $(MT_1)=115$ nM and K_i $(MT_2)=1.1$ nM at receptors expressed in CHO cells acting as MT_1/MT_2 antagonist in the cAMP assay. Interestingly, the cyclobutane carboxamide, **49b**, shows a biphasic pharmacological profile at MT_2 receptors ($K_{i\text{High}}=1$ pM, $K_{i\text{Low}}=148$ nM), but not at MT_1 receptors ($K_i=1.4$ μM), indicating the existence of a high-affinity and low-affinity state for MT_2. Ligand **49b** is an MT_1 antagonist and MT_2 antagonist/partial agonist. 5-Me, 5-Br, 6-NO_2, and 6-NH_2 substitution of the indoline benzene ring causes a substantial reduction of MT_2 affinity and selectivity. Surprisingly, the corresponding 5-OMe analog is a nonselective ligand displaying moderate affinities at both receptor subtypes (MT_1: $K_i=5.8$ nM; MT_2: $K_i=7.1$ nM). Expansion of the indoline ring in ligand **49a** by insertion of a methylene group between the indolic nitrogen and the benzene ring leads to reduced MT_1 (251 nM) and MT_2 (21 nM) binding [60]. On the contrary, relocation of the substituted nitrogen atom in the indoline ring of ligand **49a** from position 1 to position 2 is well tolerated. The resulting compound **50** is 124 times more selective for the MT_2 (2.3 nM) than for the MT_1 receptors (282 nM) [60]. In a forskolin-stimulated cAMP assay, ligand **50** is a competitive antagonist at MT_1 receptors. At the MT_2 receptor, **50** displays no intrinsic activity when tested alone. However, when added in combination with melatonin (0.01 pM–100 nM), **50** (10 nM or 100 nM) antagonized the effects of melatonin at all concentrations tested suggesting its tight binding, perhaps at a crucial portion of the MT_2 receptor affecting G-protein activation, thus requiring higher concentrations of melatonin (>100 nM) to reverse its antagonism. Another possibility could be that ligand **50** binds irreversibly to MT_2 receptors [60] (Fig. 7.6).

A series of benzothiophene analogs differing from melatonin by replacement of *N*1 with *S*, exchange of 5-OMe with *F*, and introduction of 4-fluorophenylthio moiety at C2 has been evaluated at receptors expressed in CHO cells [63]. The acetamide **51a** (MT_1: $K_i=57$ nM; MT_2: $K_i=0.87$ nM) and allyl carboxamide **51b** (MT_1: K_i=52.8 nM; MT_2: K_i=0.24 nM) display 65.5- and 220-fold selectivity toward MT_2 receptors, respectively. Both ligands are MT_1/MT_2 partial agonists.

Ligands obtained by introduction of bulky lipophilic substituents in position 7 of the tricyclic nonselective compound **10a** have been pharmacologically evaluated at melatonin receptors expressed in CHO cells [38]. The most MT_2-selective agent **52a** is substituted with a *meta*-isopropylphenyl group at C7 and shows K_i (MT_1)=13 nM and K_i (MT_2)=0.011 nM resulting in 1,200-fold MT_2 selectivity. For the *ortho-O-iso*-propylphenyl analog **52b**, binding for MT_1 (K_i>100 nM) and MT_2 (K_i=0.34 nM) is decreased, while pronounced MT_2 selectivity (>292-fold) is still present. The benzyl derivative **53a** exhibits the highest MT_2 binding (0.0085 nM) and 316-fold selectivity for MT_2. Replacement of the phenyl group in analog **53a** by a 3-thienyl moiety (analog **53b**) retains high MT_2 binding (0.0067 nM), while MT_1 affinity (0.88 nM) is ten times increased resulting in reduced MT_2 selectivity. A benzene ring annulated to the thiophene ring of analog **53b** to give analog **54** does not affect MT_1 (1.3 nM) and MT_2 (0.0060 nM) binding. Saturation of the phenyl moiety in the benzyl-substituted analog **53a** to give analog **55** causes a 3.5-fold reduction of MT_1 binding (9.2 nM), while the MT_2 affinity (0.012 nM) is virtually unchanged resulting in 799-fold MT_2 selectivity. The most MT_2-selective ligands, **52a**, **53a**, and **55**, exhibit moderate agonistic activity at MT_1 receptors as determined in the forskolin-induced cAMP accumulation assay. Interestingly, while the *meta-iso*-propylphenyl and benzyl analogs, **52a** and **53a**, behave as partial MT_2 agonists, the cyclohexylmethyl derivative **55** is a full MT_2 agonist. The latter has exhibited re-entrainment effects to a new light/dark cycle in ICR mice indicating the involvement of MT_2 receptors in the regulation of chronobiotic activity.

MT_1-Selective Ligands

Development of MT_1-selective ligands is still a challenge and only few examples of selective compounds have been reported so far. Unfortunetely, while for MT_2-selective agents selectivity ratios of>1,000 can be achieved, ligands preferentially binding to MT_1 receptors are maximally ~100 times more selective for MT_1 than for MT_2. The main structural feature generating MT_1 selectivity is a bulky hydrophobic substituent instead of the methoxy group in the position topologically equivalent to C5 of melatonin. The first MT_1-selective agents described were dimers of the nonselective MT_1/MT_2 agonist agomelatine obtained by connecting two agomelatine units via their ether oxygens by a polymethylene spacer. The optimal distance between the dimer head groups for MT_1 selectivity was determined to be three or four methylene groups [64]. Compound **56a** including the $(CH_2)_3$ linker displays 224 times higher affinity for the MT_2 (*Ki*=0.5 nM) than for the MT_1 receptors (K_i=112 nM) expressed in HEK cells acting as an antagonist at MT_1 and MT_2 receptors. In CHO cells (MT_1: K_i=3.9 nM; MT_2: K_i=149 nM), the selectivity ratio was reduced to 38 [37]. The homologous compound with a C_4 spacer, compound **56b**, shows K_i (MT_1)=3.1 nM and K_i (MT_2)=167 nM in CHO cells (54-fold MT_1 selectivity) and K_i (MT_1)=0.6 nM and K_i (MT_2)=73.2 nM in HEK cells (122-fold MT_1 selectivity) (Fig. 7.7).

An extensive series of heterodimer analogs of ligand **56b** designed by exchange of one of its agomelatine units with various aryl moieties including the equally substituted indole (melatonin), tetralin, benzofuran, and benzothiophene have been recently evaluated at receptors expressed in CHO cells [65]. Moreover, compounds obtained by further structure modifications such as variation of the amide substituent at one or both sides, replacement of one of the ethylamide side chains by acetic acid and methyl acetate, and exchange of one of the agomelatine units by a biphenyl carboxylic acid, the corresponding methyl ester, and alcohol have been reported. The most MT_1-selective ligands are biphenylcarboxylic acid, **57a** (MT_1: K_i=0.55 nM; MT_2: K_i=51.3 nM) and the structurally related alcohol **57b** (MT_1: K_i=0.09 nM; MT_2: K_i=6.53 nM) exhibiting 93-fold and 72-fold MT_1 selectivity, respectively. Ligands **57a** and **57b** act

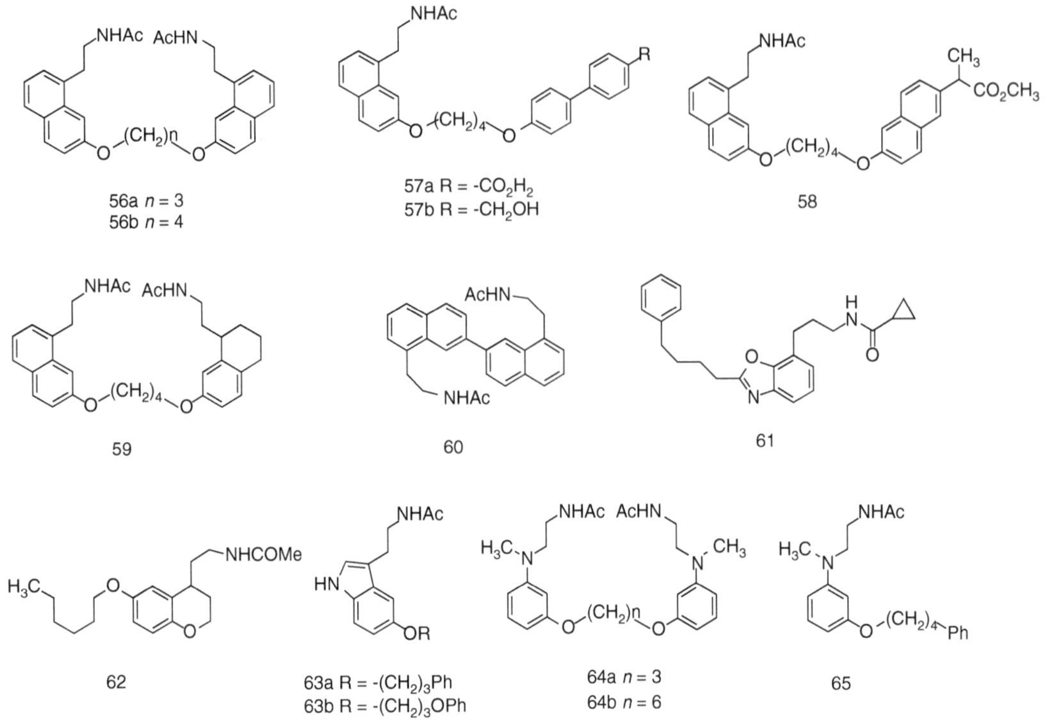

56a $n = 3$
56b $n = 4$

57a R = -CO_2H_2
57b R = -CH_2OH

58

59

60

61

62

63a R = -$(CH_2)_3Ph$
63b R = -$(CH_2)_3OPh$

64a $n = 3$
64b $n = 6$

65

Fig. 7.7 MT_1-selective ligands

as partial MT_1/MT_2 agonists in the GTPγS assay. In contrast, the less MT_1-selective ligand **58** (MT_1: K_i=0.37 nM; MT_2: K_i=4.22 nM) behaves as MT_1/MT_2 full agonist. As compounds **57a,b** and **58** lack the amide side chain attached to an aromatic ring in one part of their structures, the findings indicate that two melatonin pharmacophores are not required to achieve MT_1 selectivity. Interestingly, replacement of one of the agomelatine units in the parent compound **56b** by equally substituted indole, benzofuran, benzothiophene, and tetralin nuclei causes a substantial reduction of MT_1 selectivity from 120-fold to 21-, 10-, 5-, and 26-fold, respectively, with the tetralin analog **59** (MT_1: K_i=0.26 nM; MT_2: K_i=6.79 nM) displaying the highest binding preference for MT_1 receptors. Replacing the methyl groups in both side chains of dimeric agomelatine **56b** by cyclopropyl and allyl moieties also leads to decrease of MT_1 selectivity to ~12-fold.

Another dimeric MT_1-selective agent, ligand **60**, is a product of direct coupling of two agomelatine units via the aromatic carbon atoms. Ligand **60** shows K_i (MT_1)=5.2 nM and K_i (MT_2)=246 nM in CHO cells and acts as MT_1/MT_2 agonist [37]. Monomeric ligands, such as the 4-phenylbutyl substituted benzoxazole analog **61** [66] (CHO cells, MT_1: K_i=0.63 nM; MT_2: K_i=22 nM) and the benzopyrane derivative **62** [37] (CHO cells (MT_1: 3.4 nM; MT_2: 21.4 nM), HEK cells (MT_1: 1.2. nM; MT_2: 29 nM)), show only preference for MT_1 receptors.

The common structural feature of MT_1-selective ligands is the presence of a bulky substituent in a position corresponding to the methoxy group of melatonin. The optimal length of this substituent, as well as the nature of the terminal aromatic ring generating preferential binding for MT_1 have been explored using an extensive series of melatonin analogs obtained by replacement of the ether methyl group with arylalkyl and aryloxyalkyl moieties of different chain lengths [67]. The most MT_1-selective compounds, **63a** and **63b**, are substituted with $Ph(CH_2)_3$ and $PhO(CH_2)_3$ groups, respectively, confirming the optimal spacer length to be C_3.

Although ligands **63a** (MT_1: K_i=3.9 nM; MT_2: K_i=49 nM) and **63b** (MT_1: K_i=7.9 nM; MT_2: K_i=87 nM) show only ~10-fold selectivity toward MT_1 receptors, their MT_1 binding preference is ~3 times higher than that of the dimeric agomelatine, compound **56a** (MT_1: K_i=112 nM; MT_2: K_i=355 nM), that has been included in this study as a MT_1-selective reference ligand. These findings confirm the importance of testing multiple reference compounds having ideally different binding profiles when conducting pharmacological analysis to minimize the variability of results between different labs. Compound **63b** behaves as MT_1/MT_2 agonist in a cAMP assay at receptors expressed in CHO cells.

Another series of dimeric ligands has been designed by linking two molecules of the high-affinity nonselective MT_1/M_2 agonist **32** (MT_1: K_i=0.81 nM; MT_2: K_i–0.65 nM) via ether oxygens using polymethylene spacers $(CH_2)_n$ of different lengths (*n*=3–6, 8, 10) [68]. The compounds show MT_1 selectivity between 5-fold and 102-fold. Similar to the dimeric agomelatine series, in the most MT_1-selective ligand **64a**, the monomeric units are separated by a C_3 spacer. Ligand **64a** displays K_i (MT_1)=20.4 nM and K_i (MT_2)=2,089 nM at receptors expressed in NIH3T3 cells. The corresponding C_6 analog **64b** exhibits the highest MT_1 (3.4 nM) affinity of the whole series and is 54 times more selective for MT_1 than for MT_2 receptors. Both compounds behave as partial MT_1/MT_2 agonists in the GTPγS assay. A structurally related series of *N*-(anilinoalkyl)amides bearing 3-arylalkyloxy substituents has also been examined [69]. The phenylbutyloxy analog **65** displays the highest 78-fold selectivity toward MT_1 (MT_1: K_i=1.17 nM; MT_2: K_i=91.2 nM) acting as partial agonist at both receptor subtypes.

References

1. Reppert SM, Weaver DR, Godson C. Melatonin receptors step into the light: cloning and classification of subtypes. Trends Pharmacol Sci. 1996;17:100–2.
2. Nosjean O, Ferro M, Coge F, Beauverger P, Henlin JM, Lefoulon F, Fauchere JL, Delagrange P, Canet E, Boutin JA. Identification of the melatonin-binding site MT3 as the quinone reductase 2. J Biol Chem. 2000;275:31311–7.
3. Li P-K, Witt-Enderby PA. Melatonin receptors as potential targets for drug discovery. Drug Future. 2000;25:945–57.
4. Dubocovich ML, Yun K, Al-Ghoul WM, Benloucif S, Masana MI. Selective MT_2 melatonin receptor antagonists block melatonin-mediated phase advances of circadian rhythms. FASEB J. 1998;12:1211–20.
5. Liu C, Weaver DR, Jin X, Shearman LP, Pieschl RL, Gribkoff VK, Reppert SM. Molecular dissection of two distinct actions of melatonin on the suprachiasmatic circadian clock. Neuron. 1997;19:91–102.
6. Doolen S, Krause DN, Dubocovich ML, Duckles SP. Melatonin mediates two distinct responses in vascular smooth muscle. Eur J Pharmacol. 1998;345:67–9.
7. Hunt AE, Al-Ghoul WM, Gillette MU, Dubocovich ML. Activation of MT(2) melatonin receptors in rat suprachiasmatic nucleus phase advances the circadian clock. Am J Physiol. 2001;280:C110–8.
8. Dubocovich ML, Markowska M. Functional MT1 and MT2 melatonin receptors in mammals. Endocrine. 2005;27:101–10.
9. Hardeland R. New approaches in the management of insomnia: weighing the advantages of prolonged release melatonin and synthetic melatoninergic agonists. Neuropsychiatr Dis Treat. 2009;5: 341–54.
10. Gershell L. Insomnia market. Nature Rev Drug Discov. 2006;5:15–7.
11. Pandi-Perumal SR, Srinivasan V, Poeggeler B, Hardeland R, Cardinali DP. Drug insight: the use of melatonergic agonists for the treatment of insomnia – focus on ramelteon. Nat Clin Pract Neurol. 2007;3: 221–8.
12. Miyamoto M. Pharmacology of ramelteon, a selective MT_1/MT_2 receptor agonist: a novel therapeutic drug for sleep disorders. CNS Neurosci Ther. 2009;15: 32–51.
13. de Bodinat C, Guardiola-Lemaitre B, Mocaër E, Renard P, Muñoz C, Millan MJ. Agomelatine, the first melatonergic antidepressant: discovery characterization and development. Nat Rev Drug Discov. 2010;9: 628–42.
14. Lankford DA. Tasimelteon for insomnia. Expert Opin Investig Drugs. 2011;20:987–93.
15. Zemlan FP, Mulchahey JJ, Scharf MB, Mayleben DW, Rosenberg R, Lankford A. The efficacy and safety of the melatonin agonist β-methyl-6-chloromelatonin in primary insomnia: a randomized, placebo-controlled, crossover clinical trial. J Clin Psychiatry. 2005;66:384–90.
16. Landolt HP, Wehrle R. Antagonism of serotonergic 5-HT2A/2C receptors: mutual improvement of sleep, cognition and mood? Eur J Neurosci. 2009;29: 1795–809.
17. Rivara S, Mor M, Bedini A, Spadoni G, Tarzia G. Melatonin receptor agonists: SAR and applications to the treatment of sleep-wake disorders. Curr Top Med Chem. 2008;8:954–68.

18. Mor M, Rivara S, Pala D, Bedini A, Spadoni G, Tarzia G. Recent advances in the development of melatonin MT_1 and MT_2 receptor agonists. Expert Opin Ther Pat. 2010;20:1059–77.
19. Hardeland R. Investigational melatonin receptor agonists. Expert Opin Investig Drugs. 2010;19:747–64.
20. Sumaya IC, Masana MI, Dubocovich ML. The antidepressant-like effect of the melatonin receptor ligand luzindole in mice during forced swimming requires expression of MT_2 but not MT_1 melatonin receptors. J Pineal Res. 2005;39:170–7.
21. Li XM, Beau J, Delagrange P, Mocaer E, Lévi F. Circadian rhythm entrainment with melatonin, melatonin receptor antagonist S22153 or their combination in mice exposed to constant light. J Pineal Res. 2004;37:176–84.
22. Willis GL. The role of ML-23 and other melatonin analogues in the treatment and management of Parkinson's disease. Drug News Perspect. 2005;18: 437–44.
23. Ochoa-Sanchez R, Comai S, Lacoste B, Bambico FR, Dominguez-Lopez S, Spadoni G, Rivara S, Bedini A, Angeloni D, Fraschini F, Mor M, Tarzia G, Descarries L, Gobbi G. Promotion of non-rapid eye movement sleep and activation of reticular thalamic neurons by a novel MT2 melatonin receptor ligand. J Neurosci. 2011;31:18452–39.
24. Zlotos DP. Recent advances in melatonin receptor ligands. Arch Pharm ChemLife Sci. 2005;338: 229–47.
25. Zlotos DP. Recent progress in the development of agonists and antagonists for melatonin receptors. Curr Med Chem. 2012;19:3532–49.
26. Dubocovich ML, Cardinali DP, Delagrange P, Krause DN, Strosberg AD, Sugden D, Yocca FD. Melatonin receptors. In: Girdlestone D, editor. The IUPHAR compendium of receptor characterization and classification. 2nd ed. London: IUPHAR Media; 2000. p. 270–7.
27. Dubocovich ML, Masana MI, Iacob S, Sauri DM. Melatonin receptor antagonists that differentiate between the human Mel1aand Mel1b recombinant subtypes are used to assess the pharmacological profile of the rabbit retina ML1 presynaptic heteroreceptor. Naunyn Schmiedebergs Arch Pharmacol. 1997; 355:365–75.
28. Faust R, Garratt PJ, Trujillo Pèrez MA, Piccio VJD, Madsen C, Stenstrom A, Frolund B, Davidson K, Teh MT, Sugden D. 7-substituted-melatonin and 7-substituted-1-methylmelatonin analogues: effect of substituents on potency and binding affinity. Bioorg Med Chem. 2007;15:4543–51.
29. Leclerc V, Saıd Y, Delagrange P, Boutin JA, Renard P, Lesieur D. Synthesis of nitroindole derivatives with high affinity and selectivity for melatoninergic binding sites MT3. J Med Chem. 2002;45:1853–9.
30. Nonno R, Lucini V, Spadoni G, Pannacci M, Croce A, Esposti D, Balsamini C, Tarzia G, Fraschini F, Stankov BM. A new melatonin receptor ligand with mt1-agonist and MT2-antagonist properties. J Pineal Res. 2000;29:234–40.
31. Spadoni G, Bedini A, Guidi T, Tarzia G, Lucini V, Pannacci M, Fraschini F. Towards the development of mixed MT1-agonist/MT2-antagonist melatonin receptor ligands. Chem Med Chem. 2006;1: 1099–105.
32. Elsner J, Boeckler F, Davidson K, Sugden D, Gmeiner P. Bicyclic melatonin receptor agonists containing a ring-junction nitrogen: synthesis, biological evaluation, and molecular modelling of the putative bioactive conformation. Bioorg Med Chem. 2006;14: 1949–58.
33. El Kazzouli S, du Bellay AG, Berteina-Raboin S, Delagrange P, Caignard DH, Guillaumet G. Design and synthesis of 2-phenylimidazo[1,2-a]pyridines as a novel class of melatonin receptor ligands. Eur J Med Chem. 2011;46:4252–7.
34. Tarzia G, Diamantini G, Di Giacomo B, Spadoni G, Esposti D, Nonno R, Lucini V, Pannacci M, Fraschini F, Stankov BM. 1-(2-alkanamidoethyl)-6-methoxyindole derivatives: a new class of potent indole melatonin analogues. J Med Chem. 1997;40: 2003–10.
35. Jeanty M, Suzenet F, Delagrange F, Nosjean O, Boutin JA, Caignard DH, Guillaumet G. Design and synthesis of 1-(2-alkanamidoethyl)-6-methoxy-7-azaindolederivatives as potent melatonin agonists. Bioorg Med Chem Lett. 2011;21:2316–9.
36. Wallez V, Durieux-Poissonnier S, Chavatte P, Boutin JA, Audinot V, Nicolas J-P, Bennejean C, Delagrange P, Renard P, Lesieur D. Synthesis and structure – affinity – activity relationships of novel benzofuran derivatives as MT_2 melatonin receptor selective ligands. J Med Chem. 2002;45:2788–800.
37. Audinot V, Mailliet F, Lahaye-Brasseur C, Bonnaud A, Le Gall A, Amossé C, Dromaint S, Rodriguez M, Nagel N, Galizzi JP, Malpaux B, Guillaumet G, Lesieur D, Lefoulon F, Renard P, Delagrange P, Boutin JA. New selective ligands of human cloned melatonin MT1 and MT2 receptors. Naunyn Schmiedebergs Arch Pharmacol. 2003;367:553–61.
38. Koike T, Hoashi Y, Takai T, Nakayama M, Yukuhiro N, Ishikawa T, Hirai K, Uchikawa O. 1,6-dihydro-2H-indeno[5,4-b]furan derivatives: design, synthesis, and pharmacological characterization of a novel class of highly potent MT_2-selective agonists. J Med Chem. 2011;54:3436–44.
39. Koike T, Takai T, Hoashi Y, Nakayama M, Kosugi Y, Nakashima M, Yoshikubo S, Hirai K, Uchikawa O. Synthesis of a novel series of tricyclic dihydrofuran derivatives: discovery of 8,9-dihydrofuro[3,2-c]pyrazolo[1,5-a]pyridines as melatonin receptor (MT1/MT2) ligands. J Med Chem. 2011;54:4207–18.
40. Leeson PD, Springthorpe B. The influence of drug-like concepts on decision-making in medicinal chemistry. Nat Rev Drug Discov. 2007;6:881–90.
41. Garratt PJ, Travard S, Vonhoff S, Tsotinis A, Sugden D. Mapping the melatonin receptor. 4. Comparison of the binding affinities of a series of substituted phenylalkyl amides. J Med Chem. 1996;39:1797–805.
42. Carocci A, Catalano A, Lovece A, Lentini G, Duranti A, Lucini V, Pannacci M, Scaglione F, Franchini

C. Design, synthesis, and pharmacological effects of structurally simple ligands for MT1 and MT2 melatonin receptors. Bioorg Med Chem. 2010;18: 6496–551.

43. Tsotinis A, Vlachou M, Papahatjis DP, Calogeropoulou T, Nikas SP, Garratt PJ, Piccio V, Vonhoff S, Davidson K, Teh MT, Sugden D. Mapping the melatonin receptor. 7. Subtype selective ligands based on β-substituted N-acyl-5-methoxytryptamines and N-acyl-5-methoxy-1-methyl-tryptamines. J Med Chem. 2006; 49:3509–19.
44. Markl C, Attia MI, Julius J, Witt-Enderby PA, Zlotos DP. 1,2,3,4-tetrahydropyrazino[1,2-a]indole and 2-[(phenylmethylamino)methyl]-1H-indole analogues: probing the pharmacophore for MT_2-selective melatonin receptor ligands. Bioorg Med Chem. 2009;17:826–33.
45. Attia MI, Julius J, Witt-Enderby PA, Zlotos DP. Synthesis and pharmacological evaluation of 13a,14-dihydro-6H, 13H-pyrazino[1,2-a;4,5-a']diindole analogs as melatonin receptor ligands. Tetrahedron. 2007;63:754–60.
46. Attia MI, Witt-Enderby PA, Julius J. Synthesis and pharmacological evaluation of pentacyclic 6a,7-dihydrodiindole and 2,3-dihydrodiindole derivatives as novel melatoninergic ligands. Bioorg Med Chem. 2008;16:7654–61.
47. Rivara S, Diamantini G, Di Giacomo B, Lamba D, Gatti G, Lucini V, Pannacci M, Mor M, Spadoni G, Tarzia G. Reassessing the melatonin pharmacophore-enantiomeric resolution, pharmacological activity, structure analysis, and molecular modeling of a constrained chiral melatonin analogue. Bioorg Med Chem. 2006;14:3383–91.
48. Di Giacomo B, Bedini A, Spadoni G, Tarzia G, Fraschini F, Pannacci M, Lucini V. Synthesis and biological activity of new melatonin dimeric derivatives. Bioorg Med Chem. 2007;15:4643–50.
49. Li G, Zhou H, Jiang Y, Keim H, Topiol SW, Poda SB, Ren Y, Chandrasena G, Doller D. Design and synthesis of 4-arylpiperidinyl amide and N-arylpiperdin-3-yl-cyclopropane carboxamide derivatives as novel melatonin receptor ligands. Bioorg Med Chem Lett. 2011;21:1236–42.
50. Sun L-Q, Chen J, Mattson R, Epperson JR, Deskus JA, Li W, Takaki K, Hodges DB, Iben L, Mahle CD, Ortiz A, Molstad D, Ryan E, Yeleswaram K, Xu C, Luo G. Heterocyclic aminopyrrolidine derivatives as melatoninergic agents Bioorg. Med Chem Lett. 2003;13:4381–4.
51. Rivara S, Lodola A, Mor M, Bedini A, Spadoni G, Lucini V, Pannacci M, Fraschini F, Scaglione F, Sanchez RO, Gobbi G, Tarzia G. N-(Substituted-anilinoethyl)amides: design, synthesis, and pharmacological characterization of a new class of melatonin receptor ligands. J Med Chem. 2007;50: 6618–26.
52. Spadoni G, Bedini A, Diamantini G, Tarzia G, Rivara S, Lorenzi S, Lodola A, Mor M, Lucini V, Pannacci M, Caronno A, Fraschini F. Synthesis, enantiomeric resolution, and structure-activity relationship of a series of 10,11-dihydro-5H-dibenzo[a,d]cycloheptene MT2 receptor antagonists. Chem Med Chem. 2007; 2:1741–9.
53. Rivara S, Lorenzi S, Mor M, Plazzi PV, Spadoni G, Bedini A, Tarzia G. Analysis of structure-activity relationships for MT2 selective antagonists by melatonin MT1 and MT2 receptor models. J Med Chem. 2005; 48:4049–60.
54. Lucarini S, Bartolucci S, Bedini A, Gatti G, Orlando P, Piersanti G, Spadoni G. Synthesis and configuration determination of all enantiopure stereoisomers of the melatonin receptor ligand 4-phenyl-2-propionamidotetralin using an expedient optical resolution of 4-phenyl-2-tetralone. Org Biomol Chem. 2012;10:305–13.
55. Bedini A, Lucarini S, Spadoni G, Tarzia G, Scaglione F, Dugnani S, Pannacci M, Lucini V, Carmi C, Pala D, Rivara S, Mor M. Toward the definition of stereochemical requirements forMT2-selective antagonists and partial agonists by studying 4-phenyl-2-propionamidotetralin derivatives. J Med Chem. 2011;54:8362–72.
56. Durieux S, Chanu A, Bochu C, Audinot V, Coumailleau S, Boutin JA, Delagrange P, Caignard DH, Bennejean C, Renard P, Lesieur D, Berthelot P, Yous S. Design and synthesis of 3-phenyltetrahydronaphthalenic derivatives as new selective MT2 melatoninergic ligands. Part II. Bioorg Med Chem. 2009;17:2963–74.
57. Poissonnier-Durieux S, Ettaoussi M, Pérès B, Boutin JA, Audinot V, Bennejean C, Delagrange P, Caignard DH, Renard P, Berthelot P, Lesieur D, Yous S. Synthesis of 3-phenylnaphthalenic derivatives as new selective MT_2 melatoninergic ligands. Bioorg Med Chem. 2008;16:8339–48.
58. Bedini A, Spadoni G, Gatti G, Lucarini S, Tarzia G, Rivara S, Lorenzi S, Lodola A, Mor M, Lucini V, Pannacci M, Scaglione F. Design and synthesis of N-(3,3-diphenylpropenyl)alkanamides as a novel class of high-affinity MT_2-selective melatonin receptor ligands. J Med Chem. 2006;49:7393–403.
59. Hu Y, Ho MKC, Chan KH, New DC, Wong YH. Synthesis of substituted N-[3-(3-methoxyphenyl) propyl] amides as highly potent MT2-selective melatonin ligands. Bioorg Med Chem Lett. 2010;20:2582–5.
60. Heckman D, Attia MI, Behnam MAM, Mohsen AMY, Markl C, Julius J, Sethi S, Witt-Enderby PA, Zlotos DP. 2-[(1,3-Dihydro-2H-isoindol-2yl) methyl]-melatonin – a novel MT_2-selective melatonin receptor antagonist. Med Chem Commun. 2011;2: 991–4.
61. Chan KH, Hu Y, Ho MKC, Wong YH. Characterization of substituted phenylpropylamides as highly selective agonists at the melatonin MT2 receptor. Curr Med Chem. 2013;20:289–300.
62. Zlotos DP, Attia MI, Julius J, Sethi S, Witt-Enderby PA. 2-[(2,3-dihydro-1H-indol-1-yl)methyl]melatonin analogues: a novel class of MT2-selective melatonin receptor antagonists. J Med Chem. 2009;52:826–33.
63. Mésangeau C, Fraise M, Delagrange P, Caignard DH, Boutin JA, Berthelot P, Yous S. Preparation and pharmacological evaluation of a novel series

of 2-(phenylthio) benzo[b]thiophenes as selective MT2 receptor ligands. Eur J Med Chem. 2011;46: 1835–40.

64. Descamps-Francois C, Yous S, Chavatte P, Audinot V, Bonnaud A, Boutin JA, Delagrange P, Bennejean C, Renard P, Lesieur D. Design and synthesis of naphthalenic dimers as selective MT1 melatoninergic ligands. J Med Chem. 2003;46:1127–9.
65. Mesangeau C, Peres B, Descamps-Francois C, Chavatte P, Audinot V, Coumailleau S, Boutin JA, Delagrange P, Bennejean C, Renard P, Caignard DH, Berthelot P, Yous S. Design, synthesis and pharmacological evaluation of novel naphthalenic derivatives as selective MT1 melatoninergic ligands. Bioorg Med Chem. 2010;18:3426–36.
66. Sun LQ, Chen J, Bruce M, Deskus JA, Epperson JR, Takaki K, Johnson G, Iben L, Mahle CD, Ryan E, Xu C. Synthesis and structure–activity relationship of novel benzoxazole derivatives as melatonin receptor agonists. Bioorg Med Chem Lett. 2004;14: 3799–802.
67. Markl C, Clafshenkel WP, Attia MI, Sethi S, Witt-Enderby PA, Zlotos DP. N-acetyl-5-arylalkoxytryptamine analogs: probing the melatonin receptors for MT_1-selectivity. Arch Pharm Chem Life Sci. 2011;334:666–74.
68. Spadoni G, Bedini A, Orlando P, Lucarini S, Tarzia G, Mor M, Rivara S, Lucini V, Pannacci M, Scaglione F. Bivalent ligand approach on N-{2-[(3-methoxyphenyl) methylamino]ethyl}-acetamide: synthesis, binding affinity and intrinsic activity forMT1 and MT2 melatonin receptors. Bioorg Med Chem. 2011;19:4910–6.
69. Rivara S, Pala D, Lodola A, Mor M, Lucini V, Dugnani S, Scaglione F, Bedini A, Lucarini S, Tarzia G, Spadoni G. MT1-selective melatonin receptor ligands: synthesis, pharmacological evaluation, and molecular dynamics investigation of N-{[(3-O-substituted)anilino] alkyl}amides. Chem Med Chem. 2012;7:1954–64.

Multiple Facets of Melatonin in Immunity: Clinical Applications

8

Patricia J. Lardone, Nuria Álvarez-Sánchez,
Ana Rodríguez-Rodríguez, Juan M. Guerrero,
and Antonio Carrillo-Vico

Abstract

Nowadays, the effector capacity of melatonin in the immune system is indisputable. The almost ubiquitous distribution of melatonin receptors, its immune synthesis, and the effects of several immunological mediators on the melatonin production reinforce the concept of the melatonin/immune bidirectional circuit. Throughout the present chapter, we have highlighted that melatonin acts on the immune response by combined mechanisms which mainly involve the modulation of cytokines and the oxidative stress markers production. Overall, melatonin acts as an immune activator in basal or immunodepressed conditions, whereas it might exert a negative regulation under transient or chronic exacerbated immune response. Due to the variety of the melatonin immunomodulatory actions, it has been tested in extensive models. Thus, the clinical relevance of the several faces of melatonin on immune conditions such as infection, autoimmunity, vaccination, and immunosenescence as well as transplant and cancer is also reviewed.

Keywords

Melatonin • Pineal • Immune system • Cytokines • Inflammation • Infection
Autoimmunity • Cancer • Vaccination • Immunosenescence

Introduction

Descartes was the first to propose a physiological function of the pineal gland as a structure responsible for the environmental perception in the seventeenth century. As early as 1926, Berman reported an improvement in the resistance against infectious diseases in kittens fed for 2 years with pineal gland extracts from young bulls [1]. Therefore, the pineal-immune relationship is even prior to melatonin discover in 1958

P.J. Lardone, PhD • N. Álvarez-Sánchez, PhD
A. Rodríguez-Rodríguez, PhD • J.M. Guerrero, PhD
A. Carrillo-Vico, PhD (✉)
Bioquímica Médica y Biología Molecular-Facultad de Medicina, IBiS/Hospital Universitario Virgen del Rocio/CSIC/Universidad de Sevilla, Avda. Manuel Siurot s/n, Sevilla, 41013, Spain
e-mail: plardone@us.es; nalvarez-ibis@us.es; rodriguezana13m@gmail.com; guerrero@us.es; vico@us.es

V. Srinivasan et al. (eds.), *Melatonin and Melatonergic Drugs in Clinical Practice*,
DOI 10.1007/978-81-322-0825-9_8,

by Aaron Lerner et al. [2] in an attempt to isolate the pineal factor responsible for skin lightening of amphibians, previously described by McCord and Allen in 1917. Two events helped to consolidate the concept of the pineal gland as an active neuroendocrine organ in mammals. On one hand, Hoffman and Reiter showed that the darkness or short photoperiod induced considerable gonadal changes in the hamster, which could be completely abolished by pinealectomy. On the other hand, Axelrod and Wurtman coined the term "neuroendocrine transducer" to describe the gland as an organ that converts a light-controlled neural stimulus from the retina in an endocrine response, the melatonin production. During recent decades, the numerous and rigorous scientific analyses about the pineal gland and melatonin have changed the line of thought from skepticism and perplexity to one which has gained not only scientific respectability but also a maximum physiological interest.

Melatonin is a highly conserved indoleamine through phylogeny, being present in the same form from bacteria, unicellular eukaryotic organisms, invertebrates and vertebrates, algae, plants, and fungi, as well as in various edibles such as vegetables, fruits, herbs, and seeds [3]. Melatonin is converted in two steps from de amino acid tryptophan into serotonin and then acetylated by arylalkylamine N-acetyltransferase (EC 2.3.1.87; AA-NAT), before finally being converted into melatonin by hydroxyindole-O-methyl transferase (EC 2.1.1.4; HIOMT) [4]. The production and release of melatonin from the pineal gland follow a circadian rhythm with a nocturnal surge and the lowest level on the light phase [5]. This temporal chemical signal is involved in the synchronization of several rhythmic physiological functions, being of remarkable clinical interest in biological processes related to period and phase shifts such as sleep disturbances, jet lag, and shift work [6]. Besides the chronobiotic function, melatonin exerts cytoprotective actions by regulating oxidative stress, apoptosis, and mitochondrial homeostasis [7]. Additionally, the oncostatic [8] and immunomodulatory actions [9–11], among many others, point out the potential clinical relevance of the melatonin.

The mechanisms of action responsible for the pleiotropic effects of melatonin involve two main actions: binding to high-affinity G-protein-coupled receptors at membrane level and/or interaction with intracellular targets modulating signal transduction pathways, redox-modulated processes, or scavenging free radicals [12].

Over the last 20 years, a wide range of studies have identified melatonin in a number of extrapineal locations such as the gastrointestinal tract [13], the skin system [14], the retina and Harderian gland [15]. Original studies have also reported de novo synthesis of melatonin in the immune system (reviewed by [10]).

The immune system responses comprise a complex network of coordinated interactions involving numerous cells, proteins, and molecules to protect the host against nonself agents such as bacterias, viruses, fungi, parasites, or malignant cells which can reach the body. The immune response involves two main types of immunity: the innate or nonspecific and the acquired or specific one. The first includes mechanisms of defense, present even before the occurrence of infection, that exert a quick response and respond against microorganisms with the same way and intensity to repeated infections. This immunity only identifies specific structures shared by related groups of microorganisms, and it is unable to distinguish subtle differences among the recognized substances. The major cellular components of the innate response are macrophages, neutrophils, basophils, eosinophils, and natural killer cells (NK), in addition to various soluble factors such as the cytokines, tumor necrosis factor-alpha (TNF-α), and interleukin (IL)-1β, IL-6, and IL-8. In contrast to the innate response, the specific immunity is very refined with the magnitude of the response increasing each successive exposure to a specific microorganism. T and B lymphocytes are the main components of the specific immunity in addition to circulating proteins such as antibodies and cytokines. Specific immunity consists of humoral and cellular immunity. The first is mediated primarily by antibodies that recognize and bind to extracellular pathogens or nonself molecules, making them targets for destruction by macrophages, among other functions. Cellular immunity acts on intracellular microorganisms, and it is primarily mediated by cytotoxic T lymphocytes (CD8+) (recognize and destroy infected cells) and helper T lymphocytes (Th; CD4+) that are key elements in the regulation and coordination of the innate, humoral, and cellular responses through the production of a large variety of cytokines.

Based on the cytokine milieu, the expression of specific transcription factors, and the pattern of cytokine secretion, Th cells can differentiate mainly into four major phenotypes (Th1, Th2, Th17 (effector phenotypes), and T regulatory (Treg)) which control the excessive response of the effector's lineages. Th1 cells play a key role in the development of inflammatory processes through the production of cytokines such as interferon gamma (IFN-γ). The Th2 cells produce cytokines such as IL-4, IL-5, IL-10, and IL-13, contributing to the regulation of humoral and anti-inflammatory response. Th17 cells, a novel subset of CD4+ T cells, have been mainly identified on the basis of the RORγt transcription factor expression and the production of the IL-17 [16]. The identification of the Th17 phenotype as a member of the complex network of Th cells has reassessed the Th1/Th2 paradigm [17]. Besides the involvement in autoimmunity, Th17 cells eliminate extracellular pathogens and its relevance in inflammatory processes is becoming increasingly apparent. Thus, currently Th1 and Th17 are considered inflammatory responses, while Th2 is considered anti-inflammatory. The description of Treg cells has also updated the field of immunology, due to their remarkable functions controlling the effector cells. These cells represent a unique subpopulation CD4+ cells (mostly CD25+) with the hallmark expression of the transcription factor Foxp3 [18]. The complex modulation of the cellular network which governs the T cell response is performed by cross regulation between the different phenotypes. Thus, an increase in Th1 or Th2 cytokine promotes negative feedback regulation of the opposite phenotype. Moreover, the inflammatory (Th1/Th17) and anti-inflammatory/regulatory (Th2/Treg) differentiation is mutually exclusive [19].

Pineal-Immune Interconnection: A Bidirectional Circuit

Both the pineal gland and melatonin are constituent members of the neuroendocrine-immune system. In this line, surgical or functional pinealectomy induces regression and abnormal development in lymphoid organs [20, 21]. Pineal inactivation also promotes disturbances in the different branches of the immunity, from the innate [21, 22] to cellular and humoral [23, 24] response. The administration of melatonin to pinealectomized animals reestablished the immune competence [25, 26], highlighting the key role of the indoleamine in the pineal-mediated immune actions. Additionally, the synchronization between the melatonin production and circadian and seasonal rhythms in the immune system reinforces the pineal-immune relationship. In this regard, it is generally accepted that short photoperiods are associated with immune activation in rodents [27–30]. Seasonal variations in the immune modulatory action of melatonin have also been described in humans where daily administration of melatonin over a period of 4 years enhanced the antibody-dependent cell-mediated cytotoxicity (ADCC) in summer, but not in winter [31].

On the other hand, the pineal gland is a target for immune compounds. Thus, IFN-γ, IL-1β, granulocyte colony-stimulating factors (G-CSF), and granulocyte-macrophage colony-stimulating factor (GM-CSF) modulate the production of melatonin by the pineal gland [10]. Additionally, immune conditions such as immunization and peritonitis promote decreased production of melatonin [32, 33]. In concordance, a series of reports have suggested that inflammation acts as a negative marker on melatonin production [34–40].

The immune system is also considered one of the extrapineal sources of melatonin. The classical works from Finocchiaro et al., highlighting that human peripheral blood mononuclear cells are a putative source of melatonin [41, 42] were followed by the studies of Tan et al. and Conti et al. that identified the presence of NAT and HIOMT activities together with high concentrations of melatonin in bone marrow of rats [43], mice, and humans [44]. Rat peritoneal macrophages are also able to produce melatonin after *in vitro* incubation with tryptophan [45]. Additionally, melatonin has been identified in a wide range of immune organs and cells [46–49]. The relevant effect of melatonin on the control of IL-2/IL-2 receptor (IL-2R) has been highlighted in a series of works published by us reaching the general conclusion that endogenously synthesized melatonin is needed for a suitable stimulation of PBMC and T lymphocytes [49–52].

An important fact which also supports the relationship of melatonin with the immune system is the presence of melatonin receptors in a wide variety of organs and immune cells of many species of mammals and birds. Currently, there are enough evidences to affirm that melatonin not only interacts with membrane and intracellular targets but also this interaction mediates important regulatory effects of melatonin on the immune system (extensively reviewed in [53].

Effects of Melatonin Administration on the Immune Response

The immunomodulatory ability of melatonin is undeniable; nevertheless, the actions of melatonin are highly dependent on the immune conditions tested. Overall, melatonin increases the weight and cellularity of lymphoid organs from normal or immunodepressed rodents [54–57]. Moreover, melatonin enhances NK activity [58] and chemotaxis [59] in human immune cells. By the opposite, melatonin counteracts the exacerbated production of inflammatory cytokines, mainly TNF-α, IL-1β, or IL-6, in several experimental models of inflammation such as exercise-induced cardiac injury [60], diabetes-associated low grade of inflammation [61], traumatic brain injury [62], heatstroke-induced multiple organ dysfunction syndrome [63], ischemia-reperfusion-induced liver damage [64], neuroinflammation in experimental diabetic neuropathy [65], cerulean-induced pancreatitis [66], and lung ischemia-reperfusion injury [67], among many others (reviewed by Carrillo-Vico et al. 2013, in press). Furthermore, melatonin reduces the production of inflammatory markers in infants subjected to endotracheal intubation [68], preterm newborns with respiratory distress syndrome [69], and adults under strenuous exercise [70], as well as in Duchenne muscular dystrophy [71]. Despite the diversity of inflammatory conditions tested, the molecular mechanisms of melatonin studied always share the downregulation of the NF-κB activity. This is also underlined by many *in vitro* approaches using the mouse macrophage cell line, Raw 264.7 [72–75].

Melatonin also regulates both cellular and humoral immunity in a similar way that it modulates the innate response. Since Maestroni et al. described that reconstitution of the nighttime peak plasma melatonin completely reverted the abolished humoral and cellular response in propranolol-immunodepressed mice [21], many reports have shown how melatonin restores the humoral and cellular response in several models of immunosuppression induced by chemicals [76, 77], glucocorticoids [56], aging [78, 79], or pinealectomy [26]. Although early *in vitro* studies indirectly pointed to melatonin as a Th1 response inducer compound [80], many subsequent *in vivo* studies have reported the ability of melatonin to suppress the Th1 response in mice contact hypersensitivity [81], experimental reflux esophagitis [82], and experimental ovarian transplant [83]. Additionally, melatonin modulates the hallmark cytokines of Th1/Th2 responses, such as IFN-γ, IL-4, and IL-10, in several models indicating a bias toward Th2 response [84–87]. In concordance, pinealectomy polarized thymocytes toward Th1 response [88]. Interestingly, a preliminary study has suggested the *in vivo* inhibitory action of melatonin on the Treg cell generation in cancer patients [89]. Additionally, the *in vivo* administration of melatonin to murine subjected to experimental cancer by inoculating foregastric carcinoma cell line is associated with downregulation of CD4+CD25+ Treg and the Foxp3 expression in the tumor tissue [90].

Clinical Relevance of the Several Faces of Melatonin on Immunity

Melatonin and Sepsis

Every year, severe sepsis strikes about 750,000 US people [91]. It is the leading cause of death among patients in non-coronary intensive care units (ICU) and the tenth leading cause of death in the USA, killing a 20–50 % of patients with severe sepsis [92]. It is a heterogeneous syndrome consequence of the systemic response to the release of bacterial endotoxins, mainly lipopolysaccharide (LPS), that activate polymorphonuclear cells (PMN), monocytes, and lymphocytes, triggering both cellular and humoral immune responses. The release of cytokines, especially TNF-α, IL-1β, IL-6, IL-12, and IFN-γ, together with the generation of free radicals by PMNs and macrophages infiltrated in the tissues can lead to microvascular dysfunction and organ failure [93].

A large number of studies have highlighted the protective effect of melatonin against septic shock in experimental models [94–98]. Supporting this issue, the exposure to short photoperiods, with the subsequent increase of endogenous melatonin, augments the survival of septic Siberian hamsters and diminishes the TNF-α levels compared to animals exposed to long photoperiods [99].

Melatonin action mechanisms in sepsis are an example of the pleiotropic capacity of the molecule. For example, melatonin blocks the overproduction of proinflammatory cytokines, especially TNF-α, and increases the levels of IL-10 [95, 97, 100, 101]. In addition, melatonin increases the weight of the spleen in endotoxin-septic rats compared with control animals [102] and counteracts sepsis-caused apoptosis in spleen [95]. Moreover, melatonin neutralizes the inflammatory infiltration in different tissues of septic animals [101, 103].

Melatonin beneficial effects are not only confined to the direct modulation on the immune system. In fact, its antioxidant capacity is also responsible for the protective effect of the indoleamine through increasing the total antioxidant capacity [104] and/or reduction of the reactive oxygen species (ROS) and reactive nitrogen species (RNS) production and their deleterious effects on biomolecules in septic rodents [104–106]. Melatonin also protects upon sepsis-induced damage in mitochondria by restoring the impaired mitochondrial antioxidant systems, enhancing both GSH levels and glutathione reductase (GRd) activity, and inhibiting the nitrite formation and the induction of mitochondrial iNOS expression. Besides, melatonin reduces mitochondrial lipid peroxidation from different tissues and decreases sepsis-induced alterations in the activity of the mitochondrial respiratory chain and ATP synthesis [107, 108].

As well as in the most inflammatory conditions tested, melatonin intracellular actions in experimental models of sepsis involve the reduction of NF-κB nuclear translocation [109, 110]. Melatonin also reduces p38 MAPK and poly ADP ribose synthase (PARS) activation which is activated by DNA damage caused by ROS and RNS [109, 111]. The effects of melatonin can be, at least in part, mediated by the binding to its membrane receptors MT1 or MT2, since luzindole blocks melatonin-caused decrease in proinflammatory cytokines [100].

With regard to humans, septic patients hospitalized in the ICUs had an altered circadian rhythm of 6-sulfatoxymelatonin (aMT6) urine excretion, with loss of circadian periodicity, diminished phase amplitude, and delayed acrophase [112], but light exposure in the ICU was not responsible for the impairment in urine aMT6 excretion [113]. Additionally, nocturnal plasmatic melatonin levels inversely correlate with illness severity in ICU patients with severe sepsis [114]. The nocturnal melatonin concentration of septic patients in a state of septic shock was significantly higher than septic patients without septic shock. However, there was no significant difference for nocturnal aMT6 excretion between septic patients, with or without septic shock, and non-septic patients [115]. In a similar study, nocturnal melatonin concentrations of children with sepsis in a septic shock state were significantly higher than those of septic patients without septic shock state. The 24-h aMT6 excretion in septic patients with liver dysfunction was found significantly lower than in septic patients without liver dysfunction [116]. Therefore, the parallel measurement of serum melatonin together with the urine levels of aMT6 would be very convenient data to discard aMT6 disturbances due to hepatic dysfunction. Exogenous melatonin has also been shown to improve the clinical outcome in septic newborns by reducing lipid peroxidation, white cell count, neutrophil count, and C-reactive protein levels [117]. Moreover, melatonin reduces proinflammatory cytokine production (IL-6, IL-8, TNF-α), lipid peroxidation, and nitrite and nitrate levels in newborns suffering from respiratory distress syndrome [69].

Melatonin and Other Infections

Over the last decades, melatonin has been revealed as an important antiviral, antibiotic, and antiparasite molecule [118, 119]. Many authors have described the ability of melatonin to protect against viral infection induced by the Venezuelan equine encephalomyelitis virus (VEEV), a mosquito-borne virus of the family Togaviridae and genus Alphavirus [120]. Outbreaks occurred in northern South America from the 1920s to the 1970s with thousands of people, horses, and donkeys affected and reemerged in 1995 causing mortality of the affected people [121, 122]. The infection with VEEV causes excitation and hypermotility followed by hypomotility, paralysis, coma, and death [123]. A series of experiments carried out in mice infected with the virus demonstrated that the administration of melatonin delays the onset of the disease and reduces mortality by decreasing the viral load in blood and brain. Specifically, melatonin administration in doses of 250, 500, and 1,000 μg/kg to the infected mice reduced the mortality to 45, 40, and 16 %, respectively, compared to 100 % mortality in no melatonin-treated mice.

Melatonin pretreatment also increased the survival rate to 73 % compared to 60 % obtained with 3 days pretreatment standard [124]. Interestingly, melatonin reduced the VEEV levels in the brain of immunocompetent mice but not in immunodepressed mice, suggesting that melatonin requires the integrity of the immune system for the antiviral activity [125]. The melatonin effect was neutralized by anti-IL-1β antibodies suggesting that IL-1β production induced by melatonin treatment is a key factor involved in the rapid viral clearance [126]. In reference to the TNF-α levels, these are increased in an infection of VEEV and the melatonin administration also reduces them, contributing to control the inflammatory response occurring after VEEV infection [127]. In addition, melatonin provides protection against neural lipid peroxidation and the high levels of serum and brain nitrites [128].

Other researchers have studied the effect of melatonin in the infection of the encephalomyocarditis virus (EMCV), a highly pathogenic and aggressive virus that causes encephalitis and myocarditis in rodents. Administration of melatonin prevents paralysis and death in mice infected with sublethal doses of EMCV after acute stress [129]. Furthermore, melatonin also protects mice infected with Semliki forest virus (SFV), a classic encephalitis arbovirus that invades the central nervous system (CNS), from death. Melatonin treatment reduced viremia and significantly postponed the onset of the disease as well as protects SFV-infected mice from death [130]. Melatonin also reduces the mortality in minks infected with the Aleutian mink disease virus (AMDV) which causes a disease characterized by hypergammaglobulinemia due to the high titers of non-neutralizing anti-ADMV antibodies, with lesions in the kidney, liver, lungs, and arteries. The protective action of melatonin seemed to result from melatonin's ability to scavenge free radicals, but it could also be due to the induction of antioxidant enzymes or to the modulation of immunity [131]. Attenuated West Nile virus (WNV) is an encephalitis virus that does not invade the brain in normal conditions. However, under stressful stimulus, the WNV strain WN-25 can induce encephalitis in mice. The immunodepressive effect of stress was prevented by melatonin administration as well as the stress-related encephalitis and death of WN-25-infected mice [130]. The LP-BM5 leukemia retrovirus causes an experimental acquired immune-deficiency syndrome (AIDS). This infection inhibits the release of Th1 cytokines, stimulates the secretion of Th2 cytokines, increases hepatic lipid peroxidation, and induces vitamin E deficiency. Administration of dehydroepiandrosterone (DHEA) or melatonin, alone or in combination, prevents the reduction of B and T cell proliferation and the Th1 cytokine secretion in female C57BL/6 mice infected with the retrovirus [132]. Regarding to the human AIDS caused by immunodeficiency virus type I (HIV-1), a positive correlation between melatonin and IL-12 among the HIV-1 has been shown together with a negative correlation between melatonin and plasma HIV-1 RNA levels. Additionally, the levels of serum melatonin in HIV-1-infected individuals were significantly lower than in healthy controls [133].

Melatonin has been demonstrated as a potent free radical scavenger and antioxidant in a variety of *in vitro* and *in vivo* models of several bacterial infections, where it reduces lipid peroxidation and ROS [103]. Additionally, melatonin has a high metal binding capacity by binding iron, copper, and zinc and thereby reducing their cytoplasmic availability. Since bacteria are strongly dependent on free metals, in particular iron, for growing [134], an agent like melatonin which easily crosses the biological barriers, including bacterial cell wall, has greater importance for restricting iron-dependent bacterial growth [135]. The protective action of melatonin against bacterial infections has been evaluated in cultured medium containing *M. tuberculosis* (H37Rv strain). Addition of melatonin together with isoniazid inhibited the bacterial growth three- to fourfold than the inhibition exerted by both compounds alone. When intracellular bacterial growth was examined in inoculated monocytes, addition of either isoniazid or melatonin alone did not have any effect on macrophage mortality or viability. However, their combination resulted in a marked reduction in bacterial load. The microbicide action of melatonin is attributed to the formation of stable radicals that could modify either the isoniazid action or the binding with mycobacterial cell wall, resulting in destabilization of the cell wall causing enhanced permeability to isoniazid molecules [136]. Studies conducted in patients infected by M. tuberculosis have revealed a reduction in the plasma melatonin levels compared to control subjects. Likewise, the aMT6 level, which constitutes the major hepatic metabolite of melatonin, was lower in patients with tuberculosis than in control patients [137]. Some studies have also highlighted the presence of seasonality in the *M. tuberculosis* infection, with peaks both at the end of winter and at the beginning of the summer season [138, 139]. In this respect, some researchers have proposed that this seasonality might be related to seasonal changes in the immune system caused by annual fluctuations in the melatonin levels [137, 140]. Tryptophan limitation caused by production of IFN-γ by the host and the subsequent induction of indoleamine 2,3-dioxygenase, resulting in the depletion of tryptophan from human cells, is a key aspect of the host-parasite interaction [141, 142]. Therefore, a deficit in melatonin production promoted by tryptophan depletion would be expected. *In vitro* administration of melatonin to three Chlamydiaceae species (*Chlamydia trachomatis, Chlamydophila pneumoniae* and *Chlamydophila felis*) reduces the infection by 50 % compared with controls. The infection reduction was neutralized by pertussis toxin, an inhibitor of G proteins [143], which suggests a membrane receptor-mediated mechanism. An additional study demonstrated the *in vitro* antimicrobial activity of melatonin against multidrug-resistant gram-positive and gram-negative bacteria, methicillin-resistant Staphylococcus aureus, carbapenem-resistant Pseudomonas aeruginosa, and Acinetobacter baumannii [135]. This evidence has a clinical importance because these strains have recently emerged as primary nosocomial pathogens in hospital outbreaks.

Melatonin role in parasite infections has also been studied. In this context, some studies have shown that TNF-α, IFN-γ, and IL-12 are important for the control of *Trypanosoma cruzi* (*T. cruzi*) infection by ensuring the induction of an efficient adaptive host response [144]. These cytokines would stimulate phagocytic cells to destroy internalized parasites, mainly through nitric oxide NO generation which is especially important for the control of parasitism in the early acute phase [145]. A series of studies have reported the protective action of melatonin in experimental models of *T. cruzi* infection. Thus, melatonin reduces the blood parasitemia and the nitrite production by peritoneal macrophages in rats intraperitoneally infected with trypomastigotes of the Y strain of *T. cruzi*. The combination of melatonin and the anti-inflammatory drug meloxicam also promoted an increase in serum levels of IL-2 and IFN-γ [146]. In conjunction with DHEA, melatonin diminished the parasite load in blood and tissue [147]. After *T. cruzi* infection, the thymus, a central lymphoid organ able to generate mature T cells, undergoes a dramatic loss in size, with a consequent reduction in the number of thymocytes. A recent report has described that the combined therapy of zinc and melatonin triggers enhanced thymocyte proliferation in rats inoculated with *T. cruzi* as compared to untreated group of animals [148].

Many studies have demonstrated that *Plasmodium falciparum* (*P. falciparum*), a parasite that colonizes hepatocytes and red blood cells (RBCs) causing the deadly disease malaria, depends on intracellular calcium. Authors have set that melatonin, as well as its precursors derived from the tryptophan catabolism, induces calcium release and modulates the *P. falciparum* cell cycle [149]. Moreover, melatonin induces the ubiquitination of PfNF-YB, a transcription factor involved in *P. falciparum* cell cycle division [150]. Furthermore, melatonin is able of synchronize the *in vitro* life cycle of *P. falciparum* and *P. chabaudi in vitro* through membrane receptor-mediated mechanisms. The synchronization is also abolished *in vivo* by pinealectomy or luzindole injection. Melatonin administration restored the pinealectomy disturbances [151]. Melatonin not only causes a deleterious effect in *P. falciparum* cycle but also has an inhibitory effect on malaria development by inhibiting free radical-mediated hepatocyte apoptosis and liver damage induced by the infection itself [152].

Melatonin and Autoimmunity

Several studies have implicated both endogenous and exogenous melatonin in the development of different autoimmune diseases, including rheumatoid arthritis (RA), multiple sclerosis (MS), systemic lupus erythematosus (SLE), type 1 diabetes (T1D), and inflammatory bowel disease (IBS). However, there are also scarce data about the melatonin relationship with any other autoimmune diseases. In this sense, disturbances in circadian melatonin secretion have been described in psoriatic patients [153]. Melatonin also reduces type II collagen-induced proliferation of lymphocytes from patients with autoimmune hearing loss [154] and exerts protective effects in an experimental model of idiopathic membranous nephropathy, an autoimmune-mediated glomerulonephritis [155].

The effects of melatonin over RA, a common autoimmune disease suffered by approximately 1 % of the world population [156], seem to be controversial. Different studies using experimental models of arthritis suggest a deleterious action of both endogenous and exogenous melatonin. Thus, animals maintained in constant darkness undergo a more severe collagen-induced arthritis, with higher titers of serum anti-collagen antibodies and bigger spleen than those kept in constant light or normal photoperiod. The effect of constant darkness was counteracted by pinealectomy [157, 158]. Furthermore, melatonin administration to mice immunized with rat collagen II kept under constant light promoted a more severe arthritis when it was injected from the beginning of the immunization, whereas melatonin injection at the onset of the disease (days 30–39) did not affect the clinical signs of the disease [159]. An additional study showed a dual effect of melatonin, which increased serum anti-collagen antibodies titers together with IL-1β and IL-6 levels in serum and joints of arthritic rats, while it decreased oxidative markers in serum but not in joints. As expected, pinealectomy effects were opposed, with a reduction in antibodies, cytokine levels, and oxidative stress in joints, but elevated oxidative markers in serum [160]. In contrast to those studies supporting the deleterious effect of melatonin, a prophylactic and/or therapeutic treatment with the indoleamine reduces hind paw swelling in a similar way as indomethacin does in an adjuvant-induced arthritis model [161].

An increased incidence and severity of RA associated with higher latitudes have been showed, suggesting that the augmented melatonin production on long winter nights could be related with RA [162]. Moreover, the risk of arthritis is inversely associated with UV-B exposition [163], a radiation known to reduce the pineal synthesis of melatonin [164]. In addition, the nocturnal levels of melatonin in RA patients from northern Europe (Estonia) are higher than in RA patients from the south (Italy) [165]. RA symptoms get worse in the early morning [162], in parallel to high levels of proinflammatory cytokines and low serum concentration of cortisol [166]. Some authors have also reported a rise in serum melatonin levels at the early morning in RA patients compared with healthy controls, a positive correlation between melatonin levels and the disease activity scores, and an advance in the nocturnal peak of melatonin compared to control subjects [165, 167, 168]. However, other authors found significant lower plasmatic levels of melatonin in the RA patients [169] and increased nocturnal pineal production of melatonin induced by Freund's adjuvant in an experimental model of arthritis [170]. Supporting the melatonin action in RA, *in vitro* cultured RA synovial macrophages have high-affinity binding sites for melatonin [171] and produce high levels of IL-12 and NO after melatonin administration [172]. Additionally, synovial fluid from RA patients has relatively high levels of melatonin [171]. In the opposite sense, melatonin inhibits the excessive proliferation of RA fibroblast-like synoviocytes through the activation of the cyclin-dependent kinase inhibitors, P21 (CIP1) and P27 (KIP1), mediated by ERK [173]. Fibroblasts from synovial membranes collected from RA patients also show impaired circadian expression of timekeeping genes and proinflammatory cytokines such as TNF-α, IL-1β, and IL-6 [174]. Interestingly, a study conducted in 75 RA patients with active disease receiving daily melatonin at night during 6 months showed a slow antioxidant profile in patients, increased concentration of the erythrocyte sedimentation rate and neopterin (inflammation indicators), and no changes in pro-inflammatory cytokines (TNF-α, IL-1β, and IL-6), but these effects were not associated with any change of clinical symptoms [175].

MS is the most common neurological disease in young adults, with a worldwide prevalence of 1.1–2.5 million cases [176] and an increasing global incidence, primarily in middle-aged women. It is a progressive neurodegenerative disorder triggered by an autoimmune response against myelin [177]. Although the etiology of MS is not currently fully understood, one of the environmental factors that seems to be implicated is the latitude, since the prevalence of the disease increases in northern countries [178]. This has been associated with a reduction in daylight exposure [179, 180], because of the prevalence diminishes in mountainous areas with respect to neighboring lower areas [181]. Recently, shift work at young age has also been associated with increased incidence of MS, with a positive correlation between risk of MS and duration of shift work [182].

Although epidemiologic studies might indirectly suggest a detrimental effect of melatonin over MS, studies using the experimental autoimmune encephalomyelitis (EAE) model have reported contradictory results. Although luzindole administration [183] and constant light exposition [184] suppress EAE, pinealectomy shows an age-dependent effect on EAE. While pinealectomized newborn rats undergo extensive pathological damages and severe neurological deficit after EAE induction, pinealectomized adult rats are protected against the development of EAE [185]. Moreover, melatonin administration reduces both the severity and the duration of EAE-induced paralysis in rats through diminishing macrophage, CD4+ and CD8+ T cell infiltration in the spinal cord, as well as ICAM-1 expression in the blood vessels close to EAE lesions [186].

MS patients show impaired circadian rhythms of both melatonin and aMT6. A high percentage of patients with exacerbated MS displayed an inverse circadian rhythm of melatonin [187]. MS patients also showed alterations in aMT6 urine excretion, with lower total urine aMT6 levels than healthy controls, and a significant reduction in the night excretion of the metabolite compared to control subjects. It was normalized by IFN-β treatment [188]. A recent study has found associations between single-nucleotide polymorphisms (SNP) in two genes involved in melatonin synthesis and signaling and the risk of suffering progressive subtypes of MS in a high-risk Finnish population. The allele T of a SNP in the promoter region of tryptophan hydroxylase 2 (TPH2) was related with a higher risk of progressive MS. Moreover, a haplotype including this SNP was found to be associated with a higher risk of secondary progressive MS in males and also with disability in progressive subtypes of MS. On the other hand, two haplotypes in MTNR1B, the MT2 encoding gene, were associated with increased risk of primary or secondary progressive MS [189]. Besides melatonin actions over the course of the disease, endogenous melatonin has been related to the clinical complications of MS. Thus, serum melatonin levels inversely correlate with depression in MS patients [190]. Additionally, diurnal vision impairment related to MS was shown to be linked to melatonin circadian rhythm, and more importantly, it was improved by oral treatment with melatonin [191].

SLE is a multifactorial autoimmune disorder with a yearly incidence of 1–10 new cases per 100,000 people and an estimated prevalence around 20–150 cases per 100,000 people. The hallmark of the SLE is the formation of immune complexes in blood and tissues which cause extensive tissular damage [192]. Regarding melatonin and lupus, an uncoupling in the circadian rhythm has been described in lupus-prone mice [193]. However, melatonin levels and seasonal light variations show no association with disease activity in SLE patients from a subarctic region [194]. Melatonin administration exerts contradictory effects in murine models of SLE, being beneficial or deleterious depending on different parameters, as the timing of the administration and the gender of the animals. Melatonin administered in the morning increased the survival of lupus-prone animals, although the effect was not reproduced with evening treatment [195]. On the other hand, melatonin has been shown to be beneficial in female mice, reducing vascular lesions and inflammatory infiltration in kidneys, diminishing the titers of anti-collagen II and anti-dsDNA autoantibodies, lowering the production of proinflammatory cytokines, and augmenting the release of anti-inflammatory cytokines both in lupus-prone animals [196] and in pristane-induced lupus [197]. However, melatonin had no effect or even worsened the disease in male lupus-prone mice [196].

T1D is an autoimmune disease where the immune response destroys the pancreatic β-cells, causing a fall in insulin. Although it only accounts for 5–10 % of all cases of diabetes, its incidence is rising worldwide [198]. As most of autoimmune pathologies, a latitudinal gradient of T1D incidence has been shown, with cases increasing with latitude. It has been proposed that this relationship is associated with UV exposure and vitamin D levels [199], although melatonin involvement cannot be ruled out. Interestingly, low levels of insulin in experimental models of T1D correlate with an increased production of melatonin which is normalized by insulin administration [200, 201]. Pinealectomy of newborn nonobese diabetic (NOD) mice, a mouse model of T1D, diminishes survival significantly and induces glycosuria, whereas chronic administration of melatonin increases survival and delays the onset of the disease, maintaining normal plasmatic glucose levels [202]. Moreover, melatonin reduces proliferation of splenocytes and Th1 cells, prolonging the survival of pancreatic islet grafts in NOD mice [203]. Melatonin is not only useful for preventing the development of T1D, but it also shows protective effects against the main complication of the disease, cardiovascular disease, since it improves vascular contractile performance in diabetic rats [204] and reduces blood pressure in T1D adolescents [205].

The irritable bowel syndrome (IBS) is a functional gastrointestinal disorder associated with visceral hypersensitivity and abnormal gastrointestinal motor functions [206], whereas inflammatory bowel disease (IBD) is a group of inflammatory diseases that includes ulcerative colitis and Crohn's disease, in which both innate and adaptive immune responses seem to be implicated [207]. The relation between impaired melatonin synthesis and secretion with IBS has been suggested since urinary levels of aMT6 are lower in IBS patients than in healthy controls [208]. In the knowledge that altered melatonin levels play a role for the disease, some clinical trials have demonstrated beneficial effects of the molecule, reducing abdominal pain and distention [209, 210] and improving rectal sensibility, IBS scores, and quality of life [211, 212]. Circadian rhythmicity impairment has also been shown to be related with IBD course in experimental models. Thus, mice subjected to continuous changes in light/darkness cycle or sleep deprivation undergo a more severe colitis, with increased loss of weight and mortality, compared with control animals [213]. Furthermore, melatonin promotes favorable effects on several experimental models of colitis in rodents. It reduces visceral hyperalgia [214] and diminishes disease severity [215, 216] by acting as a radical scavenger [217], reducing lipid peroxidation and nitrosative stress [216, 218], and protecting endogenous antioxidants from depletion [219]. Moreover, melatonin modulates the immune attack to the colonic mucosa through regulating macrophage [220] and matrix metalloproteinase (MMP)-2 and MMP-9 activities [221], as well as by suppressing iNOS and cyclooxygenase (COX)-2 activities [218], proinflammatory cytokine levels [219, 222], and adhesion molecules [223]. Intracellular actions such as NF-κB inhibition and c-Jun activation have also been related with the effects of melatonin over colitis [222, 223].

Although available data regarding melatonin treatment in experimental models of colitis suggest a positive effect, to date no clinical trials have been conducted on the action of melatonin on IBD. Only three case reports have been published with different results. While melatonin treatment caused the disappearance of the clinical symptoms, which recurred when melatonin consumption was stopped, in a patient suffering from ulcerative colitis [224], the other two cases, one ulcerative colitis patient and another with Crohn's disease, experienced an exacerbation of the diseases, which remitted after stopping melatonin intake [225, 226].

Immunological Aspects of Melatonin in Cancer

Among the various functions attributed to melatonin in the control of the immune system, antitumor defense assumes a primary role. Melatonin has been demonstrated to inhibit tumor development under both *in vivo* and *in vitro* conditions. The oncostatic effects have been observed for a variety of tumor cells like breast carcinoma, ovarian carcinoma, endometrial carcinoma, human uveal melanoma cells, prostate tumor cells, and gastrointestinal tumors (reviewed by [227]). The anticarcinogenic effect of melatonin on neoplastic cells relies on its antioxidant, immunostimulating, and apoptotic properties [228]. Studies carried out in knockout mice have shown the important role of the immune system in the control of the spontaneous generation of tumors. Nearly 50 % of aged IFN-γ–/– or perforin–/– mice developed lymphomas, lung adenocarcinoma, or sarcoma [229].

In addition to stimulating the production of several cytokines that regulate immune function [10, 11], melatonin enhances immune function by direct stimulation of polymorphonuclear cells, macrophages, NK cells, and lymphocytes [55]. Recently, considerable attention has been focused on the effect of melatonin on CD4+ cells. These cells secrete IFN-γ and TNF-α that activate and regulate the cytotoxic T cell response. Melatonin treatment has been found to augment CD4+ cells in lymph nodes of rats [230]. The Th1 cells directly kill tumor cells in lymph nodes by releasing cytokines which activate "death receptors" on the tumor cell surface. Because NK cells are effective against a variety of tumors, especially leukemias and lymphomas, the regulation of NK cell activity and the enhancement of the cytolytic function of NK cells by melatonin [231] have considerable significance for possible therapeutic applications. Additionally, melatonin protects hematopoietic precursors from the toxic effect of anticancer chemotherapeutic drugs [232]. The use of adjuvant immunotherapy is an efficient method of diminishing the harmful effects associated with the systemic delivery of pharmacological doses of cytokines [233]. This evidence provided the base for the therapeutic use of melatonin as an adjuvant in combination with myelotoxic anticancer therapeutic protocols. In relation to this, melatonin protects against IL-2 toxicity and synergizes with IL-2 anticancer action in a variety of tumor types [234]. This combined strategy constitutes a novel and well-tolerated form of intervention to control tumor growth. In most patients, both performance status and quality of life are improved [235]. In this line, melatonin administration along with IL-2 and naltrexone in patients with untreatable metastatic melanoma increased Th-1 and suppressed Th-2 responses, a reportedly favorable result in anticancer treatment [236–239]. In accordance with these results, patients with IL-2 resistant advanced neoplasms responded to IL-2 therapy after the concomitant administration of melatonin [240, 241]. Patients who received both IL-2 and melatonin exhibited a significantly higher number of T lymphocytes, NK cells, and CD4+ cells than those receiving IL-2 alone. Another study using IL-2 along with melatonin and cisplatin demonstrated that it was the most effective immunotherapeutic way for treating metastatic melanoma [242]. Melatonin not only inhibited tumor growth but also suppressed significantly the toxicity of chemotherapeutic drugs and potentiated their anticancer cytotoxicity. Clinical results show that circulating melatonin tends to be depressed in patients with primary tumors of different histological types including both endocrine-dependent (mammary, endometrial, prostate cancer) and endocrine-independent tumors (lung, gastric, colorectal cancer) [207, 243]. This phenomenon appears to be transient, since patients with recidives show a normalization of melatonin [244]. However, surgical removal of the primary tumor does not lead to normalization, indicating that complex systemic changes appear to be involved in melatonin downregulation.

Melatonin in Vaccination

Vaccines are a successful attempt to establish or improve immunity to a particular disease, and thereby there is an increasing interest in improving the performance of existing vaccines. The immune-promoting activity of vaccination is determined not only by the particular antigenic component but also by the addition of suitable adjuvants capable of activating and promoting an efficient immune response against the infectious agents. Based on the immunoregulatory properties of melatonin, some *in vivo* studies have explored the use of melatonin as a vaccine agent. Thus, melatonin increased humoral response of sheeps vaccinated against *Dichelobacter nodosus* [245], the bacteria that causes ovine foot rot, a major cause of lameness in sheep [246]. The administration of melatonin was developed through subcutaneous slow-release implants (18 mg/animal following 21 days of the first dose of vaccine), and the enhancer effect on antibody titers was synergized with aluminum hydroxide. The same effect was found with a double dose of melatonin after which the titer of antibodies and the IgG levels were notably increased comparing to untreated vaccinated animals [247]. The administration of melatonin either via implants or injections also enhanced the platelet response to thrombin stimulation improving the percentage and rate of aggregation and lag time [248]. This effect was likely mediated by enhancement of thrombin-evoked Ca2+ mobilization, especially Ca2+ entry from the extracellular medium. The beneficial effect of melatonin on the immune response to vaccination against *Clostridium perfringens* type D in sheeps has also been described [249]. Interestingly, the highest increase in serum antibody levels caused by melatonin was observed when vaccination took place prepartum, suggesting that the time of immunization plays an important role in the effect of melatonin on the immune response. The powerful immune response originated after the administration of melatonin implants might be explained through two primary mechanisms: on one hand, melatonin could effectively augment the antibody response by enhancing antigen presentation to immunocompetent cells [11, 250]. On the other hand, melatonin could modulate cytokines production at the beginning of the immune response and, therefore, establishes an important cellular control. The potential role of melatonin as adjuvant has also been suggested in the use of vaccines developed against prostate cancer [251], but no study showing its effects has been published to date.

The goal of the immunization program should not only be restricted to protect from infection but also should modulate the pathology inflicted by the agent. In relation to this, melatonin administration with different immunization regimens using some *Schistosoma mansoni* antigens in hamster with schistosomiasis was evaluated [252]. Melatonin provided an excellent enhancement for the vaccine action of cercarial and soluble worm antigens, which was accompanied by a significant improvement in GSH levels. Melatonin also protected inflammation associated with Aβ vaccination [253], suggesting it can be also an effective adjuvant in the development of vaccination in immunotherapy for Alzheimer's disease (AD). Thus, the immune cell functions are strongly influenced by the antioxidant/oxidant balance, and, therefore, the antioxidant levels in these cells play a pivotal role in protecting them from oxidative stress and preserving their adequate function. The immunoregulatory and antioxidant properties of melatonin were also evidenced in an open-field vaccination procedure in sheep [254]. In this study, the coadministration of melatonin with the foot rot vaccine neutralized the rise of serum NO found in vaccinated animals. This effect could be explained by the direct reaction of melatonin on NO, or even by its known inhibitory action in the NOS expression and/or activity.

Immunological Aspects of Melatonin in Transplantation

To our knowledge, all the studies in experimental models of perfused organ transplantation have shown beneficial effects of melatonin on prolonging graft survival. Thus, melatonin treatment (200 mg/kg) inhibited immune responses to the allograft by reducing the lymphocyte proliferation capacity, preventing rejection and doubling allograft survival in a rat cardiac transplant model [255]. Similar protective effects were found in lungs with reperfusion injury after prolonged ischemia [256]. High-dose melatonin treatment significantly prolonged islet graft survival in the NOD mice by inhibiting the proliferation of T cells and the proportion of Th1 cells as well as elevating the percentage of IL-10-producing CD4 T cells [203]. The immunosuppressive effect of melatonin supplementation was also evident in a model of autologous intraperitoneal ovary transplantation in rats [257]. In line with this finding, a recent study reported a reduction in apoptosis of human ovarian grafts in melatonin-treated hosts [258]. Besides the anti-apoptotic and antioxidant properties of melatonin, another potential mechanism by which melatonin can exert beneficial effects following transplantation is the inhibition of cellular damage caused by surgical stress and ischemia-reperfusion injury (IRI). This has been demonstrated in animal models of hepatic IRI, where melatonin supplementation exerted a protective effect on the liver [259]. Specifically, melatonin reduced neutrophil recruitment, increased GSH, and decreased oxidative substances. Furthermore, the number of apoptotic cells was reduced after melatonin administration [260]. Therefore, the sum of the pleiotropic actions of melatonin may reduce graft immunogenicity following transplantation, directly improving clinical outcome. The usefulness of melatonin as an additive for increasing the quality of organ preservation solution has also been described. In a recent study, the addition of melatonin to Institute Georges Lopez (IGL-1) solution improved non-steatotic and steatotic liver graft preservation, limiting their risk against cold IRI [261]. The melatonin benefits correlated with the generation of NO (through constitutive endothelial NOS activation) and the prevention of oxidative stress and inflammatory cytokine release, including TNF-α and adiponectin. Recently, melatonin was used as one of the substances of a multidrug donor preconditioning (MDDP) which improved liver preservation and completely prevented hepatic reperfusion injury [262, 263]. This MDDP protection was provided by anti-oxidative, anti-inflammatory, and anti-apoptotic actions. The immunosuppressive potential of melatonin is also evident since immune suppressive maintenance therapy with cyclosporin a increased melatonin midnight levels [264].

Melatonin and Immunosenescence

Aging is a complex physiological process that involves a number of biochemical reactions, with molecular changes manifested in single cells as well as in the whole organism [265]. It reflects the totality progressive changes in several key physiological systems including the immune system, which is continuously remodeled over the life course, a process known as immunosenescence. Many age-related pathological conditions are directly associated with immunosenescence such as increased susceptibility to infectious diseases, neoplasias, metabolic diseases, osteoporosis, and autoimmune diseases [266]. It is interesting to note that many hormones that are associated with immune function maintenance also decline with advancing age, and the interrelationship between the endocrine system and the immune system is considered crucial of importance in normal human physiology and in mediating age-associated degenerative diseases [267, 268]. The decline in the production of a number of hormones associated with aging, such as melatonin, has been proposed to play a significant role in contributing to immunosenescence [267]. The decline of melatonin with age has been repeatedly reported [269–273], and it usually overlaps with the age-related impairment of the immune system.

Although there are many studies showing the immunomodulatory properties of melatonin, there is a lack of investigations relevant to immunosenescence where the experimental data show that melatonin exerts immunoenhancing action. Related to aging, the administration of melatonin to normal or immunocompromised mice elevated *in vitro* and *in vivo* antibody responses [235]. The severe loss of thymocytes with age is the main cause of structural thymic atrophy and thymic weight loss. According to this, melatonin administration rejuvenated degenerated thymus and redressed peripheral immune dysfunctions in aged mice [274].

In elegant, but controversial, studies of Pierpaoli's group, implantation of pineal glands from young donors into the thymus of aging recipients increased their life span [275]. Moreover, pineal grafted aged mice displayed a remarkable maintenance of thymic structure and cellularity. Pineal grafting, as well as melatonin treatment, resulted in a significant maintenance of a vigorous immunological response expressing cell-mediated transplantation immunity, as measured by a delayed-type hypersensitivity response to oxazolone [276].

This reversal of age-related thymic involution by melatonin could be attributable to increments in thymic cellularity caused by its anti-apoptotic and proliferative-enhancing effects [277]. The antioxidant ability of melatonin and its metabolites may also account for its anti-apoptotic actions on immune cells [278, 279]. In fact, melatonin is able to delay endoplasmic reticulum stress-induced apoptosis in aged leukocytes and may counteract, at the cellular level, age-related degenerative phenomena linked to oxidative stress [280]. In the same way, the age-related increase of oxidative load was reverted by melatonin, improving the general immunity in golden hamster [281]. In another study, injections of melatonin restored immune functions in experimentally immunodepressed or aging mice. Thus, melatonin was able to enhance the antibody response to a T-dependent antigen. Moreover, the enhancement of antibody response was associated with increased induction of T helper cell activity and IL-2 production [282].

In addition, an inhibitory influence of melatonin on immune parameters has also been demonstrated. Thus, melatonin has been shown to inhibit the production of proinflammatory cytokines, suggesting that the indoleamine may help to reduce acute and chronic inflammation. Indeed, melatonin was able to reduce inflammation in livers of senescence-accelerated prone mice (SAMP8) by decreasing mRNA and protein expression of TNF-α and IL-1β and increasing IL-10 [283].

Similar data were also obtained in 24-month-old rats where melatonin significantly reduced proinflammatory cytokines TNF-α, IL-1β, and IL-6 in the liver [84]. The immunomodulatory effects of melatonin in aging were also evident in the CNS, since dietary melatonin selectively reversed the lack of response to an inflammatory stimulus in the brain of aged mice [284].

Based on the experimental data that have accumulated and considering its lack of toxicity [285], high lipophilicity, and the huge capacity to prevent cell damage [286], melatonin is one of the most appealing agents to be examined in relation to age-associated deterioration in the immune system and should be considered as a potential agent to improve the quality of life in a rapidly aging population.

Conclusion

Over the present chapter, we have highlighted the pleiotropic effects of melatonin on the immune system. Despite the large number of reports pointing out melatonin as an immunomodulatory compound, the exact way by which melatonin regulates immunity still remains uncertain. While some reports support that melatonin is an immunoenhancer agent, in many other studies, anti-inflammatory actions have been described. Bearing in mind the hundreds of papers relating melatonin and the immune system, we support the idea of melatonin as an immune buffer, acting on basal or immunosuppression situations as a stimulator or being an anti-inflammatory compound against exacerbated immune responses as acute inflammation. The future implementation of working models, such as melatonin knockout animals or highly specific monoclonal antibodies, will allow determining the scope of the pathophysiological role of melatonin to tackle more ambitious clinical trials.

Acknowledgments The authors are grateful for financial support from the Instituto de Salud Carlos III, Ministerio de Economía y Competitividad (PI07/90175, RD06/0013/0001, and RD12/0043/0012), the PAIDI Program from the Andalusian Government (CTS160), and the Regional Government Ministry of Health (PI-0209-2010).

References

1. Carrillo Vico A, Guerrero JM, Lardone PJ. A wide range of melatonin actions in the immune system. In: Melatonin: present and future. New York: Nova Science Publishers, Inc; 2007. p. 59–87.
2. Lerner AB, Case JD, Takahashi Y, Lee TH, Mori V. Isolation of melatonin, the pineal factor that lightens melanocytes. J Am Chem Soc. 1958;80(10):2587.
3. Hardeland R, Poeggeler B. Non-vertebrate melatonin. J Pineal Res. 2003;34(4):233–41.
4. Axelrod J, Weissbach H. Enzymatic O-methylation of N-acetylserotonin to melatonin. Science. 1960; 131(3409):1312.
5. Zawilska JB, Skene DJ, Arendt J. Physiology and pharmacology of melatonin in relation to biological rhythms. Pharmacol Rep. 2009;61(3):383–410.
6. Rajaratnam SM, Arendt J. Health in a 24-h society. Lancet. 2001;358(9286):999–1005.
7. Hardeland R, Cardinali DP, Srinivasan V, Spence DW, Brown GM, Pandi-Perumal SR. Melatonin–a pleiotropic, orchestrating regulator molecule. Prog Neurobiol. 2011;93(3):350–84.
8. Cutando A, Lopez-Valverde A, Arias-Santiago S, DE Vicente J, DE Diego RG. Role of melatonin in cancer treatment. Anticancer Res. 2012;32(7):2747–53.
9. Radogna F, Diederich M, Ghibelli L. Melatonin: a pleiotropic molecule regulating inflammation. Biochem Pharmacol. 2010;80(12):1844–52.
10. Carrillo-Vico A, Guerrero JM, Lardone PJ, Reiter RJ. A review of the multiple actions of melatonin on the immune system. Endocrine. 2005;27(2):189–200.
11. Carrillo-Vico A, Reiter RJ, Lardone PJ, Herrera JL, Fernandez-Montesinos R, Guerrero JM, et al. The modulatory role of melatonin on immune responsiveness. Curr Opin Investig Drugs. 2006;7(5):423–31.
12. Hardeland R, Madrid JA, Tan DX, Reiter RJ. Melatonin, the circadian multioscillator system and health: the need for detailed analyses of peripheral melatonin signaling. J Pineal Res. 2012;52(2): 139–66.
13. Bubenik GA. Gastrointestinal melatonin: localization, function, and clinical relevance. Dig Dis Sci. 2002; 47(10):2336–48.
14. Slominski A, Wortsman J, Tobin DJ. The cutaneous serotoninergic/melatoninergic system: securing a place under the sun. FASEB J. 2005;19(2):176–94.
15. Iuvone PM, Tosini G, Pozdeyev N, Haque R, Klein DC, Chaurasia SS. Circadian clocks, clock networks, arylalkylamine N-acetyltransferase, and melatonin in the retina. Prog Retin Eye Res. 2005;24(4): 433–56.
16. Miossec P, Korn T, Kuchroo VK. Interleukin-17 and type 17 helper T cells. N Engl J Med. 2009;361(9): 888–98.
17. Steinman L. A brief history of T(H)17, the first major revision in the T(H)1/T(H)2 hypothesis of T cell-mediated tissue damage. Nat Med. 2007;13(2): 139–45.

18. Hong J, Li N, Zhang X, Zheng B, Zhang JZ. Induction of CD4+CD25+ regulatory T cells by copolymer-I through activation of transcription factor Foxp3. Proc Natl Acad Sci U S A. 2005;102(18):6449–54.
19. Bettelli E, Carrier Y, Gao W, Korn T, Strom TB, Oukka M, et al. Reciprocal developmental pathways for the generation of pathogenic effector TH17 and regulatory T cells. Nature. 2006;441(7090):235–8.
20. Vaughan MK, Reiter RJ. Transient hypertrophy of the ventral prostate and coagulating glands and accelerated thymic involution following pinealectomy in the mouse. Tex Rep Biol Med. 1971;29(4):579–86.
21. Maestroni GJ, Conti A, Pierpaoli W. Role of the pineal gland in immunity. Circadian synthesis and release of melatonin modulates the antibody response and antagonizes the immunosuppressive effect of corticosterone. J Neuroimmunol. 1986;13(1):19–30.
22. del Gobbo V, Libri V, Villani N, Calio R, Nistico G. Pinealectomy inhibits interleukin-2 production and natural killer activity in mice. Int J Immunopharmacol. 1989;11(5):567–73.
23. Haldar C, Singh R. Pineal modulation of thymus and immune function in a seasonally breeding tropical rodent. Funambulus pennanti. J Exp Zool. 2001; 289(2):90–8.
24. Beskonakli E, Palaoglu S, Aksaray S, Alanoglu G, Turhan T, Taskin Y. Effect of pinealectomy on immune parameters in rats with Staphylococcus aureus infection. Neurosurg Rev. 2001;24(1):26–30.
25. Rai S, Haldar C. Pineal control of immune status and hematological changes in blood and bone marrow of male squirrels (Funambulus pennanti) during their reproductively active phase. Comp Biochem Physiol C Toxicol Pharmacol. 2003;136(4):319–28.
26. Moore CB, Siopes TD. Melatonin can produce immunoenhancement in Japanese quail (Coturnix coturnix japonica) without prior immunosuppression. Gen Comp Endocrinol. 2002;129(2):122–6.
27. Vaughan MK, Vaughan GM, Reiter RJ. Effect of ovariectomy and constant dark on the weight of reproductive and certain other organs in the female vole. Microtus montanus. J Reprod Fertil. 1973;32(1):9–14.
28. Haldar C, Ahmad R. Photoimmunomodulation and melatonin. J Photochem Photobiol B. 2010;98(2): 107–17.
29. Nelson RJ. Seasonal immune function and sickness responses. Trends Immunol. 2004;25(4):187–92.
30. Haldar C, Haussler D, Gupta D. Response of CFU-GM (colony forming units for granulocytes and macrophages) from intact and pinealectomized rat bone marrow to murine recombinant interleukin-3 (rIl-3), recombinant granulocyte-macrophage colony stimulating factor (rGM-CSF) and human recombinant erythropoietin (rEPO). Prog Brain Res. 1992;91:323–5.
31. Giordano M, Vermeulen M, Palermo MS. Seasonal variations in antibody- dependent cellular cytotoxicity regulation by melatonin. FASEB J. 1993;7(11): 1052–4.
32. Markowska M, Bialecka B, Ciechanowska M, Koter Z, Laskowska H, Karkucinska-Wieckowska A, et al. Effect of immunization on nocturnal NAT activity in chicken pineal gland. Neuro Endocrinol Lett. 2000; 21(5):367–73.
33. Piesiewicz A, Kedzierska U, Adamska I, Usarek M, Zeman M, Skwarlo-Sonta K, et al. Pineal arylalkylamine N-acetyltransferase (Aanat) gene expression as a target of inflammatory mediators in the chicken. Gen Comp Endocrinol. 2012;179(2):143–51.
34. Fernandes PA, Cecon E, Markus RP, Ferreira ZS. Effect of TNF-alpha on the melatonin synthetic pathway in the rat pineal gland: basis for a 'feedback' of the immune response on circadian timing. J Pineal Res. 2006;41(4):344–50.
35. Pontes GN, Cardoso EC, Carneiro-Sampaio MM, Markus RP. Injury switches melatonin production source from endocrine (pineal) to paracrine (phagocytes) – melatonin in human colostrum and colostrum phagocytes. J Pineal Res. 2006;41(2):136–41.
36. Pontes GN, Cardoso EC, Carneiro-Sampaio MM, Markus RP. Pineal melatonin and the innate immune response: the TNF-alpha increase after cesarean section suppresses nocturnal melatonin production. J Pineal Res. 2007;43(4):365–71.
37. da Silveira Cruz-Machado S, Carvalho-Sousa CE, Tamura EK, Pinato L, Cecon E, Fernandes PA, et al. TLR4 and CD14 receptors expressed in rat pineal gland trigger NFKB pathway. J Pineal Res. 2010;49(2):183–92.
38. Tamura EK, Fernandes PA, Marcola M, da Silveira Cruz-Machado S, Markus RP. Long-lasting priming of endothelial cells by plasma melatonin levels. PLoS One. 2010;5(11):13958.
39. Carvalho-Sousa CE, da Silveira Cruz-Machado S, Tamura EK, Fernandes PA, Pinato L, Muxel SM, et al. Molecular basis for defining the pineal gland and pinealocytes as targets for tumor necrosis factor. Front Endocrinol (Lausanne). 2011;2:10.
40. da Silveira Cruz-Machado S, Pinato L, Tamura EK, Carvalho-Sousa CE, Markus RP. Glia-pinealocyte network: the paracrine modulation of melatonin synthesis by tumor necrosis factor (TNF). PLoS One. 2012;7(7):40142.
41. Finocchiaro LM, Arzt ES, Fernandez-Castelo S, Criscuolo M, Finkielman S, Nahmod VE. Serotonin and melatonin synthesis in peripheral blood mononuclear cells: stimulation by interferon-gamma as part of an immunomodulatory pathway. J Interferon Res. 1988;8(6):705–16.
42. Finocchiaro LM, Nahmod VE, Launay JM. Melatonin biosynthesis and metabolism in peripheral blood mononuclear leucocytes. Biochem J. 1991; 280:727–31.
43. Tan DX, Manchester LC, Reiter RJ, Qi WB, Zhang M, Weintraub ST, et al. Identification of highly elevated levels of melatonin in bone marrow: its origin and significance. Biochim Biophys Acta. 1999; 1472(1–2):206–14.

44. Conti A, Conconi S, Hertens E, Skwarlo-Sonta K, Markowska M, Maestroni JM. Evidence for melatonin synthesis in mouse and human bone marrow cells. J Pineal Res. 2000;28(4):193–202.
45. Martins Jr E, Ferreira AC, Skorupa AL, Afeche SC, Cipolla-Neto J, Costa Rosa LF. Tryptophan consumption and indoleamines production by peritoneal cavity macrophages. J Leukoc Biol. 2004;75(6):1116–21.
46. Jimenez-Jorge S, Jimenez-Caliani AJ, Guerrero JM, Naranjo MC, Lardone PJ, Carrillo-Vico A, et al. Melatonin synthesis and melatonin-membrane receptor (MT1) expression during rat thymus development: role of the pineal gland. J Pineal Res. 2005;39(1):77–83.
47. Naranjo MC, Guerrero JM, Rubio A, Lardone PJ, Carrillo-Vico A, Carrascosa-Salmoral MP, et al. Melatonin biosynthesis in the thymus of humans and rats. Cell Mol Life Sci. 2007;64(6):781–90.
48. Gomez-Corvera A, Cerrillo I, Molinero P, Naranjo MC, Lardone PJ, Sanchez-Hidalgo M, et al. Evidence of immune system melatonin production by two pineal melatonin deficient mice, C57BL/6 and Swiss strains. J Pineal Res. 2009;47(1):15–22.
49. Lardone PJ, Carrillo-Vico A, Naranjo MC, De Felipe B, Vallejo A, Karasek M, et al. Melatonin synthesized by Jurkat human leukemic T cell line is implicated in IL-2 production. J Cell Physiol. 2006;206(1):273–9.
50. Carrillo-Vico A, Calvo JR, Abreu P, Lardone PJ, Garcia-Maurino S, Reiter RJ, et al. Evidence of melatonin synthesis by human lymphocytes and its physiological significance: possible role as intracrine, autocrine, and/or paracrine substance. FASEB J. 2004;18(3):537–9.
51. Carrillo-Vico A, Lardone PJ, Fernandez-Santos JM, Martin-Lacave I, Calvo JR, Karasek M, et al. Human lymphocyte-synthesized melatonin is involved in the regulation of the interleukin-2/interleukin-2 receptor system. J Clin Endocrinol Metab. 2005; 90(2):992–1000.
52. Lardone PJ, Rubio A, Cerrillo I, Gomez-Corvera A, Carrillo-Vico A, Sanchez-Hidalgo M, et al. Blocking of melatonin synthesis and MT1 receptor impairs the activation of Jurkat T cells. Cell Mol Life Sci. 2010;67(18):3163–72.
53. Carrillo-Vico A, Lardone PJ, Alvarez-Sánchez N, Rodríguez-Rodríguez A, Guerrero JM. Melatonin: buffering the immune system. Int J Mol Sci. 2013; 22:8638–83.
54. Baeza I, Alvarado C, Alvarez P, Salazar V, Castillo C, Ariznavarreta C, et al. Improvement of leucocyte functions in ovariectomised aged rats after treatment with growth hormone, melatonin, oestrogens or phyto-oestrogens. J Reprod Immunol. 2009;80(1–2):70–9.
55. Currier NL, Sun LZ, Miller SC. Exogenous melatonin: quantitative enhancement in vivo of cells mediating non-specific immunity. J Neuroimmunol. 2000;104(2):101–8.
56. Haldar C, Rai S, Singh R. Melatonin blocks dexamethasone-induced immunosuppression in a seasonally breeding rodent Indian palm squirrel. Funambulus pennanti. Steroids. 2004;69(6):367–77.
57. Mori W, Aoyama H, Mori N. Melatonin protects rats from injurious effects of a glucocorticoid, dexamethasone. Jpn J Exp Med. 1984;54(6):255–61.
58. Lissoni P, Marelli O, Mauri R, Resentini M, Franco P, Esposti D, et al. Ultradian chronomodulation by melatonin of a Placebo effect upon human killer cell activity. Chronobiologia. 1986;13(4):339–43.
59. Pena C, Rincon J, Pedreanez A, Viera N, Mosquera J. Chemotactic effect of melatonin on leukocytes. J Pineal Res. 2007;43(3):263–9.
60. Veneroso C, Tunon MJ, Gonzalez-Gallego J, Collado PS. Melatonin reduces cardiac inflammatory injury induced by acute exercise. J Pineal Res. 2009;47(2): 184–91.
61. Agil A, Reiter RJ, Jimenez-Aranda A, Iban-Arias R, Navarro-Alarcon M, Marchal JA, et al. Melatonin ameliorates low-grade inflammation and oxidative stress in young Zucker diabetic fatty rats. J Pineal Res. 2013;54:381–88.
62. Tsai MC, Chen WJ, Tsai MS, Ching CH, Chuang JI. Melatonin attenuates brain contusion-induced oxidative insult, inactivation of signal transducers and activators of transcription 1, and upregulation of suppressor of cytokine signaling-3 in rats. J Pineal Res. 2011;51(2):233–45.
63. Lin XJ, Mei GP, Liu J, Li YL, Zuo D, Liu SJ, et al. Therapeutic effects of melatonin on heatstroke-induced multiple organ dysfunction syndrome in rats. J Pineal Res. 2011;50(4):436–44.
64. Kang JW, Koh EJ, Lee SM. Melatonin protects liver against ischemia and reperfusion injury through inhibition of toll-like receptor signaling pathway. J Pineal Res. 2011;50(4):403–11.
65. Negi G, Kumar A, Sharma SS. Melatonin modulates neuroinflammation and oxidative stress in experimental diabetic neuropathy: effects on NF kappaB and Nrf2 cascades. J Pineal Res. 2011;50(2): 124–31.
66. Jung KH, Hong SW, Zheng HM, Lee HS, Lee H, Lee DH, et al. Melatonin ameliorates cerulein-induced pancreatitis by the modulation of nuclear erythroid 2-related factor 2 and nuclear factor-kappaB in rats. J Pineal Res. 2010;48(3):239–50.
67. Yip HK, Chang YC, Wallace CG, Chang LT, Tsai TH, Chen YL, et al. Melatonin treatment improves adipose-derived mesenchymal stem cell therapy for acute lung ischemia-reperfusion injury. J Pineal Res. 2013;54(2):207–21.
68. Gitto E, Aversa S, Salpietro CD, Barberi I, Arrigo T, Trimarchi G, et al. Pain in neonatal intensive care: role of melatonin as an analgesic antioxidant. J Pineal Res. 2012;52(3):291–5.
69. Gitto E, Reiter RJ, Cordaro SP, La Rosa M, Chiurazzi P, Trimarchi G, et al. Oxidative and inflammatory parameters in respiratory distress syndrome of preterm newborns: beneficial effects of melatonin. Am J Perinatol. 2004;21(4):209–16.

70. Ochoa JJ, Diaz-Castro J, Kajarabille N, Garcia C, Guisado IM, De Teresa C, et al. Melatonin supplementation ameliorates oxidative stress and inflammatory signaling induced by strenuous exercise in adult human males. J Pineal Res. 2011;51(4):373–80.
71. Chahbouni M, Escames G, Venegas C, Sevilla B, Garcia JA, Lopez LC, et al. Melatonin treatment normalizes plasma pro-inflammatory cytokines and nitrosative/oxidative stress in patients suffering from Duchenne muscular dystrophy. J Pineal Res. 2010;48(3):282–9.
72. Deng WG, Tang ST, Tseng HP, Wu KK. Melatonin suppresses macrophage cyclooxygenase-2 and inducible nitric oxide synthase expression by inhibiting p52 acetylation and binding. Blood. 2006;108(2):518–24.
73. Xia MZ, Liang YL, Wang H, Chen X, Huang YY, Zhang ZH, et al. Melatonin modulates TLR4-mediated inflammatory genes through MyD88- and TRIF-dependent signaling pathways in lipopolysaccharide-stimulated RAW264.7 cells. J Pineal Res. 2012;53(4):325–34.
74. Choi EY, Jin JY, Lee JY, Choi JI, Choi IS, Kim SJ. Melatonin inhibits Prevotella intermedia lipopolysaccharide-induced production of nitric oxide and interleukin-6 in murine macrophages by suppressing NF-kappaB and STAT1 activity. J Pineal Res. 2011;50(2):197–206.
75. Huang SH, Cao XJ, Wei W. Melatonin decreases TLR3-mediated inflammatory factor expression via inhibition of NF-kappa B activation in respiratory syncytial virus- infected RAW264.7 macrophages. J Pineal Res. 2008;45(1):93–100.
76. Kim YO, Pyo MY, Kim JH. Influence of melatonin on immunotoxicity of lead. Int J Immunopharmacol. 2000;22(10):821–32.
77. Sirajudeen M, Gopi K, Tyagi JS, Moudgal RP, Mohan J, Singh R. Protective effects of melatonin in reduction of oxidative damage and immunosuppression induced by aflatoxin B1-contaminated diets in young chicks. Environ Toxicol. 2011;26(2):153–60.
78. Akbulut KG, Gonul B, Akbulut H. The effects of melatonin on humoral immune responses of young and aged rats. Immunol Invest. 2001;30(1):17–20.
79. Terron MP, Delgado J, Paredes SD, Barriga C, Reiter RJ, Rodriguez AB. Effect of melatonin and tryptophan on humoral immunity in young and old ringdoves (Streptopelia risoria). Exp Gerontol. 2009; 44(10):653–8.
80. Garcia-Maurino S, Pozo D, Carrillo-Vico A, Calvo JR, Guerrero JM. Melatonin activates Th1 lymphocytes by increasing IL-12 production. Life Sci. 1999; 65(20):2143–50.
81. Majewska M, Zajac K, Zemelka M, Szczepanik M. Influence of melatonin and its precursor L-tryptophan on Th1 dependent contact hypersensitivity. J Physiol Pharmacol. 2007;58 Suppl 6:125–32.
82. Lahiri S, Haldar C. Response of melatonin receptor MT1 in spleen of a tropical Indian rodent, Funambulus pennanti, to natural solar insolation and different photoperiodic conditions. Chronobiol Int. 2009;26(8): 1559–74.
83. Hemadi M, Shokri S, Pourmatroud E, Moramezi F, Khodadai A. Follicular dynamic and immunoreactions of the vitrified ovarian graft after host treatment with variable regimens of melatonin. Am J Reprod Immunol. 2012;67(5):401–12.
84. Kireev RA, Tresguerres AC, Garcia C, Ariznavarreta C, Vara E, Tresguerres JA. Melatonin is able to prevent the liver of old castrated female rats from oxidative and pro-inflammatory damage. J Pineal Res. 2008;45(4):394–402.
85. Kim TH, Jung JA, Kim GD, Jang AH, Ahn HJ, Park YS, et al. Melatonin inhibits the development of 2,4-dinitrofluorobenzene-induced atopic dermatitis-like skin lesions in NC/Nga mice. J Pineal Res. 2009;47(4):324–9.
86. Jaworek J, Szklarczyk J, Jaworek AK, Nawrot-Porabka K, Leja-Szpak A, Bonior J, et al. Protective effect of melatonin on acute pancreatitis. Int J Inflamm. 2012;2012:173675.
87. Raghavendra V, Singh V, Kulkarni SK, Agrewala JN. Melatonin enhances Th2 cell mediated immune responses: lack of sensitivity to reversal by naltrexone or benzodiazepine receptor antagonists. Mol Cell Biochem. 2001;221(1–2):57–62.
88. Kelestimur H, Sahin Z, Sandal S, Bulmus O, Ozdemir G, Yilmaz B. Melatonin- related alterations in Th1/Th2 polarisation in primary thymocyte cultures of pinealectomized rats. Front Neuroendocrinol. 2006;27(1):103–10.
89. Vigore L, Messina G, Brivio F, Fumagalli L, Rovelli F, DIF G, et al. Psychoneuroendocrine modulation of regulatory T lymphocyte system: in vivo and in vitro effects of the pineal immunomodulating hormone melatonin. In Vivo. 2010;24(5):787–9.
90. Liu H, Xu L, Wei JE, Xie MR, Wang SE, Zhou RX. Role of CD4+ CD25+ regulatory T cells in melatonin-mediated inhibition of murine gastric cancer cell growth in vivo and in vitro. Anat Rec (Hoboken). 2011;294(5):781–8.
91. Angus DC, Linde-Zwirble WT, Lidicker J, Clermont G, Carcillo J, Pinsky MR. Epidemiology of severe sepsis in the United States: analysis of incidence, outcome, and associated costs of care. Crit Care Med. 2001;29(7):1303–10.
92. Martin GS, Mannino DM, Eaton S, Moss M. The epidemiology of sepsis in the United States from 1979 through 2000. N Engl J Med. 2003; 348(16):1546–54.
93. Annane D, Bellissant E, Cavaillon JM. Septic shock. Lancet. 2005;365(9453):63–78.
94. Maestroni GJM. Melatonin as a therapeutic agent in experimental endotoxic shock. J Pineal Res. 1996;20(2):84–9.
95. Carrillo-Vico A, Lardone PJ, Naji L, Fernandez-Santos JM, Martin-Lacave I, Guerrero JM, et al. Beneficial pleiotropic actions of melatonin in an experimental model of septic shock in mice: regulation of pro-/anti-inflammatory cytokine network, protection against oxidative damage and anti-apoptotic effects. J Pineal Res. 2005;39(4):400–8.

96. Zhang H, Liu D, Wang X, Chen X, Long Y, Chai W, et al. Melatonin improved rat cardiac mitochondria and survival rate in septic heart injury. J Pineal Res. 2013;55:1–6.
97. Lowes DA, Webster NR, Murphy MP, Galley HF. Antioxidants that protect mitochondria reduce interleukin-6 and oxidative stress, improve mitochondrial function, and reduce biochemical markers of organ dysfunction in a rat model of acute sepsis. Br J Anaesth. 2013;110(3):472–80.
98. Escames G, Lopez LC, Tapias V, Utrilla P, Reiter RJ, Hitos AB, et al. Melatonin counteracts inducible mitochondrial nitric oxide synthase-dependent mitochondrial dysfunction in skeletal muscle of septic mice. J Pineal Res. 2006;40(1):71–8.
99. Prendergast BJ, Hotchkiss AK, Bilbo SD, Kinsey SG, Nelson RJ. Photoperiodic adjustments in immune function protect Siberian hamsters from lethal endotoxemia. J Biol Rhythms. 2003;18(1):51–62.
100. Nava F, Calapai G, Facciola G, Cuzzocrea S, Giuliani G, DeSarro A, et al. Melatonin effects on inhibition of thirst and fever induced by lipopolysaccharide in rat. Eur J Pharmacol. 1997;331(2–3):267–74.
101. Wu J-Y, Tsou M-Y, Chen T H, Chen S-J, Tsao C-M, Wu C-C. Therapeutic effects of melatonin on peritonitis-induced septic shock with multiple organ dysfunction syndrome in rats. J Pineal Res. 2008;45(1):106–16.
102. Reynolds FD, Dauchy R, Blask D, Dietz PA, Lynch D, Zuckerman R. The pineal gland hormone melatonin improves survival in a rat model of sepsis/shock induced by zymosan A. Surgery. 2003;134(3):474–9.
103. Sewerynek E, Melchiorri D, Reiter RJ, Ortiz GG, Lewinski A. Lipopolysaccharide-induced hepatotoxicity is inhibited by the antioxidant melatonin. Eur J Pharmacol. 1995;293(4):327–34.
104. Erbas O, Ergenoglu AM, Akdemir A, Yeniel AÖ, Taskiran D. Comparison of melatonin and oxytocin in the prevention of critical illness polyneuropathy in rats with experimentally induced sepsis. J Surg Res. 2013;183(1):313–20.
105. Crespo E, Macias M, Pozo D, Escames G, Martin M, Vives F, et al. Melatonin inhibits expression of the inducible NO synthase II in liver and lung and prevents endotoxemia in lipopolysaccharide-induced multiple organ dysfunction syndrome in rats. Faseb Journal. 1999;13(12):1537–46.
106. Wu CC, Chiao CW, Hsiao G, Chen A, Yen MH. Melatonin prevents endotoxin- induced circulatory failure in rats. J Pineal Res. 2001;30(3):147–56.
107. Escames G, Lopez LC, Ortiz F, Lopez A, Garcia JA, Ros E, et al. Attenuation of cardiac mitochondrial dysfunction by melatonin in septic mice. FEBS J. 2007;274(8):2135–47.
108. Escames G, Acuna-Castroviejo D, Lopez LC, Tan D-x, Maldonado MD, Sanchez-Hidalgo M, et al. Pharmacological utility of melatonin in the treatment of septic shock: experimental and clinical evidence. J Pharm Pharmacol. 2006;58(9):1153–65.
109. De Filippis D, Iuvone T, Esposito G, Steardo L, Herman AG, Pelckmans PA, et al. Melatonin reverses lipopolysaccharide-induced gastro-intestinal motility disturbances through the inhibition of oxidative stress. J Pineal Res. 2008;44(1):45–51.
110. Shang Y, Xu S-p, Wu Y, Jiang Y-x, Wu Z-y, Yuan S-y, et al. Melatonin reduces acute lung injury in endotoxemic rats. Chin Med J (Engl). 2009;122(12): 1388–93.
111. d'Emmanuele di Villa Bianca R, Marzocco S, Di Paola R, Autore G, Pinto A, Cuzzocrea S, et al. Melatonin prevents lipopolysaccharide-induced hyporeactivity in rat. J Pineal Res. 2004;36(3):146–54.
112. Mundigler G, Delle-Karth G, Koreny M, Zehetgruber M, Steindl-Munda P, Marktl W, et al. Impaired circadian rhythm of melatonin secretion in sedated critically ill patients with severe sepsis. Crit Care Med. 2002;30(3):536–40.
113. Verceles AC, Silhan L, Terrin M, Netzer G, Shanholtz C, Scharf SM. Circadian rhythm disruption in severe sepsis: the effect of ambient light on urinary 6- sulfatoxymelatonin secretion. Intensive Care Med. 2012;38(5):804–10.
114. Perras B, Kurowski V, Dodt C. Nocturnal melatonin concentration is correlated with illness severity in patients with septic disease. Intensive Care Med. 2006;32(4):624–5.
115. Bagci S, Yildizdas D, Horoz OO, Reinsberg J, Bartmann P, Mueller A. Use of nocturnal melatonin concentration and urinary 6-sulfatoxymelatonin excretion to evaluate melatonin status in children with severe sepsis. J Pediatr Endocrinol Metab. 2011;24(11–12):1025–30.
116. Bagci S, Horoz Ö, Yildizdas D, Reinsberg J, Bartmann P, Müller A. Melatonin status in pediatric intensive care patients with sepsis. Pediatr Crit Care Med. 2012;13(2):120–3.
117. Gitto E, Karbownik M, Reiter RJ, Tan DX, Cuzzocrea S, Chiurazzi P, et al. Effects of melatonin treatment in septic newborns. Pediatr Res. 2001; 50(6):756–60.
118. Bagnaresi P, Nakabashi M, Thomas AP, Reiter RJ, Garcia CR. The role of melatonin in parasite biology. Mol Biochem Parasitol. 2012;181(1):1–6.
119. Srinivasan V, Mohamed M, Kato H. Melatonin in bacterial and viral infections with focus on sepsis: a review. Recent Pat Endocr Metab Immune Drug Discov. 2012;6(1):30–9.
120. Calisher CH, Monath TP, Karabatsos N, Trent DW. Arbovirus subtyping: applications to epidemiologic studies, availability of reagents, and testing services. Am J Epidemiol. 1981;114(5):619–31.
121. Bowen GS, Calisher CH. Virological and serological studies of Venezuelan equine encephalomyelitis in humans. J Clin Microbiol. 1976;4(1):22–7.
122. Weaver SC, Salas R, Rico-Hesse R, Ludwig GV, Oberste MS, Boshell J, et al. Re-emergence of epidemic Venezuelan equine encephalomyelitis in South America. VEE Study Group. Lancet. 1996; 348(9025):436–40.

123. Bonilla E, Prasad AL, Estevez J, Hernandez H, Arrieta A. Changes in serum and striatal free amino acids after Venezuelan equine encephalomyelitis virus infection. Exp Neurol. 1988;99(3):647–54.
124. Bonilla E, Valero-Fuenmayor N, Pons H, Chacin-Bonilla L. Melatonin protects mice infected with Venezuelan equine encephalomyelitis virus. Cell Mol Life Sci. 1997;53(5):430–4.
125. Bonilla E, Rodon C, Valero N, Pons H, Chacin-Bonilla L, Garcia Tamayo J, et al. Melatonin prolongs survival of immunodepressed mice infected with the Venezuelan equine encephalomyelitis virus. Trans R Soc Trop Med Hyg. 2001;95(2):207–10.
126. Valero N, Bonilla E, Pons H, Chacin-Bonilla L, Anez F, Espina LM, et al. Melatonin induces changes to serum cytokines in mice infected with the Venezuelan equine encephalomyelitis virus. Trans R Soc Trop Med Hyg. 2002;96(3):348–51.
127. Bonilla E, Valero N, Chacin-Bonilla L, Pons H, Larreal Y, Medina-Leendertz S, et al. Melatonin increases interleukin-1beta and decreases tumor necrosis factor alpha in the brain of mice infected with the Venezuelan equine encephalomyelitis virus. Neurochem Res. 2003;28(5):681–6.
128. Valero N, MarinaEspina L, Bonilla E, Mosquera J. Melatonin decreases nitric oxide production and lipid peroxidation and increases interleukin-1 beta in the brain of mice infected by the Venezuelan equine encephalomyelitis virus. J Pineal Res. 2007;42(2):107–12.
129. Maestroni GJ, Conti A, Pierpaoli W. Role of the pineal gland in immunity. III. Melatonin antagonizes the immunosuppressive effect of acute stress via an opiatergic mechanism. Immunology. 1988;63(3):465–9.
130. Ben-Nathan D, Maestroni GJ, Lustig S, Conti A. Protective effects of melatonin in mice infected with encephalitis viruses. Arch Virol. 1995;140(2):223–30.
131. Ellis LC. Melatonin reduces mortality from Aleutian disease in mink (Mustela vison). J Pineal Res. 1996;21(4):214–7.
132. Zhang Z, Araghi-Niknam M, Liang B, Inserra P, Ardestani SK, Jiang S, et al. Prevention of immune dysfunction and vitamin E loss by dehydroepiandrosterone and melatonin supplementation during murine retrovirus infection. Immunology. 1999;96(2):291–7.
133. Nunnari G, Nigro L, Palermo F, Leto D, Pomerantz RJ, Cacopardo B. Reduction of serum melatonin levels in HIV-1-infected individuals' parallel disease progression: correlation with serum interleukin-12 levels. Infection. 2003;31(6):379–82.
134. Ward CG, Bullen JJ, Rogers HJ. Iron and infection: new developments and their implications. J Trauma. 1996;41(2):356–64.
135. Tekbas OF, Ogur R, Korkmaz A, Kilic A, Reiter RJ. Melatonin as an antibiotic: new insights into the actions of this ubiquitous molecule. J Pineal Res. 2008;44(2):222–6.
136. Wiid I, Hoal-van Helden E, Hon D, Lombard C, van Helden P. Potentiation of isoniazid activity against Mycobacterium tuberculosis by melatonin. Antimicrob Agents Chemother. 1999;43(4):975–7.
137. Ozkan E, Yaman H, Cakir E, Deniz O, Oztosun M, Gumus S, et al. Plasma melatonin and urinary 6-hydroxymelatonin levels in patients with pulmonary tuberculosis. Inflammation. 2012;35(4):1429–34.
138. Thorpe LE, Frieden TR, Laserson KF, Wells C, Khatri GR. Seasonality of tuberculosis in India: is it real and what does it tell us? Lancet. 2004;364(9445):1613–4.
139. Nagayama N, Ohmori M. Seasonality in various forms of tuberculosis. Int J Tuberc Lung Dis. 2006;10(10):1117–22.
140. Singh SS, Haldar C. Peripheral melatonin modulates seasonal immunity and reproduction of Indian tropical male bird Perdicula asiatica. Comp Biochem Physiol A Mol Integr Physiol. 2007;146(3):446–50.
141. Xie G, Bonner CA, Jensen RA. Dynamic diversity of the tryptophan pathway in chlamydiae: reductive evolution and a novel operon for tryptophan recapture. Genome Biol. 2002;3(9):1–17.
142. Pantoja LG, Miller RD, Ramirez JA, Molestina RE, Summersgill JT. Inhibition of Chlamydia pneumoniae replication in human aortic smooth muscle cells by gamma interferon-induced indoleamine 2, 3-dioxygenase activity. Infect Immun. 2000;68(11):6478–81.
143. Rahman MA, Azuma Y, Fukunaga H, Murakami T, Sugi K, Fukushi H, et al. Serotonin and melatonin, neurohormones for homeostasis, as novel inhibitors of infections by the intracellular parasite chlamydia. J Antimicrob Chemother. 2005;56(5):861–8.
144. Abrahamsohn IA. Cytokines in innate and acquired immunity to Trypanosoma cruzi infection. Braz J Med Biol Res. 1998;31(1):117–21.
145. Saeftel M, Fleischer B, Hoerauf A. Stage-dependent role of nitric oxide in control of Trypanosoma cruzi infection. Infect Immun. 2001;69(4):2252–9.
146. Oliveira LG, Kuehn CC, Santos CD, Toldo MP, do Prado Jr JC. Enhanced protection by melatonin and meloxicam combination in experimental infection by Trypanosoma cruzi. Parasite Immunol. 2010;32(4):245–51.
147. Santos CD, Toldo MP, Santello FH, Filipin Mdel V, Brazao V, do Prado Jr JC. Dehydroepiandrosterone increases resistance to experimental infection by Trypanosoma cruzi. Vet Parasitol. 2008;153(3–4):238–43.
148. Brazao V, Del Vecchio Filipin M, Santello FH, Caetano LC, Abrahao AA, Toldo MP, et al. Melatonin and zinc treatment: distinctive modulation of cytokine production in chronic experimental Trypanosoma cruzi infection. Cytokine. 2011;56(3):627–32.
149. Alves E, Bartlett PJ, Garcia CR, Thomas AP. Melatonin and IP3-induced Ca2+ release from intracellular stores in the malaria parasite Plasmodium

falciparum within infected red blood cells. J Biol Chem. 2011;286(7):5905–12.

150. Lima WR, Moraes M, Alves E, Azevedo MF, Passos DO, Garcia CR. The PfNF- YB transcription factor is a downstream target of melatonin and cAMP signalling in the human malaria parasite Plasmodium falciparum. J Pineal Res. 2013;54(2): 145–53.
151. Hotta CT, Gazarini ML, Beraldo FH, Varotti FP, Lopes C, Markus RP, et al. Calcium-dependent modulation by melatonin of the circadian rhythm in malarial parasites. Nat Cell Biol. 2000;2(7): 466–8.
152. Guha M, Maity P, Choubey V, Mitra K, Reiter RJ, Bandyopadhyay U. Melatonin inhibits free radical-mediated mitochondrial-dependent hepatocyte apoptosis and liver damage induced during malarial infection. J Pineal Res. 2007;43(4):372–81.
153. Mozzanica N, Tadini G, Radaelli A, Negri M, Pigatto P, Morelli M, et al. Plasma melatonin levels in psoriasis. Acta Derm Venereol. 1988;68(4):312–6.
154. Lopez-Gonzalez MA, Guerrero JM, Sanchez B, Delgado F. Melatonin induces hyporeactivity caused by type II collagen in peripheral blood lymphocytes from patients with autoimmune hearing losses. Neurosci Lett. 1997;239(1):1–4.
155. Wu CC, Lu KC, Lin GJ, Hsieh HY, Chu P, Lin SH, et al. Melatonin enhances endogenous heme oxygenase-1 and represses immune responses to ameliorate experimental murine membranous nephropathy. J Pineal Res. 2012;52(4):460–9.
156. McInnes IB, Schett G. The pathogenesis of rheumatoid arthritis. N Engl J Med. 2011;365(23):2205–19.
157. Hansson I, Holmdahl R, Mattsson R. Constant darkness enhances autoimmunity to type II collagen and exaggerates development of collagen-induced arthritis in DBA/1 mice. J Neuroimmunol. 1990;27(1):79–84.
158. Hansson I, Holmdahl R, Mattsson R. Pinealectomy ameliorates collagen II- induced arthritis in mice. Clin Exp Immunol. 1993;92(3):432–6.
159. Hansson I, Holmdahl R, Mattsson R. The pineal hormone melatonin exaggerates development of collagen-induced arthritis in mice. J Neuroimmunol. 1992;39(1–2):23–30.
160. Jimenez-Caliani AJ, Jimenez-Jorge S, Molinero P, Guerrero JM, Fernandez-Santos JM, Martin-Lacave I, et al. Dual effect of melatonin as proinflammatory and antioxidant in collagen-induced arthritis in rats. J Pineal Res. 2005;38(2):93–9.
161. Chen Q, Wei W. Effects and mechanisms of melatonin on inflammatory and immune responses of adjuvant arthritis rat. Int Immunopharmacol. 2002; 2(10):1443–9.
162. Cutolo M, Masi AT. Circadian rhythms and arthritis. Rheum Dis Clin North Am. 2005;31(1):115–29.
163. Arkema EV, Hart JE, Bertrand KA, Laden F, Grodstein F, Rosner BA, et al. Exposure to ultraviolet-B and risk of developing rheumatoid arthritis among women in the Nurses' Health Study. Ann Rheum Dis. 2013;72(4):506–11.
164. Brainard GC, Podolin PL, Leivy SW, Rollag MD, Cole C, Barker FM. Near- ultraviolet radiation suppresses pineal melatonin content. Endocrinology. 1986;119(5):2201–5.
165. Cutolo M, Maestroni GJ, Otsa K, Aakre O, Villaggio B, Capellino S, et al. Circadian melatonin and cortisol levels in rheumatoid arthritis patients in winter time: a north and south Europe comparison. Ann Rheum Dis. 2005;64(2):212–6.
166. Petrovsky N, Harrison LC. The chronobiology of human cytokine production. Int Rev Immunol. 1998;16(5–6):635–49.
167. Sulli A, Maestroni GJ, Villaggio B, Hertens E, Craviotto C, Pizzorni C, et al. Melatonin serum levels in rheumatoid arthritis. Ann N Y Acad Sci. 2002;966:276–83.
168. El-Awady HM, El-Wakkad AS, Saleh MT, Muhammad SI, Ghaniema EM. Serum melatonin in juvenile rheumatoid arthritis: correlation with disease activity. Pak J Biol Sci. 2007;10(9):1471–6.
169. West SK, Oosthuizen JM. Melatonin levels are decreased in rheumatoid arthritis. J Basic Clin Physiol Pharmacol. 1992;3(1):33–40.
170. Cano P, Cardinali DP, Chacon F, Reyes Toso CF, Esquifino AI. Nighttime changes in norepinephrine and melatonin content and serotonin turnover in pineal glands of young and old rats injected with Freund's adjuvant. Neuro Endocrinol Lett. 2002;23(1):49–53.
171. Maestroni GJ, Sulli A, Pizzorni C, Villaggio B, Cutolo M. Melatonin in rheumatoid arthritis: synovial macrophages show melatonin receptors. Ann N Y Acad Sci. 2002;966:271–5.
172. Cutolo M, Villaggio B, Candido F, Valenti S, Giusti M, Felli L, et al. Melatonin influences interleukin-12 and nitric oxide production by primary cultures of rheumatoid synovial macrophages and THP-1 cells. Ann N Y Acad Sci. 1999;876: 246–54.
173. Nah SS, Won HJ, Park HJ, Ha E, Chung JH, Cho HY, et al. Melatonin inhibits human fibroblast-like synoviocyte proliferation via extracellular signal-regulated protein kinase/P21(CIP1)/P27(KIP1) pathways. J Pineal Res. 2009;47(1):70–4.
174. Kouri VP, Olkkonen J, Kaivosoja E, Ainola M, Juhila J, Hovatta I, et al. Circadian timekeeping is disturbed in rheumatoid arthritis at molecular level. PLoS One. 2013;8(1):54049.
175. Forrest CM, Mackay GM, Stoy N, Stone TW, Darlington LG. Inflammatory status and kynurenine metabolism in rheumatoid arthritis treated with melatonin. Br J Clin Pharmacol. 2007;64(4):517–26.
176. Pugliatti M, Sotgiu S, Rosati G. The worldwide prevalence of multiple sclerosis. Clin Neurol Neurosurg. 2002;104(3):182–91.
177. Lassmann H, van Horssen J. The molecular basis of neurodegeneration in multiple sclerosis. FEBS Lett. 2011;585(23):3715–23.

178. Kurtzke JF. Geography in multiple sclerosis. J Neurol. 1977;215(1):1–26.
179. van der Mei IA, Ponsonby AL, Dwyer T, Blizzard L, Simmons R, Taylor BV, et al. Past exposure to sun, skin phenotype, and risk of multiple sclerosis: case–control study. BMJ. 2003;327(7410):316.
180. Islam T, Gauderman WJ, Cozen W, Mack TM. Childhood sun exposure influences risk of multiple sclerosis in monozygotic twins. Neurology. 2007; 69(4):381–8.
181. Kurtzke JF. On the fine structure of the distribution of multiple sclerosis. Acta Neurol Scand. 1967; 43(3):257–82.
182. Hedstrom AK, Akerstedt T, Hillert J, Olsson T, Alfredsson L. Shift work at young age is associated with increased risk for multiple sclerosis. Ann Neurol. 2011;70(5):733–41.
183. Constantinescu CS, Hilliard B, Ventura E, Rostami A. Luzindole, a melatonin receptor antagonist, suppresses experimental autoimmune encephalomyelitis. Pathobiology. 1997;65(4):190–4.
184. Constantinescu CS. Environmental influences in experimental autoimmune encephalomyelitis. In: Experimental models of multiple sclerosis. USA: Springer; 2005. p. 523–46.
185. Sandyk R. Influence of the pineal gland on the expression of experimental allergic encephalomyelitis: possible relationship to the acquisition of multiple sclerosis. Int J Neurosci. 1997;90(1–2): 129–33.
186. Kang JC, Ahn M, Kim YS, Moon C, Lee Y, Wie MB, et al. Melatonin ameliorates autoimmune encephalomyelitis through suppression of intercellular adhesion molecule-1. J Vet Sci. 2001;2(2):85–9.
187. Sandyk R, Awerbuch GI. Nocturnal plasma melatonin and alpha-melanocyte stimulating hormone levels during exacerbation of multiple sclerosis. Int J Neurosci. 1992;67(1–4):173–86.
188. Melamud L, Golan D, Luboshitzky R, Lavi I, Miller A. Melatonin dysregulation, sleep disturbances and fatigue in multiple sclerosis. J Neurol Sci. 2012;314(1–2):37–40.
189. Natarajan R, Einarsdottir E, Riutta A, Hagman S, Raunio M, Mononen N, et al. Melatonin pathway genes are associated with progressive subtypes and disability status in multiple sclerosis among Finnish patients. J Neuroimmunol. 2012;250(1–2): 106–10.
190. Akpinar Z, Tokgoz S, Gokbel H, Okudan N, Uguz F, Yilmaz G. The association of nocturnal serum melatonin levels with major depression in patients with acute multiple sclerosis. Psychiatry Res. 2008; 161(2):253–7.
191. Sandyk R. Diurnal variations in vision and relations to circadian melatonin secretion in multiple sclerosis. Int J Neurosci. 1995;83(1–2):1–6.
192. Tsokos GC. Systemic lupus erythematosus. N Engl J Med. 2011;365(22):2110–21.
193. Lechner O, Dietrich H, Oliveira dos Santos A, Wiegers GJ, Schwarz S, Harbutz M, et al. Altered circadian rhythms of the stress hormone and melatonin response in lupus-prone MRL/MP-fas(Ipr) mice. J Autoimmun. 2000;14(4):325–33.
194. Haga HJ, Brun JG, Rekvig OP, Wetterberg L. Seasonal variations in activity of systemic lupus erythematosus in a subarctic region. Lupus. 1999;8(4): 269–73.
195. Lenz SP, Izui S, Benediktsson H, Hart DA. Lithium chloride enhances survival of NZB/W lupus mice: influence of melatonin and timing of treatment. Int J Immunopharmacol. 1995;17(7):581–92.
196. Jimenez-Caliani AJ, Jimenez-Jorge S, Molinero P, Fernandez-Santos JM, Martin-Lacave I, Rubio A, et al. Sex-dependent effect of melatonin on systemic erythematosus lupus developed in Mrl/Mpj-Faslpr mice: it ameliorates the disease course in females, whereas it exacerbates it in males. Endocrinology. 2006;147(4):1717–24.
197. Zhou LL, Wei W, Si JF, Yuan DP. Regulatory effect of melatonin on cytokine disturbances in the pristane-induced lupus mice. Mediators Inflamm. 2010;2010:951210.
198. Daneman D. Type 1 diabetes. Lancet. 2006; 367(9513):847–58.
199. Ponsonby AL, Lucas RM, van der Mei IA. UVR, vitamin D and three autoimmune diseases–multiple sclerosis, type 1 diabetes, rheumatoid arthritis. Photochem Photobiol. 2005;81(6):1267–75.
200. Peschke E, Wolgast S, Bazwinsky I, Ponicke K, Muhlbauer E. Increased melatonin synthesis in pineal glands of rats in streptozotocin induced type 1 diabetes. J Pineal Res. 2008;45(4):439–48.
201. Peschke E, Hofmann K, Bahr I, Streck S, Albrecht E, Wedekind D, et al. The insulin-melatonin antagonism: studies in the LEW.1AR1-iddm rat (an animal model of human type 1 diabetes mellitus). Diabetologia. 2011;54(7):1831–40.
202. Conti A, Maestroni GJ. Role of the pineal gland and melatonin in the development of autoimmune diabetes in non-obese diabetic mice. J Pineal Res. 1996; 20(3):164–72.
203. Lin GJ, Huang SH, Chen YW, Hueng DY, Chien MW, Chia WT, et al. Melatonin prolongs islet graft survival in diabetic NOD mice. J Pineal Res. 2009; 47(3):284–92.
204. Reyes-Toso CF, Roson MI, Albornoz LE, Damiano PF, Linares LM, Cardinali DP. Vascular reactivity in diabetic rats: effect of melatonin. J Pineal Res. 2002; 33(2):81–6.
205. Cavallo A, Daniels SR, Dolan LM, Bean JA, Khoury JC. Blood pressure- lowering effect of melatonin in type 1 diabetes. J Pineal Res. 2004;36(4):262–6.
206. Chen CQ, Fichna J, Bashashati M, Li YY, Storr M. Distribution, function and physiological role of melatonin in the lower gut. World J Gastroenterol. 2011; 17(34):3888–98.
207. Motilva V, Garcia-Maurino S, Talero E, Illanes M. New paradigms in chronic intestinal inflammation and colon cancer: role of melatonin. J Pineal Res. 2011;51(1):44–60.

208. Radwan P, Skrzydlo-Radomanska B, Radwan-Kwiatek K, Burak-Czapiuk B, Strzemecka J. Is melatonin involved in the irritable bowel syndrome? J Physiol Pharmacol. 2009;60 Suppl 3:67–70.
209. Song GH, Leng PH, Gwee KA, Moochhala SM, Ho KY. Melatonin improves abdominal pain in irritable bowel syndrome patients who have sleep disturbances: a randomised, double blind, placebo controlled study. Gut. 2005;54(10):1402–7.
210. Thor PJ, Krolczyk G, Gil K, Zurowski D, Nowak L. Melatonin and serotonin effects on gastrointestinal motility. J Physiol Pharmacol. 2007;58 Suppl 6: 97–103.
211. Lu WZ, Gwee KA, Moochhalla S, Ho KY. Melatonin improves bowel symptoms in female patients with irritable bowel syndrome: a double-blind placebo-controlled study. Aliment Pharmacol Ther. 2005; 22(10):927–34.
212. Saha L, Malhotra S, Rana S, Bhasin D, Pandhi P. A preliminary study of melatonin in irritable bowel syndrome. J Clin Gastroenterol. 2007;41(1): 29–32.
213. Preuss F, Tang Y, Laposky AD, Arble D, Keshavarzian A, Turek FW. Adverse effects of chronic circadian desynchronization in animals in a "challenging" environment. Am J Physiol Regul Integr Comp Physiol. 2008;295(6):R2034–40.
214. Mickle A, Sood M, Zhang Z, Shahmohammadi G, Sengupta JN, Miranda A. Antinociceptive effects of melatonin in a rat model of post-inflammatory visceral hyperalgesia: a centrally mediated process. Pain. 2010;149(3):555–64.
215. Pentney PT, Bubenik GA. Melatonin reduces the severity of dextran-induced colitis in mice. J Pineal Res. 1995;19(1):31–9.
216. Cuzzocrea S, Mazzon E, Serraino I, Lepore V, Terranova ML, Ciccolo A, et al. Melatonin reduces dinitrobenzene sulfonic acid-induced colitis. J Pineal Res. 2001;30(1):1–12.
217. Winiarska K, Fraczyk T, Malinska D, Drozak J, Bryla J. Melatonin attenuates diabetes-induced oxidative stress in rabbits. J Pineal Res. 2006;40(2):168–76.
218. Dong WG, Mei Q, Yu JP, Xu JM, Xiang L, Xu Y. Effects of melatonin on the expression of iNOS and COX-2 in rat models of colitis. World J Gastroenterol. 2003;9(6):1307–11.
219. Tahan G, Gramignoli R, Marongiu F, Aktolga S, Cetinkaya A, Tahan V, et al. Melatonin expresses powerful anti-inflammatory and antioxidant activities resulting in complete improvement of acetic-acid-induced colitis in rats. Dig Dis Sci. 2011;56(3): 715–20.
220. Akcan A, Kucuk C, Sozuer E, Esel D, Akyildiz H, Akgun H, et al. Melatonin reduces bacterial translocation and apoptosis in trinitrobenzene sulphonic acid-induced colitis of rats. World J Gastroenterol. 2008;14(6):918–24.
221. Esposito E, Mazzon E, Riccardi L, Caminiti R, Meli R, Cuzzocrea S. Matrix metalloproteinase-9 and metalloproteinase-2 activity and expression is reduced by melatonin during experimental colitis. J Pineal Res. 2008;45(2):166–73.
222. Mazzon E, Esposito E, Crisafulli C, Riccardi L, Muia C, Di Bella P, et al. Melatonin modulates signal transduction pathways and apoptosis in experimental colitis. J Pineal Res. 2006;41(4):363–73.
223. Li JH, Yu JP, Yu HG, Xu XM, Yu LL, Liu J, et al. Melatonin reduces inflammatory injury through inhibiting NF-kappaB activation in rats with colitis. Mediators Inflamm. 2005;2005(4):185–93.
224. Mann S. Melatonin for ulcerative colitis? Am J Gastroenterol. 2003;98(1):232–3.
225. Calvo JR, Guerrero JM, Osuna C, Molinero P, Carrillo-Vico A. Melatonin triggers Crohn's disease symptoms. J Pineal Res. 2002;32(4):277–8.
226. Maldonado MD, Calvo JR. Melatonin usage in ulcerative colitis: a case report. J Pineal Res. 2008;45(3):339–40.
227. Srinivasan V, Pandi-Perumal SR, Brzezinski A, Bhatnagar KP, Cardinali DP. Melatonin, immune function and cancer. Recent Pat Endocr Metab Immune Drug Discov. 2011;5(2):109–23.
228. Srinivasan V, Spence DW, Pandi-Perumal SR, Trakht I, Cardinali DP. Therapeutic actions of melatonin in cancer: possible mechanisms. Integr Cancer Ther. 2008;7(3):189–203.
229. Street SE, Trapani JA, MacGregor D, Smyth MJ. Suppression of lymphoma and epithelial malignancies effected by interferon gamma. J Exp Med. 2002;196(1):129–34.
230. Castrillon PO, Esquifino AI, Varas A, Zapata A, Cutrera RA, Cardinali DP. Effect of melatonin treatment on 24-h variations in responses to mitogens and lymphocyte subset populations in rat submaxillary lymph nodes. J Neuroendocrinol. 2000;12(8): 758–65.
231. Poon AM, Liu ZM, Pang CS, Brown GM, Pang SF. Evidence for a direct action of melatonin on the immune system. Biol Signals. 1994;3(2):107–17.
232. Maestroni GJ, Conti A, Lissoni P. Colony-stimulating activity and hematopoietic rescue from cancer chemotherapy compounds are induced by melatonin via endogenous interleukin 4. Cancer Res. 1994;54(17):4740–3.
233. Akazawa T, Masuda H, Saeki Y, Matsumoto M, Takeda K, Tsujimura K, et al. Adjuvant-mediated tumor regression and tumor-specific cytotoxic response are impaired in MyD88-deficient mice. Cancer Res. 2004;64(2):757–64.
234. Miller SC, Pandi-Perumal SR, Esquifino AI, Cardinali DP, Maestroni GJ. The role of melatonin in immuno-enhancement: potential application in cancer. Int J Exp Pathol. 2006;87(2):81–7.
235. Maestroni GJ. The immunotherapeutic potential of melatonin. Expert Opin Investig Drugs. 2001;10(3): 467–76.
236. Gonzalez R, Sanchez A, Ferguson JA, Balmer C, Daniel C, Cohn A, et al. Melatonin therapy of advanced human malignant melanoma. Melanoma Res. 1991;1(4):237–43.

237. Lissoni P, Barni S, Tancini G, Rovelli F, Ardizzoia A, Conti A, et al. A study of the mechanisms involved in the immunostimulatory action of the pineal hormone in cancer patients. Oncology. 1993;50(6):399–402.
238. Lissoni P, Meregalli S, Fossati V, Paolorossi F, Barni S, Tancini G, et al. A randomized study of immunotherapy with low-dose subcutaneous interleukin-2 plus melatonin vs chemotherapy with cisplatin and etoposide as first-line therapy for advanced non-small cell lung cancer. Tumori. 1994;80(6):464–7.
239. Lissoni P, Vaghi M, Ardizzoia A, Malugani F, Fumagalli E, Bordin V, et al. A phase II study of chemoneuroimmunotherapy with platinum, subcutaneous low-dose interleukin-2 and the pineal neurohormone melatonin (P.I.M.) as a second-line therapy in metastatic melanoma patients progressing on dacarbazine plus interferon-alpha. In Vivo. 2002; 16(2):93–6.
240. Lissoni P, Rovelli F, Brivio F, Fumagalli L, Brera G. A study of immunoendocrine strategies with pineal indoles and interleukin-2 to prevent radiotherapy-induced lymphocytopenia in cancer patients. In Vivo. 2008;22(3):397–400.
241. Lissoni P, Brivio F, Fumagalli L, Messina G, Vigore L, Parolini D, et al. Neuroimmunomodulation in medical oncology: application of psychoneuroimmunology with subcutaneous low-dose IL-2 and the pineal hormone melatonin in patients with untreatable metastatic solid tumors. Anticancer Res. 2008;28(2B):1377–81.
242. Lissoni P. Biochemotherapy with standard chemotherapies plus the pineal hormone melatonin in the treatment of advanced solid neoplasms. Pathol Biol (Paris). 2007;55(3–4):201–4.
243. Bartsch C, Bartsch H. Melatonin in cancer patients and in tumor-bearing animals. Adv Exp Med Biol. 1999;467:247–64.
244. Bartsch C, Bartsch H, Fuchs U, Lippert TH, Bellmann O, Gupta D. Stage-dependent depression of melatonin in patients with primary breast cancer. Correlation with prolactin, thyroid stimulating hormone, and steroid receptors. Cancer. 1989;64(2):426–33.
245. Regodon S, Martin-Palomino P, Fernandez-Montesinos R, Herrera JL, Carrascosa-Salmoral MP, Piriz S, et al. The use of melatonin as a vaccine agent. Vaccine. 2005;23(46–47):5321–7.
246. Katz ME, Howarth PM, Yong WK, Riffkin GG, Depiazzi LJ, Rood JI. Identification of three gene regions associated with virulence in Dichelobacter nodosus, the causative agent of ovine footrot. J Gen Microbiol. 1991;137(9):2117–24.
247. Regodon S, Ramos A, Morgado S, Tarazona R, Martin-Palomino P, Rosado JA, et al. Melatonin enhances the immune response to vaccination against A1 and C strains of Dichelobacter nodosus. Vaccine. 2009;27(10):1566–70.
248. Regodon S, del Prado Miguez M, Jardin I, Lopez JJ, Ramos A, Paredes SD, et al. Melatonin, as an adjuvant-like agent, enhances platelet responsiveness. J Pineal Res. 2009;46(3):275–85.
249. Regodon S, Ramos A, Miguez MP, Carrillo-Vico A, Rosado JA, Jardin I. Vaccination prepartum enhances the beneficial effects of melatonin on the immune response and reduces platelet responsiveness in sheep. BMC Vet Res. 2012;8:84–91.
250. Pioli C, Caroleo MC, Nistico G, Doria G. Melatonin increases antigen presentation and amplifies specific and non specific signals for T-cell proliferation. Int J Immunopharmacol. 1993;15(4):463–8.
251. Connor TP. Melatonin as an adjuvant to therapeutic prostate cancer vaccines. J Pineal Res. 2008;45(2): 224.
252. Soliman MF, El Shenawy NS, El Arabi SE. Schistosoma mansoni: melatonin enhances efficacy of cercarial and soluble worm antigens in the induction of protective immunity against infection in the hamster. Exp Parasitol. 2008;119(2):291–5.
253. Jesudason EP, Baben B, Ashok BS, Masilamoni JG, Kirubagaran R, Jebaraj WC, et al. Anti-inflammatory effect of melatonin on A beta vaccination in mice. Mol Cell Biochem. 2007;298(1–2):69–81.
254. Ramos A, Laguna I, de Lucia ML, Martin-Palomino P, Regodon S, Miguez MP. Evolution of oxidative/nitrosative stress biomarkers during an open-field vaccination procedure in sheep: effect of melatonin. Vet Immunol Immunopathol. 2010;133(1): 16–24.
255. Jung FJ, Yang L, Harter L, Inci I, Schneiter D, Lardinois D, et al. Melatonin in vivo prolongs cardiac allograft survival in rats. J Pineal Res. 2004;37(1):36–41.
256. Inci I, Inci D, Dutly A, Boehler A, Weder W. Melatonin attenuates posttransplant lung ischemia-reperfusion injury. Ann Thorac Surg. 2002;73(1):220–5.
257. Sapmaz E, Ayar A, Celik H, Sapmaz T, Kilic N, Yasar MA. Effects of melatonin and oxytetracycline in autologous intraperitoneal ovary transplantation in rats. Neuro Endocrinol Lett. 2003;24(5):350–4.
258. Friedman O, Orvieto R, Fisch B, Felz C, Freud E, Ben-Haroush A, et al. Possible improvements in human ovarian grafting by various host and graft treatments. Hum Reprod. 2012;27(2):474–82.
259. Fildes JE, Yonan N, Keevil BG. Melatonin–a pleiotropic molecule involved in pathophysiological processes following organ transplantation. Immunology. 2009;127(4):443–9.
260. Baykara B, Tekmen I, Pekcetin C, Ulukus C, Tuncel P, Sagol O, et al. The protective effects of carnosine and melatonin in ischemia-reperfusion injury in the rat liver. Acta Histochem. 2009;111(1):42–51.
261. Zaouali MA, Reiter RJ, Padrissa-Altes S, Boncompagni E, Garcia JJ, Ben Abnennebi H, et al. Melatonin protects steatotic and nonsteatotic liver grafts against cold ischemia and reperfusion injury. J Pineal Res. 2011;50(2):213–21.
262. Moussavian MR, Scheuer C, Schmidt M, Kollmar O, Wagner M, von Heesen M, et al. Multidrug donor preconditioning prevents cold liver preservation and reperfusion injury. Langenbecks Arch Surg. 2011; 396(2):231–41.

263. von Heesen M, Seibert K, Hulser M, Scheuer C, Wagner M, Menger MD, et al. Multidrug donor preconditioning protects steatotic liver grafts against ischemia- reperfusion injury. Am J Surg. 2012; 203(2):168–76.
264. Cardell M, Jung FJ, Zhai W, Hillinger S, Welp A, Manz B, et al. Acute allograft rejection and immunosuppression: influence on endogenous melatonin secretion. J Pineal Res. 2008;44(3):261–6.
265. Srinivasan V, Maestroni GJ, Cardinali DP, Esquifino AI, Perumal SR, Miller SC. Melatonin, immune function and aging. Immun Ageing. 2005;2:17.
266. Castle SC. Clinical relevance of age-related immune dysfunction. Clin Infect Dis. 2000;31(2):578–85.
267. Arlt W, Hewison M. Hormones and immune function: implications of aging. Aging Cell. 2004;3(4): 209–16.
268. Karasek M. Melatonin, human aging, and age-related diseases. Exp Gerontol. 2004;39(11–12):1723–9.
269. Iguchi H. Age dependent changes in the serum melatonin concentrations in healthy human subjects and in patients with endocrine and hepatic disorders and renal failure (author's transl). Fukuoka Igaku Zasshi. 1981;72(7):423–30.
270. Girotti L, Lago M, Ianovsky O, Carbajales J, Elizari MV, Brusco LI, et al. Low urinary 6-sulphatoxymelatonin levels in patients with coronary artery disease. J Pineal Res. 2000;29(3):138–42.
271. Mishima K, Okawa M, Shimizu T, Hishikawa Y. Diminished melatonin secretion in the elderly caused by insufficient environmental illumination. J Clin Endocrinol Metab. 2001;86(1):129–34.
272. Siegrist C, Benedetti C, Orlando A, Beltran JM, Tuchscherr L, Noseda CM, et al. Lack of changes in serum prolactin, FSH, TSH, and estradiol after melatonin treatment in doses that improve sleep and reduce benzodiazepine consumption in sleep- disturbed, middle-aged, and elderly patients. J Pineal Res. 2001;30(1):34–42.
273. Luboshitzky R, Shen-Orr Z, Tzischichinsky O, Maldonado M, Herer P, Lavie P. Actigraphic sleep-wake patterns and urinary 6-sulfatoxymelatonin excretion in patients with Alzheimer's disease. Chronobiol Int. 2001;18(3):513–24.
274. Tian YM, Zhang GY, Dai YR. Melatonin rejuvenates degenerated thymus and redresses peripheral immune functions in aged mice. Immunol Lett. 2003;88(2):101–4.
275. Lesnikov VA, Pierpaoli W. Pineal cross-transplantation (old-to-young and vice versa) as evidence for an endogenous "aging clock". Ann N Y Acad Sci. 1994;719:456–60.
276. Pierpaoli W, Regelson W. Pineal control of aging: effect of melatonin and pineal grafting on aging mice. Proc Natl Acad Sci U S A. 1994;91(2):787–91.
277. Tian YM, Li PP, Jiang XF, Zhang GY, Dai YR. Rejuvenation of degenerative thymus by oral melatonin administration and the antagonistic action of melatonin against hydroxyl radical-induced apoptosis of cultured thymocytes in mice. J Pineal Res. 2001;31(3):214–21.
278. Sainz RM, Mayo JC, Uria H, Kotler M, Antolin I, Rodriguez C, et al. The pineal neurohormone melatonin prevents in vivo and in vitro apoptosis in thymocytes. J Pineal Res. 1995;19(4):178–88.
279. Espino J, Pariente JA, Rodriguez AB. Oxidative stress and immunosenescence: therapeutic effects of melatonin. Oxid Med Cell Longev. 2012;1–9.
280. Espino J, Bejarano I, Paredes SD, Barriga C, Reiter RJ, Pariente JA, et al. Melatonin is able to delay endoplasmic reticulum stress-induced apoptosis in leukocytes from elderly humans. Age (Dordr). 2011;33(4):497–507.
281. Vishwas DK, Mukherjee A, Haldar C, Dash D, Nayak MK. Improvement of oxidative stress and immunity by melatonin: an age dependent study in golden hamster. Exp Gerontol. 2013;48(2):168–82.
282. Caroleo MC, Doria G, Nistico G. Melatonin restores immunodepression in aged and cyclophosphamide-treated mice. Ann N Y Acad Sci. 1994;719:343–52.
283. Cuesta S, Kireev R, Forman K, Garcia C, Escames G, Ariznavarreta C, et al. Melatonin improves inflammation processes in liver of senescence-accelerated prone male mice (SAMP8). Exp Gerontol. 2010;45(12):950–6.
284. Sharman KG, Sharman EH, Yang E, Bondy SC. Dietary melatonin selectively reverses age-related changes in cortical cytokine mRNA levels, and their responses to an inflammatory stimulus. Neurobiol Aging. 2002;23(4):633–8.
285. Malow B, Adkins KW, McGrew SG, Wang L, Goldman SE, Fawkes D, et al. Melatonin for sleep in children with autism: a controlled trial examining dose, tolerability, and outcomes. J Autism Dev Disord. 2012;42(8):1729–37; author reply 38.
286. Reiter RJ, Tan DX, Rosales-Corral S, Manchester LC. The universal nature, unequal distribution and antioxidant functions of melatonin and its derivatives. Mini Rev Med Chem. 2013;13(3):373–84.

Melatonin and Immune Function: Clinical Significance

9

Mahaneem Mohamed, V. Srinivasan, Georges Maestroni, Ruth E. Rosenstein, and Sukru Oter

Abstract

The immune system of the body plays an important role in fighting against cancer and infectious diseases. The decreased immune function has been primarily attributed to the increased incidence of neoplastic and infectious diseases in the elderly. Alteration in circadian rhythmicity of various subsets of lymphocyte population in cancer patients suggests impaired integration of nervous, endocrine, and immune responses in neoplastic disease. The photoperiodic regulation of immune function with enhancement during short photoperiods and inhibition during long photoperiods is supported by the seasonal outbreak of some infectious diseases. The pineal biomolecule melatonin could be a very useful resource for inhibiting neoplastic growth as its immunomodulatory role may stimulate several immune mechanisms. Melatonin stimulates natural killer cells which are known to attack and destroy cancerous cells. It also influences T-helper 1

M. Mohamed, MD, MSc, PhD (✉)
Department of Physiology, School of Medical Sciences, Universiti Sains Malaysia, Kubang Kerian, Kelantan 16150, Malaysia
e-mail: mahaneem@kck.usm.my

V. Srinivasan, MSc, PhD, MAMS
Sri Sathya Sai Medical Educational and Research Foundation, An International Medical Sciences Research Study Center, Prasanthi Nilayam, 40-Kovai Thirunagar Extn, Goldwins, Coimbatore, TN 641014, India

National Health Service, Department of Mental Health, Psychiatric Service of Diagnosis and Treatment, Hospital "G. Mazzini", ASL 4, Teramo, Italy

Department of Neuroscience and Imaging, University "G.D' Annunzio", Chieti 66013, Italy
e-mail: sainivasan@yahoo.com, venkataramanujamsrinivasan6@gmail.com

G. Maestroni, PhD
Department of Pharmacology, University of Insubria, Medical School, Via OttorniRossi, 9, Varese 21100, Italy
e-mail: maestro.grand@ngi.it

R.E. Rosenstein, PhD
Department of Human Biochemistry, School of Medicine/CEFyBO, University of Buenos Aires/CONICET, Paraguay 2155, 5th floor, Buenos Aires 1121, Argentina
e-mail: ruthr@fmed.uba.ar

S. Oter, MD, PhD
Department of Physiology, Gulhane Military Medical Academy, Gulhane Askeri Tip Akademisi, Fizyoloji Anabilim Dali, General Tevfik Saglam Caddesi, Etlik, Ankara 6010, Turkey
e-mail: oters@gata.edu.tr

V. Srinivasan et al. (eds.), *Melatonin and Melatonergic Drugs in Clinical Practice*, DOI 10.1007/978-81-322-0825-9_9, © Springer India 2014

cells, B lymphocytes, and release of cytokines from immunoregulatory cells. The immunomodulatory role for melatonin and its application in the control of infectious and neoplastic diseases is supported by the synthesis of melatonin by lymphocytes and thymus.

Keywords
Melatonin • Immune mechanism • Lymphocytes • Innate immunity • Adaptive immunity • Cancer • Infectious diseases

Abbreviations

AFMK	N^1-acetyl-N^2-formyl-5-methoxykynuramine
CCL	Chemokine ligand
COX2	Cyclooxygenase-2
CSF	Cerebrospinal fluid
DPSCs	Dental pulp stem cells
GH	Growth hormone
GSH	Glutathione
hESCs	Human embryonic stem cells
HIV	Human immunodeficiency virus
HLA	Human leukocyte antigen
hMSCs	Human mesenchymal stem cells
IFN	Interferon
Ig	Immunoglobulin
IL	Interleukin
M-CSF	Macrophage colony-stimulating factor
NFκB	Nuclear factor kappa B
NK	Natural killer
NR1F1	Nuclear receptor subfamily 1 group F, member 1
$O2^{-\bullet}$	Superoxide anion (radical)
OSCSCs	Oral squamous carcinoma stem cells
RAR	Retinoic acid receptor
ROR	RAR-related orphan receptor-α
SCF	Stem cell factor
TCR	T-cell receptor
TGF-β	Transforming (or tumor) growth factor
TNF-α	Tumor necrosis factor-α
TSH	Thyroid-stimulating hormone

Introduction

Based on epidemiological studies, individual longevity is determined by the level of immunity [1]. The existence of "immunological risk phenotypes" that predict the individual life span has also been identified [2]. A steady decline in immune function that increases with aging, which is termed as "immunosenescence," predisposes an individual to increased susceptibility to infectious diseases, proliferative or neurodegenerative diseases, or a combination of any of these disease states [3]. A standard set of guidelines is provided by SENIEUR protocol among the various screening approaches recommended for studying the decline in immune function in relation to aging [4]. Immunogerontological studies show inconsistencies in age-related changes in both nonspecific and specific immune functions [5, 6]. Interrelationship between the endocrine and immune systems [7] and influences of nutritional status of individuals [6] are considered primary determinants of immune function and variability of immunosenescence seen in different individuals of the same chronological age [8]. The age-associated decline in the levels of various hormones like estrogens, dehydroepiandrosterone, growth hormone (GH), and the pineal hormone melatonin has been suggested as a contributory factor for immunosenescence [7]. Among these hormones, involvement of melatonin in modulating immune responses is of paramount importance [9]. The individual's susceptibility to infectious or proliferative diseases depends upon his own immunocompetent status. The variations in the degree of susceptibility to infectious or proliferative diseases among individuals of the same chronological age are attributed to the degree of variations in immunocompetency. This is determined by the interplay of various factors such as the environmental, genetic, and nutritional status and the hormonal levels. The immuno-neuroendocrine axis also affects the susceptibility of an individual to various diseases [10]. In understanding the competency of immune mechanism among individuals of the same age, the importance of psychoneuroimmunology is gaining much recognition [11]. In this chapter, the immunomodulatory role of melatonin in relation to aging, infectious, and proliferative diseases, namely, cancer, with the aim of understanding its therapeutic significance for treating these disease states is discussed.

Immunity and Aging

The interrelationship between the endocrine and immune systems is important in mediating age-associated degenerative diseases. Aging causes changes in humoral immunity as reflected by decreased number of B lymphocytes and increased levels of immunoglobulin (Ig)A and IgG [12]. There is reduction in CD27+ memory cells and CD5+ B cells with low levels of T cells which occurs with aging [13]. In the elderly, a decline in organ-specific autoantibodies together with an increase of non-organ-specific antibodies has been reported [14]. Therefore, the reduced humoral responsiveness and altered antibody-mediated defense mechanisms observed in the elderly are caused by the intrinsic primary cell deficit. Furthermore, the involution of the thymus with age results in alteration of gene expression leading to immunosenescence at cellular, molecular, and genetic levels [3]. Thymic weight loss and atrophy with severe loss of thymocytes occur with aging [15].

Other than age-related changes in the immune mechanisms, the changes are also reflected in the endocrine and nervous mechanisms as these systems interact with the immune system. Bidirectional connections among the immune systems with the endocrine and nervous systems mediated by chemokines/cytokines are important for maintaining body homeostasis [16, 17]. A decrease in peripheral B-cell compartment and an increase in activated T-cell compartment were found to be associated with a decrease of thyroid-stimulating hormone (TSH) secretion [16]. Based on these findings, it is suggested that the hypothalamus-pituitary axis plays an immunomodulatory role and influences cellular immune responses by releasing various hormones and neuropeptides [16, 17]. Therefore, it is observed that there are two distinct immune cellular compartments: the diurnal compartment (lymphocyte subsets with acrophase during daytime; CD8, CD16, T-cell receptor [TCR]-γδ-bearing cells) and the nocturnal compartment (lymphocytes subsets with acrophase during night; CD4, CD20, CD25, human leukocyte antigen [HLA]-DR). The time-qualified changes in the levels of activities of these lymphocytes show distinct variations in the young and middle-aged persons when compared to the elderly. These changes are most likely the physiological mechanism for triggering and regulating immune responses [18]. In another study, severe alterations of circadian rhythmicity of variation of TCR-γδ-bearing cells have been found in the elderly subjects [17]. As these cells represent the true immune surveillance cells, their altered circadian rhythmicity is likely to contribute to the increased incidence of cancer seen among the elderly [19]. There is also an observation on circadian variations for the levels of other lymphocytes. The circadian rhythm of CD25 is phase-advanced, while the circadian rhythm of total T cells is phase-delayed in the elderly subjects. In the late morning, the T suppressor/cytotoxic lymphocytes, the natural killer (NK) cells, and the levels of TCR-δ1 are higher and show a clear circadian rhythmicity. It is speculated that TCR-δ1 cells are specialized for mycobacterial immunity or destruction of "stressed" autologous cells (acute leukemia cells) [20]. Increased T-cell activity seen in this study is suggested to be the cause for increased frequency of autoimmune response seen in the elderly [21]. The alterations of these lymphocytes reflect the patterns of circadian rhythmicity and also severely impair the operation of the immune system in aging [17]. When correlation between lymphocyte subpopulations and hormonal changes in the blood is studied, the levels of melatonin and cortisol remain normal in all three categories of subjects (young, middle, and elderly) studied. However, in elderly subjects of above 80 years, melatonin levels are low [21].

Immunity and Cancer

Changes in cytokine microenvironment and decreased functional activities of both innate and adaptive immunities, particularly deficits in the activities of both T and B cells, occur with aging [22]. NK cells are the main components of the innate immune system, being responsible for inhibiting metastasis growth and cancer. Some studies have demonstrated decreased functional ability of human NK cells with age [23, 24]. NK cells of aged individuals show decreased production of interferon (IFN)-γ and chemokines in response to interleukin (IL)-2 and IL-6 [24]. However, another study has shown that the ability of human NK cells to synthesize chemokines in response to IL-6 stimulation is preserved in normal healthy individuals of over 90 years [25]. The preservation of NK-cell cytotoxic capacity in peripheral blood of centenarians has also been demonstrated [26]. Studies on polymorphonuclear leukocytes of elderly individuals show a decrease in intracellular chemotactic and phagocytic activity [25, 27]. Functional alterations in the capacity of NK-cell activity and granulocytic activity with decreased anion superoxide ($O_2^{-\bullet}$) production have been demonstrated in the granulocytes of aged centenarians [28]. Decreased production of $O_2^{-\bullet}$ in granulocytes is attributed to a reduction of the signal transduction mechanism [29]. The attenuation of Fc-mediated $O_2^{-\bullet}$ generation and phagocytosis seen in the elderly is a major factor for the decline of neutrophil function of elderly individuals [27, 30]. Regarding the function of monocyte, decreased generation of $O_2^{-\bullet}$ and diminished levels of IL-2 have been reported in the elderly [31].

In addition, increased production of proinflammatory mediators such as IL-1, IL-6, and IL-8 has been reported in individuals with pathological aging [32]. An increase of IL-6, the "cytokine of gerontologists" [33], has been reported even in healthy elderly individuals of more than 85 years [34–36]. This increase of IL-6 seen in elderly individuals is one of the major contributory factors for age-associated diseases and increased mortality [37, 38]. Cytometric phenotypic analytical studies reveal that the ability of T cells to promote B-cell activation and antibody production is much compromised in elderly individuals [39]. In addition, decreased T lymphocytes and B lymphocytes have been reported in the elderly [40]. Reduction of CD27+ memory B cells, with low T-cell numbers, also occurs in aged individuals [41]. Significant decrease of cellular immunity, as reflected by a decrease in the number of CD3+, CD4+, and CD8+ cells and naive T lymphocytes CD4+ and CD45RA, occurs in the elderly [42]. T-cell alteration in aging is associated with a decrease in the number of naive cells, causing decline in specific immunization response in old-age group [43]. A large increase of dysfunctional cytomegalovirus-specific CD8+ T cells is common in the elderly [44]. Longitudinal studies undertaken in a Swedish population (OCTO studies) suggest that a pattern of immune parameters with low CD4+ cells, high CD8+ cells, and low IL-2 production is predictive of increased mortality rates [45–47].

Aging, Immunity, and Cancer

Understanding the function of the immune system in aging may provide insights into the complex relationship between immunity and cancer. Studies on knockout mice reveal the role of the immune system in controlling the spontaneous generation of tumors. Among aged knockout mice (IFN-$\gamma^{-/-}$ perforin mice), it is found that 50 % of them develop lymphomas, lung adenocarcinoma, or sarcoma [48], which may indicate the importance of healthy functioning of the immune system in preventing the development of tumors. NK cells of the innate immune system play an important role in inhibiting cancerous growth and metastatic tumors. This has been revealed by a prospective study undertaken on 3500 middle-aged and elderly Japanese over 11 years wherein it was noted that the incidence of cancer was higher in individuals who had lower NK cytotoxic activity [49]. Similar findings of lower levels of NK cells in patients with gastric carcinoma correlated with increased tumor size, metastases, and worse prognosis were reported [50]. Unlike the other cells of the immune system, the number of NK cells is actually increased in healthy aged individuals when compared to young or middle-aged persons [31, 32]. The increase of NK cells or NK-cell receptors on T cells is suggested to be of beneficial in curbing the growth of neoplastic cells through its immune surveillance mechanism [51].

The importance of immune surveillance mechanisms in arresting neoplastic growth has been demonstrated in an experimental study. Crossing of tumor suppressor heterozygous $p53^{+/-}$ onto a perforin$^{-/-}$ mice causes reduction in the age of onset of lymphomas with increased frequency of lymphomas, suggesting that the tumor suppressor deficits associated with increase in age are exaggerated by the absence of immune surveillance mechanism [52]. The importance of perforins in suppressing spontaneous lymphomas is also indicated by this study [52].

It has recently been reported that NK cells preferentially target stem cells. Increased NK-cell function was seen when these cells were cultured with primary oral squamous carcinoma stem cells (OSCSCs) when compared to more differentiated OSCSCs. Inhibition of differentiation or reversion of cells to the less-differentiated phenotypes by blocking nuclear factor kappa B (NFκB) or targeted knockdown of cyclooxygenase-2 (COX2) significantly augments NK-cell function. NK cells also cause lysis of human mesenchymal stem cells (hMSCs), human embryonic stem cells (hESCs), and dental pulp stem cells (DPSCs) than their differentiated counterparts. NK-cell-mediated lysis of these cells, namely, OSCSCs, hMSCs, and DPSCs, is prevented by total population of monocytes. This might show that the cytotoxic function of immune effectors is largely suppressed by tumor microenvironment by a number of distinct effectors and secretors. Hence, it is advised that the patients with cancer may benefit from repeated allogenic NK-cell transplantation at the site of tumor for specific elimination of cancer stem cells [53].

A newly synthesized indoleamine derivative Ey-6 kills MC38 tumor cells in a dose-dependent manner (25, 50, 100 μM) with calreticulin induction. Ey-6 treatment altered the tumor cell microenvironment favorable to antitumor immune responses by inducing the secretion of IFN-γ from MC38 cells, which is considered as an important mechanism for inducing antitumor responses. Ey-6 is a novel chemotherapeutic agent that can manipulate the host immunity favorable to eliminate tumor cells by attacking only tumor cells and not attacking normal antigen-presenting cell and dendritic cell maturation [54]. Recent development of immunological newer tools has made possible the attack on cancer cells with specificity of the immune system. Immunotherapy has been done against melanoma, prostate cancer, colorectal cancer, and hematological malignancies [55].

In the tumor microenvironment, there is always a delicate balance between antitumor immunity and tumor-oriented proinflammatory activity, and modulation of immune cell microenvironment and inflammatory processes represents a novel method of target for therapeutic intervention in the control of malignant diseases. Recently, it was reported that a tumor-derived chemokine ligand (CCL), namely, CCL-5, is highly expressed in cancer and plays a critical role in immune escape of colorectal cancer. High levels of CCL-5 expression in human and murine colon cancer cells are associated with high apoptosis of CD8+ T cells and infiltration of T_{reg} cells. RNA interference-mediated knockdown of CCL-5 delayed tumor growth in immunocompetent syngeneic hosts without any effect on tumor growth in immunodeficient hosts. Hence, controlling the expression of CCL-5 will help in increasing CD8+ T cells and for lysis of tumor cells [56]. As cancer medical therapy is currently based on the use of high doses of cyclophosphamide or anthracyclines which not only kill tumor cells but also inhibit T-cell function or macrophages, the use of immunotherapy for arresting specifically the neoplastic growth without affecting normal bone marrow cells, or antigen-presenting cells, has become crucial for effective management and control of cancer [55].

Immunity and Infections

Human beings are constantly exposed to a variety of bacterial and viral infections but are endowed with intrinsic mechanisms to protect themselves against these infections. In this aspect, coordinated actions of innate and adaptive immune mechanisms play an important role. Immunosenescence is associated with greater incidence of infection, as there is a decline in the ability to raise primary immune response against pathogenic antigens [40]. There is a progressive decline in the function of both the adaptive and innate immune systems [30, 57]. Age-related deficiencies of the adaptive immune system include atrophy of the thymus, restriction in the production of naive T cells, and replicative senescence of peripheral T-cell pool [30]. These changes of the adaptive immunity contribute to increased susceptibility of the elderly to novel viral infections such as influenza [58]. Infectious diseases like influenza and pneumonia are major health problems and leading causes of death in the elderly [12].

Class I-restricted CD8+ cells are essential for fighting against infectious agents and form part of the "immunological clock," and reduction in their numbers predicts lack of protection against pathogenic microorganisms. Age-related thymic involution with decreased output of new cells predisposes elderly individuals to a variety of new infectious diseases like pneumonia and urinary tract, skin, and soft tissue infections and infections from viral origin [12]. The antibodies IgA and IgG generally give greater protection against bacterial and viral infections, and increased levels of these antibodies have been reported in healthy old centenarians [39]. The subclasses IgG1, IgG2, and IgG3 are increased, whereas IgM is not increased. IgG1 and IgG3 are involved in the humoral responses to viral infections, whereas IgM is involved with antigens present on the bacteria surface [24]. In addition to age-related reductions in the level of autoantibodies and B cells, the ability of T cells to promote B-cell activation and antibody production is also greatly decreased in elderly people [39]. Besides these changes, innate immune mechanism is very much impaired in the aged people. Both macrophages and granulocytes provide primary resistance to infectious diseases caused by viral and bacterial infections. Regarding granulocytes, accumulated evidence suggests decreased efficiency in the functional activities of these cells such as phagocytosis, chemotaxis, and O_2^- production in the elderly as compared with younger individuals [24].

The ability of mononuclear cells to produce proinflammatory cytokines such as IL-1, IL-6, IL-8, and tumor necrosis factor-α (TNF-α) is also very much increased in the elderly [58]. Plasma IL-6 levels increase from 50 to 60 years and continue to increase till the person reaches the extreme age limit [58]. Although the increase in IL-6 levels is suggested as the most powerful predictor of morbidity and mortality in the elderly, it is also found in healthy centenarians. It is suggested that the increase in IL-6 with increase in age is the consequence of the successful adaptation to several stress factors, including infections which occur throughout life [12, 22].

The fact that the immunosenescence is responsible for increased prevalence and severity of infectious diseases has been supported by several studies [59–61]. Recently, a study conducted in 17 centenarians (the age group from 100 to 105) revealed that IL-22 levels increased in all these healthy centenarians. IL-22 is a proinflammatory cytokine produced by activated T lymphocytes and NK cells. It belongs to proinflammatory cytokine family of IL-10 and stimulates the production of acute phase reactants and thereby promotes antimicrobial defense [62]. Another IL that has recently been advocated for fighting against microbial agents is IL-15. IL-15 has been shown to play a major role in the development of inflammatory and protective immune responses to microbial invaders and parasites by modulating immune cells of both the innate and adaptive systems [63].

The search for administration of suitable substances that can promote both innate and adaptive immunities in the elderly for improving the quality of life has been ongoing for a number of years, and recent studies have pointed out the use of dietary phenols. Numerous studies have reported curative properties of dietary polyphenols such as curcumin, genistein, resveratrol, and epigallocatechin in cancer [64]. Micronutrients like zinc, selenium, and vitamin E have been shown to have immunoenhancing properties. Zinc deficiency has been associated with increased bacterial infections and used for human immunodeficiency virus (HIV)-infected individuals [65]. Use of trace elements and vitamins has been suggested for immunoenhancement in the elderly to fight against infections and cancer [66]. The decline in the production of different hormones like growth hormone, estrogens, dehydroepiandrosterone, and melatonin has been suggested as a possible contributory factor of immunosenescence [7]. Hence, hormone replacement therapy for enhancing immune mechanism of the elderly has been suggested [12]. In this aspect, melatonin, a natural antioxidant with immunoenhancing properties, has been suggested as a possible therapeutic agent to be used in the elderly to fight against cancer and infections [8].

Immunomodulatory Role of Melatonin

The role of melatonin in immunomodulation has been explored by one of the authors of this chapter (GM), who is the first in demonstrating that inhibition of melatonin synthesis resulted in inhibition of both cellular and humoral immunities [67]. A decrease in cellularity of the thymus and spleen with depressed autologous mixed lymphocyte reaction is noted in mice kept in constant light or injected with β-adrenergic blockers, procedures which block melatonin synthesis. These mice are also unable to mount primary antibody responses to sheep erythrocytes [67]. Late afternoon injection of melatonin increases both the primary and secondary responses to sheep red blood cells [68]. Maestroni et al. postulated that stimulating effects of melatonin on immune mechanisms are both direct and through opioidergic pathways [69]. The effect of melatonin in correcting the immunodeficiency status induced by propranolol (β-adrenergic blockers) is abolished by injection of the opioid antagonist naltrexone, showing the involvement of the opioidergic pathways in mediating the immune modulatory functions of melatonin [69].

Removal of the pineal gland (pinealectomy) abolishes both humoral and cellular responses in white turkey poults (birds), whereas melatonin replacement therapy restores both humoral and cellular responses in these birds. These findings show the importance of melatonin for the functions of the immune system [70]. Immunoenhancing action of melatonin is attributed to its direct effects on immunocompetent cells like lymphocytes, NK cells, and granulocyte-macrophage cells. The existence of specific melatonin binding sites in lymphoid cells provides an anatomical basis for the direct effects of melatonin on the regulation of the lymphoid system. High-affinity melatonin binding sites and their signal transduction pathways are identified in human lymphocytes by using I^{125}-melatonin as a ligand [71, 72]. Melatonin through its actions on MT1 melatonin receptors blocks the inhibitory effects of prostaglandin E2 on IL-2 production in human lymphocytes [73]. Moreover, melatonin increases the production of monocytes and macrophages. The enhanced monocyte production induced by melatonin is suggested to be due to its direct action on melatonin receptors on progenitor cell [90]; to the increased sensitivity of monocytes to stimulants such as IL-3, IL-4, and IL-6; or to the granulocyte-macrophage colony-stimulating factor

[74, 75]. The stimulatory effect of melatonin on monocyte/macrophage production in rodents has been confirmed by another study [76].

Melatonin is suggested to regulate hemopoietic cell proliferation by acting on bone marrow stromal cells that contain receptors for κ-opioid cytokine peptides. By activating these receptors and releasing opioid peptides from these stromal cells, melatonin may regulate hemopoietic cell proliferation [77]. In addition to increased lymphocytes and monocyte series, melatonin administration increases the circulating number of NK cells and spontaneous NK-cell activity [78]. The melatonin-induced increase in the NK-cell number is due to the increased production of cytokines like IL-2, IL-6, and IFN-γ from T cells [79].

Action of Melatonin on the Thymus and T Lymphocytes

The thymus, as a primary lymphoid organ, has profound effects on the immune system and is often referred as the "organ of youth in mammals." The process of thymic involution is considered as one of the remarkable feature occurring with age [80]. In the earliest study conducted on pineal influence on thymus growth, it was noticed that pinealectomy in young mice caused accelerated involution of the thymus [81]. The loss of thymocytes with age is the main cause for thymic atrophy and weight loss. The reversal of age-associated thymic involution by melatonin was studied. The thymic cell number of a 2-month-old mice was 12.6×10^7, and at 24 month's age the number was reduced to 7.3×10^7 in the control population. However, when mice were treated with melatonin, the cell number was 9.1×10^7 at 24 months, showing that melatonin was able to arrest the fall in thymocyte numbers. In addition, it was demonstrated that melatonin prevents thymocyte apoptosis mediated by dexamethasone [82]. This protective effect of melatonin on thymocytes is attributed to its antiapoptotic action on the thymus [83]. This reversal of age-associated thymic involution by melatonin adds further support to the findings that melatonin can be used as a potential therapeutic agent for correcting the immunodeficiency state associated with aging and other immunocompromised states [8].

There is much debate to ascertain whether melatonin favors proinflammatory T-helper (Th)1 or anti-inflammatory Th2 response. The Th1/Th2 balance is significant for an appropriate immune response [84]. Administration of melatonin to mice causes the release of proinflammatory Th1 cytokines such as IFN-γ and IL-2. However, melatonin increases the production of IL-10 when it is injected to antigen-primed mice, indicating that melatonin can activate anti-inflammatory Th2 immune response [85]. The relevance of Th1 versus Th2 cytokine expression plays a crucial role in the regulation of cellular immune response [86]. In turn, these responses play a critical role in determining the susceptibility to infectious diseases and progress of inflammatory disorders [75, 87, 88]. Decreased serum levels of melatonin and IL-12 in a cohort of 77 HIV-infected individuals have been reported suggesting the possibility that impairment of immune response may have been a causal factor for reported decrease of serum melatonin levels [89]. Melatonin favors Th1 lymphocyte response in immunodeficiency conditions [90]. It is suggested that Th1 responses are readily transformed into Th2 dominance through depletion of intracellular glutathione (GSH) [91]. GSH in reduced form is the most important cellular antioxidant. Depletion of GSH from antigen-presenting cells in vivo causes reduced Th1 activity and increased Th2 activity [92]. The presence of high levels of oxidized GSH resulted in polarization to type Th2 cells [92]. Thus, the immune activity status can have either Th1 or Th2 characteristics, depending on the relative antioxidant status of the cells. Melatonin increases cytokine production like IL-2, IL-6, and IFN-γ in Th1 cells and thereby enhances NK-cell activity [93].

More recently melatonin has been shown to promote a time-dependent decrease of retinoic acid receptor (RAR)-related orphan receptor (ROR)-α (also known as NR1F1; nuclear receptor subfamily 1, group F, member 1) levels suggesting a role for the ROR-α transcriptional activity. Interestingly, ROR-α acts as a "molecular switch" implicated in the mutually exclusive

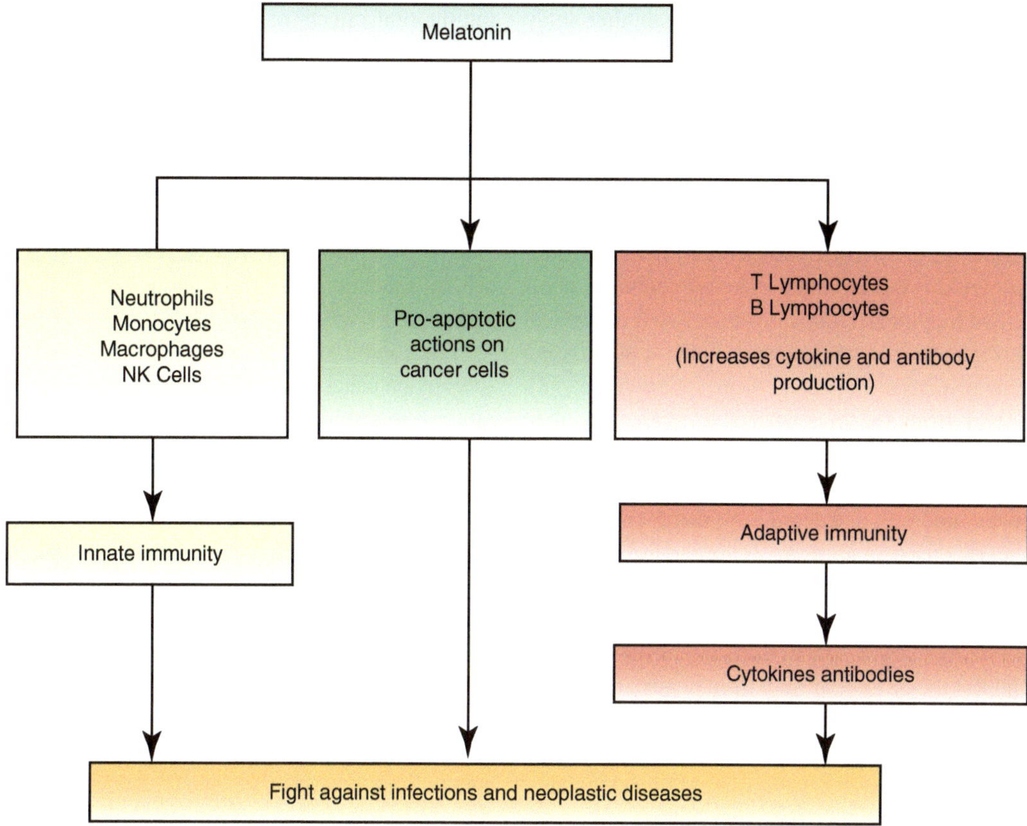

Fig. 9.1 Stimulatory effects of melatonin on innate and adaptive immune mechanisms

generation of Th1 and T_{reg} cells, both involved in the harm/protection balance of immune conditions such as autoimmunity or acute transplant rejection. Therefore, the identification of melatonin as a natural modulator of ROR-α gives it a tremendous therapeutic potential for a variety of clinical disorders [94].

Melatonin, Immunity, and Cytokines

Melatonin influences the immune system by regulating the production of cytokines from immunocompetent cells, and it enhances the production of IL-2, IL-6, and IFN-γ from cultured human mononuclear cells [93, 95, 96]. Melatonin increases the production of IL-1, IL-6, TNF-α, and reactive oxygen species by activating monocytes [93]. Melatonin upregulates gene expression of transforming growth factor (TGF)-β, macrophage colony-stimulating factor (M-CSF), TNF-α, stem cell factor (SCF), IL-1β, and IFN-γ which in turn increases their production [88]. Immunoenhancing effects of melatonin are attributed to its antiapoptotic action on certain cells, antioxidant actions, and on its influence in enhancing the production of cytokines [8]. A schematic diagram showing the beneficial effects on melatonin on immune mechanisms (both innate immunity and adaptive immunity) is presented in Fig. 9.1.

Effects of Melatonin on Infections and Immunity: Direct Evidences

Injections of melatonin to Siberian hamsters 4 h before the onset of darkness (in order to lengthen the endogenous melatonin profile) mimicked the effects of short days on febrile response to a simulated infection, emphasizing the importance of the duration of melatonin secretion in controlling host response to infection [97]. In another study on Siberian hamsters, it is noted that exposure to short days increases the number of circulating leukocytes and several lymphocyte populations. The short day exposure also attenuates both the magnitude and the duration of two major consequences of bacterial infection, i.e., anorexia and cachexia [97]. Since the effect of the short photoperiod on circulating leukocyte count is abolished by pinealectomy, it is concluded that pineal hormone melatonin is responsible for attenuating the adverse responses to bacterial infection [98]. Apart from the beneficial role of melatonin in combating bacterial and viral infections through its immunomodulatory mechanisms which has been already discussed, its metabolite in the neural tissue, namely, N[1]-acetyl-N[2]-formyl-5-methoxykynuramine (AFMK), is also effective in stimulating neutrophils and fighting against infections [99, 100]. Both melatonin and AFMK inhibit the release of IL-8 from neutrophils; however, AFMK is much more effective than melatonin in this aspect. Moreover, the production of TNF-α by neutrophils is also inhibited by melatonin. As IL-8 and TNF-α contribute to inflammation [101], the inhibition of them by melatonin and AFMK is essential for combating against chronic inflammation [100].

Melatonin, Immunity, and Anticarcinogenic Effects

The development of carcinogenesis is protected by endogenous mechanisms which can be categorized into immune and nonimmune-dependent mechanisms. Immunosurveillance is one of the major processes whereby cancerous cells are detected and destroyed. NK cells play an important role in immunosurveillance against virus-infected cells and neoplasia. The influence of melatonin on NK-cell number and functional activity has already been discussed. The activation of monocytes and macrophages by melatonin is another mechanism through which melatonin exerts its anticarcinogenic effects. In addition to melatonin's stimulatory effect on CD4+ cells, Th1 cells are also important for the antitumoral effects of melatonin.Th1 cells have the ability to kill the tumor cells by releasing cytokines that activate "death receptors" on tumor cell surface [102]. In addition to its effects of activating immune mechanisms, melatonin also has the ability to directly inhibit the cancer growth. This has been demonstrated in a recent study on hepatocarcinoma HepG2 cell lines in which melatonin addition induces cell cycle arrest [103–105].

The combination of melatonin with immunotherapy on cancer patients has been tried in some studies. In a study conducted on 24 patients with advanced cell tumors (lung cancer, 9 patients; colorectal cancer, 7 patients; gastric cancer, 3 patients; breast cancer, 2 patients, hepatocarcinoma, 1 patient; pancreatic cancer, 1 patient; unknown tumor, 1 patient), melatonin was given along with IL-2. Melatonin was administered 7 days before the injection of IL-2. Progress was found only in 6/24 patients, while stability was reported in 14/24 patients. This study shows melatonin combination with IL-2 in treating conditions with advanced neoplasms [106]. Similarly, administration of low subcutaneous dose of IL-2 with melatonin was found beneficial in causing tumor regression and prolonging the survival of cancer patients with metastatic colorectal cancer [107]. The interrelationship between melatonin and the immune system in cancer was also studied in 42 patients with advanced gastrointestinal cancer (colorectal, pancreatic, gastric cancer). The circadian rhythm of plasma melatonin is observed to be altered with peak melatonin level reaching at 0800–0900 h with 5–7 h delay with respect to average peak time in healthy controls. The study of TNF-α rhythm and soluble TNF-α receptors (type 1 and type 2) in these patients indicated an interrelationship between the neuroendocrine network and cytokine network [108]. Based upon the neurohormonal studies carried out on lung cancer patients, in which overall increased serum levels of cortisol and altered cortisol rhythm were found, it was suggested that chronic treatment of advanced cancer patients with melatonin can normalize cortisol rhythm and this effect could stabilize the disease. As melatonin possesses a strong antiapoptotic property, it can play an important role as a system regulator in immunoenhancement and has a potential value to be used as an adjuvant tumor immunotherapeutic agent [109].

Conclusions

The incidence of infectious diseases and neoplastic diseases is higher in elderly individuals. There is also seasonal outbreak of some infectious diseases. The immune system plays a major role in the ability of the host organism to combat infectious and/or neoplastic diseases. Both innate and adaptive immunities have distinct roles. The greater incidence of infectious diseases and neoplastic diseases seen in the elderly is attributed to many factors such as the nutritional status of the individual and environmental conditions but, most importantly, the immune status of the elderly. As age advances there is drastic reduction in immune capability of the body, known as immunosenescence, which is suggested to be the main reason for the greater occurrence of these diseases in the elderly. Immune mechanisms are regulated by a complex neuroendocrine network in which melatonin is very important. Melatonin has a stimulatory role on innate, cellular, and humoral immunity. The beneficial role of melatonin in immune modulation has been shown in experimental studies on various animals. The anticarcinogenic effect of melatonin is exerted partly through its immunomodulatory mechanism. Recent studies on lung cancer patients suggest that there is disordered hormonal secretion pattern and circadian variations of various lymphocyte subpopulations revealing impaired integration among the nervous, endocrine, and immune systems in neoplastic disease. Treatment with melatonin can restore these disturbed functions found in cancer patients and can be of therapeutic value as a "chronotherapeutic agent" in treating cancer. Moreover, because of its antiapoptotic nature with immunoenhancement properties, melatonin has a potential value for being used as an adjunct tumor immunotherapeutic agent. In addition, the photoperiodic changes of melatonin secretion and its correlation with seasonal infections are also gaining much attention. The synthesis of melatonin by the lymphocytes and thymus supports the immunomodulatory role of melatonin. This may suggest the possibility of using melatonin as an adjunct therapy in the control and management of infectious diseases and cancer.

References

1. Wikby A, Ferguson F, Forsey R, Thompson J, Strindhall J, Lofgren S, et al. An immune risk phenotype, cognitive impairment, and survival in very late life: impact of allostatic load in Swedish octogenarian and non octogenarian humans. J Gerontol A Biol Sci Med Sci. 2005;60:556–65.
2. Pawelec G, Ouyang Q, Colonna-Romono G, Candore G, Lio D, Caruso C. Is human immunosenescence clinically relevant? Looking for immunological risk phenotypes. Trends Immunol. 2002;23:330–2.
3. Tarazona R, Solana R, Ouyang Q, Pawelec G. Basic biology and clinical impact of immunosenescence. Exp Gerontol. 2002;37:183–9.
4. Ligthart GJ, Corberand JX, Fournier C, Galanaud P, Hiljmans W, Kennes B, et al. Admission criteria for immunogeronto-logical studies in man: the SENIEUR protocol. Mech Ageing Dev. 1984;28:47–55.
5. Fietta A, Merlini C, Dos Santos C, Rovida S, Grassi C. Influence of aging on some specific and nonspecific mechanisms of the host defense system in 146 healthy subjects. Gerontology. 1994;40:237–45.
6. Ahluwalia N. Aging, nutrition and immune function. J Nutr. 2004;8(1):2–6.
7. Arit W, Hewison M. Hormones and immune function: implications of aging. Aging Cell. 2004;3:209–16.
8. Srinivasan V, Maestroni GJM, Cardinali DP, Esquifino AI, Pandi-Perumal SR, Miller SC. Melatonin, immune function and aging. Immun Aging. 2005;2:17. http://www.immunityageing.com/content/2/1/17. Accessed on 24 Apr 2012.
9. Nelson RJ. Seasonal immune function and sickness responses. Trends Immunol. 2004;25:187–92.
10. Reichlin S. Neuroendocrine-immune interactions. N Engl J Med. 1993;329:1246–53.
11. Srinivasan V. Psychoneuroimmunology. Indian J Clin Pract. 1995;5(11):39–41.
12. Ginaldi L, Loreto MF, Corsi MP, Modesti M, Martinis M. Immuno-senescence and infectious diseases. Microbes Infect. 2001;3:851–7.
13. Colonna-Romano G, Bulati M, Aquino A, Scialabba G, Candore G, Lio D, et al. B cells in the aged: CD27, CD5, and CD 40 expression. Mech Ageing Dev. 2003;124:389–93.

14. Weksler ME, Szabo P. The effect of age on the B-cell response. J Clin Immunol. 2000;20:240–9.
15. Tian YM, Zhang GY, Dai YR. Melatonin rejuvenates thymus and redresses peripheral immune functions in aged mice. Immunol Lett. 2003;88:101–4.
16. Mazzoccoli G, DeCata A, Carughi S, Greco A, Inglese M, Perfetto F, et al. A possible mechanism for altered immune response in the elderly. In Vivo. 2010;24(4):471–87.
17. Mazzoccoli G, Inglese M, De Cata A, Carughi S, Dagostino MP, Marzulli N, et al. Neuroendocrine-immune interactions in healthy aging. Geriatr Gerontol. 2011;11:98–106.
18. Mazzoccoli G, Sothern RB, De Cata A, Giuliani F, Fontana A, Copetti M, et al. A timetable of 24-hour patterns for human lymphocyte subpopulations. J Biol Regul Homeost Agents. 2011;25(3):387–95.
19. Mazzoccoli G, Vendemiale G, De Cata A, Tarquini R. Change of γδ TCR-expressing T cells in healthy aging. Int J Immunopathol Pharmacol. 2011;24:201–9.
20. Bensussan A, Lagabrielle JF, Degos L. TcRγδ bearing lymphocyte clones with lymphokine activated killer activity against autologous leukemic cells. Blood. 1989;15:135–9.
21. Mazzoccoli G, Vendemiale M, La Viola A, De Cata A, Carughi A, Greco A, et al. Circadian variations of cortisol, melatonin, and lymphocyte subpopulations in geriatric age. Int J Immunopathol Pharmacol. 2010;23(1):289–96.
22. Hakim FT, Flomerfelt FA, Boyiadzis M, Gress RE. Aging, immunity and cancer. Curr Opin Immunol. 2004;16:151–6.
23. Borrego F, Alonso MC, Galiani MD, Carracedo J, Ramirez R, Ostos B, et al. NK phenotypic markers and IL2 response in NK cells from elderly people. Exp Gerontol. 1999;34:253–65.
24. Ginaldi L, De Martinis M, D'Ostillo A, Marini L, Loreto MF, Quaglino D. The immune system in the elderly: III. Innate immunity. Immunol Res. 1999;20: 117–26.
25. Mariani E, Meneghetti A, Neri S, Ravaglia G, Forti P, Cattini L, et al. Chemokine production by natural killer cells from nonagenarians. Eur J Immunol. 2002;32:1524–9.
26. Krishnaraj R. Senescence and cytokine modulate the NK cell expression. Mech Ageing Dev. 1997;96: 89–101.
27. Fulop Jr T, Foris G, Worum I, Paragh G, Leovey A. Age related variations of some polymorphonuclear leukocytes functions. Mech Ageing Dev. 1985;29: 1–8.
28. Miyagi C, Watanabe H, Toma H, Akisaka M, Tomiyama K, Sato Y, et al. Functional alteration of granulocytes, NK cells, and natural killer cells in centenarians. Hum Immunol. 2000;61:908–16.
29. Lipschitz DA, Udupa KB, Boxer LA. The role of calcium in the age related decline of neutrophil function. Blood. 1988;71:659–65.
30. Lord JM, Butcher S, Killampali V, Lascelles D, Salmon M. Neutrophil ageing and immunosenescence. Mech Ageing Dev. 2001;122:1521–35.
31. Castle SC. Clinical relevance of age related immune dysfunction. Clin Infect Dis. 2000;31:578–85.
32. Franceschi C, Bonafe M, Valensin S, Olivieri F, De Luca M, Ottaviani E, et al. Inflam-aging. An evolutionary perspective on immune-senescence. Ann N Y Acad Sci. 2000;908:244–54.
33. Ershler WB. Interleukin-6: a cytokine for gerontologists. J Am Geriatr Soc. 1993;41:176–81.
34. Mysliwska J, Bryl E, Foerster J, Mysliwski A. Increase of interleukin-6 and decrease of interleukin-2 production during the ageing process are influenced by the health status. Mech Ageing Dev. 1998;100: 313–28.
35. Straub RH, Miller LE, Scholmerich J, Zietz B. Cytokines and hormones as possible links between endocrinosenescence and immunosenescence. J Neuroimmunol. 2000;109:10–5.
36. Forsey RJ, Thompson JM, Ernerudh J, Hurst JL, Strindhall J, Johansson B, et al. Plasma cytokine profiles in elderly humans. Mech Ageing Dev. 2003;124: 487–93.
37. Ferrucci L, Harris TB, Guralnik JM, Tracy RP, Corti MC, Cohen HJ, et al. Serum IL-6 level and the development of disability in older patients. J Am Geriatr Soc. 1999;106:506–12.
38. Harris TB, Ferrucci L, Tracy RP, Corti MC, Wacholder C, Ettinger Jr WH, et al. Associations of elevated interleukin-6 and C-reactive protein levels with mortality in the elderly. Am J Med. 1999;106:506–12.
39. Cossarizza A, Ortolani C, Monti D, Franceschi C. Cytometric analysis of immuno-senescence. Cytometry. 1997;27:297–313.
40. Fagnoni FF, Vescovini RR, Passeri GG, Bologna G, Pedrazzoni M, Lavagetto G, et al. Shortage of circulating of naive CD8(+) T cells provide new insights on immunodeficiency in aging. Blood. 2000;95: 2860–8.
41. Breitbart E, Wang X, Leka LS, Dallal GE, Meydani SN, Stollar BD. Altered memory B cell homeostasis in human aging. J Gerontol A Biol Sci Med Sci. 2002;57:B304–11.
42. Pawelec G, Effros RB, Caruso C, Ramarque E, Barnett Y, Solana R. T cells and aging. Front Biosci. 1999;4:D216–69.
43. Linton PJ, Haynes L, Tsui L, Zhang X, Swain S. From naive to effector-alterations with aging. Immunol Rev. 1997;160:9–18.
44. Quyang Q, Wagner WM, Zheng W, Wikby A, Remarque EJ, Pawelec G. Dysfunctional CMV-specific CD8+ cells accumulate in the elderly. Exp Gerontol. 2004;39:607–13.
45. Ferguson FG, Wikby A, Maxson P, Olsson J, Johansson B. Immune parameters in longitudinal study of a very old population of Swedish people: a comparison between survivors and non-survivors. J Gerontol A Biol Sci Med Sci. 1995;50:B378–82.
46. Wikby A, Maxson P, Olsson J, Johansson B, Fergusson FG. Changes in CD8 and CD4 lymphocyte subsets, T cell proliferation responses and non survival in the very old: the Swedish longitudinal OCTO-immune study. Mech Ageing Dev. 1998;102:187–98.

47. Olsson J, Wikby A, Johansson B, Lofgren S, Nilsson BO, Fergusson FG. Age related changes in peripheral blood T-lymphocytes subpopulations and cytomegalovirus infections in the very old: the Swedish longitudinal OCTO immune study. Mech Ageing Dev. 2000;121:187–201.
48. Street SE, Trapani JA, MacGregor D, Smyth MJ. Suppression of lymphoma and epithelial malignancies affected by interferon-γ. J Exp Med. 2002;196: 129–34.
49. Imai K, Matsuyama S, Miyaki S, Suga K, Nagachi K. Natural cytotoxic activity of peripheral blood lymphocytes and cancer incidence; an 11 year follow up study of a general population. Lancet. 2000;356:1795–9.
50. Takeuchi H, Maehara Y, Tokunaga Y, Koga T, Kakeji Y, Sugimachi K. Prognostic significance of natural killer cell activity in patients with gastric carcinoma: a multivariate analysis. Am J Gastroenterol. 2001;96:574–8.
51. Bonafe M, Valensin S, Gianni W, Marigliano V, Franceschi C. The unexpected contribution of immunosenescence to the levelling off of cancer incidence and mortality in the oldest old. Crit Rev Oncol Hematol. 2001;39:227–33.
52. Smyth MJ, Thia KY, Street SE, MacGregor D, Godfrey D, Trapani J. Perforin-mediated cytotoxicity is critical for surveillance of spontaneous lymphoma. J Exp Med. 2000;192:755–60.
53. Jewett A, Tseng HC, Arasteh A, Saddat S, Christensen RE, Cacalano RA. Natural killer cells preferentially target cancer stem cells: role of monocytes in protection against NK cell mediated lysis of cancer stem cells. Curr Drug Deliv. 2011;9(1):5–16.
54. Oh SJ, Ryu CK, Baek SY, Lee H. Cellular mechanism of newly synthesized indoleamine derivative-induced immunological death of tumor cell. Immune Netw. 2011;11(6):383–9.
55. Pandoffi F, Cianci R, Pagliari D, Casciano F, Bagala C, Astone A, et al. The immune response to tumors as a tool toward immunotherapy. Clin Dev Immunol. 2011. http://www.hindawi.com/journals/cdi/2011/894704/. Accessed on 15 Apr 2012.
56. Chang LY, Lin YC, Mahalingam J, Huang CT, Chen TW, Kang CW, et al. Tumor-derived chemokine CCL-5 enhances TGF-β-mediated killing of CD8+ T cells in colon cancer by T-regulatory cells. Cancer Res. 2012;72(5):1092–102.
57. Butcher S, Chahal H, Lord JM. Ageing and the neutrophil: no appetite for killing? Immunology. 2000; 100:411–6.
58. Rajagopalan S, Yoshikawa TT. Tuberculosis in the elderly. Z Gerontol Geriatr. 2000;33:374–80.
59. Wick G, Grubeck-Loebenstein B. Primary and secondary alterations of immune reactivity in the elderly: impact of dietary factors and disease. Immunol Res. 1997;160:171–84.
60. Weiskopf D, Weinberger D, Grubeck-Lobenstein B. The aging of the immune system. Transpl Int. 2009;22(11):1041–50.
61. Ponnappan S, Ponnappan U. Aging and immune function: molecular mechanisms to inventions. Antioxid Redox Signal. 2011;14(8):1551–85.
62. Basile G, Paffumi I, D'Angelo AG, Figliomreni P, Cucinotta MD, Pace E, et al. Health centenarians show high levels of interleukin-22. Arch Gerontol Geriatr. 2011;54(3):459–61.
63. Perera RY, Lichy JH, Waldman TR, Perera LP. The role of interleukin-15 in inflammation and immune responses. Microbes Infect. 2012;14(3):247–61.
64. Ghiringhelli F, Rebe C, Hichami A, Delmas D. Immunomodulation and anti-inflammatory roles of polyphenols as anticancer agents. Anticancer Agents Med Chem. 2012;12(8):852–73.
65. Khanna KW, Markan RB. A perspective on cellular immunity in the elderly. Clin Infect Dis. 1999;28: 710–3.
66. Chandra RK. Effect of vitamin and trace element supplementation on immune responses and infections in the elderly subjects. Lancet. 1992;340:1124–7.
67. Maestroni GJ, Conti A, Pierpaoli W. Role of the pineal gland in immunity. Circadian synthesis and release of melatonin modulates the antibody response and antagonizes the immunosuppressive effect of corticosterone. J Neuroimmunol. 1986;13:19–30.
68. Maestroni GJ, Conti A, Pierpaoli W. Role of the pineal gland in immunity: II. Melatonin enhances the antibody response via an opiatergic mechanism. Clin Exp Immunol. 1987;8:384–91.
69. Maestroni GJ, Conti A, Pierpaoli W. The pineal gland and the circadian, opiatergic, immunoregulatory role of melatonin. Ann N Y Acad Sci. 1987;496:67–77.
70. Moore CB, Siopes TD. Effect of melatonin supplementation on the ontogeny of immunity in the large White turkey poult. Poult Sci. 2002;81:1898–903.
71. Gonzalez-Haba MG, Garcia-Maurino S, Calvo JR, Goberna R, Guerrero JM. High affinity binding of melatonin by human circulating T lymphocytes (CD4+). FASEB J. 1995;9:1331–5.
72. Garcia-Perganeda A, Pozo D, Guerrero JM, Calvo JR. Signal transduction for melatonin in human lymphocytes: involvement of a pertussis toxin sensitive G-protein. J Immunol. 1997;159:3774–81.
73. Carrillo-Vico A, Garcia-Maurino S, Calvo JR, Guerrero JM. Melatonin counteracts the inhibitory effect of PGE-2 on interleukin-2 production in human lymphocytes via its mt1 membrane receptor. FASEB J. 2003;17:755–7.
74. Maestroni GJ, Conti A, Lissoni P. Colony stimulating activity and hematopoietic rescue from cancer chemotherapy compounds are induced by melatonin via endogenous interleukin-4. Cancer Res. 1994;54: 4740–3.
75. Maestroni GJ, Covacci V, Conti A. Hematopoietic rescue via T cell dependent endogenous granulocyte-macrophage colony-stimulating factor induced by the pineal neurohormone melatonin in tumor bearing mice. Cancer Res. 1994;54:2429–32.
76. Kaur C, Ling EA. Effects of melatonin on macrophages/microglia in post natal rat brain. J Pineal Res. 1999;26:158–68.
77. Maestroni GJ. The immunotherapeutic potential of melatonin. Expert Opin Investig Drugs. 2001;10: 467–76.

78. Angeli A, Gatti G, Sartori ML, Ponte D, Carignola R. Effect of exogenous melatonin on human natural killer cell (NK) cell activity. In: Gupta D, Attansio A, Reiter RJ, editors. An approach to the immunomodulatory role of the pineal gland. Tubingen: Brain Research Promotion; 1988. p. 145–56.
79. Currier NL, Sun LZ, Miller SC. Exogenous melatonin: quantitative enhancement in vivo of cells mediating non-specific immunity. J Neuroimmunol. 2000; 104:101–8.
80. Gruver AL, Hudson LL, Sempowski GD. Immunosenescence of ageing. J Pathol. 2007;211: 144–56.
81. Csaba G, Barath P. Morphological changes of thymus and thyroid gland after post-natal extirpation of pineal body. Endocrinol Exp. 1975;9:59–67.
82. Hoijman E, Rocha-Viegas L, Keller-Sarmiento MI, Rosenstein RE, Pecci A. Involvement of Bax protein in the prevention of glucocorticoid-induced thymocytes apoptosis by melatonin. Endocrinology. 2004; 145(1):418–25.
83. Tian TM, Li PP, Jiang XF, Zhang GY, Dai YR. Rejuvenation of degenerative thymus by oral melatonin administration and the antagonistic action of melatonin against hydroxyl radical induced apoptosis of cultured thymocytes in mice. J Pineal Res. 2001; 31:214–21.
84. Raghavendra V, Singh V, Kulkarni SK, Agrewala JN. Melatonin enhances Th2 cell mediated: lack of sensitivity to reversal by naltrexone or benzodiazepine receptor antagonists. Mol Cell Biochem. 2001;221: 57–62.
85. Calcagni E, Elenkov I. Stress system activity, innate, and T helper cytokines, and susceptibility to immune related diseases. Ann N Y Acad Sci. 2006;1069:62–76.
86. Chaouat G. The Th1/Th2 paradigm still important in pregnancy? Semin Immunopathol. 2007;29:95–113.
87. Srinivasan V, Spence DW, Trakht I, Pandi-Perumal SR, Cardinali DP, Maestroni GJ. Immunomodulation by melatonin: its significance for seasonally occurring diseases. Neuroimmunomodulation. 2008;15:93–101.
88. Liu F, Ng TB, Fung MC. Pineal indoles stimulate the gene expression of immuno-modulating cytokines. J Neural Transm. 2001;108:397–405.
89. Nunnari G, Nigro L, Palermo F, Leto D, Pomerantz RJ, Cacopardo B. Reduction of serum melatonin levels in HIV-1 infected individuals parallel disease progression: correlation with serum interleukin-12 levels. Infection. 2003;31:379–82.
90. Kidd P. Th1/Th2 balance: the hypothesis, its limitations and implications for health and disease. Altern Med Rev. 2003;8:223–46.
91. Peterson JD, Herzenberg LA, Vasquez K, Waltenbaugh C. Glutathione levels in antigen-presenting cells modulates Th1 versus Th2 receptor patterns. Proc Natl Acad Sci U S A. 1998;95:3071–6.
92. Murata Y, Shimamura T, Hamuro J. The polarization of Th1/Th2 balance is dependent on the intracellular thiol redox status of macrophages due to its distinctive cytokine production. Int Immunol. 2002;14:201–12.
93. Garcia-Maurino S, Gonzalez-Haba MG, Calvo JR, Rafil-el-Idrissi M, Sanchez-Margalet V, Goberna R, et al. Melatonin enhances IL-2, IL-6, and IFNγ production by human circulating CD4+ cells: a possible nuclear receptor mediated mechanism involving T helper type1 lymphocytes, and monocytes. J Immunol. 1997;159:574–81.
94. Lardone PJ, Guerrero JM, Fernandez-Santos JM, Martin-Laeve I, Carrillo-Vico A. Melatonin synthesized by T lymphocytes as a ligand of the retinoic acid related orphan receptor. J Pineal Res. 2011;51(4):454–62.
95. Garcia-Maurino S, Pozo D, Carrillo-Vico A, Calvo JR, Guerrero JM. Melatonin activates Th1 lymphocytes by increasing IL-12 production. Life Sci. 1999; 65:2143–50.
96. Morrey KM, McLachlan JA, Serkin CD, Bakouche O. Activation of human monocytes by the pineal hormone melatonin. J Immunol. 1994;153:2671–80.
97. Bilbo SD, Nelson RJ. Melatonin regulates energy balance and attenuates fever in Siberian hamsters. Endocrinology. 2002;143:2527–33.
98. Wen JC, Dhabbar FS, Prendergast BJ. Pineal dependent and independent effect of photoperiod on immune function in Siberian Hamsters (Phodopus sungorus). Horm Behav. 2007;51:31–9.
99. Silva SO, Rodriguez MR, Carvalho SR, Catalani LH, Campa A, Ximenes VF. Oxidation of melatonin and its catabolites, N-acetyl-N-formyl 5 methoxykynuramine by activated leukocytes. J Pineal Res. 2004;37:171–5.
100. Silva SO, Rodriguez MR, Xieminas VF, Bueno-da-silva AE, Amarantes-Mendes GP, Campa A. Neutrophils as specific target for melatonin and kynuramine: effects on cytokine release. J Neuroimmunol. 2004;156:146–52.
101. Adams DH, Llyod AR. Chemokines: leukocyte recruitment and activation cytokines. Lancet. 1997; 349:490–5.
102. Knutson KL, Disis ML. Tumor-antigen specific T helper cells in cancer immunity and immunotherapy. Cancer Immunol Immunother. 2005;54:721–8.
103. Martin-Renedo J, Mauriz JL, Jorquera F, Ruiz-Andres O, Gonsalez P, Gonsalez-Gallego J. Melatonin induces cell cycle arrest and apoptosis in hepatocarcinoma HepG2 cell line. J Pineal Res. 2008;45:532–40.
104. Ozdemir F, Deniz O, Kayner K, Arslan M, Kavgaci H, Yildiz B, et al. The effect of melatonin on human hepatoma (Hep G2) cell line. Bratisl Lek Listy. 2009;110:276–9.
105. Srinivasan V, Pandi-Perumal SR, Brzezinski A, Bhatnagar KP, Cardinali DP. Melatonin, immune function and cancer. Recent Pat Endocr Metab Immune Drug Discov. 2011;5:109–23.
106. Lissoni P, Brivio F, Ardizzoia A, Tancini G, Barni S. Subcutaneous therapy with low-dose interleukin-2 plus the neurohormone melatonin in metastatic gastric cancer patients with low performance status. Tumori. 1993;79:401–4.

107. Barni S, Lissoni P, Cazzaniga M, Ardizzoia A, Meregalli S, Fossati V, et al. A randomized study of low-dose subcutaneous interleukin-2 plus melatonin versus supportive care alone in metastatic colon-cancer patients progressing under 5-fluorouracil and folates. Oncology. 1995;52:243–5.

108. Muc-Wierzgon M, Nowakowska-Zajdel E, Zubelewicz B, Wierzgon J, Kokot T, Klala K, et al. Circadian fluctuations of melatonin, tumor necrosis factor α and its soluble receptors in the circulation of patients with advanced gastrointestinal cancer. J Exp Clin Cancer Res. 2003;22:171–8.

109. Jung B, Ahmad N. Melatonin in cancer management: progress and promise. Cancer Res. 2006;66:9789–93.

Circadian Variation of Immune Mechanisms in Lung Cancer and the Role of Melatonin

10

Gianluigi Mazzoccoli

Abstract

New cancer immunotherapeutic strategies rely on recent advances in the knowledge of the mechanisms responsible for antitumor immunity. Immune parameters in humans show temporal variations related to circadian changes of total lymphocytes and specific lymphocyte subsets in the peripheral blood, with an inverse relationship of the total number of lymphocytes to plasma cortisol concentration and a direct correlation to plasma melatonin levels. Immune responses are characterized by nyctohemeral variations and are physiologically controlled by neuroendocrine pathways. The discoveries of the antitumor cytokine network underlay innovative anticancer immunotherapeutic approach, taking into account neuroendocrine and neuroimmune status of cancer patients. Lung cancer patients present anomalies of proportions and circadian variations of lymphocyte subsets, as well as of hormones and cytokines that may impair the interplay among different lymphocyte subpopulations and neuroendocrine system components, decisive for an efficient immune response. A chronobiologic strategy of correctly timed circadian stage-dependent sampling and/or dosing schedule taking in consideration circadian rhythmicity in biochemical, physiological, and behavioral processes will be critical in any attempts to successfully optimize and personalize decision-making when evaluating immunomodulatory effects determined by biological response modifiers and adoptive immunotherapy protocols, in addition to neuroendocrine endogenous molecules, such as the pineal indole melatonin.

Keywords

Circadian rhythmicity • Immune system • Melatonin • Lung cancer • Chronobiology

G. Mazzoccoli, MD
Division of Internal Medicine and Chronobiology Unit, Department of Medical Sciences, IRCCS Scientific Institute and Regional General Hospital "Casa Sollievo Della Sofferenza" Opera Di Padre Pio Da Pietrelcina, Cappuccini Avenue, S. Giovanni Rotondo, 71013 FG, Italy
e-mail: g.mazzoccoli@operapadrepio.it

V. Srinivasan et al. (eds.), *Melatonin and Melatonergic Drugs in Clinical Practice*,
DOI 10.1007/978-81-322-0825-9_10, © Springer India 2014

Abbreviations

CCL20	Chemokine (C–C motif) ligand 20
CCR6	Chemokine (C–C motif) receptor 6
CTLA-4	Cytotoxic T-lymphocyte antigen 4
EGF	Epidermal growth factor
Foxp3	Forkhead transcription factors
GH	Growth hormone
GITR	Glucocorticoid-induced TNF-α receptor
GVHD	Graft-versus-host disease
HSCT	Hematopoietic stem cell transplantation
IFN	Interferon
IGF	Insulin-like growth factor
IL	Interleukin
LAK	Lymphokine-activated killer cells
MHC	Major histocompatibility complex
MLT-R	Melatonin receptors
NAT	*N*-acetyl-transferase
NK	Natural killer
PD-1	Programmed death-1
PKC	Protein kinase C
TCR	T-cell receptors
TNF	Tumor necrosis factor
TRH	Thyrotropin-releasing hormone
TSH	Thyroid-stimulating hormone

Introduction

A major advance for the treatment of neoplastic disease could derive from harmless and widely applicable immunotherapy strategies. An example is represented by the antibody drug ipilimumab which promotes broad T-cell function by blocking a surface protein called cytotoxic T-lymphocyte antigen 4 (CTLA-4), prolonging survival in 20–30 % of patients, but often accompanied by severe or even fatal autoimmune side effects. A new class of cancer drug that boosts T cells in a more targeted fashion blocking a protein called programmed death-1 (PD-1) has been found capable to reduce tumor mass in a variety of cancers, including lung cancer.

Previous cancer immunotherapies were typically founded on empirical criteria, elaborated independently of the evaluation of immune cell subset differentiation and endogenous cytokine production and based on an artificial manipulation of anticancer immunity through the administration of in vitro-activated immune cells or genetically engineered biological drugs without taking into consideration the immune status of the individual cancer patient. The efficacy of the immunotherapeutic strategies depends on the host immunobiological response and requires the definition of antitumor immune mechanisms and immune status of cancer patients before the start of treatments [1].

Virtually every body function in humans has been shown to display circadian rhythmicity in healthy individuals, with known times of highest and lowest values in relation to an individual's sleep–wake schedule, which is usually the dominant synchronizer for the body clock [2, 3]. Thus, prominent circadian patterns have been documented for nearly all aspects of human physiology, including variation of circulating lymphocyte subpopulations, as well as most analytes and variables detected in the blood and urine. In spite of a large body of literature documenting daily 24 h cycles in nearly all physiological variables, however, this variation is widely disregarded in medical practice even today. Nevertheless, a diurnal curve with variables measured at different time points can provide more information than a single determination obtained during a single office visit. Thus, relationships among physiological variables determined at only a single time point may be misleading due to variations in the 24 h timing of high and low values among variables, in addition to any possible alterations in circadian rhythms with age or health status [4].

Lymphocyte cell surface CD4 and CD8 coreceptors both express only transiently at a very early stage during thymus ontogeny, whereas in mature circulating cells, expression of either coreceptor is mutually exclusive, and conventional CD3+ T cells usually express either CD4+brightCD8- or CD4-CD8bright phenotypes. A small fraction of peripheral T cells co-express CD4 and low levels of CD8 (CD4+CD8dim). These cells have been associated with mucosal-related lymphocytes, but their ontogenetic origin is not clear. CD4+CD8dim T cells are rare in peripheral blood, can bear the morphology of large granular lymphocytes, can express natural killer (NK)-associated antigens, and can have cytotoxic activity. NK cells are large granular lymphocytes that express neither α/β or γ/δ TCR (T-cell receptors) nor CD3 on their surface, can lyse a number of different tumor cells, and may be stimulated by interferon gamma (IFN-γ), interleukin (IL) 2, IL-12, and IL-18 [5].

The expression of the CD4 and CD8 molecules by mature T cells has been considered mutually exclusive as mentioned above, with only immature T cells expressing both these proteins simultaneously in the thymus, but significant numbers of double positive CD4+CD8+ T lymphocytes have been detected in peripheral blood and secondary lymphoid tissues. The CD8+ lymphocytes are heterogeneous in subphenotypes and functions and include T cells that express high-density CD8 (CD4-CD8+bright) and T cells that express low-density CD8 (CD4+CD8dim+). CD4+ T lymphocytes expressing CD8dim represent cytotoxic effector populations and contain high amounts of perforin, which explains their greater cytolytic capacity [5].

Circulating CD4+CD8+dim cells may represent activated cells. This suggestion stems from in vitro studies showing that mitogen activation of CD4+CD8- or CD4-CD8+ cells produced a subset of CD4+CD8+ cells. Prolonged culture of these CD4+CD8+ cells resulted in reversion to the original phenotype, indicating that dual expression of CD4 and CD8 represented a transitional phenotype. However, the maturation/activation status and proliferative potential of the small population of circulating CD4+CD8+ lymphocytes found in healthy individuals have not been assessed.

A distinct subset of CD3+CD4-CD8- T lymphocytes expresses a CD3-associated heterodimer made up of the protein encoded by the TCR gamma-gene and a second glycoprotein termed TCR delta. TCR gamma-delta (γδTCR) is expressed on CD3+ thymocytes during fetal ontogeny before the appearance of TCR alpha-beta (αβTCR), on CD3+CD4-CD8- adult thymocytes, and on a subset (1–10 %) of CD3+ cells in adult peripheral lymphoid organs and the peripheral blood [6, 7].

Lymphocyte Subpopulations Oscillate with a Circadian Pattern

Circadian rhythms in a number of leukocyte subtypes and the expression of cell surface molecules that trigger immune responses have been documented in experimental animals [8]. In humans significant circadian rhythms have been evidenced in the following subsets: CD3+ and CD4+, with peaks in the middle of the night; CD20+ borderline significant, with a peak at the beginning of the dark span; and CD8+, CD8+dim, CD16+, and γδTCR-expressing cells, with peaks near midday, in antiphase to CD3+ and CD4+ cells. A borderline-significant 12 h rhythm in HLA-DR+ with two peaks every 24 h, one in the morning and the other in the evening, may reflect the presence of this molecule on two subsets (e.g., CD8+ vs. CD4+) that show opposing circadian rhythmicity [9–11].

These opposing circadian variations most likely indicate a temporal (i.e., circadian) organization of cellular immune function. Levels of T cytotoxic lymphocytes and natural killer and γδTCR-bearing cells are minimal at night and rise to a maximum around noon, and this teleologically stated behavior might be useful to prepare the organism for the demands of the active period and the challenges of infectious agents, whereas the higher nocturnal levels of CD4+ lymphocytes might relate to their regulatory function [12–14]. The different changes of lymphocyte subsets may be responsible for time-dependent variations of magnitude and/or expression of immune responses. Circadian rhythmicity characterizes T-cell responses to phytohemagglutinin, tetanus toxoid, lipopolysaccharide, and concanavalin A. Furthermore, phenomenons mediated by cellular immunity, such as allograft survival, are influenced by the circadian time of transplantation, and contact hypersensitivity responses or joint pain due to inflammation in rheumatoid arthritis and osteoarthritis are greatest late at night and early in the morning, respectively [15].

Naive T lymphocytes need to be activated and subsequently differentiate into effector cells to perform their immune functions. Regulation of T-cell responses involves diverse strategies of activation and inhibition to optimize recognition of infected or transformed cells while preventing tissue damage as a result of autoreactivity and chronic inflammation. TCR-CD3-dependent responses are regulated by constitutive or inducible expression of costimulatory and inhibitory receptors, such as CD28+ and its CTLA-4 counterpart. In recent years, however, it has become evident that the expression of NK-cell receptors of the NKG2 family (e.g., NKG2D and CD94/NKG2 receptors) on CD8+αβ+ effector T cells may represent another means to regulate cytolytic functions in the tissue microenvironment, effectively controlling antigen-specific killing. NKG2D is one of the most widely distributed "NK-cell receptors," being expressed at the surface of all CD8+αβ+ T cells, γδ T cells, NK cells, as well as on certain activated CD4+ T cells. NKG2D is a potent costimulator of TCR-mediated effector functions and upregulates antigen-specific T-cell-mediated cytotoxicity directed against cells or tissues expressing stress-induced NKG2D ligands (NKG2DLs), particularly under conditions of suboptimal TCR engagement [16–18].

The physiological role of T lymphocytes expressing γδTCR, the molecular and structural properties of γδTCR, and the relationship between CD3+αβ T lymphocytes, CD16+ cells, and CD3+γδ T lymphocytes are still a matter of investigation. The periphery of the immune system, as opposed to the central lymphoid organs, contains heterogeneously distributed B and T cells whose phenotype, repertoire, developmental origin, and function are highly divergent. It appears that, in contrast to the bulk of T and B lymphocytes, certain γδ and αβ T cells found in the periphery do not depend on the thymus or bone marrow for their development but arise from different, nonconventional lineages.

In addition to divergent lineages that are targeted to different organs guided by a space/time sequence of tissue-specific homing receptors, local induction or selection processes may be important in the diversification of peripheral lymphocyte compartments. The different compartmentalization of lymphocytes in space and in time has major functional consequences and leads to a partial fragmentation of immunoregulatory circuits at the local level [19]. The CD8+dim T cytotoxic lymphocytes, CD16+ (NK) cells, and the γδTCR-expressing cells show evident coordination of timing and a clear circadian rhythmicity of variation with higher levels during the photoperiod, and as documented in the scientific literature, they share costimulators and ligands, suggesting that the cytotoxic cell compartment is tightly connected in time and perhaps function. The surface molecules and mechanisms involved in the activation of γδTCR+ cells are similar to those of αβTCR+ cells, and activated γδTCR+ cells have strong cytotoxic effector activity using both death receptor/death ligand and cytolytic granule pathways and produce various cytokines, frequently including tumor necrosis factor (TNF)-α and IFN-γ. Most CD3+γδ-expressing T-cell lines mediate cytotoxicity against a broad spectrum of tumor cell targets, although the functional significance of this observation remains unclear. One hypothesis is that γδTCR-expressing cells recognize subtle alterations in host cells that may be associated with neoplastic transformation. These cells might thus represent the true immune surveillance cells [20].

The lymphocyte subsets in the peripheral blood change with circadian rhythmicity but with different 24 h patterns among subpopulations, thereby revealing a temporal organization for lymphocyte functions essential in triggering immune responses. The 24 h chronograms and their respective peak times in relation to sleep–wake spans (and statistically identified by acrophases or orthophases) can potentially serve as useful references and as a possible guide to sampling and/or applying medical techniques at appropriate time(s) within a 24 h period during experimental, diagnostic, and/or therapeutic procedures [15].

Circadian Rhythmicity in the Cross Talk Among Organ Systems

The host immune defense plays an important role especially in earlier phases of neoplastic disease, and lymphocytes are an essential component of specific immune responses that produce tumor rejection [21]. Effector cells that exert antitumor effects are represented by tumor-infiltrating lymphocytes (TIL), populations of antigen-specific major histocompatibility complex-restricted T cells, usually CD8+dim cytotoxic T cells, NK (CD16+) cells, and γδTCR-expressing cells, that have been identified and isolated from TIL in various types of cancer and that may function by similar routes of activation in physiological and pathological conditions and by the same pattern of circadian rhythmicity [22].

The neuroendocrine and immune systems work in tight connection, with reciprocal influences, modulatory processes, and feedback and feed-sideward mechanisms and with enhancing and/or suppressing effects that regulate the fine-tuning of fundamental functions that allow body defense and homeostasis [23]. Circadian rhythmicity represents the background of a stage where immune cells, neuroendocrine hormones, monoamines, and cytokine/chemokines play their parts as actors in a mysterious and fascinating opera directed by time. The circadian variation of lymphocyte subsets is related to hormones such as cortisol, monoamines such as epinephrine and melatonin, and cytokines and chemokines, since immune cells have surface membrane receptors for these substances, and circadian rhythmicity may allow the occurrence of timed windows of maximal scheduled interaction among key lymphocyte subsets, immunomodulating hormones, and cytokines/chemokines [24–28]. Several studies have put in evidence reciprocal influences among the hypothalamus, pituitary, thyroid, adrenal, pineal gland, and immune system. Cortisol has a well-recognized influence on immune function, inducing significant immunosuppression, characterized by the reduced cellular and humoral response of monocytes and B and T lymphocytes.

Melatonin, a hormone secreted by the pineal gland, is able to influence the secretion of many endocrine glands and modulates the function of the immune system, and its production is under the control of the nervous system. The pineal hormone directly stimulates activated helper T lymphocytes and plays an immunomodulatory influence on the thymic function mediated by thyrotropin-releasing hormone (TRH) and thyroid-stimulating hormone (TSH). Relationships between the hypothalamic–pituitary–thyroid axis and immune system are demonstrated by the presence of receptors for TSH and thyroid hormones, T4 and T3, on immune cells and on the alterations of the immune system function observed in hyper- or hypothyroidism. The immunostimulatory role of growth hormone (GH) and insulin-like growth factor (IGF)1 has been highlighted. GH and IGF1 have an important role in stimulating lymphocyte production and function. IGF1 is one of the most important growth factors for normal cell proliferation, and it acts as an endocrine hormone via the blood and as paracrine and autocrine growth factor locally. GH stimulates the biosynthesis of IGF1 in the liver and in other organs and tissues, and an autocrine or paracrine GH/IGF1 system has been evidenced in lymphoid tissues, capable of influencing lymphopoiesis and immune function. Immune responses show temporal variations, related to circadian changes of total lymphocytes and specific lymphocyte subsets in the peripheral blood, of antibodies and cell-mediated immune responses, with an inverse relationship to plasma cortisol concentration [23, 26]. As stated above, there are different circadian variations of the total number of circulating immune cells and of specific lymphocyte subpopulations. The total number of circulating lymphocytes changes with circadian rhythmicity in antiphase with cortisol, and this rhythm of variation is recognizable for the changes of melatonin, TRH, TSH, GH, total T cells, T-helper/inducer subset, CD4/CD8 ratio, B cells and activated T cells, total B cells, and T-activated lymphocytes with expression of the α chain of IL-2 receptor. The levels of T suppressor/cytotoxic lymphocytes, NK cells, and γδTCR-expressing cells are higher around noon. These opposing circadian variations resemble a temporal organization of cellular immune function [23]. The immune and neuroendocrine systems interact and modulate one another functionally sharing a set of receptors and ligands: immune cells synthesize neuroendocrine hormones which are biologically active and produced in physiologically significant quantities and possess functional receptors for these hormones which modulate immune response. Body homeostasis is maintained by a perfect integration among the nervous, endocrine, and immune systems involving different glands and organs and guided by a spatiotemporal sequence of tissue-specific events, chemokine–cytokine/receptor interaction, and regulatory processes. Besides temporal organization, there is the possibility for differential regulation since various immune inducers stimulate different hormones from lymphocytes and the particular responses elicited will correspond to the lymphocyte subset being induced or hormone being produced. There are different correlations among lymphocyte subpopulation, and hormone time-related variations and circadian rhythmicity may be responsible for physiological timed windows of interaction among the hypothalamus, pituitary, thyroid, adrenal, and pineal glands and the immune system, and this phenomenon may explain different ways of interaction.

Relationships between lymphocyte subsets and TRH, TSH, and thyroxine seem to be influenced by the presence of melatonin, and they are positive only in the photoperiod, when melatonin, TRH, and TSH levels are very low. TRH enhances the proliferation of splenic and thymic lymphocytes in rats, and its administration in humans led to increased secretion of IL-2 into the blood. TSH has been shown to have a variety of immune-regulating cytokine-like activities that can affect the magnitude of antibody and cell-mediated responses of peripheral lymphocytes. TRH and TSH enhance lymphocyte activity, but the major concern is to know whether their effects on immune responses are direct or are related to their regulation of the secretion of thyroid hormones. Enhanced lymphoid responses, achieved with high levels of T3 and T4, but low levels of TSH and TRH – and with the converse in hypothyroid conditions – strengthen the possibility that levels of thyroid hormones modulate lymphocyte reactivity independently of TSH and TRH levels. Thyroid hormones play critical roles in differentiation, growth, and metabolism, but their participation in immune system regulation has not been completely elucidated. An important role is played by thyroid hormones in regulating lymphocyte reactivity via the regulation of protein kinase C (PKC) content in lymphocytes, which could be involved in altered responsiveness to mitogen-induced stimulation of proliferative responses. An inhibitory action of the pineal gland on hypothalamic–pituitary–thyroid axis (with reduced thyroid response to TSH in the presence of elevated melatonin levels) has been evidenced in vitro, in hamsters and rats and in humans, so that melatonin may play a modulatory action on hypothalamic–pituitary–thyroid axis, functioning as a servomechanism that diminishes or increases responses when stimuli are, respectively, too strong or too low [29, 30]. This mechanism, called feed-sideward, could also act in the interaction among the immune system and neuroendocrine hormones to prevent overstimulation of immune cells and overboosting of immune response.

GH is known to stimulate immune responses indirectly by regulating production of IGF1 but may have a direct effect as well [31]. Receptors for both GH and IGF1 are found on all hematopoietic cells in the bone marrow and on B- and T-cell subsets in secondary lymphoid tissues. Administration of GH or its proximal mediator IGF1 can reverse thymic involution in aging mice and accelerate immune recovery in immune-compromised animals, including hematopoietic stem cell transplantation (HSCT). GH is produced by thymocytes, thymic epithelial cells, and mature lymphocytes; it appears to stimulate T lymphocytes and NK cells, but data of the literature are sparse and contrasting. IGF1 treatment enhances T-cell reconstitution after syngeneic HSCT and when administered after allogeneic HSCT, it produces an increased number of thymic precursors, peripheral T cells, myeloid populations, and B cells and does not exacerbate graft-versus-host disease (GVHD) morbidity and mortality. GH is secreted mostly at night, and a negative correlation has been evidenced in the photoperiod and in the scotoperiod between GH serum levels and B cells (lymphocyte subset characterized by circadian variation with acrophase at night). This may be an important finding considered that specific humoral immune response seems to be decreased by elevated levels of GH and this effect could be counteracted by IGF1 that is characterized by more steady serum levels and has two major effects on B-cell development: it acts as a differentiation factor to potentiate pro-B to pre-B-cell maturation, and it also acts as a B-cell proliferation cofactor to synergize with IL-7.

The relationships between lymphocyte subpopulations and cortisol must be considered with particular attention because, as precedently referred, the total number of circulating lymphocytes changes with circadian rhythmicity in antiphase with this hormone so that the correlation may be influenced by this effect and in the photoperiod may result positive for lymphocyte subsets characterized by circadian variation with acrophase at night (CD4) and negative for lymphocyte subsets characterized by circadian variation with acrophase at noon (CD8). The circadian variation of lymphocyte subsets has been related to cortisol and epinephrine influence on cell redistribution to the bone marrow and mobilization and migration to the lymphoid and nonlymphoid organs and peripheral tissues. The phenomenon of circadian rhythmicity in lymphocyte subpopulation changes may be more complex and may involve other hormones as TRH, TSH, GH, and IGF1 and monoamines as melatonin, chemokines, and cytokines as IL-2, and immune system function may be related to circadian rhythmicity with timed interactions among key lymphocyte subsets, immunomodulating hormones, and cytokines/chemokines as well [23, 26, 32].

Melatonin and Circadian Patterns in Host–Tumor Relationships

The host immune defense influences the appearance and the development of malignant neoplastic diseases acting upon the promotion or the control of malignant cells. In this regard, the lymphocytes play a key role in the immune surveillance, are an essential component of the biological host reaction, and are the basic elements in the immunotherapy of cancer. The activation and development of an adaptive immune response is initiated by the engagement of a TCR by an antigenic peptide major histocompatibility complex (MHC), and the outcome of this engagement is determined by both positive and negative signals determining costimulation and co-inhibition. Tumor-infiltrating lymphocytes (TIL) are populations of antigen-specific MHC-restricted T cells, usually CD8+ cytotoxic T cells, whose response may be stimulated by a T-helper 1 cytokine milieu. This includes IFN-γ, IL-2 and IL-12, γδTCR+ cells (that are homogeneously composed of non-MHC-restricted cytolytic cells), NK cells (large granular lymphocytes that express neither α/β or γ/δ T-cell receptor nor CD3 on their surface, can lyse a number of different tumor cells, and may be stimulated by IFN-γ, IL-2, IL-12, and IL-18), and the lymphokine-activated killer cells (LAK), a mixed population of peripheral blood lymphocytes that develop non-MHC-restricted lytic activity for malignant cells after culture in vitro with high concentrations of IL-2 [21].

An effective T-cell-mediated immune surveillance is capable of monitoring the genetic integrity of mammalian cells, and T lymphocytes are an essential component of the specific immune responses that produce tumor rejection especially in the earlier phases of neoplastic disease. The function and activity of T cells (i.e., activation, proliferation, acquisition of memory, and cytolytic function versus induction of anergy, ignorance, and programmed cell death) are ultimately governed by the balance between positive and negative signaling within T cells, conferred through interactions between various T-cell co-regulatory receptors and ligands. This balance is maintained through direct mechanisms, such as the inhibition of tumor growth by antitumor cytotoxic T-cell activity, and by cytokine-mediated lysis of tumor cells, or by indirect mechanisms, such as the promotion of tumor growth by regulatory T cells that suppress antitumor T-cell responses and by humoral immune responses that increase chronic inflammation in the tumor microenvironment.

Cancer can alter immunity through direct invasion and replacement of normal lymphoid tissue and through the production of humoral factors that interfere with immune function or causing cachexia and malnutrition, which increases the severity of the immunodeficiency. Neoplastic tissue can downregulate antitumor T-cell-mediated immunity through the tumor-associated B7-H1 molecule by interacting with the T-cell ligand PD-1, thereby resulting in tumor-reactive T-cell apoptosis or impairments in cytokine production and cytotoxicity of activated antitumor T cells.

Another mechanism may be represented by a severe alteration of the physiological time structure of the human organism. Body homeostasis is maintained by numerous rhythmic biological functions presenting different phases, and this phenomenon is particularly evident when the rhythms that characterize the working of the multiple elements interconnected in the immune system are considered. A complete loss of rhythmicity or a change of phase and/or amplitude may alter the physiological array of rhythms with the onset of chrono-disruption or internal desynchronization.

Chronic circadian disruption promotes tumor growth by altering the circadian rhythms of function of the innate immune system upholding cancer growth, as NK-cell function is modulated by circadian mechanisms and plays a key role in tumor cell lysis. On the other hand, there is evidence that prolonged subjection to unstable work or lighting schedules, particularly in rotating shift-workers, is associated with an increased risk of immune-related diseases, including several cancers [33].

There are controversial results about the profile of T cytotoxic lymphocytes and NK cells in cancer patients [1]; anyway in lung cancer patients, severe alterations of the relative percentages and the circadian rhythmicity of the lymphocyte subsets have been documented [34, 35]. CD8, CD8bright (T-helper subset), and γδTCR (cytolytic cells which have been proposed to bridge the innate and adaptive immune responses and to lyse tumor target cells)- and Vδ2TCR-expressing cells are significantly diminished, whereas CD16 and CD25 (activated T cells with expression of alpha chain of IL-2 receptor) are significantly increased, and this increase is paralleled by increased IL-2 serum levels. CD3-, CD8-, CD8bright-, CD8dim-, CD20-, and HLA-DR-bearing lymphocytes showed loss of normal circadian rhythmicity in the cancer patients [36–38]. The decrease of T suppressor subpopulation has been observed in other types of cancer (gastric cancer, colorectal carcinoma, urological cancer, breast cancer); an increase of NK cells in the peripheral blood is a frequent report in cancer patients, and a high proportion of NK in TIL seems to be related to a more favorable prognosis, whereas the increase of CD4+CD25+ T cells seems to be associated with a poor prognosis. CD4+CD25+ T cells contain T regulatory cells that suppress antigen-specific T-cell immune responses and might hamper effective immune surveillance of emerging cancer cells and impede effective immune responses to established tumors. CD4+CD25+ T regulatory cells constitute 5–10 % of peripheral blood CD4+ lymphocytes and may express CD25 (the alpha chain of the IL-2 receptor), CTLA-4, a glucocorticoid-induced TNFα receptor (GITR), and a member of the forkhead transcription factors (Foxp3). Higher levels of T regulators have been reported in the peripheral blood of patients with several types of tumors (malignant melanoma, Hodgkin lymphoma, and ovarian, gastric, lung, breast, pancreatic, and colorectal cancers) and appear also in the tumor microenvironment. T-helper 17 (Th17) cells have been found in tumor tissues, and interleukin 17A (IL-17A)-deficient mice are more susceptible to developing lung melanoma, whereas adoptive T-cell therapy with tumor-specific Th17 cells is able to prevent tumor development. Furthermore, Th17 cells prop up C–C motif ligand 20 (CCL20) chemokine production by tumor tissues, and tumor-bearing chemokine (C–C motif) receptor 6 (CCR6)-deficient mice did not respond to Th17 cell therapy so that Th17 cells support a protective inflammation that promotes the activation of tumor-specific CD8(+) T cells. Immunotherapy by means of Th17 cells induces an outstanding activation of tumor-specific CD8(+) T cells, which are essential for the antitumor outcome. Th17 cells endorse dendritic cell recruitment into the tumor tissues and boost CD8 alpha(+) dendritic cells containing tumor material in draining lymph nodes [39]. A transcription factor involved in Th17 differentiation is represented among the others by RORα [40], which is upregulated in Th17 cells, and deficiency or suppression of

RORα transcriptional activity completely abolishes IL-17 production [41]. RORα has been suggested as a mediator of nuclear melatonin signaling, and the identification of melatonin as a natural modulator of RORα suggests the involvement of the pineal hormone in the molecular switch implicated in the mutually exclusive generation of Th17 and Treg cells [42]. Melatonin serum levels have been reported to be decreased in lung cancer patients with advanced disease [43], but the rhythm of secretion seems to be maintained until the later stages of disease [44]. The pineal gland plays a physiological anticancer role, and most antitumor immunostimulating effects of the pineal gland are referred to its most-studied hormone, melatonin, which acts on specific receptors (MLT-R) expressed either on the cell surface or at the nuclear site. Nuclear MLT-R is involved in the control of DNA expression and apoptotic mechanisms, and these actions could explain the great number of biological effects played by the pineal hormone. Melatonin is an indole hormone, synthesized starting from tryptophan through different enzymatic pathways but in particular N-acetyl-transferase (NAT). Light inhibits NAT activation; thus, melatonin production during the day is low, whereas the increased production of melatonin during the night determines a well-documented circadian rhythm, with high levels during the night and low during the day. Melatonin plays an anticancer activity through at least five fundamental mechanisms: (1) a direct antiproliferative action on tumors expressing MLT-R; (2) an inhibition of epidermal growth factor (EGF) receptor, which exerts an essential role in stimulating cancer cell proliferation; (3) an anticancer immunostimulatory action consisting of a stimulation of T-lymphocyte response to IL-2 by activating a specific MLT-R on Th lymphocytes and IL-2-induced IL-12 secretion by dendritic cells; (4) an inhibitory effect on tumor neoangiogenesis; and (5) an antioxidant activity, which may amplify the cytotoxic potency of cancer chemotherapies. Melatonin may also exert important palliative effects in the treatment of cancer patients, including an anticachectic activity due to an inhibition of TNF-α, which plays a role in the pathogenesis of cancer cachexia; an antiasthenic action; and a thrombopoietic activity, which makes melatonin useful in the treatment of cancer-related thrombocytopenia due to previous chemotherapies or radiotherapies or to cancer growth itself [1].

In lung cancer patients cortisol serum levels are reported significantly elevated with loss of circadian rhythmicity [45–47]. The increase in overall cortisol levels, possibly indicating increased stress levels, and loss of rhythm may represent a marker of altered function of the regulatory mechanisms of neuroendocrine secretion in the presence of advanced neoplastic disease. Increased cortisol levels may also possibly be involved in a two-way relationship with the changes of lymphocyte subpopulations, determining a decrease in CD8 and γδTCR-expressing cells, that normally show the same acrophase when cortisol serum levels reach their zenith (near awakening). In lung cancer patients GH serum levels are increased, but the nyctohemeral pattern of secretion is lost, and this determines an unbalanced relationship between GH secretion and IGF-1 serum levels [48, 49]. A global disorder of the neuroendocrine axes has to be considered and may also explain the increase of TRH levels and the decrease of TSH levels observed in lung cancer patients. An important causal factor may be represented by the altered time structure of GH and TRH secretion evidenced in lung cancer patients, but another explanation may be represented by hormone resistance, and the changes in the TRH/TSH axis and GH/IGF-1 axis function in the patients suffering from cancer may be mediated by the inflammatory cytokines. IL-2 serum levels are increased in lung cancer patients, maybe following immune activation and maybe representative of a global increase of the other cytokine/chemokines that mediate inflammation [50, 51].

Conclusion

The nervous, endocrine, and immune systems have well-established and very close interrelationships that contribute to maintain body homeostasis and involve the production and secretion of a variety of cellular mediators known as regulatory molecules (hormones, cytokines, chemokines, integrins, and others). Among these factors, the main players are melatonin, cortisol, and immune cells, which are a rich source of cytokines and other active molecules. The hormone melatonin serves as a chemical messenger of darkness in all species studied to date and is an important component of the timing systems for circadian rhythms. The daily external environmental cycle of a light span followed by a dark span synchronizes circadian rhythms by providing a signal that is sent to the pineal gland to produce melatonin during darkness and inhibit its production during light. As a multitasking molecule, melatonin spreads widely throughout all body tissues and functions as a signal molecule via receptor-dependent and independent means to modulate the physiology and molecular biology of cells for general and local coordination of intercellular relationships and to synchronize their biological rhythms. The alterations of neuroendocrine and immune system function evidenced in lung cancer patients need to be addressed to implement immunotherapeutic strategies, and their correction could be a powerful tool in the treatment of this neoplastic disease.

References

1. Lissoni P, Rovelli F. Principles of psychoneuroendocrinoimmunotherapy of cancer. Immunotherapy. 2012;4(1):77–86.
2. Reppert SM, Weaver DR. Coordination of circadian timing in mammals. Nature. 2002;418(6901):935–41.
3. Mazzoccoli G. The timing clockwork of life. J Biol Regul Homeost Agents. 2011;25(1):137–43.
4. Mazzoccoli G, Giuliani F, Sothern RB. A method to evaluate dynamics and periodicity of hormone secretion. J Biol Regul Homeost Agents. 2011;25(2):231–8.
5. Lambert C, Ibrahim M, Iobagiu C, Genin C. Significance of unconventional peripheral CD4+CD8dim T cell subsets. J Clin Immunol. 2005; 25:418–27.
6. Matis LA, Cron R, Bluestone JA. Major histocompatibility complex-linked specificity of gamma delta receptor-bearing T lymphocytes. Nature. 1987; 330:262–4.
7. Matis LA, Bluestone JA. Specificity of gamma delta receptor bearing T cells. Semin Immunol. 1991; 3:75–80.
8. Pelegrí C, Vilaplana J, Castellote C, Rabanal M, Franch A, Castell M. Circadian rhythms in surface molecules of rat blood lymphocytes. Am J Physiol Cell Physiol. 2003;284:C67–76.
9. Suzuki S, Toyabe S, Moroda T, Tada T, Tsukahara A, Iiai T, Minagawa M, Maruyama S, Hatakeyama K, Endoh K, Abo T. Circadian rhythm of leucocytes and lymphocytes subsets and its possible correlation with the function of the autonomic nervous system. Clin Exp Immunol. 1997;110(3):500–8.
10. Mazzoccoli G, Bianco G, Correra M, Carella AM, Balzanelli M, Giuliani A, Tarquini R. Circadian variation of lymphocyte subsets in healthy subjects. Recenti Prog Med. 1998;89(11):569–72.
11. Mazzoccoli G, Correra M, Bianco G, De Cata A, Balzanelli M, Giuliani A, Tarquini R. Age-related changes of neuro-endocrine-immune interactions in healthy humans. J Biol Regul Homeost Agents. 1997; 11(4):143–7.
12. Arjona A, Boyadjieva N, Sarkar DK. Circadian rhythms of granzyme B, perforin, IFN-gamma, and NK cell cytolytic activity in the spleen: effects of chronic ethanol. J Immunol. 2004;172:2811–7.
13. Arjona A, Sarkar DK. Circadian oscillations of clock genes, cytolytic factors, and cytokines in rat NK cells. J Immunol. 2005;174:7618–24.
14. Arjona A, Sarkar DK. Are circadian rhythms the code of hypothalamic-immune communication? Insights from natural killer cells. Neurochem Res. 2008; 33(4):708–18.
15. Mazzoccoli G, Sothern RB, De Cata A, Giuliani F, Fontana A, Copetti M, Pellegrini F, Tarquini R. A timetable of 24-hour patterns for human lymphocyte subpopulations. J Biol Regul Homeost Agents. 2011; 25(3):387–95.
16. Maasho K, Opoku-Anane J, Marusina AI, Coligan JE, Borrego F. Source. Naive CD8+ T cells costimulatory receptor for human cutting edge: NKG2D is a costimulatory receptor for human naive CD8+ T cells. J Immunol. 2005;174:4480–4.
17. Cerboni C, Ardolino M, Santoni A, Zingoni A. Detuning CD8+ T lymphocytes by down-regulation of the activating receptor NKG2D: role of NKG2D ligands released by activated T cells. Blood. 2009; 113:2955–64.
18. Maccalli C, Scaramuzza S, Permiani G. TNK cells (NKG2D+ CD8+ or CD4+ T lymphocytes) in the control of human tumors. Cancer Immunol Immunother. 2009;58:801–8.
19. von Andrian UH, Mempel TR. Homing and cellular traffic in lymph nodes. Nat Rev Immunol. 2003; 3:867–78.
20. Kabelitz D, Wesch D, He W. Perspectives of gamma delta T cells in tumor immunology. Cancer Res. 2007;67:5–8.
21. Parmiani G. Tumor-infiltrating T, cells-friend or foe of neoplastic cells? N Engl J Med. 2005;353:2640–1.
22. Mazzoccoli G, Balzanelli M, Giuliani A, De Cata A, La Viola M, Carella AM, Bianco G, Tarquini R.

Lymphocyte subpopulations anomalies in lung cancer patients and relationship to the stage of disease. In Vivo. 1999;13(3):205–9.
23. Mazzoccoli G, Muscarella LA, Fazio VM, Piepoli A, Pazienza V, Dagostino MP, Giuliani F, Polyakova VO, Kvetnoy I. Antiphase signalling in the neuroendocrine-immune system in healthy humans. Biomed Pharmacother. 2011;65(4):275–9.
24. Dimitrov S, Benedict C, Heutling D. Cortisol and epinephrine control opposing circadian rhythms in T cell subsets. Blood. 2009;113:5134–43.
25. Lange T, Dimitrov S, Born J. Effects of sleep and circadian rhythm on the human immune system. Ann N Y Acad Sci. 2010;1193:48–59.
26. Mazzoccoli G, De Cata A, Greco A, Carughi S, Giuliani F, Tarquini R. Circadian rhythmicity of lymphocyte subpopulations and relationship with neuroendocrine system. J Biol Regul Homeost Agents. 2010;24(3):341–50.
27. Dimitrov S, Lange T, Born J. Selective mobilization of cytotoxic leukocytes by epinephrine. J Immunol. 2010;184(1):503–11.
28. Bollinger T, Bollinger A, Naujoks J, Lange T, Solbach W. The influence of regulatory T cells and diurnal hormone rhythms on T helper cell activity. Immunology. 2010;131(4):488–500.
29. Mazzoccoli G, Giuliani A, Carughi S, De Cata A, Puzzolante F, La Viola M, Urbano N, Perfetto F, Tarquini R. The hypothalamic-pituitary-thyroid axis and melatonin in humans: possible interactions in the control of body temperature. Neuro Endocrinol Lett. 2004;25(5):368–72.
30. Mazzoccoli G, Carughi S, Sperandeo M, Pazienza V, Giuliani F, Tarquini R. Neuro-endocrine correlations of hypothalamic-pituitary-thyroid axis in healthy humans. J Biol Regul Homeost Agents. 2011;25(2): 249–57.
31. Mazzoccoli G, Giuliani F, Inglese M, Marzulli N, Dagostino MP, De Cata A, Greco A, Carughi S, Tarquini R. Chronobiologic study of the GH-IGF1 axis and the aging immune system. J Appl Biomed. 2010;8(4):213–26.
32. Mazzoccoli G, Sothern RB, Pazienza V, Piepoli A, Muscarella LA, Giuliani F. Chronobiologic study of neuro-endocrine axis hormone sequence signalling in healthy men. Biomed Aging Pathol. 2011;1: 129–37.
33. Logan RW, Zhang C, Murugan S, O'Connell S, Levitt D, Rosenwasser AM, Sarkar DK. Chronic shift-lag alters the circadian clock of NK cells and promotes lung cancer growth in rats. J Immunol. 2012;188(6): 2583–91.
34. Mazzoccoli G, Grilli M, Carughi S, Puzzolante F, De Cata A, La Viola M, Giuliani A, Urbano N, Tarquini R, Perfetto F. Immune system alterations in lung cancer patients. Int J Immunopathol Pharmacol. 2003; 16(2):167–74.
35. Mazzoccoli G, Fontana A, Copetti M, Pellegrini F, Piepoli A, Muscarella LA, Pazienza V, Giuliani F, Tarquini R. Stage dependent destructuration of neuro-endocrine-immune system components in lung cancer patients. Biomed Pharmacother. 2011;65(1): 69–76.
36. Mazzoccoli G, Vendemiale G, De Cata A, Carughi S, Tarquini R. Altered time structure of neuro-endocrine-immune system function in lung cancer patients. BMC Cancer. 2010;10:314.
37. Mazzoccoli G, Sothern RB, Parrella P, Muscarella LA, Fazio VM, Giuliani F, Polyakova V, Kvetnoy IM. Comparison of circadian characteristics for cytotoxic lymphocyte subsets in non-small cell lung cancer patients versus controls. Clin Exp Med. 2012;12: 181–94.
38. Mazzoccoli G, Tarquini R, Durfort T, Francois JC. Chronodisruption in lung cancer and possible therapeutic approaches. Biomed Pharmacother. 2011;65(7): 500–8.
39. Martin-Orozco N, Muranski P, Chung Y, Yang XO, Yamazaki T, Lu S, Hwu P, Restifo NP, Overwijk WW, Dong C. T helper 17 cells promote cytotoxic T cell activation in tumor immunity. Immunity. 2009;31(5): 787–98.
40. Jetten AM. Retinoid-related orphan receptors (RORs): critical roles in development, immunity, circadian rhythm, and cellular metabolism. Nucl Recept Signal. 2009;7:e003.
41. Solt LA, Kumar N, Nuhant P, Wang Y, Lauer JL, Liu J, Istrate MA, Kamenecka TM, Roush WR, Vidović D, Schürer SC, Xu J, Wagoner G, Drew PD, Griffin PR, Burris TP. Suppression of TH17 differentiation and autoimmunity by a synthetic ROR ligand. Nature. 2011;472:491–4.
42. Lardone PJ, Guerrero JM, Fernández-Santos JM, Rubio A, Martín-Lacave I, Carrillo-Vico A. Melatonin synthesized by T lymphocytes as a ligand of the retinoic acid-related orphan receptor. J Pineal Res. 2011;51:454–62.
43. Hu S, Shen G, Yin S, Xu W, Hu B. Melatonin and tryptophan circadian profiles in patients with advanced non-small cell lung cancer. Adv Ther. 2009;26(9):886–92.
44. Mazzoccoli G, Carughi S, De Cata A, La Viola M, Giuliani A, Tarquini R, Perfetto F. Neuroendocrine alterations in lung cancer patients. Neuro Endocrinol Lett. 2003;24(1–2):77–82.
45. Mazzoccoli G, Carughi S, De Cata A, La Viola M, Vendemiale G. Melatonin and cortisol serum levels in lung cancer patients at different stages of disease. Med Sci Monit. 2005;11(6):CR284–8.
46. Mazzoccoli G, Francavilla M, De Petris MP, Giuliani F, Sothern RB. Comparison of whole body circadian phase evaluated from melatonin and cortisol secretion profiles in healthy humans. Biomed Aging Pathol. 2011;1:112–22.
47. Mazzoccoli G, Giuliani F, Sothern RB. Determination of whole body circadian phase in lung cancer patients: melatonin vs. cortisol. Cancer Epidemiol. 2012;36(1): e46–53.

48. Mazzoccoli G, Giuliani A, Bianco G, De Cata A, Balzanelli M, Carella AM, La Viola M, Tarquini R. Decreased serum levels of insulin-like growth factor (IGF)-I in patients with lung cancer: temporal relationship with growth hormone (GH) levels. Anticancer Res. 1999;19(2B):1397–9.
49. Mazzoccoli G, Sothern RB, Pazienza V, Piepoli A, Muscarella LA, Giuliani F, Tarquini R. Circadian aspects of growth hormone-insulin-like growth factor axis function in patients with lung cancer. Clin Lung Cancer. 2012;13(1):68–74.
50. Mazzoccoli G, Pazienza V, Piepoli A, Muscarella LA, Giuliani F, Sothern RB. Alteration of hypothalamic-pituitary-thyroid axis function in non-small-cell lung cancer patients. Integr Cancer Ther. 2012;11(4): 327–36.
51. Mazzoccoli G, Vinciguerra M, Muscarella LA, Fazio VM, Parrella P, Tarquini R. Hormone and cytokine circadian alteration in non small cell lung cancer patients. Int J Immunopathol Pharmacol. 2012;25(3): 691–702.

Melatonin and Melatonergic Drugs for Therapeutic Use in Breast Cancer

11

Emilio J. Sanchez-Barcelo, Maria D. Mediavilla Aguado, and Samuel Cos Corral

Abstract

Melatonin-estradiol interactions at the cellular level explain the effects of melatonin on breast carcinogenesis. The objective of this chapter is to review the mechanisms supporting the usefulness of melatonin in breast cancer therapy, particularly its properties of selective estrogen receptor modulator (SERM) and selective estrogen enzyme modulator (SEEM), since these properties are probably the best explanation of its oncostatic effects on hormone-dependent breast cancer. Currently, perhaps the most widespread idea about the usefulness of melatonin in the management of breast cancer is that it could be considered as a complement to conventional treatments. Thus, as an adjuvant of SERMs, melatonin could enhance their antiestrogenic actions, whereas in association with SEEMs, melatonin could reduce the osteoporosis induced by these drugs, potentiate their effects, and add its own antiaromatase actions. Melatonin could be used for the relief of some of the symptoms frequently associated with the cancerous process or of those arising during cancer treatment (depression, anxiety, sleep disturbances, cognitive dysfunction, etc.). As an adjuvant to chemotherapy treatments (anthracyclines, taxanes, platinum drugs, etc.), melatonin protects against or mitigates the side effects of these drugs and, in some cases, potentiates their oncostatic effects. Administered in conjunction with radiotherapy, melatonin acts as an antioxidant radioprotector. Furthermore, melatonin may prevent breast cancer caused by chronodisruption.

Keywords

Melatonin • Breast cancer • Estradiol • SEEM • SERM • Antiestrogen • Antiaromatase

E.J. Sanchez-Barcelo, PhD, MD (✉)
M.D. Mediavilla Aguado, PhD, MD
S. Cos Corral, PhD, MD
Department of Physiology and Pharmacology, and
Research Institute "Marqués de Valdecilla" (IFIMAV),
University of Cantabria, Avd. Herrera Oria s/n, 39011
Santander, Spain
e-mail: barcelo@unican.es; mediavid@unican.es;
coss@unican.es

V. Srinivasan et al. (eds.), *Melatonin and Melatonergic Drugs in Clinical Practice*,
DOI 10.1007/978-81-322-0825-9_11, © Springer India 2014

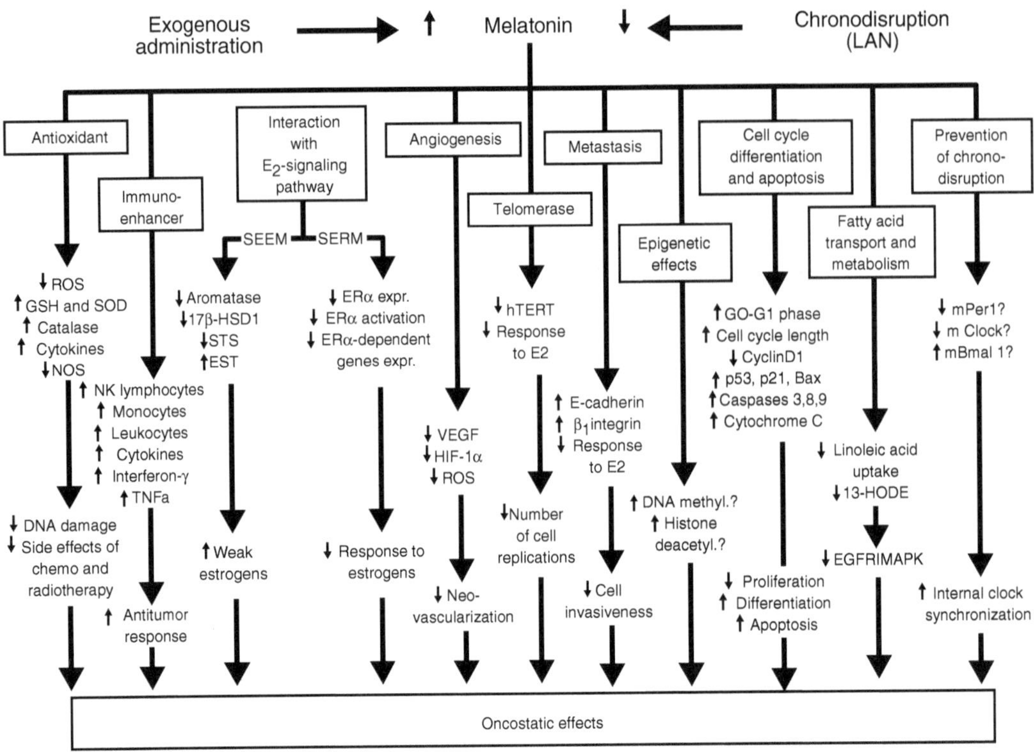

Fig. 11.1 Summary of the possible mechanisms involved in the oncostatic effects of melatonin (See more information in Mediavilla et al. [1])

Introduction

During the latter half of the last century, several studies were carried out to assess the oncostatic properties of melatonin against different neoplasias including breast cancer, leukemia, colorectal cancer, melanoma, prostate cancer, and pancreatic cancer [1]. From these studies, the most promising results were obtained in breast cancer cells expressing estrogen receptors [2]. The former hypothesis on the possible role of melatonin in breast cancer stated that if this molecule downregulates the gonadal estrogens, any reduction in melatonin synthesis, whatever its cause, could lead to a relative increase in estrogen levels which would, in turn, increase the turnover of breast epithelial cells and aggravate the risk of malignant transformation [3]. However, the melatonin-estradiol (E_2) interactions at the cellular level, rather than changes in estradiol concentration, are currently considered as the explanation of the effects of melatonin on breast cancer [2, 4, 5]. In this chapter we will review the mechanisms supporting the usefulness of melatonin on breast cancer therapy, emphasizing its value as an adjuvant to other conventional oncostatic drugs (antiestrogens and antiaromatases) as well as to oncologic therapies (chemo- and radiotherapy).

Mechanisms of Breast Cancer Inhibition by Melatonin

The possible mechanisms of melatonin's oncostatic actions are summarized in Fig. 11.1 from Mediavilla et al. [1]. Most, but not all, of these mechanisms have been studied in the context of hormone-dependent breast tumors, particularly those based on the relationships of melatonin with the estrogen-signaling pathway. We will focus this review fundamentally on melatonin's antiestrogenic effects, which is probably the main explanation of its oncostatic effects on breast cancer. Other oncostatic mechanisms of melatonin which are of interest in breast cancer treatment will be commented on brief, and for more information about these subjects, the reader is referred to the above mentioned review [1].

Melatonin as Both a SERM (Selective Estrogen Receptor Modulator) and a SEEM (Selective Estrogen Enzyme Modulator)

Drugs which are able to interact with the estrogen-signaling pathway are classified in two groups: those interfering with the actions of the endogenous estrogens at the level of the estrogen receptors (ER) are called SERMs (i.e., tamoxifen and its derivates), whereas drugs modulating the activity of the enzymes involved in the synthesis and transformation of steroids are called SEEMs (i.e., formestane, exemestane, letrozole).

Melatonin interacts with the ER behaving like a SERM. Thus, in estrogen-sensitive MCF-7 human breast cancer cells, melatonin, at physiological concentrations (1 nM), counteracts the E_2-induced cell proliferation and invasiveness, increases the sensitivity to antiestrogens such as tamoxifen, and downregulates the E_2-induced expression of growth factors and proto-oncogenes [6–13]. Interestingly, unlike other SERMs, such as tamoxifen or its derivates, melatonin neither binds to the ER nor changes its affinity nor interferes with the binding of E_2 to its receptor [4, 14–16]. What melatonin does is to decrease the expression of ERα and to inhibit the binding of the E_2-ER complex to the estrogen response element (ERE) in DNA [14–17]. These effects depend on melatonin binding to specific membrane receptors, particularly the MT1 receptors, coupled to Gi proteins [17–20]. The activation of these receptors led the inhibition of the adenylate cyclase (AC), thus decreasing the activity of the cAMP/PKA signaling pathway [21]. The overexpression of the MT1 receptors enhances the response of MCF-7 cells to the antiestrogenic effects of melatonin and alterations of MT1 genes have been found in primary human breast tumors and breast cancer cell lines [22–25].

The opposing regulation of cAMP intracellular concentration by E_2 and melatonin is probably the key to understanding how melatonin modulates E_2-induced ERα transactivation [4]. E_2 increases cAMP in target breast cancer cells [26]. This increase in cAMP results from enhanced AC activity by a mechanism which does not involve genomic actions of the steroid [26]. What melatonin does, through its binding to MT1 membrane receptors, is to decrease cAMP, thus counteracting the E_2-induced ERα transcriptional activity by interacting with the cAMP signaling cascade [17, 27, 28].

Melatonin also has antiestrogenic actions which are not dependent on its binding to MT1 receptors, but rather on its properties as an endogenous calmodulin (CaM) antagonist able to bind to and inactivate the Ca^{2+}/CaM complex [29, 30]. CaM plays an important role in the ligand-dependent transcriptional activation of ERα (although not of the ERβ), by facilitating its association with coactivators and binding to the ERE [31–34]. In the absence of CaM, the conformation of ERα is altered facilitating its association with corepressors rather than with coactivators. Melatonin, by inactivating the Ca^{2+}/CaM complex, inhibits the E_2-induced transactivation of the ER dependent on CaM, this being one of the mechanisms by which this indoleamine may interact with the E_2-signaling pathway on mammary cancer cells [30, 35]. Interestingly, as indicated above, CaM binds exclusively to ERα. Consequently, since the antiestrogenic effects of melatonin are, at least in part, dependent on its ability to inactivate CaM, melatonin may be considered basically as a specific inhibitor of E_2-induced ERα-mediated transcriptional activation, since it does not inhibit ERβ-mediated transactivation [35]. In fact, the sensitivity of MCF-7 human breast cancer cells to melatonin depends on the ERα:ERβ ratio and this sensitivity is abolished by ERβ overexpression [35].

The role of retinoic acid-related orphan receptors alpha (RORα) in melatonin antiestrogenic effects is controversial [36]. Recently, Hill's group demonstrated that the E_2-induced transcriptional activity of ERα is significantly enhanced by the overexpression of RORα and that this effect can be repressed by melatonin via activation of its MT1 receptors or by inhibiting CaM [37].

Not only ovaries but other tissues, including the adipose tissue and skin, vascular endothelium, aortic smooth muscle, some brain areas, as well as osteoblasts and chondrocytes, can all synthesize estrogens. These extra-ovarian sources of estrogens deserve special consideration in postmenopausal women whose ovaries have ceased to function, and plasmatic concentration of E_2 is very low. Postmenopausal women suffering hormone-dependent breast cancer show higher E_2 concentrations in the tumor tissue than in plasma [38]. The local synthesis of E_2 in the adipose mammary tissue explains the growth of E_2-dependent mammary tumors in postmenopausal patients, and consequently, this fact has led directly to the design of anticancer drugs with the synthesis of estrogens as their target, the so-called SEEMs.

The main precursors for the local synthesis of estrogens are dehydroepiandrosterone (DHEA) and its sulfate conjugate. Enzymes involved in the synthesis and interconversion of steroid hormones are the following: (a) the 17β-hydroxysteroid dehydrogenase (17β-HSD) enzyme family, including reductant and oxidative isoforms. The reductant isoforms (e.g., 17β-HSD type 1) catalyze the conversion of the relatively weak estrone (E_1), androstenedione and 5-androstenedione, into the more potent E_2, testosterone and 5-dihydrotestosterone, while the oxidative isoforms (e.g., 17β-HSD type 2) catalyze the formation of steroids of low activity; (b) P-450 aromatase, which transforms androgens into estrogens; (c) estrogen sulfatase (STS), which converts estrogen sulfates into E_1 and E_2; and (d) estrogen sulfotransferases (EST) which catalyzes the conversion of estrogens into their inactive sulfates [39]. In breast adenocarcinomas, local estrogen production is biased toward the formation of active E_2 because the activity of 17β-HSD type 1, STS, and aromatase is higher than that of 17β-HSD type 2 and EST [40]. Studies carried out in our laboratory demonstrate that melatonin inhibits the expression and activity of P450 aromatase, 17β-HSD type 1 and STS, enzymes involved in the synthesis or transformation of biologically active estrogens from androgens or estrogens with lower biological activity. Conversely, melatonin increases the expression and activity of EST, which catalyzes the conversion of estrogens into inactive sulfate conjugates. Thus, the SEEM properties of melatonin could reverse the increased expression of aromatase, 17β-HSD type 1, and STS which is characteristic of mammary cancer tissue and which is responsible for the elevated concentrations of E_2 in tumors [41–46]. The antiaromatase effects of melatonin depend on its binding to MT1 receptors and have been demonstrated not only in vitro but in vivo as well [41–47]. Figure 11.2 summarizes the effects of melatonin on the enzymes involved in the local production and transformation of steroids in human breast carcinoma tissue.

Melatonin is, as far as we know, the only molecule which possesses both SERM and SEEM properties. This double mechanism of action, and the specific inhibition of ERα, confers to melatonin unique potential advantages for the treatment of these neoplasias.

Figure 11.3, from Sanchez-Barcelo et al. (2012) depicts the SERM and SEEM effects of melatonin, which may explain its effects on estrogen-dependent tumors, such as most mammary adenocarcinomas [48].

Other Mechanisms of Breast Cancer Inhibition by Melatonin

Modulation of the cell cycle and the induction of apoptosis are two goals in the control of tumor growth. Melatonin increases the duration of the cell cycle in MCF-7 human breast cancer cells by expanding the G1phase, thus reducing cell proliferation and allowing the repair of damaged DNA [49]. This extended G1 phase may be explained, at least in part, by melatonin-dependent upregulation of p53 and p21 expression and downregulation of cyclin D1 [9, 11, 50]. Melatonin, which has been shown to protect normal cells from apoptosis, was found to induce apoptosis in various cancer cells including MCF-7 human breast

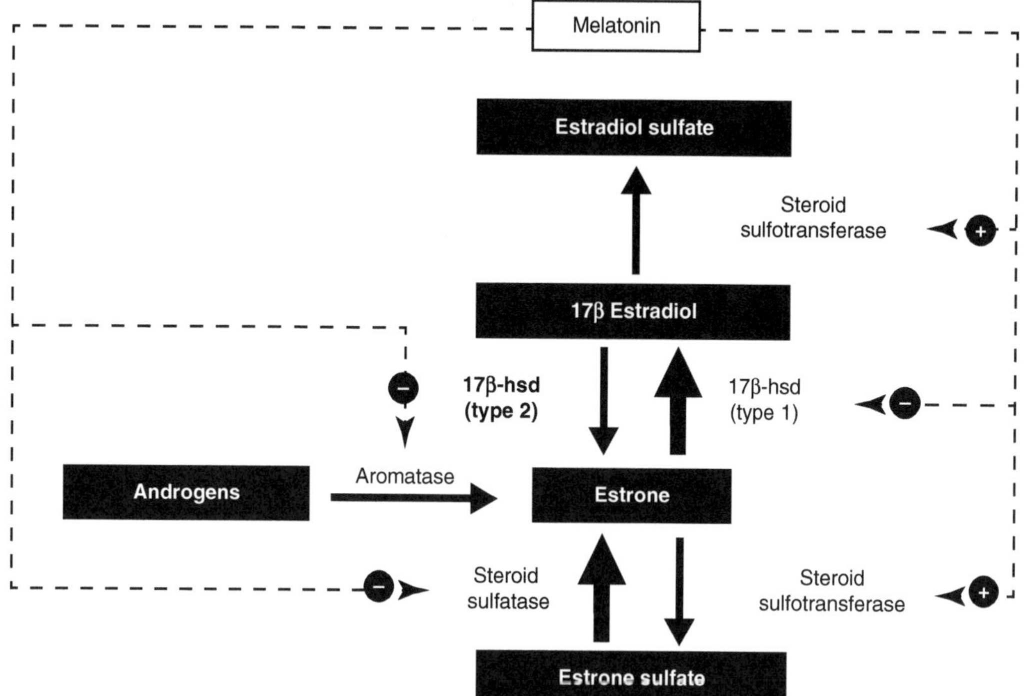

Fig. 11.2 Effects of melatonin on the enzymatic mechanisms involved in the synthesis and transformation of estrogens in human breast cancer cells. The "sulfatase pathway" is quantitatively higher than the "aromatase pathway." Melatonin inhibits aromatase, sulfatase, and 17β-HSD1while increases activity of sulfotransferase (Composed with data from [4, 39, 41–45])

cancer cells [9, 51, 52]. However, the lack of effects of melatonin on apoptosis has also been reported [53].

Telomerase activity is observed in 85–90 % of all cancers, whereas it is absent in most differentiated tissues [54]. The existence of an imperfect ERE on the promoter of hTERT (the telomerase subunit which is the major determinant of its enzyme activity) explains why E_2 upregulates telomerase activity in MCF-7 cells (ERα positive), but has no effect on cells lacking the ERα [55]. Studies in vitro and in vivo showed that melatonin inhibits the E_2-induced hTERT expression [56, 57].

Oxidative stress may play a role in all steps of carcinogenesis (initiation, progression, and metastasis) [58]. Many of the carcinogenic effects of E_2 in breast tissue depend on the oxidative stress induced by estrogens metabolites [59]. Consequently, antioxidants have been considered protective against cancer. Melatonin and its metabolites are able to both scavenge free radicals and radical-related reactants and stimulate the expression of antioxidative enzymes and reduce the expression of pro-oxidants [60, 61]. Accordingly, the anticarcinogenic actions of melatonin would be dependent, at least in part, on its antioxidative and free radical scavenging activity [62].

The inhibition of the *angiogenesis* is one cancer treatment strategy that is now widely investigated. Patients with tumors may have abnormally high levels of VEGF, an important endogenous proangiogenic molecule, which correlates with rapid tumor growth, early metastasis, and poor prognosis [63]. Melatonin's antiangiogenic properties, inhibiting VEGF, have been described in clinical and experimental studies [64–67]. This data makes further research on the angiogenic properties of melatonin of significant importance, as such research is likely to result in beneficial clinical applications in the field of oncological therapy.

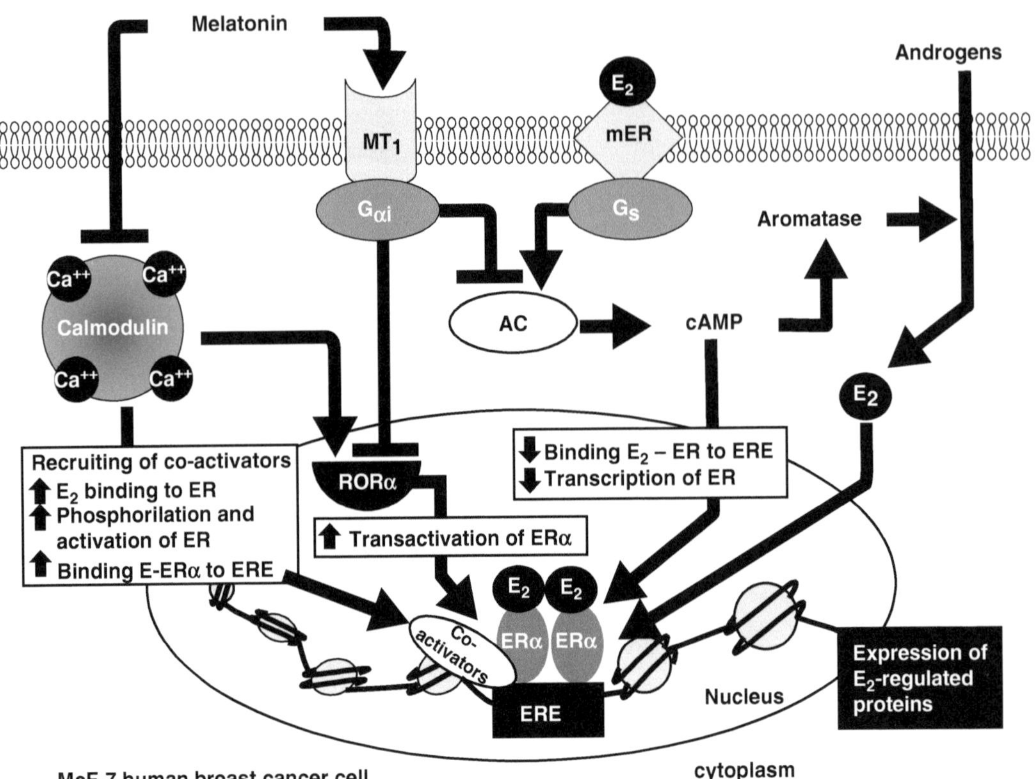

Fig. 11.3 Summary of the mechanisms involved in melatonin's SERM and SEEM actions. As a SERM, melatonin inhibits three pathways which potentiate the estradiol-induced transactivation of the ERα: (a) one dependent on the cAMP cascade, which is activated by membrane ER and inhibited by the activation of MT_1 melatonin receptors; (b) the second dependent on calmodulin, a calcium binding protein inhibited by melatonin; and (c) the third, dependent on the melatonin-induced inhibition of RORα, either by activation of MT_1 or by its effects as a CaM antagonist. As a SEEM, melatonin, through the activation of MT1 receptors and the inhibition of the cAMP-pathway, inhibits the expression and activity of P450 aromatase in epithelial breast cells as well as in adipocytes, reducing the local synthesis of E_2. Furthermore (not shown) melatonin also inhibits estrogen sulfatase while increases the activity of sulfotransferase (Modified from Sanchez-Barcelo et al. [48])

Chronodisruption, defined as a critical loss of time order at different levels of an organism, including gene expression in individual cells, is considered to be potentially carcinogenic [68]. Since light is the main synchronizer of the mammalian circadian system, changes in the pattern of light exposure, such as exposure to light at night (LAN), are frequently the cause of chronodisruption. Experimental studies have demonstrated that LAN enhances the growth of mammary tumors and also underscored the relationship between LAN-induced changes in melatonin secretion and the growth of chemically induced mammary tumors [69, 70]. The clear implication is that melatonin could be one of the links between circadian disruption and cancer development.

Melatonin (1–10 nM), in vitro, reduces the *invasiveness* of different clones of MCF-7 human breast cancer cells and blocks the stimulatory effects of E_2 on cell invasiveness [6, 7]. The anti-invasive response to melatonin is enhanced by the overexpression of the MT1 receptor and inhibited by the administration of luzindole, an MT1/MT2 receptor antagonist [71].

Melatonin is considered to be an *immunoenhancer* agent, since it stimulates the production of natural killer cells, monocytes and leukocytes, as well as the production of cytokines including interleukin (IL-2, IL-6, IL-12), interferon-gamma, and TNFα by binding to specific membrane and nuclear receptors present in these cells [72]. However, there are as yet no experimental studies on the oncostatic potential of melatonin specifically focused on its immunoenhancing properties.

Epigenetic alterations are considered as an important mechanism involved in tumorigenesis. Epigenetic regulation of gene expression involves basically two classes of molecular mechanisms: histone modifications and DNA methylation. Recent studies with microarray of DNA methylation and gene expression profiling in MCF-7 human breast cancer cell lines treated with physiologic doses of melatonin (1 nM) provide detailed insights into the DNA methylation patterns induced by melatonin and suggest a potential mechanism of the anticancer effect of aberrant DNA methylation in melatonin-treated breast cancer cells [73].

Clinical Uses of Melatonin in Breast Cancer Therapy

Almost all the clinical studies on the usefulness of melatonin in cancer treatment have been carried out by Lissoni et al. in Italy during the last two decades. Several reviews have evaluated the published information concerning the clinical uses of melatonin in oncology [74–76]. However, for different reasons, it is difficult to obtain definitive conclusions about melatonin's effects from these studies. Among these reasons are as follows: the fact that it is not clear whether the same patients have been included in different trials from the same group; the heterogeneity of the tumors grouped in every trial, the terminal status of most of the patients included in the trials; the different treatments (melatonin alone or associated with other standard therapies); and the nature of the studies (mostly nonrandomized).

At present, perhaps the most widespread idea about the usefulness of melatonin in the management of breast cancer is that it could be considered as a complement to conventional treatments, rather than as a specific anticancer drug [2]. In summary, the main clinical uses of melatonin in breast cancer would be the following:

1. Because of its SERM and SEEM properties and its lack of negative side effects, melatonin could be an excellent adjuvant to drugs used for cancer prevention and treatment. Specifically used in conjunction with SERMs (tamoxifen, raloxifene, etc.), melatonin could enhance their antiestrogenic actions [43]. Administered with antiaromatase drugs (anastrozole, letrozole, exemestane, etc.), melatonin could reduce the osteoporosis induced by these drugs as well as potentiate their effects and add its own antiaromatase actions [2].
2. Prevention of breast cancer associated with chronodisruption. Since the abolition of night shift work and the reduction of nocturnal lighting to prevent the inhibition of melatonin synthesis induced by LAN seems unrealistic, the administration of exogenous melatonin could achieve a certain degree of protection against breast cancer caused by light-induced chronodisruption. Since melanopsin, the retinal ganglion cell photopigment involved in the circadian phototransduction, is sensible to light in the blue range (460–480 nm) by filtering this wavelength band, it would be possible to avoid or reduce the risk of melatonin suppression by exposure to LAN [77]. Some optical devices based on this idea have been already patented [48].
3. Melatonin could be used for the relief of some of the symptoms frequently associated with the cancerous process or those arising during cancer treatment (depression, anxiety, sleep disturbances, cognitive dysfunction, etc.). Currently, a double-blind randomized, placebo-controlled clinical trial (MELODY) is being done to investigate whether oral melatonin (6 mg/daily) ameliorates these symptoms in women with breast cancer [78].
4. Melatonin could be used as an adjuvant of chemotherapy treatments (anthracyclines, taxanes, platinum drugs, etc.) since it protects against or lessens the side effects of these

drugs and, in some cases, potentiates their oncostatic effects. It may be therefore possible to increase the dosage or frequency of chemotherapy treatment if given in combination with melatonin [2, 79, 80]. A recent meta-analysis, which includes 33 studies carried out between 1996 and 2007, and comprising a population of 2,446 cases, documented that melatonin decreased neurotoxicity, myelosuppression, asthenia, cachexia, and diarrhea in chemotherapy patients with different kinds of tumors [81].

5. In conjunction with radiotherapy, melatonin, acting as an antioxidant radioprotector, allows for the use of higher doses of radiation, thus resulting better therapeutic value from such treatments [82, 83]. Topical applications of melatonin emulsions have been proposed to prevent local radiation injuries [84].

Melatonergic Drugs

Although the functions of melatonin in the body are numerous and extensive, its role in entraining circadian rhythms to the light–dark cycle is probably the best known. Probably for this reason, the effort of most laboratories has been focused upon developing melatonergic drugs for the treatment of circadian pathologies (i.e., sleep disturbances or seasonal affective disorders) rather than for breast cancer therapy. Among the melatonergic compounds patented in the last years, the most successful, up to now, have been agomelatine and ramelteon, both basically designed for treatment of depression and sleep troubles [85]. However, evidence of the oncostatic properties of melatonin in hormone-dependent breast cancer is stimulating research for synthetic molecules useful in breast cancer therapy. Recently, two benzofuran MT_1/MT_2 melatonin receptor agonists (S23219-1 and S23478-1) have been tested for their in vitro and in vivo antitumoral activity, and it has been determined that these compounds are more effective than melatonin in inhibiting proliferation and promoting apoptosis of MCF-7 cells as well as in inducing regression of NMU-induced rat mammary tumors [86].

Conclusion

Melatonin is a natural compound with multiple properties and low toxicity which confers to this molecule unique utility in the prevention and treatment of hormone-dependent breast cancer, particularly in combination with other oncostatic drugs (antiestrogens and antiaromatases), as well as an adjuvant therapy to counteract the side effects of chemotherapy and radiotherapy and to increase the efficacy of these treatments. Despite the strength of the experimental results describing: (a) the ability of melatonin to reduce the growth of chemically induced rat mammary adenocarcinomas, (b) its capacity to inhibit the proliferation and invasiveness of MCF-7 human breast cancer cells, and (c) the relevance of light-induced suppression of nocturnal melatonin as a factor favoring the growth of rat mammary tumors, clinical trials to clarify the possible value of melatonin in the therapy of human breast cancer are still scarce.

References

1. Mediavilla MD, Sanchez-Barcelo EJ, Tan DX, Manchester L, Reiter RJ. Basic mechanisms involved in the anti-cancer effects of melatonin. Curr Med Chem. 2010;17:4462–81.
2. Sanchez-Barcelo EJ, Mediavilla MD, Alonso-Gonzalez C, Reiter RJ. Melatonin uses in oncology: breast cancer prevention and reduction of the side effects of chemotherapy and radiation. Expert Opin Investig Drugs. 2012;21:819–31.
3. CohenCohen M, Lippman M, Chabner B. Role of pineal gland in aetiology and treatment of breast cancer. Lancet. 1978;2:814–6.
4. Sánchez-Barceló EJ, Cos S, Mediavilla D, Martínez-Campa C, González A, Alonso-González C. Melatonin-estrogen interactions in breast cancer. J Pineal Res. 2005;38:217–22.
5. Schernhammer ES, Giobbie-Hurder A, Gantman K, Savoie J, Scheib R, Parker LM, et al. A randomized controlled trial of oral melatonin supplementation and breast cancer biomarkers. Cancer Causes Control. 2012;23:609–16.
6. Cos S, Fernández R, Güézmes A, Sánchez-Barceló EJ. Influence of melatonin on invasive and metastatic properties of MCF-7 human breast cancer cells. Cancer Res. 1998;58:4383–90.
7. Mao L, Yuan L, Slakey LM, Jones FE, Burow ME, Hill SM. Inhibition of breast cancer cell invasion by

melatonin is mediated through regulation of the p38 mitogen-activated protein kinase signaling pathway. Breast Cancer Res. 2010;12(6):R107.

8. Wilson ST, Blask DE, Lemus-Wilson AM. Melatonin augments the sensitivity of MCF-7 human breast cancer cells to tamoxifen in vitro. J Clin Endocrinol Metab. 1992;75:669–70.
9. Cucina A, Proietti S, D'Anselmi F, Coluccia P, Dinicola S, Frati L, et al. Evidence for a biphasic apoptotic pathway induced by melatonin in MCF-7 breast cancer cells. J Pineal Res. 2009;46:172–80.
10. Mediavilla MD, Güezmez A, Ramos S, Kothari L, Garijo F, Sánchez Barceló EJ. Effects of melatonin on mammary gland lesions in transgenic mice overexpressing N-ras proto-oncogene. J Pineal Res. 1997; 22:86–94.
11. Mediavilla MD, Cos S, Sánchez-Barceló EJ. Melatonin increases p53 and p21WAF1 expression in MCF-7 human breast cancer cells in vitro. Life Sci. 1999;65:415–20.
12. Molis TM, Spriggs LL, Jupiter Y, Hill SM. Melatonin modulation of estrogen-regulated proteins, growth factors, and proto-oncogenes in human breast cancer. J Pineal Res. 1995;18:93–103.
13. Ram PT, Kiefer T, Silverman M, Song Y, Brown GM, Hill SM. Estrogen receptor transactivation in MCF-7 breast cancer cells by melatonin and growth factors. Mol Cell Endocrinol. 1998;141:53–64.
14. Molis TM, Walters MR, Hill SM. Melatonin modulation of estrogen receptor expression in MCF-7 human breast cancer cells. Int J Oncol. 1993;3:687–94.
15. Molis TM, Spriggs LL, Hill SM. Modulation of estrogen receptor mRNA expression by melatonin in MCF-7 human breast cancer cells. Mol Endocrinol. 1994;8:1681–90.
16. Rato AG, Pedrero JG, Martinez MA, del Rio B, Lazo PS, Ramos S. Melatonin blocks the activation of estrogen receptor for DNA binding. FASEB J. 1999; 13:857–68.
17. Kiefer T, Ram PT, Yuan L, Hill SM. Melatonin inhibits estrogen receptor transactivation and cAMP levels in breast cancer cells. Breast Cancer Res Treat. 2002;71:37–45.
18. Baldwin WS, Barrett JC. Melatonin: receptor-mediated events that may affect breast and other steroid hormone-dependent cancers. Mol Carcinog. 1998;21:149–55.
19. Jones MP, Melan MA, Witt-Enderby PA. Melatonin decreases cell proliferation and transformation in a melatonin receptor-dependent manner. Cancer Lett. 2000;151:133–43.
20. Ram PT, Day J, Yuan L, Dong C, Kiefer TL, Lai L, et al. Involvement of the mt1 melatonin receptor in human breast cancer. Cancer Lett. 2002;179: 141–50.
21. Lai L, Yuan L, Chen Q, Dong C, Mao L, Rowan B, et al. The Galphai and Galphaq proteins mediate the effects of melatonin on steroid/thyroid hormone receptor transcriptional activity and breast cancer cell proliferation. J Pineal Res. 2008;45:476–88.
22. Collins A, Yuan L, Kiefer TL, Cheng Q, Lai L, Hill SM. Overexpression of the MT1 melatonin receptor in MCF-7 human breast cancer cells inhibits mammary tumor formation in nude mice. Cancer Lett. 2003;189:49–57.
23. Yuan L, Collins AR, Dai J, Dubocovich ML, Hill SM. MT(1) melatonin receptor overexpression enhances the growth suppressive effect of melatonin in human breast cancer cells. Mol Cell Endocrinol. 2002; 192:147–56.
24. Dillon DC, Easley SE, Asch BB, Cheney RT, Brydon L, Jockers R, et al. Differential expression of high-affinity melatonin receptors (MT1) in normal and malignant human breast tissue. Am J Clin Pathol. 2002;118:451–8.
25. Lai L, Yuan L, Cheng Q, Dong C, Mao L, Hill SM. Alteration of the MT1 melatonin receptor gene and its expression in primary human breast tumors and breast cancer cell lines. Breast Cancer Res Treat. 2009;118:293–305.
26. Aronica SM, Kraus WL, Katzenellenbogen BS. Estrogen action via the cAMP signaling pathway: stimulation of adenylate cyclase and cAMP-regulated gene transcription. Proc Natl Acad Sci U S A. 1994;91:8517–21.
27. Cardinali DP, Bonanni Rey RA, Mediavilla MD, Sánchez-Barceló E. Diurnal changes in cyclic nucleotide response to pineal indoles in murine mammary glands. J Pineal Res. 1992;13:111–6.
28. Godson C, Reppert SM. The Mel1a melatonin receptor is coupled to parallel signal transduction pathways. Endocrinology. 1997;138:397–404.
29. Benítez-King G, Ríos A, Martínez A, Antón-Tay F. In vitro inhibition of Ca2+/calmodulin-dependent kinase II activity by melatonin. Biochim Biophys Acta. 1996;1290:191–6.
30. Dai J, Inscho EW, Yuan L, Hill SM. Modulation of intracellular calcium and calmodulin by melatonin in MCF-7 human breast cancer cells. J Pineal Res. 2002;32:112–9.
31. Bouhoute A, Leclercq G. Modulation of estradiol and DNA binding to estrogen receptor upon association with calmodulin. Biochem Biophys Res Commun. 1995;208:748–55.
32. Castoria G, Migliaccio N, Nola E, Auricchio F. In vitro interaction of estradiol receptor with Ca2+ calmodulin. Mol Endocrinol. 1988;2:167–74.
33. García Pedrero JM, Del Rio B, Martínez-Campa C, Muramatsu M, Lazo PS, Ramos S. Calmodulin is a selective modulator of estrogen receptors. Mol Endocrinol. 2002;16:947–60.
34. Li L, Sacks DB. Functional interactions between calmodulin and estrogen receptor-alpha. Cell Signal. 2007;19:439–43.
35. del Río B, García Pedrero JM, Martínez-Campa C, Zuazua P, Lazo PS, Ramos S. Melatonin, an endogenous-specific inhibitor of estrogen receptor alpha via calmodulin. J Biol Chem. 2004;279:38294–302.
36. Kiefer TL, Lai L, Yuan L, Dong C, Burow ME, Hill SM. Differential regulation of estrogen receptor

alpha, glucocorticoid receptor and retinoic acid receptor alpha transcriptional activity by melatonin is mediated via different G proteins. J Pineal Res. 2005;38:231–9.
37. Dong C, Yuan L, Dai J, Lai L, Mao L, Xiang S, et al. Melatonin inhibits mitogenic cross-talk between retinoic acid-related orphan receptor alpha (RORalpha) and ERalpha in MCF-7 human breast cancer cells. Steroids. 2010;75:944–51.
38. van Landeghem AA, Poortman J, Nabuurs M, Thijssen JH. Endogenous concentration and subcellular distribution of estrogens in normal and malignant human breast tissue. Cancer Res. 1985;45: 2900–6.
39. Pasqualini JR. The selective estrogen enzyme modulators in breast cancer: a review. Biochim Biophys Acta. 2004;1654:123–43.
40. Suzuki T, Miki Y, Nakamura Y, Moriya T, Ito K, Ohuchi N, et al. Sex steroid-producing enzymes in human breast cancer. Endocr Relat Cancer. 2005;12: 701–20.
41. Cos S, Martínez-Campa C, Mediavilla MD, Sánchez-Barceló EJ. Melatonin modulates aromatase activity in MCF-7 human breast cancer cells. J Pineal Res. 2005;38:136–42.
42. Cos S, González A, Güezmes A, Mediavilla MD, Martínez-Campa C, Alonso-González C, et al. Melatonin inhibits the growth of DMBA-induced mammary tumors by decreasing the local biosynthesis of estrogens through the modulation of aromatase activity. Int J Cancer. 2006;118:274–8.
43. Cos S, González A, Martínez-Campa C, Mediavilla MD, Alonso-González C, Sánchez-Barceló EJ. Melatonin as a selective estrogen enzyme modulator. Curr Cancer Drug Targets. 2008;8:691–702.
44. González A, Martínez-Campa C, Mediavilla MD, Alonso-González C, Sánchez-Mateos S, Hill SM, et al. Effects of MT1 melatonin receptor overexpression on the aromatase-suppressive effect of melatonin in MCF-7 human breast cancer cells. Oncol Rep. 2007;17:947–53.
45. González A, Alvarez-García V, Martínez-Campa C, Mediavilla MD, Alonso-González C, Sánchez-Barceló EJ, et al. In vivo inhibition of the estrogen sulfatase enzyme and growth of DMBA-induced mammary tumors by melatonin. Curr Cancer Drug Targets. 2010;10:279–86.
46. Martínez-Campa C, González A, Mediavilla MD, Alonso-González C, Alvarez-García V, Sánchez-Barceló EJ, et al. Melatonin inhibits aromatase promoter expression by regulating cyclooxygenases expression and activity in breast cancer cells. Br J Cancer. 2009;101:1613–9.
47. Gonzalez A, Cos S, Martinez-Campa C, Alonso-Gonzalez C, Sanchez-Mateos S, Mediavilla MD, Sanchez-Barcelo EJ. Selective estrogen enzyme modulator actions of melatonin in human breast cancer cells. J Pineal Res. 2008;45:86–92.
48. Sanchez-Barcelo EJ, Mediavilla MD, Alonso-Gonzalez C, Rueda N. Breast cancer therapy based on melatonin. Recent Pat Endocr Metab Immune Drug Discov. 2012;6:108–16.
49. Cos S, Blask DE, Lemus-Wilson A, Hill AB. Effects of melatonin on the cell cycle kinetics and "estrogen-rescue" of MCF-7 human breast cancer cells in culture. J Pineal Res. 1991;10:36–42.
50. Cini G, Neri B, Pacini A, Cesati V, Sassoli C, Quattrone S, et al. Antiproliferative activity of melatonin by transcriptional inhibition of cyclin D1 expression: a molecular basis for melatonin-induced oncostatic effects. J Pineal Res. 2005;39:12–20.
51. Jou MJ, Peng TI, Yu PZ, Jou SB, Reiter RJ, Chen JY, et al. Melatonin protects against common deletion of mitochondrial DNA-augmented mitochondrial oxidative stress and apoptosis. J Pineal Res. 2007;43: 389–403.
52. Sanchez-Hidalgo M, Guerrero JM, Villegas I, Packham G, de la Lastra CA. Melatonin, a natural programmed cell death inducer in cancer. Curr Med Chem. 2012;19:3805–21.
53. Cos S, Mediavilla MD, Fernández R, González-Lamuño D, Sánchez-Barceló EJ. Does melatonin induce apoptosis in MCF-7 human breast cancer cells in vitro? J Pineal Res. 2002;32:90–6.
54. Moon IK, Jarstfer MB. The human telomere and its relationship to human disease, therapy, and tissue engineering. Front Biosci. 2007;12:4595–620.
55. Kyo S, Takakura M, Kanaya T, Zhuo W, Fujimoto K, Nishio Y, et al. Estrogen activates telomerase. Cancer Res. 1999;59:5917–21.
56. Leon-Blanco MM, Guerrero JM, Reiter RJ, Calvo JR, Pozo D. Melatonin inhibits telomerase activity in the MCF-7 tumor cell line both in vivo and in vitro. J Pineal Res. 2003;35:204–11.
57. Martínez-Campa CM, Alonso-González C, Mediavilla MD, Cos S, González A, Sanchez-Barcelo EJ. Melatonin down-regulates hTERT expression induced by either natural estrogens (17beta-estradiol) or metalloestrogens (cadmium) in MCF-7 human breast cancer cells. Cancer Lett. 2008;268:272–7.
58. Klaunig JE, Wang Z, Pu X, Zhou S. Oxidative stress and oxidative damage in chemical carcinogenesis. Toxicol Appl Pharmacol. 2011;254:86–99.
59. Cavalieri E, Frenkel K, Liehr JG, Rogan E, Roy D. Estrogens as endogenous genotoxic agents – DNA adducts and mutations. J Natl Cancer Inst Monogr. 2000;27:75–93.
60. Galano A, Tan DX, Reiter RJ. Melatonin as a natural ally against oxidative stress: a physicochemical examination. J Pineal Res. 2011;51:1–16.
61. Rodriguez C, Mayo JC, Sainz RM, Antolín I, Herrera F, Martín V, et al. Regulation of antioxidant enzymes: a significant role for melatonin. J Pineal Res. 2004; 36:1–9.
62. Karbownik M, Lewinski A, Reiter RJ. Anticarcinogenic actions of melatonin which involve antioxidative processes: comparison with other antioxidants. Int J Biochem Cell Biol. 2001;33:735–53.
63. Salven P, Mänpää H, Orpana A, Alitalo K, Joensuu H. Serum vascular endothelial growth factor is often

elevated in disseminated cancer. Clin Cancer Res. 1997;3:647–51.

64. Lissoni P, Barni S, Meregalli S, Fossati V, Cazzaniga M, Esposti D, Tancini G. Modulation of cancer endocrine therapy by melatonin: a phase II study of tamoxifen plus melatonin in metastatic breast cancer patients progressing under tamoxifen alone. Br J Cancer. 1995;71:854–6.
65. Alvarez-García V, González A, Alonso-González C, Martínez-Campa C, Cos S. Regulation of vascular endothelial growth factor by melatonin in human breast cancer cells. J Pineal Res. 2012. doi:10.1111/jpi.12007. Epub ahead of print.
66. Cui P, Luo Z, Zhang H, Su Y, Li A, Li H, et al. Effect and mechanism of melatonin's action on the proliferation of human umbilical vein endothelial cells. J Pineal Res. 2006;41:358–62.
67. Dai M, Cui P, Yu M, Han J, Li H, Xiu R. Melatonin modulates the expression of VEGF and HIF-1 alpha induced by CoCl2 in cultured cancer cells. J Pineal Res. 2008;44:121–6.
68. Filipski E, Lévi F. Circadian disruption in experimental cancer processes. Integr Cancer Ther. 2009; 8:298–302.
69. Blask DE, Brainard GC, Dauchy RT, Hanifin JP, Davidson LK, Krause JA, et al. Melatonin-depleted blood from premenopausal women exposed to light at night stimulates growth of human breast cancer xenografts in nude rats. Cancer Res. 2005;65:11174–84.
70. Cos S, Mediavilla D, Martínez-Campa C, González A, Alonso-González C, Sánchez-Barceló EJ. Exposure to light-at-night increases the growth of DMBA-induced mammary adenocarcinomas in rats. Cancer Lett. 2006;235:266–71.
71. Hill SM, Frasch T, Xiang S, Yuan L, Duplessis T, Mao L. Molecular mechanisms of melatonin anticancer effects. Integr Cancer Ther. 2009;8:337–46.
72. Carrillo-Vico A, Calvo JR, Abreu P, Lardone PJ, García-Mauriño S, Reiter RJ, et al. Evidence of melatonin synthesis by human lymphocytes and its physiological significance: possible role as intracrine, autocrine, and/or paracrine substance. FASEB J. 2004;18:537–9.
73. Lee SE, Kim SJ, Yoon HJ, Yu SY, Yang H, Jeong SI, et al. Genome-wide profiling in melatonin-exposed human breast cancer cell lines identifies differentially methylated genes involved in the anticancer effect of melatonin. J Pineal Res. 2012. doi:10.1111/j.1600-079X.2012.01027.x. Epub ahead of print.
74. Mills E, Wu P, Seely D, Guyatt G. Melatonin in the treatment of cancer: a systematic review of randomized controlled trials and meta-analysis. J Pineal Res. 2005;39:360–6.
75. Panzer A, Viljoen M. The validity of melatonin as an oncostatic agent. J Pineal Res. 1997;22:184–202.
76. Sanchez-Barcelo EJ, Mediavilla MD, Tan DX, Reiter RJ. Clinical uses of melatonin: evaluation of human trials. Curr Med Chem. 2010;17:2070–95.
77. West KE, Jablonski MR, Warfield B, Cecil KS, James M, Ayers MA, et al. Blue light from light-emitting diodes elicits a dose-dependent suppression of melatonin in humans. J Appl Physiol. 2011;110:619–26.
78. Hansen MV, Madsen MT, Hageman I, Rasmussen LS, Bokmand S, Rosenberg J, et al. The effect of MELatOnin on depression, anxietY, cognitive function and sleep disturbances in patients with breast cancer. The MELODY trial: protocol for a randomised, placebo-controlled, double-blinded trial. BMJ Open. 2012;2:e000647. doi:10.1136/bmjopen-2011-000647.
79. Hara M, Yoshida M, Nishijima H, Yokosuka M, Iigo M, Ohtani-Kaneko R, et al. Melatonin, a pineal secretory product with antioxidant properties, protects against cisplatin-induced nephrotoxicity in rats. J Pineal Res. 2001;30:129–38.
80. Nahleh Z, Pruemer J, Lafollette J, Sweany S. Melatonin, a promising role in taxane-related neuropathy. Clin Med Insights Oncol. 2010;4:35–41.
81. Block KI, Koch AC, Mead MN, Tothy PK, Newman RA, Gyllenhaal C. Impact of antioxidant supplementation on chemotherapeutic toxicity: a systematic review of the evidence from randomized controlled trials. Int J Cancer. 2008;123:1227–39.
82. Shirazi A, Ghobadi G, Ghazi-Khansari M. A radiobiological review on melatonin: a novel radioprotector. J Radiat Res. 2007;48:263–72.
83. Shirazi A, Mihandoost E, Mohseni M, Ghazi-Khansari M, Rabie Mahdavi S. Radio-protective effects of melatonin against irradiation-induced oxidative damage in rat peripheral blood. Phys Med. 2013;29:65–74.
84. Vasin MV, Ushakov IB, Kovtun VY, Komarova SN, Semenova LA. Effect of melatonin, ascorbic acid, and succinic acid on the cumulative toxic effect of repeated treatment with gammafos (amifostine). Bull Exp Biol Med. 2004;137:450–2.
85. Sanchez-Barcelo EJ, Martinez-Campa CM, Mediavilla MD, Gonzalez A, Alonso-Gonzalez C, Cos S. Melatonin and melatoninergic drugs as therapeutic agents: Ramelteon and Agomelatine, the two most promising melatonin receptor agonists. Recent Pat Endocr Metab Immune Drug Discov. 2007; 1:142–51.
86. Mao L, Cheng Q, Guardiola-Lemaître B, Schuster-Klein C, Dong C, Lai L, et al. In vitro and in vivo antitumor activity of melatonin receptor agonists. J Pineal Res. 2010;49:210–21.

Melatonin and Malaria: Therapeutic Avenues

12

V. Srinivasan, Mahaneem Mohamed, Rahimah Zakaria, Asma Hayati Ahmad, and Rozieyati Mohamed Saleh

Abstract

Malaria, one of the most deadly diseases of our time, affects more than 200 million people across the globe and is responsible for about one million deaths annually. Besides *Plasmodium falciparum* which is the main cause for malarial infection in human beings, *Plasmodium knowlesi* from Malaysia also remains as the most virulent parasite spreading fast not only in Malaysia but also in different parts of the world. Global malaria eradication program by use of insecticide spraying has resulted in good response in the past. Treatment of malaria-infected patients with antimalarial drugs has helped to eliminate malarial infections successfully, but with increased resistance displayed by malarial parasites to these drugs, there is resurgence of malaria caused both by drug resistance and by infection caused by new malarial species like *Plasmodium knowlesi*. Recent advances on molecular studies on malarial parasites reveal that the pineal hormone

V. Srinivasan, MSc, PhD, MAMS (✉)
Sri Sathya Sai Medical Educational and Research Foundation, An International Medical Sciences Research Study Center, Prasanthi Nilayam, 40-Kovai Thirunagar Extn, Goldwins, Coimbatore, Tamilnadu 641014, India

National Health Service, Department of Mental Health, Psychiatric Service of Diagnosis and Treatment, Hospital "G. Mazzini", ASL 4, Teramo, Italy

Department of Neuroscience and Imaging, University "G.D' Annunzio", Chieti 66013, Italy
e-mail: sainivasan@yahoo.com, venkataramanujamsrinivasan6@gmail.com

M. Mohamed, MD, MSc, PhD
R. Zakaria, MBBS, MSc, PhD (Physiology)
A. Hayati Ahmad, MBBS, MSc
Department of Physiology, School of Medical Sciences, Universiti Sains Malaysia, Kubang Kerian, Kelantan 16150, Malaysia
e-mail: mahaneem@kck.usm.my; rahimah@kck.usm.my; asma@kck.usm.my

R. Mohamed Saleh, DPhil
School of Heath Sciences, Universiti Sains Malaysia, Health Campus, Kubang Kerian, Kelantan 16150, Malaysia
e-mail: rozieyati@kk.usm.my

V. Srinivasan et al. (eds.), *Melatonin and Melatonergic Drugs in Clinical Practice*, DOI 10.1007/978-81-322-0825-9_12, © Springer India 2014

melatonin acts as a cue for growth and development of *Plasmodium falciparum*. Same may be true for *Plasmodium knowlesi* also. Hence, treatment modalities that can effectively block the action of melatonin on *Plasmodium* species during nighttime by way of using either bright light therapy or use of melatonin receptor blocking can be considered as useful approaches for eliminating malarial infection in man.

Keywords
Malaria • Antimalarial drugs • *Plasmodium knowlesi* • Melatonin • Luzindole

Abbreviations

AFMK	*N*(1)-acetyl-*N*(2)-formyl-5-methoxykynuramine
cAMP	Cyclic adenosine monophosphate
DDT	Dichloro-diphenyl-trichloroethane
EM	Erythrocyte membrane
P	*Plasmodium*
Pcalp	*Plasmodium* calpain
PCT	Parasite clearance times
PfPK7	*Plasmodium falciparum* protein kinase 7
PKA	Protein kinase A
PLC	Phospholipase C
PRR	Parasite reduction ratio
PVM	Parasitophorous membrane
RBC	Red blood cell
SERA	Serine repeat antigen (multigene family)
TBD	Transmission-blocking drugs
UPS	Ubiquitin-proteosome protein degradation system

Introduction

Malaria, one of the deadliest infectious diseases, is caused by a group of parasites from the genus *Plasmodium*. It consists of five different species, namely, *P. falciparum*, *P. vivax*, *P. malariae*, *P. ovale*, *and P. knowlesi*, *P falciparum* being the most lethal [1]. Symptoms and signs of malaria include high fever, headache, vomiting, chillness, shaking, and anemia. The control and management of malaria mainly involves chemotherapy. The classical antimalarial drugs include artemisinin, pyronaridine, lumefantrine, piperaquine, chloroquine, mefloquine, pyrimethamine, and atovaquone [2]. However, since there is increased resistance to these drugs, there is a need for the development and application of new innovative approaches and introduction of novel drugs with greater efficacy to control and eradicate this disease [3]. The drugs that target the hepatic and sexual forms of the malaria parasite include artemisinin [4], primaquine [5], and artemisinin combination therapies [6]. As *Plasmodium* sporozoites reach the mammalian liver within minutes after being released into the host's blood by the infected female *Anopheles* mosquito, the drugs that act on the parasitic stages in the liver are suggested to eliminate the cryptic hypnozoite infection reservoirs [2]. In the absence of transmission-blocking drugs (TBD), primaquine is the only available effective antimalarial drug that has gametocytocidal property [7]. Screening of asexual blood stages of *P. falciparum* is considered more successful than molecular-target-based approaches, and new drug developments are based on this line of approach. The ongoing strategy for development of TBD rests primarily on blood schizonticides that act effectively against late stage of gametocytes [7]. The goal of antimalarial drug therapy should be directed to reduce the disease and death incidences by targeting blood stage parasites. In the case of *P. falciparum*, it requires elimination of all persistent asexual blood stage forms and the long-lasting mature stage V, i.e., *P. falciparum* gametocytes, responsible for transmission of malaria [8]. Studies conducted on BALB/c mice showed that luzindole, the antagonist of melatonin receptor, inhibited the number of trophozoites [9].

Molecular Biology of *Plasmodium* Life Cycle

The sporozoites are injected into humans by a female *Anopheles* mosquito and are taken up into the liver to infect the hepatocytes. These parasites develop to form exoerythrocytic schizonts which give rise to several thousands of merozoites. With the rupture of liver cells, merozoites are released into the bloodstream where they invade erythrocytes. The intraerythrocytic merozoites replicate synchronously and some develop into male and female gametocytes. These constitute the later stages of *P. falciparum* infection. The gametocytes are then taken up into the female mosquito gut during a blood meal. The male gametocytes are activated (exflagellation) and form gametes which fuse with the female gametes to form diploid ookinetes. These ookinetes migrate to the midgut of the insect and pass through the gut wall to form oocysts. Following meiotic division, sporozoites are formed which then migrate to the salivary glands of the mosquito, ready to be transmitted into humans [10].

Of the various stages outlined above, residence in the human erythrocyte is essential for the life cycle for all *Plasmodium* that infect man, and it is this phase of the life cycle that causes disease manifestations such as fever, anemia, and neurological manifestations [11]. With the introduction of new genetic and molecular tools and imaging technology, many exciting discoveries have been made regarding the biology of growth and development of *Plasmodium*. Genome sequencing projects have been successfully completed for *P. falciparum* and other species [12–14]. It is suggested that progression of the malaria parasite life cycle involves interplay between the parasite's changing environment and its own built-in genetic program [15]. Examination of the *P. falciparum* proteome detected more than 900 proteins in gametocytes. Of these, 315 are found exclusively in gametocytes. Nearly 97 proteins identified are gamete specific [16]. The absence of sex chromosomes in malarial parasites plus the presence of gametocyte-specific and sex-specific genes found dispersed amongst 14 chromosomes raises many unsolved questions regarding the molecular mechanism that triggers gametogenesis of malarial parasites. The only known fact is that all merozoites from a sexually committed schizont will become either male or female [17, 18]. Factors that influence gametocyte development include host red blood cell (RBC) age and hypoxia [7]. The first molecular markers of gametocytes, namely, Pfs16 and Pfg27/25, are expressed within 24 h after their commitment and differentiation of sexual stages at the cellular level [7]. Some studies suggest that potential signalling pathways in the parasite are essential in triggering gametocytogenesis such as phorbol ester-inducing pathways [19] and the cyclic adenosine monophosphate (cAMP) signalling pathway [20]. It is suggested that G-protein-dependent signalling system may mediate the switch to sexual development in response to environmental factors [15].

Intraerythrocytic Phase of *Plasmodium falciparum*

The intraerythrocytic phase is the most lethal form of human malaria parasite and is the primary cause of malaria morbidity and mortality. Arrest of the RBC stage of *Plasmodium* life cycle is therefore considered as the main pharmaceutical target [21]. The RBC cycle of *P. falciparum* occurs over a period of 48 h and consists of three stages of development known as ring, trophozoite, and schizont. Schizonts give rise to a number of merozoites that are released into the circulation at a specific time of day [22, 23]. Evidences support the role of host circadian system and the pineal hormone melatonin in the synchronous maturation and survival of *Plasmodium* in the host [24].

Ubiquitin-Proteosome System and Its Importance

Malarial parasite's emergence from host erythrocytes, egress, involves a coordinated event of rupture of parasitophorous membrane (PVM) and the erythrocyte membrane (EM). Many proteases such as aspartic proteases, cysteine proteases, and a series of serine repeat antigens (SERAs) are involved in this process [25]. Proteases like Pcalp in *P. falciparum* are essential for optimal growth of the parasite and cell cycle progression [26]. These proteases are the targets of antimalarial drugs due to their involvement in parasite development and invasion [27]. The most important protease system in *P. falciparum* is the ubiquitin-proteosome protein degradation system (UPS) which is responsible for degrading unwanted or misfolded proteins and thereby plays an important role in cell cycle regulation. The UPS pathway in *P. falciparum* (http://sites.huji.ac.iL/malaria/maps/proteaUbiqpath.html) is suggested to perform functions specific to pathogenesis or virulence [25]. Recent studies show that the pineal hormone melatonin upregulates genes related to UPS which is inhibited by luzindole, a melatonin antagonist [28]. The effects of melatonin on UPS transcription modulation are mediated by a protein kinase known as PfPK7 (*Plasmodium falciparum* protein kinase 7), a *P. falciparum* orphan kinase that causes increase in cytosolic calcium and upregulation of UPS genes [28]. The signalling pathways in *Plasmodium* are fundamental to the development of new drugs for malaria control. Nearly 20–30 % of the drug discovery program in most pharmaceutical companies focuses on protein kinases [29]. Kinase inhibitors such as genistein and tyrphostin block *P. falciparum* cell cycle [30]. Treatment with melatonin induces increases in cAMP production and protein kinase A (PKA) in both *P. falciparum* and *P. chabaudi* (rodent malaria parasite), but the extent of melatonin-induced activation of the cAMP/PKA signalling pathway is lower in *P. falciparum* than in *P. chabaudi* [31].

Malaria Eradication Programs

The Global Malarial Eradication Program was launched by the World Health Organization in 1955 and has been effective [32] in eradicating malaria. However, more people are at risk of suffering from malaria now than at any other time [33]. It is estimated that more than two billion people are at risk of being infected with malaria [34]. Hence, there is urgent need for effective implementation of global fight through multifaceted approach to control malaria. Some of the suggested methods include the use of vector control programs like spraying with dichloro-diphenyl-trichloroethane (DDT), insecticide-impregnated bed nets to protect against infection by mosquitoes, and medicines for prevention and to treat infection [33]. Developing an effective human malaria vaccine will be helpful not only to serve those living in malaria endemic areas but also to eradicate the disease globally [35]. The first vaccine developed by GlaxoSmithKline, namely, RTS,S, has been effective in reducing the risk of clinical malaria and in preventing episodes of severe malaria for at least 18 months [36]. But serious doubts have been raised over long-term prophylaxis by vaccination since malarial parasites develop various sophisticated mechanisms to avoid the host immune system [33]. With this in mind, the Bill & Melinda Gates Foundation (2007) introduced an agenda with the final goal of eradicating malaria by making extinct all species of *Plasmodium* that cause malaria infection in man [37]. Besides the four *Plasmodium* species that cause malaria in humans, a fifth species known as *Plasmodium knowlesi*, originally described as a parasite of long-tailed macaque monkeys, also infects humans in certain regions in Malaysia [38]. Unlike other *Plasmodium* species, *P. knowlesi* has a daily replication cycle, and untreated *P. knowlesi*-malaria infections may reach potentially lethal levels of parasitemia [39]. A recent prospective clinical study conducted in the Sarawak region of Malaysia reveals that approximately 10 % of the patients infected with *P. knowlesi* had severe signs and symptoms, and 1–2 % of cases had a fatal outcome [40]. All lethal cases of *P. knowlesi* developed prominent abdominal signs and symptoms, associated with kidney liver dysfunction with concurrent hyperparasitemia [41]. Besides Sarawak, cases of *P. knowlesi* are now reported throughout Peninsular Malaysia and the cases are increasing year after year [42]. The vector for *P. knowlesi* is *Anopheles cracens* [43].

Therapeutic procedures using chloroquine were found effective in treating patients with *P. knowlesi* infections [44].

Antimalarial Drugs

The four principal purposes for antimalarial drug therapy are the following: (1) to treat malaria illness, (2) to prevent malaria infection and disease, (3) to eliminate dormant malaria parasites from the liver, and (4) to prevent malaria transmission [8]. Successful malaria control and elimination programs rely mainly on drug-based treatment and prevention procedures rather than insecticides as used in the mid-twentieth century. Due to the advent of resistant parasites, priority should be given to the use of new and innovative antimalarial drugs to replace less efficacious older drugs [8]. Speed of action is considered as one of the main determinant of antimalarial compound efficacy and is also a "crucial clinical parameter" to determine the in vivo parasite clearance times (PCT) [2]. The drug with immediate onset of action is artemisinin with an in vitro parasite reduction ratio (PRR) higher than 8. Of the various antimalarial compounds tested, mefloquine, chloroquine, artemisinin, and pyrimethamine induce reduction in the number of viable parasites to virtually zero levels after 72 h of treatment [2]. Drugs like artemisinin and its derivatives artesunate and halofantrine induce the greatest reduction. Artemether contains endoperoxidase bond that is required for antimalarial properties [45]. Drugs like atovaquone, triazolopyrimidine, and pyridine act by directly impairing malaria parasite mitochondrial function [46]. All endoperoxides whether natural, semisynthetic, or synthetic (artemisinin, dihydroartemisinin, artesunate, and the ozonids OZ 277, OZ439) are the most potent antimalarials that are currently used against asexual blood stages. They act by alkylating heme and other vital biomolecules [45, 47] as well as by degrading phospholipids in parasite membranes [48]. This later action of endoperoxides has a major impact on all replicating stages of *Plasmodium* life cycle like asexual blood stage, liver schizont, oocyst, and microgametogenesis, and these have been demonstrated [49].

Transmission-Blocking Drugs (TBD)

Eradicating malaria also depends on approaches that prevent transmission of parasite between humans and mosquitoes. Reduction of gametocytes in their mature forms (stage V) should be the key targets for TBD. Clinical studies have shown that primaquine eliminates gametocytes effectively when used alone [50] or in combination with sulfadoxine-pyrimethamine and artesunate [51]. The most severe "bottleneck" identified during the process of transmission is the oocyte stage in the mosquito hemocoel, which is the main target for drug intervention. *P. berghei* ookinete production in vitro was the most practical approach to identify the molecules that target the early development of *Plasmodium* parasites in the mosquito. Of the 46 molecules tested at a concentration of 10 μM, the most potent molecules identified were cycloheximide and atovaquone [49]. Drugs like thiostrepton and pyronaridine, although less effective in inhibiting ookinete production, inhibited *P. falciparum* exflagellation by more than 80 % similar to sulfamethoxazole and mefloquine [49]. Although the design of drugs that act on ookinete are attractive, it requires a compound that has a half-life matching that of gametocytes. While this is possible with a majority of malaria species (with gametocytes of short half-life), it is difficult with *P. falciparum* since its mature gametocytes survive up to 3 weeks. Moreover, targeting oocytes with drugs or vaccines will be more difficult because exposure of oocytes to drugs or selective delivery of drugs to oocytes is impossible and will only result in the development of drug resistance [7].

Modulation of Malaria Parasite Replication Cycle by Melatonin

Involvement of melatonin in modulating the life cycle of *P. falciparum* has been the subject of investigation for a long time. In vitro studies show that incubating malarial parasites with different doses of melatonin ranging from 10 to 100 nM and examining different stages of malarial parasites result in reduction in the percentage of cells with ring and trophozoite stage but increase of mature schizont stage (two times higher) [9]. As host melatonin secretion is high during the dark hours of the night, it is inferred that host melatonin secretion occurring at nighttime (melatonin secretion begins at around 7:00 PM to 9:00 PM and reaches maximum around 2:00 AM to 4:00 AM) acts to synchronize the *Plasmodium* cell cycle. The increase of parasitemia caused by melatonin was completely abolished by melatonin receptor antagonist luzindole, and from this it was concluded that melatonin is the "host-derived signal" for release of billions of malarial parasites into the blood [9]. Recent genome analytical studies showed that both calcium and cAMP are essential for coordinating the events of maturation and development of intraerythrocytic stages of *Plasmodium* [52].

As mentioned above, PfPK7 plays a crucial role in melatonin transduction pathway. Ample evidences have been documented for involvement of melatonin in regulating UPS and signalling pathways in *Plasmodium* [28]. Melatonin modifies the life cycle of *P. falciparum* by upregulating the genes related to UPS. The effect of melatonin on UPS was completely blocked by melatonin antagonist luzindole indicating thereby the presence of melatonin receptors on the surface of *Plasmodium* membrane and their involvement in mediating melatonin modulatory action on *Plasmodium*'s growth and development [28]. Not only melatonin but its precursors *N*-acetylserotonin, tryptamine, serotonin, and melatonin metabolite *N*(1)-acetyl-*N*(2)-formyl-5-methoxykynuramine (AFMK) also modulate the intraerythrocytic *P. falciparum* cell cycle [53, 54]. The ability of melatonin and other tryptophan derivatives to synchronize *P. falciparum* cultures is blocked by inhibition of phospholipase C (PLC) and melatonin receptors [53, 54]. Moreover, the effects of melatonin on Ca^{2+} release and synchronized progression through the cell cycle are blocked by PLC inhibitor U73122 [53, 54]. As has been pointed out in the earlier paragraph, melatonin increases both cAMP and PLC that causes Ca^{2+} mobilization. This action of melatonin is essential for synchronization of malarial parasite's cell cycle [55]. Thus the existence of classical PLC-dependent intracellular Ca^{2+} release pathway in *P. falciparum* and its stimulation by melatonin has been shown to be the main mechanism for parasitic development and release in the human host [56].

Involvement of Melatonin in Other Parasites

In unicellular organisms melatonin is invariably associated with nighttime and functions mainly as a "darkness signal" [57]. *Trypanosoma cruzi*, a flagellated protozoan parasite, synthesizes and responds to melatonin, and melatonin is essential for regulating its life cycle and its parasitic ability [58]. Similarly, an endogenous circadian pacemaker has been described in the nematode *Caenorhabditis elegans* [59]. In this species melatonin seems to act as a neuromodulator regulating locomotor activity through distinct receptor pathway [60]. It is suggested that microfilaria *Wuchereria bancrofti* that are released into a host's bloodstream during nighttime are cued by the host secretion of melatonin [61]. From these examples it is clear that these organisms have endogenous circadian rhythms that are self-sustained but synchronized to the24-h day by an environmental time cue regulated by melatonin [61].

Therapeutic Interventions Against Actions of Melatonin on *P. falciparum*

From the foregoing discussions on effects of melatonin in modulating *P. falciparum* replication cycle, it is evident that inhibition or suppression of nocturnal melatonin secretion in the host or prevention of melatonin action on *P. falciparum* by using melatonin receptor antagonists or agents that inhibit PLC activation in malarial parasites can help to prevent the development of later asexual stages of *Plasmodium* [62]. Luzindole, the common MT1 and MT2 melatonin receptor antagonist, can be employed to prevent the development of asexual stages of malarial parasites in man. Luzindole can be administered to the host in the late evening around 6:00 PM, and blood can be examined for the presence of asexual stages of malarial parasites, namely, *P. falciparum* or *P. knowlesi*, through serial blood samples drawn during nighttime (every 2 or 3 h). Once the complete elimination of asexual stages of *Plasmodium* in the host's blood is confirmed, the drug (luzindole) can be administered for the duration of 1 month. The dose and the number of days to be administered have to be worked out only after conducting pilot study on malaria-infected patients (*P. falciparum* or *P. knowlesi*). To compensate for the melatonin deficiency induced in the host by luzindole at night, melatonin at physiological doses (0.25–0.5 mg) can be administered during the daytime for the entire period of treatment.

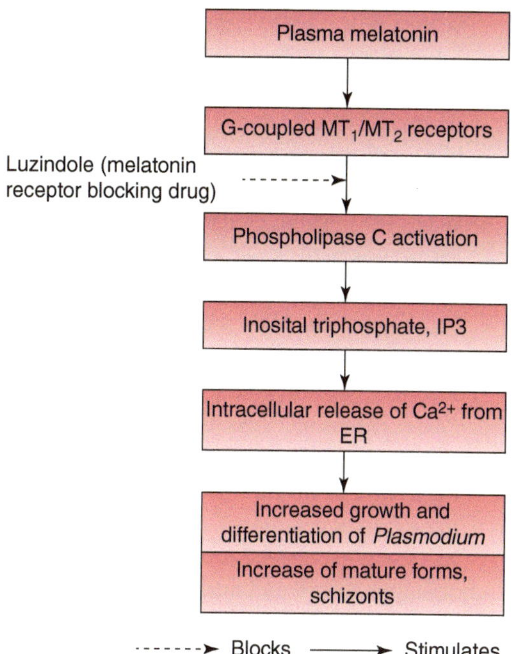

Fig. 12.1 Schematic diagram showing stimulatory effects of melatonin on *Plasmodium* cell cycle (growth, differentiation, and development)

Melatonin Antagonism via Bright Light Application

Exposure to bright light during nighttime causes either reduction in plasma melatonin levels or complete suppression of plasma melatonin depending upon the intensity of the light applied. Exposure of human beings to 2,500 lx at around 2:00 AM causes complete suppression of plasma melatonin concentration [63]. Circadian changes of plasma melatonin levels of the host constitute a key signal that causes synchronous maturation and development of *Plasmodium* [9], and malarial parasites have intrinsic ability to sense plasma melatonin levels [56]. Therefore, complete suppression of plasma melatonin at night can be helpful in desynchronizing *plasmodium* growth and development and arrest the parasitic cell cycle and development of gametocytes in the host [62]. A light mask treatment, using light applied through the eyelids during sleep, will deliver light of required intensities without affecting the patient's sleep at night [64]. A patent (US 2012/0041520 A1) of a system for delivering bright light through eye lids has recently been approved [65]. A schematic diagram showing stimulatory effects of melatonin on *Plasmodium* cell cycle (growth, differentiation, and development) is summarized in Fig. 12.1.

Conclusion

Human malaria is caused mainly by infection with *Plasmodium falciparum* and *Plasmodium malariae* [66]. Now *Plasmodium knowlesi*, a malaria parasite from Malaysia, is fast spreading throughout the globe and causes great concern for effective eradication of malaria from Malaysia as well as from the entire globe [38, 39, 42]. Malarial infection caused by all these species causes variable clinical symptoms such as fever, chills, headache, muscular aches, abdominal pain, cough, and diarrhea and affects several important organs of the body like cerebral tissue, heart, liver, and kidney [67]. Malarial infection also increases the generation of reactive oxygen species in the tissues and decreases the antioxidative enzymes like catalase, glutathione peroxidase, and superoxide dismutase [68]. Eradication of malaria requires institution of antimalarial drugs that can act both at the asexual and gametocyte stages of malarial parasites in the human blood as well as those that can curb the development of gametocytes within mosquito vectors. The use of TBD is much needed today for malaria eradication programs [7]. The endoperoxides, whether natural or synthetic (artemisinin or its derivatives dihydroartemisinin), are the most potent antimalarial drugs that are currently used against asexual blood stages [45]. Although the design of drugs that act on ookinete is attractive, it is difficult to achieve since it requires a compound that has half-life that matches that of gametocytes [7].

Recent studies have shown that melatonin secreted at nighttime synchronizes the *Plasmodium* cell cycle. Both intracellular calcium and cAMP are essential for coordinating the events of maturation and development of intraerythrocytic stages of *Plasmodium* [52]. Melatonin regulates *Plasmodium* cell cycle by acting on cAMP and intracellular Ca^{2+} release [56]. Hence, use of drugs that block the action of melatonin on *Plasmodium* or procedures like bright light that can suppress the nocturnal plasma levels of melatonin completely will be effective methods for arresting the growth and development of asexual stages of malarial parasite [62]. Melatonin is an effective antioxidant that has been shown to be effective in preventing oxidative stress-induced hepatic damage and apoptosis seen in Swiss mice infected with malarial parasites [69]. But the beneficial effects of melatonin in malaria-infected animal species [70] cannot be applied to human cases since in humans, the beneficial actions of melatonin will be much overshadowed by its action in promoting malarial growth and development. Hence, use of melatonin antagonists or the procedures that suppress plasma melatonin levels completely will only be helpful in preventing growth and spread of malarial infections caused by *P. falciparum*, *P. malariae*, or *P. knowlesi* infection in human beings.

References

1. WHO, World Malaria Report: 2010, WHO Press, Geneva, Switzerland, 2010.
2. Sanz LM, Crespo B, De-Cozar C, Ding XC, Llergo JL, Burrows JN, et al. P. falciparum in vitro killing rates allow to discriminate between different anti-malarial mode-of-action. PLoS One. 2012;7(2):e30949.
3. Alonso PL, Djimde A, Kremsner P, Magill A, Najera J, Plowe CV, et al. malERA Consultative Group on Drugs. A research agenda for malaria eradication: drugs. PLoS Med. 2011;8(1):e1000402. doi:10.1371/journal.pmd1000402.
4. Piyaphanee W, Krudsood S, Tangpukdee N, Thanachartwet W, Silachamroon U, et al. Emergence and clearance of gametocytes in uncomplicated Plasmodium falciparum malaria. Am J Trop Med Hyg. 2006;74:432–5.
5. Shekalaghe S, Drakeley C, Gosling R, Ndaro A, van Meegeren M, Enevold A. Primaquine clears submicroscopic Plasmodium falciparum gametocytes that persist after treatment with sulphadoxine-pyrimethamine and artesunate. PLoS One. 2007;2:e.1023. doi: 10.1371/journal.pone.0001023.
6. Bousema T, Okell I, Shekalaghe S, Griffin JT, Omar S, Sawa P, et al. Revisiting the circulation time of Plasmodium falciparum gametocyte: molecular detection methods to estimate the duration of gametocyte carriage and the effect of gametocytocidal drugs. Malar J. 2010;9:136.
7. Sinden RE, Carter R, Drakeley C, Leroy D. The biology of sexual development of Plasmodium: the design and implementation of transmission-blocking strategies. Malar J. 2012;11:70.
8. Breman JG, Brandling-Bennett AD. The challenge of malaria eradication in the twenty-first century: research linked to operations is the key. Vaccine. 2011;29:D97–103.
9. Hotta CT, Gazarini ML, Beraldo FH, Varotti FP, Lopes C, Markus RP, et al. Calcium-dependent modulation by melatonin of the circadian rhythm in malarial parasites. Nat Cell Biol. 2000;2:466–8.
10. Beier J. Malaria parasite development in mosquitoes. Annu Rev Entomol. 1998;43:519–43.
11. Schofield L. Intravascular infiltrates and organ-specific inflammation in malaria pathogenesis. Immunol Cell Biol. 2007;85:130–7.
12. Gardner MJ, Hall N, Fung E, White O, Berriman M, Hyman RW, et al. Genome sequence of the human malaria parasite Plasmodium falciparum. Nature. 2002;419(6906):512–9.
13. Pain A, Bohme U, Berry AE, Mungall K, Finn RD, Jackson AP, et al. The genome of simian and human malaria parasite Plasmodium knowlesi. Nature. 2008;455(7214):799–803.
14. Carlton J. The Plasmodium vivax genome sequencing project. Trends Parasitol. 2003;19(5):227–31.
15. Baker DA. Malaria gametocytogenesis. Mol Biochem Parasitol. 2010;172:57–65.
16. Lasonder E, Ishihama Y, Andersen JS, Vermunt AM, Pain A, Sauerwein RW, et al. Analysis of the Plasmodium falciparum proteome by high-accuracy mass spectrometry. Nature. 2002;419:537–42.
17. Smith TG, Lourenco P, Carter R, Walliker D, Landford-Cartwright LC. Commitment to sexual differentiation in the human malarial parasite, Plasmodium falciparum. Parasitology. 2000;121(Pt5):127–33.

18. Silvestrini F, Alano P, Williams JL. Commitment to the production of male and female gametocytes in the human malarial parasite Plasmodium falciparum. Parasitology. 2000;121(Pt 5):465–71.
19. Trager W, Gill GS. Plasmodium falciparum gametocyte formation in vitro: its stimulation by phorbol diesters and by 8-bromo cyclic adenosine monophosphate. J Protozool. 1989;36:451–4.
20. Inselburg J. Stage-specific inhibitory effect of cyclic AMP on asexual maturation and gametocyte formation of Plasmodium falciparum. J Parasitol. 1983;69:592–7.
21. Kappe SH, Vaughen SM, Boddey JA, Cowman AF. That was then, but this is now: malaria research in the time of an eradication agenda. Science. 2010;328(5980):862–6.
22. Garcia CR, Markus RP, Madeira L. Tertian and quartan fevers: temporal regulation in malarial infection. J Biol Rhythms. 2001;16:436–43.
23. Bannister L, Mitchell G. The ins, outs, and roundabouts of malaria. Trends Parasitol. 2003;19:209–13.
24. Hotta CT, Markus RP, Garcia CR. Melatonin and N-acetylserotonin cross the red blood cell membrane and evoke calcium mobilization in malarial parasites. Braz J Med Biol Res. 2003;36:1583–7.
25. Lilburn TG, Cai H, Zhou Z, Wang Y. Protease-associated cellular networks in malaria parasite Plasmodium falciparum. BMC Genomics. 2011;12(S5):59.
26. Russo I, Oksman A, Vaupel B, Goldberg DE. A calpain unique to alveolates is essential in Plasmodium falciparum reveals an involvement in pre-5-phase development. Proc Natl Acad Sci U S A. 2009;106(5):1554–9.
27. Blackman MJ. Malarial proteases and host cell egress: an 'emerging' cascade. Cell Microbiol. 2008;10(10):1925–34.
28. Koyama FC, Ribeiro RY, Garcia JL, Azevedo MF, Charabarti D, Garcia CRS. Ubiquitin proteosome system and the atypical kinase PfPK7 are involved in melatonin signaling in Plasmodium falciparum. J Pineal Res. 2012. doi:10.1111/j.1600-079X.2012.00981.x.
29. Cohen P. Protein kinases-the major drug targets of the twenty first century. Nat Rev Drug Discov. 2002;1:309–15.
30. Gazharini ML, Garcia RL. Interruption of the blood stage cycle of malaria parasite, Plasmodium chabaudi by protein tyrosine kinase inhibitors. Braz J Med Biol Res. 2003;36:1465–9.
31. Gazarini ML, Beraldo FH, Almeida FM, Bootman FM, deSilva AM, Garcia CRS. Melatonin triggers PKA activation in the rodent malarial parasite Plasmodium chabaudi. J Pineal Res. 2011;50:64–70.
32. WHO. Making a difference. The World Health Report. Health Millions. 1999;25:3–5.
33. Wells TNC, Alonso PL, Gutteridge WE. New medicines to improve control and contribute to the eradication of malaria. Nat Rev. 2009;8:879–91.
34. Snow RW, Guerra CA, Noor AM, Myint HY, Hay SI. The global distribution of clinical episodes of Plasmodium falciparum malaria. Nature. 2005;434:214–7.
35. Saleh JA, Yusuph H, Zailani SB, Ali B. Malaria vaccine: the pros and cons. Niger J Med. 2010;19(1):8–13.
36. Guinovart C, et al. Insights into long lasting protection induced by RTS.S/A502A malaria vaccine: further results from a phase IIb trial in Mozambican children. PLoS One. 2009;4:e5165.
37. Robert I, Enserink M. Did they really say eradication? Science. 2007;318:1544–5.
38. Singh B, Kim Sung L, Matusop A, Radhakrishnan A, Shamsul SS, Cox-Singh J, et al. A large focus of naturally acquired Plasmodium knowlesi infections in human beings. Lancet. 2004;363:1017–24.
39. Sabbatani S, Fiorino S, Manfredi R. Plasmodium knowlesi: from Malaysia, a novel health care threat. Infez Med. 2012;1:5–11.
40. Daneshvar C, Davis TME, Cox-Singh J, Rafa'ee MZ, Zakaria SK, Divis PC, et al. Clinical and laboratory features of human Plasmodium knowlesi infection. Clin Infect Dis. 2009;49:852–60.
41. Cox-singh J, Hiu J, Lucas SB, Divis PC, Zulkarnaen M, Chandran P, et al. Severe malaria-a case of fatal Plasmodium knowlesi infection with post-mortem findings: a case report. Malar J. 2010;9:1–7.
42. Vythilingam I. Plasmodium knowlesi in humans: a review on the role of its vectors in Malaysia. Trop Biomed. 2010;27(1):1–12.
43. Vythilingam I, NoorAzian YM, Huat TC, Ida Jiram A, Yusri YM, Azahari AH, et al. Plasmodium knowlesi in humans, macaques and mosquitoes in Peninsular Malaysia. Parasit Vectors. 2008;1:26. doi:10.1186/1756-3305-1-26.
44. Daneshwar C, Davis TME, Cox-Singh J, Rafa'ee MZ, Zakaria SK, Divis PC, et al. Clinical and parasitological response to oral chloroquine and primaquine in uncomplicated human Plasmodium knowlesi infections. Malar J. 2010;9:238–44.
45. O'Neill PM, Barton VE, Ward SA. The molecular mechanism of action of artemisinin-the debate continues. Molecules. 2010;15:1705–21.
46. Gujjar R, Marwaha A, El Mazouni F, White J, White KL, Creason S, et al. Identification of a metabolically stable triazolopyrimidine-based dihydroorotate dehydrogenase inhibitor with anti malarial activity in mice. J Med Chem. 2009;52:1864–72.
47. Klonis N, Crespo Ortis MP, Bottova I, Abu-Baker N, Kenney S, Rosenthal PJ, et al. Artemisinin activity against Plasmodium falciparum requires haemoglobin uptake and digestion. Proc Natl Acad Sci U S A. 2011;108:11405–10.
48. Kumura N, Furukawa H, Onyango AN, Izumi M, Nakajima S, Ito H, et al. Different behaviour of artemisinin and tetraoxane in the oxidative degradation of phospholipid. Chem Phys Lipids. 2009;160:114–20.
49. Delves M, Plouffe D, Scheurer C, Meister S, Wittlin S, Winzeler EA, et al. The activities of current antimalarial drugs on the life cycle stages of Plasmodium. PLoS Med. 2012;9(2):e1001169.
50. Wilairatana P, Tangpukdee N, Krudsood S. Longterm primaquine administration to reduce Plasmodium falciparum gametocyte transmission in hypoendemic areas. Southeast Asian J Top Med Public Health. 2010;41:1306–11.

51. Shekalaghe SA, Drakeley C, van den Bosch S, ter Braak R, van den Bijllardt W, Mwanziva C, et al. A cluster randomized trial of mass drug administration with a gametocytocidal drug combination to interrupt malaria transmission in a low endemic area in Tanzania. Malar J. 2011;10:247.
52. Hardeland R, Cardinali DP, Srinivasan V, Spence DW, Brown GM, Pandi-Perumal SR. Melatonin-A pleiotropic, orchestering regulator molecule. Prog Neurobiol. 2011;93(3):350–84.
53. Florens L, Washburn MP, Raine JD, Anthony RM, Grainger M, Haynes JD, et al. A proteomic view of the Plasmodium falciparum life cycle. Nature. 2002;419:520–6.
54. Beraldo FH, Garcia CRS. Products of tryptophan metabolism induce Ca^{2+} release and modulate the cell cycle of Plasmodium falciparum malarial parasites. J Pineal Res. 2005;39:224–30.
55. Beraldo AH, Mikoshiba K, Garcia CR. Human malarial parasite Plasmodium falciparum displays a capacitative entry: 2 aminoethyl diphenylborinate blocks the signal transduction pathway of melatonin on P. falciparum cell cycle. J Pineal Res. 2007;43:360–4.
56. Alves E, Barlett PJ, Garcia CRS, Thomas A. Melatonin and IP_3 release from intracellular stores in the Malaria Parasite Plasmodium falciparum within increased red blood cells. J Biol Chem. 2011;286(7):5905–12.
57. Balzer I, Hardeland R. Photoperiodism and effects of indoleamines in a unicellular algae. Gonyaulax polyedra. Science. 1991;253:795–7.
58. Macías M, Rodríguez-Cabezas MN, Reiter RJ, Osuna A, Acuña-Castroviejo D. Presence and effects of melatonin in Trypanosoma cruzi J Pineal Res. 1999;27(2):86–94.
59. Saigusa T, Ishizaki S, Watabiki S, Ishil N, Tanakadate A, Tamai V, et al. Circadian behavioural rhythm in Caenorhabditis elegans. Curr Biol. 2002;12:R46–7.
60. Tanaka D, Furusawa K, Kameyama K, Okamoto H, Doi M. Melatonin signalling regulates locomotion behaviour and homeostatic states through distinct pathways in Caenorhabditis elegans. Neuropharmacology. 2007;53:157–68.
61. Sack RL. Host melatonin secretion is timing signal for the release of W. bancrofti. Med Hypotheses. 2009;73:147–9.
62. Srinivasan V, Ahmed AH, Mohamed M, Zakariah R. Melatonin effects on Plasmodium falciparum life cycle; a new avenue for therapeutic approach. Recent Pat Endocr Metab Immune Drug Discov. 2012;6(2):139–47.
63. Lewy AJ, Wehr TA, Goodwin FK, Newsome DA, Markey SP. Light suppresses melatonin secretion in humans. Science. 1980;210:1267–9.
64. Ando K, Kripke DF, Cole RJ, Elliott JA. Light mask 500 lux treatment for delayed sleep phase syndrome. Prog Neuropsychopharmacol Biol Psychiatry. 1999;23:15–24.
65. Colbaugh ME, Timothy A. System and method for delivering electromagnetic radiation to the eyeball of a subject. US 2012/0041520 A1 dated, 16 Feb 2012.
66. Garcia CRS, De Azevedo MF, Wunderlich G, Budu A, Young JA, Bannister L. Plasmodium in the post-genomic era: new insights into the molecular cell biology of malaria parasites. Int Rev Cell Mol Biol. 2008;266:85–156.
67. Abate K. Modern day malaria: an overview of this lingering threat. Adv Nurse Pract. 2008;16:67–8.
68. Siddiqui NJ, Pandey VC. Studies on hepatic oxidative stress and anti oxidative defense system during arteether treatment of Plasmodium yoelii nigeriensis infected mice. Mol Cell Biochem. 1999;196:169–73.
69. Guha M, Maity P, Choubey V, Mitra K, Reiter RJ, Bandyopadhyay U. Melatonin inhibits free-radical mediated mitochondrial-dependent hepatocyte apoptosis and liver damage induced during malarial infection. J Pineal Res. 2007;43:372–81.
70. Srinivasan V, Spence DW, Moscovitch A, Pandi-Perumal SR, Trakht I, Brown GM, et al. Malaria: therapeutic implications of melatonin. J Pineal Res. 2010;48:1–8.

Melatonin's Role in Human Reproduction: Recent Studies

13

Rahimah Zakaria, Amnon Brzezinski, and V. Srinivasan

Abstract

Melatonin, *N*-acetyl-5-methhoxytryptamine, is a molecule with diverse physiological function. It affects reproductive functions in a wide variety of species. This chapter describes the roles of melatonin on various reproductive parameters. Melatonin has an inhibitory influence on hypothalamic GnRH secretion. Melatonin acts as antioxidant and reduces oxidative stress-induced testicular dysfunctions and poor oocytes quality in many experimental animals. During fetal life, melatonin regulates circadian rhythm and has been suggested to play a role in the regulation of fetal REM and NREM sleep. In adults, melatonin regulates the time of parturition in both humans and nonhuman primates. Many studies have suggested that melatonin could be an effective treatment for preeclampsia, due to its antioxidant properties as well as its antihypertensive and anticonvulsive actions.

Keywords

Melatonin • GnRH • Parturition • Oocyte • Testes • Preeclampsia

R. Zakaria, MBBS, MSc, PhD (Physiology) (✉)
Department of Physiology,
School of Medical Sciences, Universiti Sains Malaysia,
Kubang Kerian, Kelantan 16150, Malaysia
e-mail: rahimah@kck.usm.my

A. Brzezinski, MD
Department of Obstetrics and Gynecology,
Hadassah Hebrew-University Medical Center,
Ein-Kerem, Jerusalem 91120, Israel
e-mail: amnonbrz@gmail.com

V. Srinivasan, MSc, PhD, MAMS
Sri Sathya Sai Medical Educational
and Research Foundation, An International Medical
Sciences Research Study Center, Prasanthi Nilayam,
40-Kovai Thirunagar Extn, Goldwins, Coimbatore,
TN 641014, India

National Health Service, Department
of Mental Health, Psychiatric Service of Diagnosis
and Treatment, Hospital "G. Mazzini",
ASL 4, Teramo, Italy

Department of Neuroscience and Imaging,
University "G.D' Annunzio", Chieti 66013, Italy
e-mail: sainivasan@yahoo.com,
venkataramanujamsrinivasan6@gmail.com

V. Srinivasan et al. (eds.), *Melatonin and Melatonergic Drugs in Clinical Practice*,
DOI 10.1007/978-81-322-0825-9_13, © Springer India 2014

Introduction

The report of human pineal gland tumor that altered pubertal development by Huebner [1] in 1898, almost 70 years before the identification of melatonin, suggests that some factor of pineal origin may be capable of influencing reproductive function. This finding has led many researchers to examine the association between the pineal and the reproductive status in a variety of species but with limited success in demonstrating a functional relationship [2, 3].

Wurtman et al. [4] first reported that exogenous administration of melatonin reduces the weight of the ovaries of female rats in 1963. Since then, abundant evidence has been adduced that the pineal gland, acting via melatonin, affects reproductive function in a wide variety of species [5]. There is growing evidence that the pattern of melatonin secretion, mediated by photoperiod, directly influences reproductive function. The major physiological role of melatonin is to encode the daily light/dark (LD) cycle. The onset and offset of pineal melatonin secretion synchronize to dusk and dawn, respectively, and therefore, the duration of the melatonin signal varies in proportion to the length of the night. This variation in melatonin signal duration is used to synchronize neuroendocrine rhythms with the annual variation in day-length in seasonal mammals. Additionally, fetal and newborn animals use the maternal melatonin signal to entrain endogenous circadian rhythms prior to the availability of direct photic information. The efficacy of exogenous melatonin in modifying particular reproductive functions has been found to differ markedly among species, depending on the age of the animal, the time of melatonin administration relative to the prevailing LD cycle, or phase of the estrus cycle [6].

A seasonal distribution in human natural conception and birth rates has been reported by epidemiological studies in several geographical areas [7]. Suppression in the pituitary-ovarian activity [8] and reduction in the conception rate have been reported to take place during the dark winter near the Arctic Circle [9]. These observations and the data from studies in mammals inspired reproductive physiologists to search for a role for the pineal gland and melatonin in human sexual maturation (i.e., puberty) and reproduction [10, 11]. Roles of melatonin on reproductive functions are summarized in Fig. 13.1.

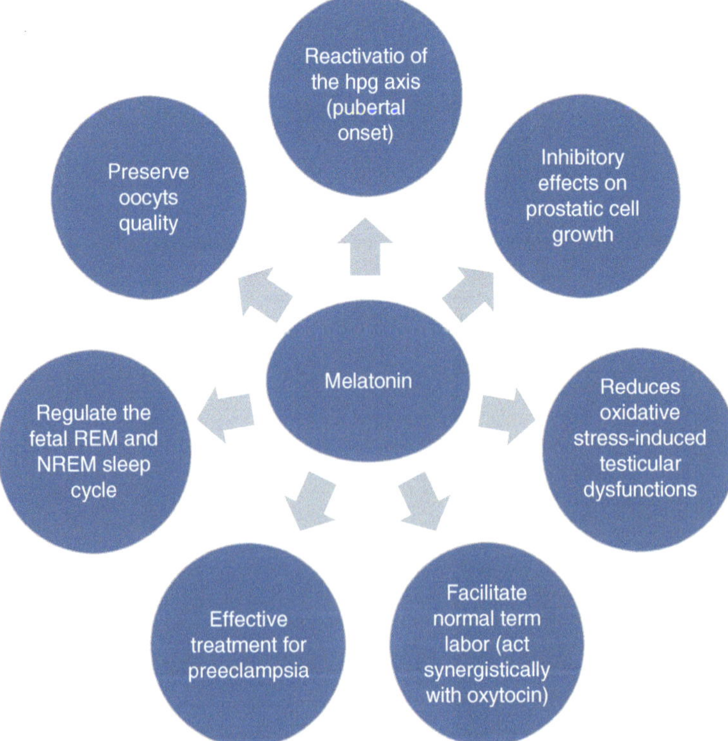

Fig. 13.1 Schematic diagram showing *possible* effects of melatonin on reproductive functions

Melatonin and Puberty

It has been suggested that melatonin is involved in the modulation of human pubertal development. The hypothalamo-pituitary-gonadal (HPG) axis, which is active during fetal life and the first year of life, remains quiescent until the age of 10 years. Reactivation of the hypothalamic-pituitary axis is because of the progressive increase in the amplitude and frequency of gonadotropin-releasing hormone (GnRH) pulses and, hence, the pulsatile secretion of luteinizing hormone (LH) and follicle-stimulating hormone (FSH) [12]. Similar to endogenous HPG hormones, the amplitude of the endogenous melatonin rhythm varies across the lifespan [13–17]. The onset of a circadian melatonin rhythm in human infants appears only after 9 weeks of age. A peak in melatonin secretion is established between 3 and 5 years of age, with a subsequent decline to adult levels by 15–18 years of age. Amplitude remains relatively stable until old age, when a marked decline has been demonstrated, due to a general weakening of the circadian system [18].

It has been suggested that nocturnal melatonin secretary pattern has an inhibitory influence on hypothalamic secretion of GnRH in humans [19]. It has been postulated that before puberty melatonin concentrations are too high to allow hypothalamic activation. But at 9 or 10 years of age, the decline in serum melatonin below the threshold value (approximately 500 pmol/l = 115 pg/ml) forms the triggering signal of GnRH and thereafter the onset of pubertal changes occur [20]. The functional significance of a decline in melatonin as it relates to the onset of puberty remains debatable [21, 22] because other factors coincide with pubertal stage may contribute to melatonin amplitude.

Previous study reported that melatonin levels decreased as a function of age [14], and when age was accounted for, the puberty-related decline of melatonin disappeared [23]. Later study by Waldhauser et al. [24] and Crowley et al. [22] found the reduction in melatonin concentration with age is not caused by increase in body mass but is temporally related to sexual maturation. Furthermore, Young and colleagues argued that the pineal gland secretes the same amount of melatonin across puberty, and the change in melatonin levels measured during this developmental period is accounted for by increasing body mass and associated diffusion of melatonin in larger body habitus [25]. This latter study, however, did not measure pubertal stage, and evidence from several studies does not support this finding [26–28].

Sex is another factor that may contribute to melatonin amplitude during puberty. Studies of adults reported that women secrete more melatonin compared to men [29, 30]. Several studies of adults [31] and adolescents [23, 26, 28, 32], however, do not find these sex differences or find a difference accounted for by the youngster's age [33]. The recent studies by Cain et al. [29] and Crowley et al. [22] showed lower melatonin amplitude across pubertal maturation; pre- and early pubertal youngsters showed higher melatonin amplitude compared to their late- and postpubertal peers. This melatonin decline was similar between boys and girls, but overall, girls secreted more melatonin compared to boys. Of the factors examined, Tanner stage and sex explained the salivary melatonin amplitude decline during this developmental period, but age and BMI did not. The significance of females secreting more melatonin than males during adolescence and adulthood is unknown; however, the sex difference in melatonin amplitude may contribute to sleep disorders (e.g., insomnia) where prevalence rates differ by sex [22, 29].

Puberty stage predicts melatonin amplitude better than chronological age [22, 28], and it is suggested that sexual maturation and the reactivation of the HPG axis may explain melatonin amplitude more precisely than age during this developmental period. Waldhauser and colleagues [34] reported an inverse relationship between melatonin and LH secretion in children and young adults and suggested that melatonin may be a gonadotropin inhibitor.

Evidence obtained from human pathological studies also suggests that high nocturnal melatonin levels seen in children has a suppressive effect on, pulsatile secretion of GnRH, ovarian function and pubertal development [21]. More recent data show that melatonin may act indirectly to inhibit GnRH secretion through a novel neurohormone called gonadotropin-inhibitory hormone (GnIH) [35, 36], which further supports a role of melatonin in the reactivation of the HPG axis.

High nocturnal melatonin secretion has been reported in children with delayed puberty when compared with age-matched controls [37], whereas low levels of melatonin have been reported in children with precocious puberty [21]. Studies of patients with precocious puberty, for example, showed lower melatonin levels in patients compared to normal controls [21, 24, 38]. Other studies, however, did not replicate this finding [39, 40], and pituitary-gonadal suppression by a GnRH agonist does not alter [41] or decreases [24] circulating melatonin levels in patients with precocious puberty.

It has been demonstrated that in boys having a precocious puberty, melatonin concentration was higher compared to age-matched children of normal puberty age, while boys with delayed puberty had lower melatonin concentration [42]. Moreover, hypothalamic amenorrhea was associated with high melatonin concentrations [43]. On the basis of all these observations, it is suggested that melatonin may be part of the cascade of events preceding the awakening of HPG axis at puberty [44].

The mechanism by which melatonin inhibits the reproductive axis until puberty remains unclear. There have nevertheless been some suggestive findings which merit further investigation. These include the following: (1) Evidence that melatonin is involved in the control of pulsatile secretion of LH [45] and a negative correlation between nocturnal serum melatonin and LH concentrations has been documented [34]. (2) Women with high blood melatonin levels have been shown to have functional hypothalamic amenorrhea with decreased GnRH/LH pulsatile secretion [41, 45]. In addition, amenorrheic athletes who displayed irregularities in hypothalamic-pituitary-ovarian axis functioning were found to have increase in the nocturnal peak amplitude and duration of melatonin [46, 47]. (3) Melatonin at 10 nM has been shown to downregulate GnRH gene expression in a cyclical manner over a 24 h period in GnRH-secreting neurons [48]. (4) Melatonin levels in the human preovulatory follicular fluid have been found to be significantly higher than in peripheral serum [49, 50]. Iodomelatonin binding sites have been identified in human granulose cells from preovulatory follicles [51, 52].

Melatonin and Testicular Function

There is evidence that melatonin may modulate testicular and sperm functions. Since melatonin binding sites were detected in the reproductive system of different species [53, 54], it seems reasonable to assume that melatonin exerts its actions via direct interaction with the steroidogenic cells of the reproductive organs.

In rats and mice, melatonin was found to have an inhibitory effect on Leydig cells [55, 56]. The epididymis is important for the maturation and storage of spermatozoa before their passage into the female reproductive tract. High-affinity [^{125}I] iodomelatonin binding sites have been identified in the rats' epididymis [57]. A functional interaction between testosterone and melatonin has been identified in the rat epididymis. This is based on the observation that testosterone reversed the decrease of specific 2-[^{125}I] iodomelatonin binding to the epididymis of castrated rats [58]. Mel1a and Mel1b receptor mRNAs are expressed in epithelial cells of rat epididymis suggesting that melatonin has a role in the regulation of epididymal physiology [58]. High-affinity specific G-protein-coupled melatonin receptors have been identified in the cytosol of human prostate glandular epithelial cells [59]. These receptors are believed to mediate the inhibitory effects of melatonin on prostatic cell growth [60].

Melatonin levels in seminal plasma are depressed in infertile patients exhibiting poor motility, leukocytospermia, varicocele, and nonobstructive azoospermia, all of which are conditions associated with oxidative stress in the male tract [61]. Moreover, the intraperitoneal injection of melatonin has been shown to alleviate oxidative stress in the testes following the experimental induction of a left-sided varicocele [62].

Melatonin acts as antioxidant and reduces oxidative stress-induced testicular dysfunctions in many experimental animals [63–66]. Intraperitoneal administration of melatonin for 5 days had been shown to be a potentially beneficial agent to reduce testicular damage in adult diabetic rats, probably by decreasing oxidative stress [63]. In addition, melatonin improved histopathological changes in testicular tissue induced by hyperlipidemia in mice [64]. Melatonin is a potent antioxidant agent in preventing testicular post ischemic reperfusion injury, as shown by changed abnormal sperm rate to normal [65] and ameliorating fluoride-induced reproductive organ toxicity in male rats [66].

Several studies have shown that sperm is negatively affected by oxidative stress caused by inflammatory processes, and it has been shown that melatonin or its metabolites are able to protect sperm from oxidative damage [67]. Additional studies have shown that human seminal fluid contains melatonin [68], and spermatozoa express melatonin receptors [69]. Furthermore, Fujinoki demonstrated that melatonin is able to stimulate flagellar motility [70].

Melatonin and Human Conception/Pregnancy

Seasonal trends in human reproduction have been reported. Among people living in the Arctic, pituitary-gonadal function and conception rates are lower in the dark winter months than in the summer [71]. In these northerly regions, the photoperiod is likely to affect human conception [7]. Further, during the dark periods of the winter season, increases in serum melatonin concentration in humans have been shown to correlate with reduced activity of the anterior pituitary-ovarian axis [72]. Conversely, nocturnal plasma LH levels are higher in the summer than in the winter [73].

Several trials have reported that endogenous melatonin levels decrease with age [74], inducing a decrease in oocyte quality in women near the end of their reproductive life. Melatonin administration was shown to be able to preserve oocytes quality by increasing melatonin intrafollicular concentrations. Indeed, high melatonin levels in the follicular fluid lead to a reduction of intrafollicular oxidative damage. Reduction of the oxidative stress increases fertilization and pregnancy rates in women who failed to become pregnant due to poor oocyte quality [75].

The role, if any, of melatonin during human pregnancy is unclear. It has been suggested that the diurnal maternal rhythm serves as a signal for the fetus to entrain the LD rhythms in newborns after delivery. It has been reported that serum melatonin levels during human pregnancy are higher than in a nonpregnant state [76]. Nocturnal melatonin concentration reportedly rises after 24 weeks of gestation and reaches a peak at 32 weeks of gestation. These high levels decline to nonpregnant levels on the second day of puerperium [77]. It has also been reported that nighttime melatonin levels were significantly higher in twin pregnancies after 28 weeks of gestation as compared with singleton pregnancies [76].

Maternal Melatonin and Fetal Development

In animal studies, maternal pinealectomy has been shown to reduce fetal plasma melatonin concentration and to abolish the fetal melatonin rhythm [78]. Melatonin, a small molecule, is transferred from maternal circulation to that of the fetus through the placenta. In one study, oral administration of 3 mg of melatonin to pregnant women led to marked increases in the serum levels of melatonin in the umbilical vein, changes which correlated with those in the umbilical vein [78]. This finding, therefore, is an evidence of a circadian rhythm of plasma melatonin exists in the fetal circulation [79]. Melatonin receptors have been identified in human fetal SCN [80, 81].

Generation and maintenance of circadian clock function depend on clock genes and their protein products (brain and muscle ARNT-like protein-1 (Bmal-1), period (Per1-3) and cytochrome (cry1-2) genes) [82]. Maternal melatonin suppression or its replacement has been shown to affect both MT_1 gene and clock genes, suggesting that maternal melatonin has a role in modulating fetal clock gene function via MT_1 in the fetal SCN [82]. In addition to circadian rhythm regulation in the fetus, it has been suggested that melatonin plays a role in the regulation of REM and NREM sleep. In the human fetus, REM and NREM sleep are distinguished at 30 weeks of gestation [82]. Given the hypnotic effect of melatonin, maternal melatonin may be one of the factors that regulate the fetal REM and NREM cycle [83, 84].

Melatonin and Complications of Pregnancy

It has been found that patients with severe preeclampsia exhibit significantly lower nighttime serum melatonin levels than individuals with mild preeclampsia or normal pregnant women after 32 weeks of gestation [76]. Although the pathophysiology of preeclampsia is still unclear, elevated oxidative stress is considered to be one of the possible precipitating factors [85, 86]. Because melatonin has significant antioxidant properties [87–89], it has been postulated that the elevated levels of melatonin during pregnancy may be one of the factors which reduce oxidative damage from ROS in the placenta and systemic endothelial cells [90]. Melatonin has been found useful against oxidized low-density lipoprotein (LDL)-induced inhibition of NO production in the endothelium of human umbilical arteries [91], and hence, it is likely that by inhibiting LDL oxidation melatonin may protect against oxidized LDL-induced impairment of endothelial function in preeclamptic women [90].

Many studies have suggested that melatonin could be an effective treatment for preeclampsia, due to its antioxidant properties [92]. Furthermore, other important properties have been described for melatonin, such as antihypertensive [93] and anticonvulsive [94] actions. Therefore, melatonin could be able to exert its beneficial effects on several parameters that are altered in preeclampsia.

Melatonin and the Timing of Parturition

In some mammalian species, melatonin has been shown to be the photoperiodic mediator regulating time of parturition. Rats give parturition predominantly during the daytime, even when the light-dark cycles are reversed [95–97]. Pinealectomy abolished the daytime delivery in rats, whereas melatonin replacement therapy restored the daytime birth pattern [98].

On the other hand, both term and preterm human parturition has been reported to the late nighttime and early morning hours [99–102]. There are reports that in humans, the initiation of labor exhibits a circadian pattern with a maximum between 24:00 and 05:00 h [103]. The expression of functional melatonin receptors in the human myometrium both in nonpregnant and pregnant women has been documented [104]. Melatonin augmented the contractile force of human myometrial strips through a synergism with α-adrenergic receptors [105]. During the time of transition from myometrial quiescence to labor a significant increase in gap junctions has been found [106]. Gap junctions serve to coordinate individual myometrial cell contractions into powerful labor-inducing forces. Melatonin at physiological concentrations has been shown to modulate the strength of affinity between gap junctions [75, 107]. Therefore, melatonin might be part of the mechanisms underlying the initiation of parturition. In nonhuman primates, the phasing of nocturnal parturition has been shown to also be shifted by reversal of the light/dark cycles [108], pointing to a light-sensitive clock mechanism underlying this reproductive event. In addition, data from both humans and nonhuman primates show nocturnally peaking uterine contractions in late pregnancy [109, 110].

High myometrial contractions during the day in rodents are consistent with inhibitory effects of nocturnal melatonin in this species, while high uterine contractions at night in humans and nonhuman primates [109, 110] are consistent with stimulatory effects of nocturnal melatonin on this organ. Thus, melatonin would appear to be anti-contractile (i.e., tocolytic) in terms of its effects on the rat uterus but uterotonic to human uterus [111].

It would seem rational to believe that the circadian rhythm of parturition in mammals is set to its appropriate nocturnal or diurnal phase by the central circadian oscillator located in the hypothalamic SCN as this structure is not only linked to the retina for entrainment to light, but via both neural and hormonal efferents, it can direct a variety of behavioral and physiological rhythms [112]. In fact, the circadian timing of birth in the rat has been demonstrated to require an intact SCN [112]. Takayama et al. [98] showed that female rats whose endogenous melatonin was eliminated by pinealectomy had no disturbances in estrous cyclicity or in their ability to become pregnant, but they failed to deliver their young exclusively during the daytime, which is the normal phase for rats. Instead, the animals gave birth randomly across the 24-h light-dark cycle. Melatonin has been shown to be effective in restoring the daytime birth pattern when it was administered in the evening, but it was unsuccessful when given in the morning or continuously [111].

Human myometrium regulates the expression of receptors for both melatonin and oxytocin in parallel as a function of gestational stage. Thus, strongly suggest that signaling through the MT_2 melatonin receptor may actively contribute to labor by serving to temporally "gate" the cellular events which underlie the well-known amplification of uterine contractions at night [109]. By acting synergistically with oxytocin and potentially other pro-contractile factors, melatonin may facilitate the coordinated and forceful contractions of the pregnant uterus necessary for normal term labor [113].

Conclusion

The report of human pineal gland tumor that altered pubertal development by Huebner [1] in 1898 and the discovery of melatonin by Lerner and colleagues in 1958 [114] heralded a new field of research on melatonin's role in human reproduction. To date, scientific evidence has been provided to support melatonin's roles in human reproduction such as puberty, testicular function, pregnancy outcome and complications, fetal development, and parturition.

Melatonin may have some modulatory effects on human diseases that are related to the reproductive system. For example, lighting during the night of sufficient intensity apparently reduces circulating melatonin levels and resets the circadian pacemaker of the SCN. This phenomenon has been related to increased risk of breast cancer [115] perhaps by down-regulating gonadal synthesis of steroids, by acting on receptor sites within the neuroendocrine reproductive axis or altered estrogen receptor function. Melatonin supplementation could be an effective treatment to achieve pregnancy especially in cases related to poor quality of oocyte in older mothers [75]. On the other hand, their real therapeutic efficacy could be relevant in women having high risk to undergo through pregnancy complication such as PCOS patients especially prone to develop gestational diabetes, premature delivery with the increased risk for the infant to suffer of RDS, and in women having an increased risk of preeclampsia. Therefore, in the right circumstances, it is possible that by reinforcing and optimizing our temporal organization, melatonin may have substantial benefits for reproductive health.

References

1. Huebner O. Tumor des Glandula pinealis. Dtsch Med Wochenschr. 1898;24(pt 2):214–5.
2. Kitay JI, Altschule MD. The pineal gland. Cambridge: Harvard University Press; 1954.
3. Thieblot L, Le Bars H. Le Glande Pineale ou Epiphyse. Paris: Maloine; 1955.
4. Wurtman RJ, Axelrod J, Chu EW. Melatonin, a pineal substance: its effect on the rat ovary. Science. 1963;141:277–80.
5. Reiter RJ. The melatonin rhythm. Both a clock and calendar. Experientia. 1993;49:654–64.
6. Johnston JD, Messager S, Barrett P, Hazlerigg DG. Melatonin action in the pituitary: neuroendocrine synchronizer and developmental modulator? J Neuroendocrinol. 2003;15:405–8.
7. Rojansky N, Brzezinski A, Schenker JG. Seasonality in human reproduction: an update. Hum Reprod. 1992;7:735–45.
8. Kaupipila A, Kivela A, Pakarinen A, Vakkuri O. Inversed seasonal relationship between melatonin and ovarian activity in humans in a region with a strong seasonal contrast in luminosity. J Clin Endocrinol Metab. 1987;65:823–8.
9. Sanhal B. Seasonal birth pattern in Sweden in relation to birth order and maternal age. Acta Obstet Gynecol Scand. 1978;57:393–7.
10. Brzezinski A, Wurtman RJ. The pineal gland: it's possible role in human reproduction. Obstet Gynecol Surv. 1988;43:197–207.
11. Brzezinski A. Melatonin in humans. N Engl J Med. 1997;336:186–95.
12. Sizonenko PC. Physiology of puberty. J Endocrinol Invest. 1989;12:59–63.
13. Waldhauser F, Steger H. Changes in melatonin secretion with age and pubescence. J Neural Transm. 1986;21(Suppl):183–97.

14. Waldhauser F, Weiszenbacher G, Tatzer E, Gisinger B, Waldhauser M, Schemper M, Frisch H. Alterations in nocturnal serum melatonin levels in humans with growth and aging. J Clin Endocrinol Metabol. 1988;66(3):648–52.
15. Iguchi H, Kato K, Ibayashi H. Age-dependent reduction in serum melatonin concentrations in healthy human subjects. J Clin Endocrinol Metabol. 1982;55:27–9.
16. Sack RL, Lewy AJ, Erb DL, Vollmer WM, Singer CM. Human melatonin production decreases with age. J Pineal Res. 1986;3:379–88.
17. Zhao ZY, Xie Y, Fu YR, Bogdan A, Touitou Y. Aging and the circadian rhythm of melatonin: a cross-sectional study of Chinese subjects 30–110 yr of age. Chronobiol Int. 2002;19:1171–82.
18. Carlomagno G, Nordio M, Chiu TT, Unfer V. Contribution of myo-inositol and melatonin to human reproduction. Eur J Obstet Gynecol Reprod Biol. 2011;159:267–72.
19. Buchanan KL, Yellon SM. Delayed puberty in the male Djungarian hamster: effect of short photoperiod or melatonin treatment on the Gn-RH neuronal system. Neuroendocrinology. 1991;54:96–102.
20. Silman RE. Melatonin and the human gonadotrophin-releasing hormone pulse generator. J Endocrinol. 1991;128:7–11.
21. Cavallo A. Melatonin and human puberty: current perspectives. J Pineal Res. 1993;15(3):115–21.
22. Crowley SJ, Acebo C, Carskadon MA. Human puberty: salivary melatonin profiles in constant conditions. Dev Psychobiol. 2012;54(4):468–73.
23. Cavallo A. Plasma melatonin rhythm in normal puberty: interactions of age and pubertal stages. Neuroendocrinology. 1992;55(4):372–9.
24. Waldhauser F, Boepple PA, Schemper M, Mansfield MJ, Crowley Jr WF. Serum melatonin in central precocious puberty is lower than in age-matched prepubertal children. J Clin Endocrinol Metabol. 1991;73(4):793–6.
25. Young IM, Francis PL, Leone AM, Stovell P, Silman RE. Constant pineal output and increasing body mass account for declining melatonin levels during human growth and sexual maturation. J Pineal Res. 1988;5(1):71–85.
26. Cavallo A, Dolan LM. 6-Hydroxymelatonin sulfate excretion in human puberty. J Pineal Res. 1996;21(4):225–30.
27. Fideleff HL, Boquete H, Fideleff G, Albornoz L, Lloret SP, Suarez M, Cardinali DP. Gender-related differences in urinary 6-sulfatoxymelatonin levels in obese pubertal individuals. J Pineal Res. 2006;40(3):214–8.
28. Salti R, Galluzzi F, Bindi G, Perfetto F, Tarquini R, Halberg F, Cornelissen G. Nocturnal melatonin patterns in children. J Clin Endocrinol Metabol. 2000;85:2137–44.
29. Cain SW, Dennison CF, Zeitzer JM, Guzik AM, Khalsa SB, Santhi N, Duffy JF. Sex differences in phase angle of entrainment and melatonin amplitude in humans. J Biol Rhythms. 2010;25(4):288–96.
30. Wetterberg L, Bratlid T, von Knorring L, Eberhard G, Yuwiler A. A multinational study of the relationships between nighttime urinary melatonin production, age, gender, body size, and latitude. Eur Arch Psychiatry Clin Neurosci. 1999;249:256–62.
31. Burgess HJ, Fogg LF. Individual differences in the amount and timing of salivary melatonin secretion. PLoS One. 2008;3(8):e3055.
32. Griefahn B, Brode P, Blaszkewicz M, Remer T. Melatonin production during childhood and adolescence: a longitudinal study on the excretion of urinary 6-hydroxymelatonin sulfate. J Pineal Res. 2003;34(1):26–31.
33. Penny R. Melatonin excretion in normal males and females: increase during puberty. Metabolism. 1982;31:816–23.
34. Waldhauser F, Weiszenbacher G, Frisch H, Zeitlhuber U, Waldhauser M, Wurtman RJ. Fall in nocturnal serum melatonin during prepuberty and pubescence. Lancet. 1984;1(8373):362–5.
35. Tsutsui K. A new key neurohormone controlling reproduction, gonadotropin-inhibitory hormone (GnIH): biosynthesis, mode of action and functional significance. Prog Neurobiol. 2009;88(1):76–88.
36. Ubuka T, Bentley GE, Ukena K, Wingfield JC, Tsutsui K. Melatonin induces the expression of gonadotropin-inhibitory hormone in the avian brain. Proc Natl Acad Sci U S A. 2005;102(8):3052–7.
37. Cohen HN, Hay ID, Anneswley TM, Beastall GH, Wallace AM, Spooner R, Thomson JA, Eastwold P, Klee GG. Serum immunoreactive melatonin in boys with delayed puberty. Clin Endocrinol. 1982;17:291–7.
38. Commentz JC, Helmke K. Precocious puberty and decreased melatonin secretion due to a hypothalamic hamartoma. Horm Res. 1995;44(6):271–5.
39. Cavallo A. Plasma melatonin rhythm in disorders of puberty: interactions of age and pubertal stages. Horm Res. 1991;36(1–2):16–21.
40. Ehrenkranz JR, Tamarkin L, Comite F, Johnsonbaugh RE, Bybee DE, Loriaux DL, Cutler Jr GB. Daily rhythm of plasma melatonin in normal and precocious puberty. J Clin Endocrinol Metabol. 1982;55(2):307–10.
41. Berga SL, Jones KL, Kaufmann S, Yen SS. Nocturnal melatonin levels are unaltered by ovarian suppression in girls with central precocious puberty. Fertil Steril. 1989;52(6):936–41.
42. Silman RE, Leone RM, Hooper RJ, Preece MA. Melatonin, the pineal gland and human puberty. Nature. 1979;282(5736):301–3.
43. Arendt J. Melatonin and the mammalian pineal gland. 1st ed. London: Chapman & Hall; 1995. p. 17.
44. Brzezinski A. Melatonin and human reproduction: why the effect is so elusive? In: Pandi-Perumal SR, Cardinali Melatonin DP, editors. From molecules to therapy. New York: Nova; 2007. p. 219–25.

45. Brzezinski A, Lynch HJ, Wurtman RJ, Seibel MM. Possible contribution of melatonin to the timing of the luteinizing hormone surge. N Engl J Med. 1987;316:1550–1.
46. Laughin GA, Loucks AB, Yen SCC. Marked augmentation of nocturnal melatonin secretion in amenorrheic athletes but not in cycling atheletes. Unaltered by opiodergic or dopaminergic blockade. J Clin Endocrinol Metab. 1991;73:1321–6.
47. Aleandri V, Spina V, Morini A. The pineal gland and reproduction. Hum Reprod Update. 1996;3:225–35.
48. Roy D, Belsham DD. Melatonin receptor activation regulates GnRH gene expression and secretion in GT1-7Gn-RH neurons. Signal transduction mechanisms. J Biol Chem. 2002;277:251–8.
49. Brzezinski A, Siebel MM, Lynch HJ, Deng MH, Wurtman RJ. Melatonin in human preovulatory follicular fluid. J Clin Endocrinol Metab. 1987;64: 865–7.
50. Ronnberg L, Kauppila A, Leppaluoto J, Marikainen H, Vakkuuri O. Circadian and seasonal variation in human preovulatory follicular fluid melatonin concentration. J Clin Endocrinol Metab. 1990;71:492–6.
51. Ayre EA, Wang ZP, Brown GM, Pang SF. Localization and characterization of [^{125}I] iodomelatonin binding sites in duck gonads. J Pineal Res. 1994;17:39–47.
52. Ayre EA, Pang SF. 2-[^{125}I] Iodomelatonin binding sites in the testis and ovaries: putatitive melatonin receptors in the gonads. Biol Signals. 1994;3:71–84.
53. Cagnacci A, Volpe A. Influence of melatonin and photoperiod on animal and human reproduction. J Endocrinol Invest. 1996;19:382–411.
54. Yu ZH, Chow PH, Pang SF. Identification and characterization of 2[125I]-iodomelatonin binding sites in the rat epididymis. J Pineal Res. 1994;17:195–201.
55. Ng TB, Lo L. Inhibitory actions of pineal indoles on steroidogenesis in isolated rat Leydig cells. J Pineal Res. 1988;5:229–43.
56. Persengiev S, Kehajova J. Inhibitory actions of melatonin and structurally related compounds on testosterone production by mouse leydig cells in vitro. Cell Biochem Funct. 1991;9:281–6.
57. Shiu SYW, Yu ZH, Chow PH, Pang SF. Putative melatonin receptors in the male reproductive tissues. Front Horm Res. 1996;21:90–100.
58. Shiu SYW, Li L, Wong JTY, Pang SF. Biology of G-protein coupled melatonin receptors in the epididymis and prostate of mammals. Chin Med J. 1997;110:648–55.
59. Laudon M, Gilad E, Matzkin H, Braf Z, Zisapel N. Putatitive melatonin receptors in benign prostate tissue. J Clin Endocrinol Metab. 1996;81:1336–42.
60. Gilad E, Laudon M, Matzkin H, Pick E, Sofer M, Braf Z, Zisapel N. Functional melatonin receptors in the human prostate epithelial cells. Endocrinology. 1996;137:1412–7.
61. Awad H, Halawa F, Mostafa T, Atta H. Melatonin hormone profile in infertile males. Int J Androl. 2006;29:409–13.
62. Semercioz A, Onur R, Ogras S, Orhan I. Effects of melatonin on testicular tissue nitric oxide level and antioxidant enzyme activities in experimentally induced left varicocele. Neuro Endocrinol Lett. 2003;24:86–90.
63. Guneli E, Tugyan K, Ozturk H, Gumustekin M, Cilaker S, Uysal N. Effect of melatonin on testicular damage in streptozotocin-induced diabetes rats. Eur Surg Res. 2008;40:354–60.
64. Zhang K, Lv Z, Jia X, Huang D. Melatonin prevents testicular damage in hyperlipidaemic mice. Andrologia. 2012;44:230–6.
65. Koksal M, Oğuz E, Baba F, Ali Eren M, Ciftci H, Demir ME, Kurcer Z, Take G, Aral F, Ocak AR, Aksoy N, Ulas T. Effects of melatonin on testis histology, oxidative stress and spermatogenesis after experimental testis ischemia-reperfusion in rats. Eur Rev Med Pharmacol Sci. 2012;16: 582–8.
66. Rao MV, Bhatt RN. Protective effect of melatonin on fluoride-induced oxidative stress and testicular dysfunction in rats. Res Rep Fluoride. 2012;45(2): 116–24.
67. du Plessis SS, Hagenaar K, Lampiao F. The in vitro effects of melatonin on human sperm function and its scavenging activities on NO and ROS. Andrologia. 2010;42:112–6.
68. Bornman MS, Oosthuizen JM, Barnard HC, Schulenburg GW, Boomker D, Reif S. Melatonin and sperm motility. Andrologia. 1989;21:483–5.
69. van Vuuren RJ, Pitout MJ, van Aswegen CH, Theron JJ. Putative melatonin receptor in human spermatozoa. Clin Biochem. 1992;25:125–7.
70. Fujinoki M. Melatonin-enhanced hyperactivation of hamster sperm. Reproduction. 2008;136:533–41.
71. Puolakka J, Jarvinen PA, Kauppila A. Changing pattern of childbirth in northern Finland over the past three decades. In: Fortune circumpolar health. Seattle and London: University of Washington Press; 1985. p. 181 5.
72. Kauppilla A, Kivela A, Pakarinen A, Vakkuri O. Inverse seasonal relationship between melatonin and ovarian activity in humans in a region with a strong seasonal contrast in luminosity. J Clin Endocrinol Metab. 1987;65:823–8.
73. Kivela A, Kauppila A, Ylostalo P, Vakkuri O. Seasonal, menstrual and circadian secretion of melatonin gonadotrophins and prolactin in women. Acta Physiol Scand. 1988;132:321–7.
74. Reiter RJ, Tan DX, Fuentes-Broto L. Melatonin: a multitasking molecule. Prog Brain Res. 2010;181: 127–51.
75. Tamura H, Takasaki A, Miwa I, et al. Oxidative stress impairs oocyte quality and melatonin protects oocytes from free radical damage and improves fertilization rate. J Pineal Res. 2008;44:280–7.

76. Nakamura Y, Tamura H, Kashida S, Takayama H, Yagamata Y, Karube A, Sugino N, Kato H. Changes of serum melatonin level and its relationship to feto-placental unit during pregnancy. J Pineal Res. 2001;30:29–33.
77. Kivela A. Serum melatonin during human pregnancy. Acta Endocrinol (Copenh). 1991;124:233–7.
78. Yellon SM, Longo LD. Effect of maternal pinealectomy and reverse photoperiod n the circadian melatonin in the sheep and fetus during the last trimester of pregnancy. Biol Reprod. 1988;39:1093–9.
79. Munoz-Hoyos A, Jaldo-Alba F, Molina-Carballo A, Rodriguez-Cabezas T, Molina-Font JA, Acuna-Castroviejo D. Absence of plasma melatonin circadian rhythm during the first 72 h of life in human infants. J Clin Endocrinol Metab. 1993;77:699–703.
80. Reppert SM, Weaver DR, Rivkees SA, Stopa EC. Putative melatonin receptor in a human biological clock. Science. 1998;242:78–81.
81. Thomas I, Pervis CC, Drew JE, Abramovich DR, Williams LM. Melatonin receptors in human fetal brain: 2-[^{125}I] iodomelatonin binding site and MT1 gene expression. J Pineal Res. 2002;33:218–24.
82. Hawkins GA, Meyers DA, Bleeker ER, Pack AI. Identification of coding polymorphisms in human circadian rhythm genes Per 1, Per2, Per3, clock, AmtI, Cry1, Cry2, and timeless in multiethnic screening panel. DNA Seq. 2007;10:1.
83. Okatani Y, Okamura K, Hayashi K, Wakatsuki A, Tamura S, Sagara Y. Maternal-fetal transfer of melatonin in pregnant women near term. J Pineal Res. 1998;25:129–34.
84. Mirmiran M, Maas YG, Ariagno RL. Development of fetal and neonatal sleep and circadian rhythms. Sleep Med Rev. 2003;7:321–34.
85. Fait V, Sela S, Ophir E, Khoury S, Nissimov J, Tkach M, Hirsch Y, Khotaba S, Tarasowa L, Oettinger M. Hyperemesis gravidarum is associated with oxidative stress. Am J Perinatol. 2002;19:93–8.
86. Myatt L, Cui X. Oxidative stress in placenta. Histochem Cell Biol. 2004;122:369–82.
87. Reiter RJ. Interaction of the pineal hormone melatonin with oxygen centered free radicals: a brief review. Braz J Med Biol Res. 2003;26:1141–55.
88. Srinivasan V. Melatonin, oxidative stress and neurodegenerative diseases. Indian J Expt Biol. 2002;40:668–79.
89. Srinivasan V, Pandi-Perumal SR, Maestroni GJ, Esquifino AJ, Hardeland R, Cardinali DP. Role of melatonin in neurodegenerative diseases. Neurotox Res. 2005;7:293–318.
90. Tamura H, Nakamura Y, Terron MP, Flores LJ, Manchester LC, Tan DX, Sugino N, Reiter RJ. Melatonin and pregnancy in the human. Reprod Toxicol. 2008;25:291–303.
91. Wakatsuki A, Okatani Y, Ikenouse N, Shinohara K, Watanabe K, Fukaya T. Melatonin protects against oxidized low density lipoprotein induced inhibition of nitric oxide production in human umbilical artery. J Pineal Res. 2001;31:281–8.
92. Milczarek R, Klimek J, Zelewski L. Melatonin inhibits NADPH-dependent lipid peroxidation in human placental mitochondria. Horm Metab Res. 2000;32:84–5.
93. Simko F, Paulis L. Melatonin as a potential antihypertensive treatment. J Pineal Res. 2007;42:319–22.
94. Pagni CA, Zenga F. Posttraumatic epilepsy with special emphasis on prophylaxis and prevention. Acta Neurochir Suppl. 2005;93:27–34.
95. Plaut SM, Grota LJ, Ader R, Graham CW. Effects of handling and the light–dark cycle on time of parturition in the rat. Lab Anim Care. 1970;20:447–53.
96. Boer K, Lincoln DW, Swaab DF. Effects of electrical stimulation of the neurohypophysis on labour in the rat. J Endocrinol. 1975;65:163–76.
97. Lincoln DW, Porter DG. Timing of the photoperiod and the hour of birth in rats. Nature. 1976;260: 780–1.
98. Takayama H, Nakamura Y, Tamura H, Yamaagata Y, Harada A, Nakata M, Sugino N, Kato H. Pineal gland (melatonin) affects the parturition time, but not luteal function and fetal growth, in pregnant rats. Endocr J. 2003;50:37–43.
99. Glattre E, Bjerkedal T. The 24-hour rhythmicity of birth: a population study. Acta Obstet Gynecol Scand. 1983;62:31–6.
100. Cooperstock M, England JE, Wolfe RA. Circadian incidence of labor onset hour in preterm birth and chorioamnionitis. Obstet Gynecol. 1987;70: 852–5.
101. Lindow SW, Jha RR, Thompson JW. 24-hour rhythm to the onset of preterm labour. BJOG. 2000;107:1145–8.
102. Vatish M, Steer PJ, Blanks AM, Hon M, Thornton S. Diurnal variation is lost in preterm deliveries before 28 weeks of gestation. BJOG. 2010;117:765–7.
103. Longo LD, Yellon SM. Biological time keeping during pregnancy and the role of circadian rhythms during parturition. In: Kunzel W, Jensen A, editors. The endocrine control of the fetus. Berlin: Springer; 1988. p. 173–92.
104. Schlabritz-Loutsevitch N, Hellner N, Middendorf R, Muller D, Olcese J. The human myometrium as a target for melatonin. J Clin Endocrinol Metab. 2003;88:908–13.
105. Martensson LG, Andersson RG, Berg G. Melatonin together with noradrenaline augments contractions of human myometrium. Eur J Pharmacol. 1996;316:273–5.
106. Salomonis N, Cotte N, Zambon AC, Pollard KS, Vranizan K, Doniger SW, Dolganov G, Conklin BR. Identifying genetic networks underlying myometrial transition to labor. Genome Biol. 2005;6:R12.1–R16.
107. Olecese J. Melatonin effects on uterine physiology. In: Pandi-Perumal SR, Cardinali DP, editors. Melatonin: from molecules to therapy. New York: Nova; 2007. p. 205–25.
108. Ducsay CA, Yellon SM. Photoperiod regulation of uterine activity and melatonin rhythms in the pregnant rhesus macaque. Biol Reprod. 1991;44:967–74.

109. Zahn V, Hattensperger W. Circadian rhythm of pregnancy contractions. Z Geburtshilfe Perinatol. 1993;197:1–10.
110. Farber DM, Giussani DA, Jenkins SL, Mecenas CA, Winter JA, Wentworth RA, Nathanielsz PW. Timing of the switch from myometrial contractures to contractions in late-gestation pregnant rhesus monkeys as recorded by myometrial electromyogram during spontaneous term and androstenedione-induced labor. Biol Reprod. 1997;56:557–62.
111. Olcese J. Circadian aspects of mammalian parturition: a review. Mol Cell Endocrinol. 2012;349: 62–7.
112. Reppert SM, Weaver DR. Coordination of circadian timing in mammals. Nature. 2002;418:935–41.
113. Sharkey JT, Puttaramu R, Word RA, Olcese J. Melatonin synergizes with oxytocin to enhance contractility of human myometrial smooth muscle cells. J Clin Endocrinol Metab. 2009;94:421–7.
114. Lerner AB, Case JD, Takahashi Y, Lee Y, Mori W. Isolation of melatonin, the pineal gland factor that lightens melanocytes. J Am Chem Soc. 1958; 80:2587.
115. Stevens RG. Circadian disruption and breast cancer: from melatonin to clock genes. Epidemiology. 2005;16:254–8.

Melatonin: An Introduction to Its Physiological and Pharmacological Effects in Humans

14

Bruno Claustrat

Abstract

Melatonin is a methoxyindole that, under normal environmental conditions, is synthesized and secreted principally by the pineal gland at night. The endogenous rhythm of secretion is generated by the suprachiasmatic nuclei and entrained to the light/dark cycle. Light is able to either suppress or synchronize melatonin production depending on the light schedule. The nycthemeral rhythm of this hormone can be evaluated by repeated measurement of plasma or saliva melatonin levels or urine levels of 6-sulphatoxymelatonin, the main hepatic metabolite.

Secretion of melatonin adjusts to night length, and its primary physiological function is to convey information concerning the daily cycle of light and darkness to body structures. This information is used for the organization of functions that respond to changes in the photoperiod, such as seasonal rhythms. However, in temperate areas under field conditions, there is only limited evidence for a relationship between seasonal rhythmicity of physiological functions in humans and possible alterations in the melatonin message. In addition, daily melatonin secretion, which is a very robust biochemical signal of night, can be used for the organization of circadian rhythms. Although the evidence for possible functions of this hormone in humans is mainly based on correlative observations between physiological effects and changes in melatonin secretion, there is some evidence that melatonin stabilizes and strengthens the coupling of circadian rhythms, especially of core temperature and sleep-wake rhythms. The

B. Claustrat, PhD
Hormone Laboratory, Hospices Civils de Lyon,
59 Bd Pinel, Bron 69677, France

INSERM, U846 Chronobiology Group,
Hospices Civils de Lyon, 59 bd Pinel,
18 Avenue du Doyen Lépine, Bron 69500, France
e-mail: bruno.claustrat@chu-lyon.fr

V. Srinivasan et al. (eds.), *Melatonin and Melatonergic Drugs in Clinical Practice*,
DOI 10.1007/978-81-322-0825-9_14, © Springer India 2014

circadian organization of other physiological functions, such as immune and antioxidant defenses, hemostasis, and glucose regulation, also depends on the melatonin signal.

The difference between the physiological and pharmacological effects of melatonin is not always clear, but is based upon the dose, and not the duration, of the hormone message. A pharmacological dose provides supraphysiological levels of melatonin, while a "physiological" dose provides plasma levels of the same order of magnitude as a nocturnal peak. However, when a low melatonin dose is given using a simple capsule, a narrow hormone signal is achieved, which does not mimic endogenous secretion. It is admitted that a "physiological" dose provides plasma melatonin levels of the same order of magnitude as a nocturnal peak. Since the regulatory system of melatonin secretion is complex, involving central and autonomic pathways, there are many pathophysiological situations in which melatonin secretion can be disturbed. The resulting change could increase predisposition to a disease, add to the severity of symptoms, or modify the course and outcome of the disorder. Since melatonin receptors are very widely distributed in the body, putative therapeutic indications of this compound are multiple. Great advances in therapeutics could be made by performing multicenter trials in large series of patients in order to establish the efficacy of melatonin and the absence of long-term toxicity.

Keywords
Melatonin • Human • Circadian rhythms • Physiology • Pathophysiology

Introduction

Melatonin was isolated and characterized from the bovine pineal by the dermatologist Aaron Lerner in 1958 [1] and is the main hormone secreted by the pineal gland. Secondary sources are retina, gut, skin, platelets, bone marrow, and probably other structures, but their systemic contribution is insignificant [2–7]. Melatonin (*N*-acetyl-5-methoxytryptamine), an indole compound, is synthesized from serotonin and this and the fact that it lightens the frog's skin by contracting melanophores led to its name (i.e., melanophore-contracting hormone; Greek: μελας = black; τουος = tension, in the sense of contraction).

Although melatonin has been extensively detected in the animal kingdom, more recently, it has also been found in different structures in higher plants (leaves, fruits, and seeds), but the levels are too low to provide a significant melatonin supply for humans. Melatonin is also present in lower phyla, including bacteria [8]. Due to its being directly derived from an amino acid, the ubiquitous molecule melatonin was probably one of the first compounds which appeared on earth to coordinate some basic events of life.

The main physiological functions of melatonin are related to its hormonal properties, although it may also exhibit autocrine or paracrine properties, for example, in the retina or the gut [9]. The pineal gland was initially shown to be an active neuroendocrine transducer of environmental information in animals, especially in photoperiodic species. For many years, this data was extrapolated to humans. Today, some understanding of the role of melatonin in human physiology and disease has emerged, but many of its functions and effects remain underestimated. This review will focus on data about melatonin in humans, as an introduction to the following chapters.

Biochemical Aspects and Regulation

Biosynthesis

Melatonin is synthesized from tryptophan, which is taken up from the circulation and transformed into serotonin, which is then converted into melatonin by a two-step process involving the sequential activities of two enzymes, serotonin-N-acetyltransferase (NAT), the limiting enzyme in the synthesis of melatonin, and hydroxyindole-*O*-methyltransferase (HIOMT) [10]. The mRNAs encoding these enzymes are expressed in the pineal with a day/night rhythm (for review, see [11]). Melatonin synthesis is initiated by the binding of norepinephrine to adrenergic β1-receptors, which leads to activation of pineal adenylate cyclase, an increase in cyclic AMP (cAMP) levels, and de novo synthesis of NAT. The cAMP-induced gene transcription repressor (ICER), an isoform of the cAMP-responsive element modulator (CREM), is activated in conjunction with NAT expression and represents a mechanism that limits the nocturnal production of melatonin [12]. Melatonin synthesis depends upon tryptophan availability, as it is reduced after acute tryptophan depletion [13]; other nutritional factors might also influence melatonin synthesis, for example, folate status [14] and levels of vitamin B6, a coenzyme in tryptophan decarboxylation that can stimulate melatonin production in prepubertal children, but not in adults [15, 16]. Fluvoxamine, a serotonin uptake inhibitor, also increases the amplitude and duration of the plasma melatonin peak [17].

Secretion

Melatonin displays high lipid and water solubility (octanol/water partition coefficient of ≈13), which facilitates its passage across cell membranes [18]. After its release into the circulation, it gains access to various fluids, tissues, and cellular compartments (saliva, urine, cerebrospinal fluid, preovulatory follicle, semen, amniotic fluid, and milk). As melatonin is not stored in the pineal, its plasma profile faithfully reflects pineal activity [19]. Secretion occurs at night, maximum plasma levels being reached at around 03:00–04:00 a.m., varying with chronotype, whereas diurnal levels are undetectable or low in rested subjects. This nycthemeral rhythm displays the largest amplitude observed for a hormone rhythm. Nocturnal melatonin production rates, estimated by deconvolution analysis of daily plasma melatonin concentration profiles, are between 10 and 80 μg/night, the lowest value for a hormone secretion [20].

The plasma melatonin profile displays great intersubject heterogeneity. Nonetheless, it is very reproducible from day to day in the same subject and represents one of the most robust circadian rhythms. In the absence of renal or hepatic abnormality, it provides a good evaluation of melatonin secretion [21]. In some subjects, nocturnal secretion is extremely low or even absent. The effects of low melatonin secretion on vulnerability to rhythmic organization and morbidity are unknown. At the present time, no polymorphism of enzymes can explain this heterogeneity. Blood melatonin is bound mainly to albumin (70 %) and, to a lesser extent, to orosomucoid [22]. Circulating melatonin can reach all body tissues and can cross the blood-brain barrier to modulate brain activity. A PET study showed that radioactivity in the brain was maximum 6–8 min after intravenous injection of ^{11}C-melatonin [23].

After maturation during the first year of life, rhythmic melatonin production reaches its highest levels at the age of 3–6 years, and then the nocturnal peak drops progressively by 80 % to adult levels. This change is temporally linked to the appearance of sexual maturity and is not simply the consequence of increasing body size and constant melatonin production due to the lack of pineal growth during childhood [24]. Data on normal precocious puberty treated by gonadotropin-releasing hormone analogues suggest that the reduction in melatonin production at normal puberty is not likely to be dependent on pubertal gonadotropin or sex steroids [25]. Although melatonin may modulate steroidogenesis, especially progesterone production, no clear consensus has emerged about melatonin changes that may occur during the ovarian cycle. While changes in the circadian pattern of melatonin secretion immediately preceding the LH surge cannot be excluded, melatonin secretion may not be necessary for menstrual cyclicity to occur [26, 27]. The transient increase in melatonin secretion during menopause could be related to the dramatic decrease in the estrogen environment [28]. On aging, the melatonin rhythm is progressively dampened, with a tendency to a phase advance, and can be completely abolished in advanced age [29]. The question whether impaired melatonin secretion with advancing age is related to increasing pineal calcification remains unanswered. Finally, the decrease in melatonin secretion that is reinforced in elderly insomniacs is the rationale for treatment with this hormone [30]. These data will be discussed in another chapter

Metabolism

In the brain, melatonin is oxidized into *N1-acetyl-N2*-formyl-5-methoxykynuramine (AFMK) by the reaction of melatonin with reactive oxygen species (ROS) [31]. AFMK displays an in vitro antioxidant capacity and is the last melatonin-related compound involved in the process by which melatonin and its metabolites successively scavenge ROS, referred as the free radical scavenging cascade.

The liver, which clears more than 90 % of circulating melatonin, is the primary site of metabolism. Melatonin is first hydroxylated to 6-hydroxymelatonin (6OH-melatonin) by CYP1A2. There are wide interindividual differences (10–200-fold) in CYP1A2 activity [32], which are related to single-nucleotide polymorphisms in the *CYP1A2* gene that are associated with increased inducibility, decreased activity or inducibility, or even loss of activity of the CYP1A2 enzyme. Since this cytochrome is important in the metabolism of many commonly used drugs, the interaction of melatonin with substrate compounds results in changes in melatonin bioavailability. For example, caffeine intake dramatically increases melatonin bioavailability due to inhibition of first-pass hepatic metabolism. Melatonin has been proposed as an alternative probe drug to caffeine to assess CYP1A2 activity [33]. On the other hand, polycyclic aromatic hydrocarbons in cigarette smoke induce cytochrome CYP1A2 expression and reduce intake of exogenous melatonin, but do not affect endogenous nocturnal levels [34]. 6OH-melatonin is excreted in the urine as sulfate and, to a lesser extent, as glucuronide conjugate [35]. Urine 6-sulfatoxymelatonin (aMT6S) excretion closely parallels the plasma melatonin profile [36]. About 1 % of melatonin remains unchanged in the urine. 3-hydroxymelatonin, which is also detected in the urine, could represent a biomarker of OH°radical generation. In addition to lower pineal secretory activity, patients with liver cirrhosis show decreased melatonin clearance, with a consequent delayed rise in the plasma melatonin peak and increased daytime levels of this hormone [37]. In addition, in patients with chronic renal failure, daytime melatonin and aMT6S levels are increased and melatonin rhythmicity blunted [38].

Regulation of Melatonin Secretion (Fig. 14.1)

Like other circadian rhythms in mammals (such as drinking and feeding, sleep-wake cycle, temperature, cortisol, or corticosterone), the melatonin rhythm is generated by an endogenous clock located in the suprachiasmatic nuclei (SCN) of the hypothalamus. These results were obtained in animals, mainly rodents and monkeys, and extended to humans [39, 40] and confirmed by pathophysiological observations in patients [41].

The light/dark cycle is the main zeitgeber of the regulatory system of melatonin secretion. The melatonin rhythm is entrained to the dark period. The photic information is transmitted to the central pacemaker via retinohypothalamic fibers: during the day, in the presence of light, the output from the retinohypothalamic tract

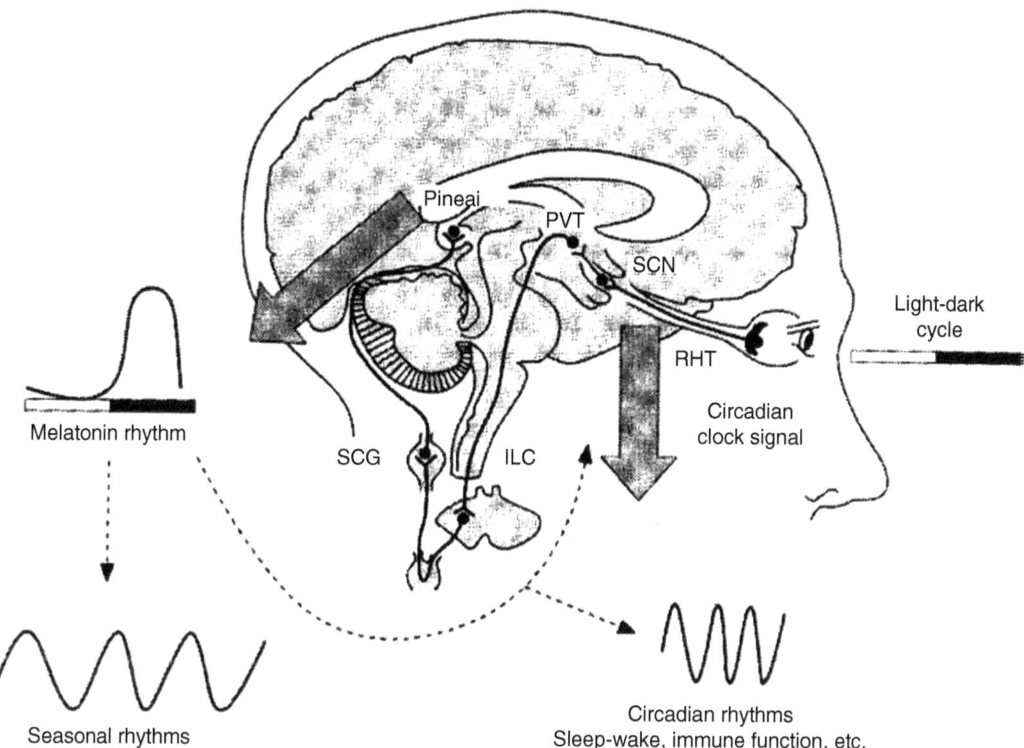

Fig. 14.1 Control of melatonin secretion. Photic information is conveyed to the suprachiasmatic nuclei (*SCN*), principally through the retinohypothalamic tract (*RHT*), and synchronizes the activity of the circadian oscillator to exactly 24 h. Neuronal efferent pathways from the SCN directly distribute circadian information to different brain areas, including the pineal gland, which generates the melatonin rhythm. The neural route for environmental lighting control of melatonin secretion includes the paraventricular nuclei of the hypothalamus (*PVT*), the intermediolateral column of the thoracic chord gray (*ILC*) and the superior cervical ganglion (*SCG*). The generated melatonin rhythm might be used by the SCN to distribute its rhythmic information. Melatonin can feedback at the level of the SCN, as well as that of the retina itself. A melatonin-driven circadian rhythm of sensitivity to melatonin may exist in the structure(s) involved in seasonality (Reprinted from Cardinali and Pevet [72])

inhibits melatonin synthesis. Artificial light of sufficient intensity and duration administered at night suppresses melatonin production [42]. Light intensities of 2,000–2,500 lx for 2 h (02:00–04:00 a.m.) completely suppress melatonin secretion, whereas domestic light intensities (50–300 lx) have a modest suppressive effect [43]. In addition, after exposure to light for several consecutive nights, melatonin secretion escapes the inhibitory effect and progressively shifts (phase delay) to the morning. Full spectrum bright light is routinely used, but the most effective wavelengths are in the range of 446–477 nm [44, 45]. Because the action spectrum derived from irradiance response curves does not correspond to either scotopic or photopic action spectra, new photoreceptors have been hypothesized [44, 45]. Blue-enriched light leads to faster reaction times in tasks associated with sustained attention, and the cognitive improvement is related to lower salivary melatonin levels [46]. In addition, there is no significant difference in melatonin suppression between all color vision-deficient, protanopic, deuteranopic, and control subjects [47]. Retinal ganglion cells innervating the SCN show an intrinsic response to light. These melanopsin-containing cells are involved in the photic entrainment of circadian rhythms [48]. Furthermore, this system sends photic information not only to the endogenous clock in the SCN but also to other brain areas involved in nonimage forming responses to light, including pupil constriction and induction of sleep [49]

The neural pathway from the SCN to the pineal gland first passes through the upper part of the cervical spinal cord, where synaptic connections are made with preganglionic cell bodies of the superior cervical ganglia (SCG) of the sympathetic chains [50, 51], and then neural cells in the SCG send projections to the pineal gland. The main neurotransmitter regulating the pineal gland is norepinephrine, which is released at night in response to stimulatory signals originating in the SCN. The data obtained in animals have been confirmed in humans using different drugs [52]. β1-adrenergic blockers suppress nocturnal melatonin secretion, as do the α2-blocker clonidine and α-methyl-para-tyrosine, which reduces presynaptic catecholamine synthesis. Conversely, melatonin secretion is reinforced by drugs which increase synaptic catecholamine availability, such as monoamine oxidase inhibitors or tricyclic antidepressants. In addition to norepinephrine, the sympathetic endings of the SCG release neuropeptide Y. Nerve fibers innervating the pineal gland originate in perikarya located in the parasympathetic sphenopalatine and otic ganglia and the trigeminal ganglion, the sensory ganglion of the fifth cranial nerve [51]. Two peptides, vasoactive intestinal peptide (VIP) and peptide histidine isoleucine (PHI), appear to be important in parasympathetic innervation, whereas substance P (SP), calcitonin gene-related peptide (CGRP), and pituitary adenylate cyclase-activating peptide (PACAP) are present in cell bodies of the trigeminal ganglion [51]. These neurotransmitters involved in the control of the pineal activity are only able to modulate the effect of norepinephrine. In animals, VIP, PACAP, and opioids via σ receptors stimulate melatonin secretion, whereas GABA, neuropeptide Y, dopamine, and glutamate inhibit melatonin production. Whether the above mechanisms are relevant to melatonin secretion in humans remains to be elucidated. Activation of GABA receptors by benzodiazepines and enhancement of endogenous GABAergic tone by sodium valproate [53] reduce melatonin levels at night, whereas dopaminergic agonists and antagonists and opioid receptor-blocking agents have no marked effect on melatonin levels. Other drugs, such as dihydropyridine calcium antagonists or prostaglandin inhibitors, probably alter melatonin secretion. These data and many others strongly warrant an investigation of any other drugs taken by patients before evaluation of melatonin secretion.

The suppression of melatonin production by exposure to low-frequency electromagnetic fields (EMF) has been invoked as a possible mechanism by which exposure to these fields may result in an increased incidence of cancer. More recent data do not report a distinct influence of EMF on the melatonin levels [54].

Melatonin Rhythm: A Marker of the Circadian Clock

Melatonin can be considered as a reliable output (the hour hand) of the endogenous clock. There is a close relationship between the plasma melatonin peak and the minimum core temperature, including entrained conditions and constant routine protocols. In contrast to the temperature rhythm, the melatonin rhythm is not very sensitive to masking effects, except that exerted by light. Consequently, Lewy and Sack recommended evaluating the onset of the plasma melatonin profile under dim light (50 lx, "Dim Light Melatonin Onset", D.L.M.O.) [55]. Evaluation of the plasma melatonin pattern requires repeated blood sampling. A maximum 1-h interval is needed to obtain reliable values for onset, offset, acrophase, and the area under the curve. The melatonin profile can be simultaneously determined with temperature and sleep recordings and provides an excellent diagnostic element for detecting circadian rhythm sleep disorders. Moreover, saliva and urine sampling offers a useful alternative for outpatient explorations and laboratory or field studies but requires waking the patient [56]. Finally, posture should be controlled during investigations [57].

Physiological Role of Melatonin

Melatonin secretion is related to the duration of darkness. Its main function is to mediate dark signals, with possible implications in the control of circadian rhythmicity and seasonality. The melatonin message, which is generated at night, is read differently in nocturnal animals and in humans. In this sense, melatonin is not the universal hormone for sleep.

Clinical observations meeting the classical concept in endocrinology of hormone deficiency and replacement are not available to illustrate the physiological properties of melatonin. Pinealectomized patients, in whom the circulating melatonin rhythm is abolished, do not provide a pure situation of melatonin suppression due to the possible side effects of surgery and/or radiation therapy, especially on adjacent structures. Furthermore, the pineal gland is not essential for life, and some effects of melatonin are probably subtle. In addition, light given to suppress melatonin secretion should be administered at night, which is not compatible with the study of sleep modulation by this hormone.

Chazot et al. [58] grouped together recurrent symptoms observed after pinealectomy as "pinealoprive syndrome"; these mainly consisted of hemicranial headache or unilateral orbital cephalalgia with or without sympathetic abnormality and disturbance of vision, but afternoon sleepiness, mood disorders, visual and auditory hallucinations, and convulsive seizures were also recorded. These observations meet the hypothesis of a stabilizing role for the pineal gland. However, Krieg et al. [59] claimed that pinealectomy itself does not cause specific sleep impairment, whereas craniotomy does.

Are Seasonal Physiological Events Related to Seasonal Variation in Melatonin Secretion?

The role of melatonin in seasonal changes in the physiology and behavior of various photoperiodic species has been extensively documented. The seasonal changes in the number of hours per day that melatonin is secreted mediate the temporal coupling of reproductive activity to seasonal changes in day length. In 1963, Wurtman et al. [60] reported that exogenous administration of melatonin reduces the weight of the ovaries of female rats. Since then, abundant evidence has been adduced that the pineal gland, acting via melatonin, affects reproductive performance in a wide variety of species. These observations stimulated a search for a role for the pineal gland and melatonin in human reproduction. Clinical experience related to this issue has yielded inconclusive and sometimes conflicting results [26, 61].

For a long time, humans were claimed to be poorly sensitive to photoperiod variations, as no difference was found between the duration of nocturnal melatonin secretion in summer and winter in temperate zones. However, studies conducted under appropriate natural or controlled laboratory conditions showed that humans also exhibit changes in the daily melatonin profile. For example, the melatonin rhythm was phase delayed during winter compared with the summer in shift workers living in Antarctica [62]. In temperate latitudes (40–50°N), data on the influence of the photoperiod are less clear. Wehr [63] showed that, under laboratory conditions, the duration of nocturnal melatonin secretion increased with decreased duration of artificial light and that sleep responded to this change in day length. They proposed that the circadian pacemaker consists of two component oscillators, one entrained to dusk controlling onset of melatonin secretion and one entrained to dawn and controlling the offset. The dusk- and dawn-entrained components of the circadian pacemaker are considered to control evening and morning transitions in melatonin secretion and to adjust the timing of these transitions in seasonal changes in day length [64]. The response to these seasonal changes is abolished by modern artificial lighting, as no summer-winter differences in melatonin, cortisol, thyrotropin, and rectal temperature profiles were observed in men exposed to either natural or artificial light in an urban environment [65]. In contrast, the seasonal alterations in the natural photoperiod at high latitudes have a repercussion on melatonin secretion in humans. Although there is no direct evidence that changes in duration of melatonin secretion mediate the effect of the photoperiod, as occurs in animal models, a response to this seasonal message is likely. In Finland, Kauppila et al. [66] observed a 2-h extension of melatonin secretion in winter compared with the summer and that a decrease in plasma ovarian steroids paralleled the winter increase in melatonin secretion, in agreement with a variation in rate of conception during the year observed at high latitudes, increased fertility being associated with longer days. In temperate areas, the influence of photoperiod on reproduction is less clear. Finally, nutritional and environmental (artificial light and blunting of seasonal changes in temperature) factors could be responsible for the progressive decline in the seasonality of human reproduction [67].

Seasonal affective disorders (SAD) of the winter type are characterized by recurrent depressive episodes during the short photoperiod. Changes in the duration and/or phase of melatonin secretion during this period were initially hypothesized to play a role in the pathogenesis of SAD and prompted its treatment with phototherapy [68]. Although phototherapy is an effective treatment for SAD and might act on some biological rhythms, there is no clear evidence that the observed beneficial effect of this treatment results from changes in melatonin profile [69, 70].

Circadian Effects: Melatonin, the Endogenous Synchronizer

The time of melatonin secretion adjusts to the light/dark cycle. The general opinion is that melatonin, by providing the organism with night information, is an endogenous synchronizer than can stabilize circadian rhythms, reinforce them, and maintain their mutual phase relationship [71, 72].

Major physiological functions (e.g., regulation of blood pressure, immune response, and hemostasis), cell regulation (multiplication), and biochemical mechanisms (respiratory chain and antioxidant defenses) include a circadian component, and melatonin receptors are widely distributed throughout the body. Physiological phenomena that display nycthemeral variation are mainly influenced. The direct effect of melatonin on the temperature rhythm is a good example: melatonin reinforces the nocturnal decrease in central temperature, an event which facilitates sleep propensity [73]. Since melatonin receptors have been identified in the peripheral vasculature, the decreased central temperature may be the result of peripheral vasodilation due to melatonin receptor stimulation [74].

The arguments put forward for the influence of melatonin on the cortisol rhythm and sleep-wake cycle are more indirect. The cortisol and melatonin rhythms remain phase locked after phase-shifting manipulation. In addition, a direct modulatory effect of melatonin on cortisol secretion cannot be excluded, since melatonin receptors have been demonstrated in the primate adrenal gland and physiological doses of melatonin inhibit the in vitro ACTH-stimulated cortisol production [75]. Temperature nadir, sleepiness, and melatonin excretion peaks coincide, and this temporal relationship remains during a 72-h sleep deprivation [76]. Also, there is a close correlation between melatonin suppression and the enhancement of alertness by light exposure at night [77]. When melatonin secretion is shifted to the morning after a repeated nocturnal administration of bright light, nocturnal alertness is improved and diurnal sleep, which is synchronous with melatonin secretion, displays a physiological architecture. Furthermore, there is a clear relationship between the durations of sleep and melatonin secretion. Aeschbach et al. [78] observed a longer biological night in long sleepers than in short sleepers, and the former showed longer nocturnal periods of high plasma melatonin levels, increased cortisol levels, low body temperature, and increasing sleepiness.

Maternal melatonin, which crosses the placenta, is one of the maternal rhythmic signals capable of synchronizing the fetal biological clock, while, in the newborn, the pronounced daily melatonin rhythm in the milk might take over. In infancy, the imbalance in sleep distribution between night and day becomes progressively more marked with age; at around 3–4 months, an age that corresponds to melatonin rhythm maturation, the infant remains awake during most of the daytime and most of its sleep is concentrated during the night [79]. Taken as a whole, these data support the idea that, under physiological conditions, melatonin is involved in the circadian regulation, especially the sleep-wake cycle.

The existence of a phase-response curve (PRC) of pineal melatonin secretion to the administration of exogenous melatonin (chronobiotic effect) provides an indirect argument that the effect of melatonin on the activity-rest cycle is indirectly mediated by its effect on the phase of the sleep-wake cycle [80, 81]. When melatonin is given in the late afternoon or the evening, a phase advance in the plasma melatonin profile is observed, whereas a phase delay is seen following melatonin administration from early morning to noon [80]. Such a phase shift has been obtained with a single low-dose melatonin injection providing a hormone signal of a similar magnitude to the physiological nocturnal melatonin peak [81]. There is a possibility that melatonin works by a direct feedback effect on the clock; melatonin binding sites have been identified in the SCN, and melatonin can alter the electrical or metabolic activity of the SCN. Consequently, the main rhythms (sleep-wake, temperature, and cortisol) controlled by the circadian system can be manipulated by melatonin administration.

Current evidence shows that the pineal plays an important role in modulating the immune response (for review, see [82]), since functional inhibition (constant light condition) or pharmacological inhibition (propranolol administration) of melatonin synthesis in mice is associated with suppressed humoral and cellular immunological responses. Interactions between the pineal gland and the immune system are bidirectional, since interleukins and cytokines (interferon gamma) affect melatonin synthesis and release [83]. In addition, melatonin scavenging of NO or free radicals in lymphoid cells has been described and could explain the melatonin-modulated circadian variation in experimental chronic inflammation. This kind of approach raises new questions regarding the mechanism of chronic inflammation, in disorders such as rheumatoid arthritis and nocturnal asthma, diseases that present rhythmic symptoms over a 24-h period [84, 85]. It is clear that melatonin provides a functional link between the neuroendocrine and immune-hematopoietic systems.

The validity of melatonin as an oncostatic agent seems well established, and the antitumor mechanisms of melatonin have been identified: these include its antiproliferative actions, its immunostimulatory effects on host anticancer defenses, and its antioxidant activity. However, there are isolated reports of stimulation of tumor growth, especially if melatonin is administered in the morning, indicating a circadian-stage dependency of its antitumor action [86]. In the past, very few patients with advanced disease have been studied in open studies. A controlled trial showed the possibility of improving the effects of chemotherapy, in terms of both survival and quality of life, by concomitant administration of melatonin and cisplatinium etoposide in metastatic non-small cell lung cancer [87].

Sites and Mechanisms of Action of Melatonin

Thanks to its easy passage across cell membranes and the very wide distribution of its receptors, melatonin displays pleiotropic functions [88]. Besides exerting biological activity via specific membrane receptors, melatonin interacts with nuclear receptors and intracellular proteins, such as calmodulin or tubulin-associated proteins, and has direct or indirect antioxidant effects, which participate in many general functions [89].

Receptors

A melatonin receptor nomenclature was recently proposed by the International Union of Pharmacology (IUPHAR) [90]. Two subtypes, MT1 and MT2, of mammalian melatonin receptors have been cloned. Both subtypes are members of the seven-transmembrane G protein-coupled receptor family. The MT1 receptor is coupled to different G proteins that mediate adenylyl cyclase inhibition and phospholipase Cβ activation, while the MT2 receptor is also coupled to inhibition of adenylyl cyclase and, additionally, inhibits the soluble guanylyl cyclase pathway. MT1 and MT2 polymorphisms have been found in humans and may be associated with sleep disorders [91]. A binding protein originally thought to represent a third membrane receptor (MT3) turned out to be the primarily cytosolic enzyme quinone reductase 2 (QR2).

Some effects of melatonin cannot be explained by membrane receptors or radical scavenging. Melatonin appears to be the natural ligand for the orphan nuclear hormone receptor superfamily RZR/ROR. Melatonin nuclear receptors are involved in the immunomodulator effect of melatonin [92].

Antioxidant Activity

Melatonin is a potent free radical scavenger, being more potent than vitamin E, the reference in the field [93]. It directly scavenges the highly toxic hydroxyl radical and other ROS. Melatonin also displays antioxidative properties, as it increases levels of several antioxidative enzymes, including superoxide dismutase, glutathione peroxidase, and glutathione reductase. On the other hand, it inhibits the pro-oxidative enzyme nitric oxide synthase. Since there is considerable experimental evidence that oxidative stress is a significant component of certain brain diseases, the ability of melatonin to protect against neurodegeneration has been tested in a multitude of models [94]. The first positive results were obtained in vitro with high doses of melatonin [95]. There is now experimental evidence that the levels of endogenously melatonin produced can act as a physiological antioxidant [96]. Furthermore, the antioxidant defense system displays a daily rhythm that is abolished by pinealectomy in the rat or by light in humans. Few data on the protective effects of melatonin against free radicals are available in humans. Controlled trials are difficult to set up, because the life of the patients involved in such studies is at stake. The first positive results were obtained in septic newborns and showed that very high melatonin doses (20 mg per subject) significantly reduced serum levels of lipid peroxidation products and inflammation markers, increased the survival rate, and improved the clinical outcome [97]. Similarly, the increased blood levels of malondialdehyde and nitrite/nitrate observed in asphyxiated newborns were reduced by melatonin treatment (total dose of 80 mg per infant); three of the ten asphyxiated newborns not given melatonin, and none of the ten who received it died within 72 h after birth [98]. Despite ethical difficulties, these results of major interest should be replicated in a larger number of patients.

Pharmacological and Therapeutic Considerations

The difference between the physiological and pharmacological effects of melatonin is not always clear, but is based upon the dose, and not the duration, of the hormone message. It is accepted that a "physiological" dose provides plasma melatonin levels of the same order of magnitude as a nocturnal peak (equal to, or lower than, 100 pg/ml or 400 pM) [90]. Oral administration of 0.5 mg or more, quickly released in the body, does not mimic the endogenous profile, but leads to supraphysiological levels over a short time. Although in vitro studies suggest that high melatonin doses desensitize receptors, efficacy is maintained in humans after repeated administration, and no tolerance or rebound symptoms are reported after withdrawal. The MT1 and MT2 receptors are differentially regulated in vitro, the MT1 receptor being activated by physiological melatonin concentrations and the MT2 receptor by supraphysiological levels, and this might explain inconsistent or contradictory effects observed depending on melatonin dose and metabolism.

In order to mimic endogenous secretion, a controlled-release melatonin preparation (Circadin®, 2 mg) has been developed for treatment of insomnia related to aging. However, the resulting plasma melatonin levels are several times higher than a physiological nocturnal peak. As far as we know, only a buccal transmucosal patch has been able to provide moderate melatonin levels for a chosen time, but its development was abandoned by the pharmaceutical company 15 years ago [99]. In addition, oral administration of a simple melatonin capsule provides a heterogeneous hormone signal as a consequence of high first-pass hepatic metabolism and variable catabolism by CYP1A2, and this variability is greater in elderly adults [100]. In addition, considering the PRC, the turning point from phase delay to phase advance is around 3 p.m., opposite the melatonin acrophase. A high melatonin dose given around noon could lead to spillover of high plasma melatonin levels from the phase-delay to the phase-advance portion of the melatonin PRC, resulting in the absence of the phase-shifting effect of melatonin or a variable result among subjects, depending on their individual melatonin metabolism. Finally, since melatonin receptors display a very wide distribution in the body, the putative therapeutic indications of this compound are multiple. Theses aspects will be treated in subsequent chapters.

Concluding Remarks

Although melatonin was discovered more than 50 years ago, its physiological role in humans needs further investigation. However, continuous progress has reinforced the idea that melatonin plays the role of a universal endogenous synchronizer, even for physiological functions for which circadian organization does not appear of paramount importance at first sight. The influence of melatonin on hemostasis, glucose homeostasis, phosphocalcic metabolism, blood pressure, immune system, and antioxidant defenses deserves attention. In addition, the availability of selective antagonists that could be used in humans could help in understanding the physiological importance of melatonin.

Alterations to the 24-h melatonin profile are associated with a large variety of pathological situations. Some of the changes might be responsible for the development of a major disease, while others may be a consequence of an existing disorder, since due to its complex regulation melatonin secretion is nonspecifically disturbed in most pathophysiological situations. In both situations, the resulting alteration in melatonin secretion could favor predisposition to disease, increase the severity of symptoms, or modify the course and outcome of the disorder.

The evaluation of melatonin secretion should be extended to situations in which dramatic disturbances of endogenous rhythms and immune and antioxidant defenses are patent, e.g., in patients admitted to intensive care units. Study conditions (light environment, drug intake, and comparison with control groups) should be strictly controlled. In these situations, great therapeutic advances could be achieved with melatonin by developing multicenter trials in large series of patients in order to definitively establish its efficacy and absence of long-term toxicity.

References

1. Lerner AB, Case JD, Takakashi Y, et al. Isolation of melatonin, the pineal gland factor that lightens melanocytes. J Am Chem Soc. 1958;80:2587.
2. Liu C, Fukuhara C, Wessel 3rd JH, et al. Localization of Aa-nat mRNA in the rat retina by fluorescence in situ hybridization and laser capture microdissection. Cell Tissue Res. 2004;315:197–201.
3. Bubenik GA. Gastrointestinal melatonin: localization, function, and clinical relevance. Dig Dis Sci. 2002; 47:2336–48.
4. Slominski A, Pisarchik A, Semak I, et al. Serotoninergic and melatoninergic systems are fully expressed in human skin. FASEB J. 2002;16:896–8.
5. Champier J, Claustrat B, Besancon R, et al. Evidence for tryptophan hydroxylase and hydroxy-indol-O-methyl-transferase mRNAs in human blood platelets. Life Sci. 1997;60:2191–7.
6. Cardinali DP, Ladizesky MG, Boggio V, et al. Melatonin effects on bone: experimental facts and clinical perspectives. J Pineal Res. 2003;34:81–7.
7. Stefulj J, Hortner M, Ghosh M, et al. Gene expression of the key enzymes of melatonin synthesis in extrapineal tissues of the rat. J Pineal Res. 2001;30:243–7.
8. Hardeland R. Melatonin and 5 methoxytryptamine in non-metazoans. Reprod Nutr Dev. 1999;39:399–408.
9. Tan DX, Manchester LC, Hardeland R, et al. Melatonin: a hormone, a tissue factor, an autocoid, a paracoid, and an antioxidant vitamin. J Pineal Res. 2003;34:75–8.
10. Klein DC, Moore RY. Pineal N-acetyltransferase and hydroxyindole-O-methyltrans-ferase: control by the retinohypothalamic tract and the suprachiasmatic nucleus. Brain Res. 1979;174:245–62.
11. Bernard M, Guerlotté J, Grève P, et al. Melatonin synthesis pathway: circadian regulation of the genes encoding the key enzymes in the chicken pineal gland and retina. Reprod Nutr Dev. 1999;39:325–34.
12. Stehle JH, Foulkes NS, Molina CA, et al. Adrenergic signals direct rhythmic expression of transcriptional repressor CREM in the pineal gland. Nature. 1993; 365:314–20.
13. Zimmermann RC, McDougle CJ, Schumacher M, et al. Effects of acute tryptophan depletion on nocturnal melatonin secretion in humans. J Clin Endocrinol Metab. 1993;76:1160–4.
14. Fournier I, Ploye F, Cottet-Emard JM, Brun J, Claustrat B. Folate deficiency alters melatonin secretion in rats. J Nutr. 2002;132:2781–4.
15. Munoz-Hoyos A, Amoros-Rodriguez I, Molina-Carballo A, et al. Pineal response after pyridoxine test in children. J Neural Transm Gen Sect. 1996; 103:833–42.
16. Luboshitzky R, Ophir U, Nave R, et al. The effect of pyridoxine administration on melatonin secretion in normal men. Neuro Endocrinol Lett. 2002;23: 213–7.
17. Skene DJ, Bojkowski CJ, Arendt J. Comparison of the effects of acute fluvoxamine and desipramine administration on melatonin and cortisol production in humans. Br J Clin Pharmacol. 1994;37:181–6.
18. Pardridge WM, Mietus LJ. Transport of albumin-bound melatonin through the blood–brain barrier. J Neurochem. 1980;34:1761–3.
19. Reiter RJ. Pineal melatonin: cell biology of its synthesis and of its physiological interactions. Endocr Rev. 1991;12:151–80.
20. Geoffriau M, Claustrat B, Veldhuis J. Estimation of frequently sampled nocturnal melatonin production in humans by deconvolution analysis: evidence for episodic or ultradian secretion. J Pineal Res. 1999;27: 139–44.
21. Grof E, Grof P, Brown GM, Arato M, Lane J. Investigations of melatonin secretion in man. Prog Neuropsychopharmacol Biol Psychiatry. 1985;9: 609–12.
22. Morin D, Simon N, Depres-Brummer P, et al. Melatonin high-affinity binding to alpha-1-acid glycoprotein in human serum. Pharmacology. 1997;54: 271–5.
23. Le Bars D, Thivolle P, Vitte PA, et al. PET and plasma pharmacokinetic studies after bolus intravenous administration of ^{11}C melatonin in humans. Nucl Med Biol. 1991;18:357–62.
24. Waldhauser F, Ehrhart B, Förster E. Clinical aspects of the melatonin action: impact of development, aging, and puberty, involvement of melatonin in psychiatric disease and importance of neuroimmunoendocrine interactions. Experientia. 1993;49:671–81.
25. Waldhauser F, Boepple PA, Schemper M, et al. Serum melatonin in central precocious puberty is lower than in age-matched prepubertal children. J Clin Endocrinol Metab. 1991;73:793–6.
26. Brzezinski A, Lynch HJ, Wurtman RJ, Seibel MM. Possible contribution of melatonin to the timing of the luteinizing hormone surge. N Engl J Med. 1987; 316:1550–1.
27. Berga SL, Yen SSC. Circadian pattern of plasma melatonin concentrations during four phases of the human menstrual cycle. Neuroendocrinology. 1990; 51:606–12.
28. Okatani Y, Morioka N, Wakatsuki A. Changes in nocturnal melatonin secretion in perimenopausal women: correlation with endogenous estrogen concentrations. J Pineal Res. 2000;28:111–8.
29. Iguchi H, Kato KI, Ibayashi H. Age-dependent reduction in serum melatonin concentrations in healthy human subjects. J Clin Endocrinol Metab. 1982; 55:27–9.
30. Haimov I, Laudon M, Zisapel N, et al. Sleep disorders and melatonin rhythms in elderly people. Br Med J. 1994;309:167.
31. Hirata F, Hayaishi O, Tokuyama T, Senoh S. In vitro and in vivo formation of two new metabolites of melatonin. J Biol Chem. 1974;249:1311–3.

32. Gunes A, Dahl ML. Variation in CYP1A2 activity and its clinical implications: influence of environmental factors and genetic polymorphisms. Pharmacogenomics. 2008;9:625–37. Review.
33. Härtter S, Korhonen T, Lundgren S, Rane A, Tolonen A, Turpeinen M, Laine K. Effect of caffeine intake 12 or 24 hours prior to melatonin intake and CYP1A2*1F polymorphism on CYP1A2 phenotyping by melatonin. Basic Clin Pharmacol Toxicol. 2006;99:300–4.
34. Ursing C, von Bahr C, Brismar K, Röjdmark S. Influence of cigarette smoking on melatonin levels in man. Eur J Clin Pharmacol. 2005;61:197–201.
35. Francis PL, Leone AM, Young IM, et al. Gas chromatographic-mass spectrometric assay for 6-hydroxymelatonin sulfate and 6-hydroxymelatonin glucuronide in urine. Clin Chem. 1987;33:453–7.
36. Arendt J, Bojkowski C, Franey C, et al. Immunoassay of 6-hydroxymelatonin sulfate in human plasma and urine: abolition of the urinary 24-hour rhythm with Atenolol. J Clin Endocrinol Metab. 1985;60: 1166–73.
37. Iguchi H, Kato KI, Ibayashi H. Melatonin serum levels and metabolic clearance rate in patients with liver cirrhosis. J Clin Endocrinol Metab. 1982;54:1025–7.
38. Ludemann P, Zwernemann S, Lerchl A. Clearance of melatonin and 6-sulfatoxymelatonin by hemodialysis in patients with end-stage renal disease. J Pineal Res. 2001;31:222–7.
39. Edgar DM, Dement WC, Fuller CA. Effect of SCN lesions on sleep in squirrel monkeys: evidence for opponent processes in sleep-wake regulation. J Neurosci. 1993;13:1065–79.
40. Moore RY. The fourth C.U. Ariens Kappers lecture. The organization of the human circadian timing system. Prog Brain Res. 1992;93:99–115.
41. Cohen RA, Albers HE. Disruption of human circadian and cognitive regulation following a discrete hypothalamic lesion: a case study. Neurology. 1991;41:726–9.
42. Lewy AJ, Wehr TA, Goodwin FK, et al. Light suppresses melatonin secretion in humans. Science. 1980;210:1267–9.
43. Bokjowski CJ, Aldhous ME, English J, et al. Suppression of nocturnal plasma melatonin and 6-sulphatoxymelatonin by bright and dim light in man. Horm Metab Res. 1987;19:437–40.
44. Thapan K, Arendt J, Skene D. An action spectrum for melatonin suppression: evidence for a novel non-rod, non-cone photoreceptor system in humans. J Physiol. 2001;535:261–7.
45. Brainard GC, Hanifin JP, Greeson JM, et al. Action spectrum for melatonin regulation in humans: evidence for a novel circadian photoreceptor. J Neurosci. 2001;21:6405–12.
46. Chellappa SL, Steiner R, Blattner P, Oelhafen P, Götz T, Cajochen C. Non-visual effects of light on melatonin, alertness and cognitive performance: can blue-enriched light keep us alert? Prog Brain Res. 2011;190:119–33.
47. Ruberg FL, Skene DJ, Hanifin JP, et al. Melatonin regulation in humans with color vision deficiencies. J Clin Endocrinol Metab. 1996;81:2980–5.
48. Berson DM, Dunn FA, Takao M. Phototransduction by retinal ganglion cells that set the circadian clock. Science. 2002;295:1070–3.
49. Hughes S, Hankins MW, Foster RG, Peirson SN. Melanopsin phototransduction: slowly emerging from the dark. Prog Brain Res. 2012;199:19–40.
50. Moore RY. The innervation of the mammalian pineal gland. In: Reiter RJ, editor. The pineal and reproduction. Basel: Karger; 1978. p. 1–29.
51. Moller M, Baeres FMM. The anatomy and innervation of the mammalian pineal gland. Cell Tissue Res. 2002;309:139–50.
52. Cagnacci A. Melatonin in relation to physiology in adult humans. J Pineal Res. 1996;21:200–13.
53. Monteleone P, Tortorella A, Borriello R, et al. Suppression of nocturnal plasma melatonin levels by evening administration of sodium valproate in healthy humans. Biol Psychiatry. 1997;41:336–41.
54. Warman GR, Tripp HM, Warman VL, Arendt J. Circadian neuroendocrine physiology and electromagnetic field studies: precautions and complexities. Radiat Prot Dosimetry. 2003;106:369–73.
55. Lewy AJ, Sack RL. The dim light melatonin onset as a marker for circadian phase position. Chronobiol Int. 1989;6:93–102.
56. Nowak R, McMillen IC, Redman J, Short RV. The correlation between serum and salivary melatonin concentrations and urinary 6-hydroxymelatonin sulphate excretion rates: two non-invasive techniques for monitoring human circadian rhythmicity. Clin Endocrinol (Oxf). 1987;27:445–52.
57. Deacon S, Arendt J. Posture influences melatonin concentrations in plasma and saliva in humans. Neurosci Lett. 1994;167:191–4.
58. Chazot G, Claustrat B, Broussolle E, Lapras C. Headache and depression: recurrent symptoms in adult pinealectomized patients. In: Nappi G et al., editors. Headache and depression: serotonin pathways as a common clue. New York. Raven; 1991. p. 299–303.
59. Krieg SM, Slawik H, Meyer B, Wiegand M, Stoffel M. Sleep disturbance after pinealectomy in patients with pineocytoma WHO°I. Acta Neurochir. 2012; 154:1399–405.
60. Wurtman RJ, Axelrod J, Chu EW. Melatonin, a pineal substance: its effect on the rat ovary. Science. 1963;141:277–80.
61. Srinivasan V, Spence WD, Pandi-Perumal SR, Zakharia R, Bhatnagar KP, Brzezinski A. Melatonin and human reproduction: shedding light on the darkness hormone. Gynecol Endocrinol. 2009;25: 779–85.
62. Yoneyama S, Hashimoto S, Honma K. Seasonal changes of human circadian rhythms in Antarctica. Am J Physiol. 1999;277:1091–7.

63. Wehr TA. The durations of human melatonin secretion and sleep respond to changes in daylength (photoperiod). J Clin Endocrinol Metab. 1991;73:1276–80.
64. Wehr TA, Aeschbach D, Ducan Jr WC. Evidence for a biological dawn and dusk in the human circadian timing system. J Physiol. 2001;535:937–51.
65. Wehr TA, Giesen HA, Moul DE, et al. Suppression of men's responses to seasonal changes in day length by modern artificial lighting. Am J Physiol. 1995;269:173–8.
66. Kauppila A, Kivela A, Pakarinen A, Vakkuri O. Inverse seasonal relationship between melatonin and ovarian activity in humans in a region with a strong seasonal contrast in luminosity. J Clin Endocrinol Metab. 1987;65:823–8.
67. Wehr TA. Photoperiodism in humans and other primates: evidence and implications. J Biol Rhythms. 2001;16:348–64.
68. Lewy AJ, Sack RL, Miller LS, Hoban TM. Antidepressant and circadian phase shifting effects of light. Science. 1987;235:352–4.
69. Wehr TA, Jacobsen FM, Sack DA, et al. Phototherapy of seasonal affective disorder: time of day and suppression of melatonin are not critical for antidepressant effects. Arch Gen Psychiatry. 1986;43:870–5.
70. Wirz-Justice A, Graw P, Krauchi K, et al. Light therapy in seasonal affective disorder is independent of time of day or circadian phase. Arch Gen Psychiatry. 1993;50:929–37.
71. Armstrong SM. Melatonin: the internal zeitgeber of mammals? Pineal Res Rev. 1989;7:157–202.
72. Cardinali DP, Pevet P. Basic aspects of melatonin action. Sleep Med Rev. 1998;2:175–90.
73. Strassmann RJ, Qualls CR, Lisansky EJ, Peake GT. Elevated rectal temperature produced by all-night bright light is reversed by melatonin infusion in men. J Appl Physiol. 1991;71:2178–82.
74. Van der Helm-van Mil AH, van Someren EJ, van den Boom R, et al. No influence of melatonin on cerebral blood flow in humans. J Clin Endocrinol Metab. 2003;4:5989–94.
75. Torres-Farfan C, Richter HG, Rojas-Garcia P, et al. mt1 Melatonin receptor in the primate adrenal gland: inhibition of adrenocorticotropin-stimulated cortisol production by melatonin. J Clin Endocrinol Metab. 2003;88:450–8.
76. Akerstedt T, Froberg JE, Friberg Y, Wetterberg L. Melatonin excretion, body temperature and subjective arousal during 64 hours of sleep deprivation. Psychoneuroendocrinology. 1979;4:219–25.
77. Cajochen C, Zeitzer JM, Czeisler CA, Dijk DJ. Dose–response relationship for light intensity and ocular and electroencephalographic correlates of human alertness. Behav Brain Res. 2000;115:75–83.
78. Aeschbach D, Sher L, Postolache TT, et al. A longer biological night in long sleepers than in short sleepers. J Clin Endocrinol Metab. 2003;88:26–30.
79. Rivkees SA. Developing circadian rhythmicity in infants. Pediatrics. 2003;112:373–81.
80. Lewy AJ, Ahmed S, Latham Jackson JM, Sack RL. Melatonin shifts human circadian rhythms according to a phase-response curve. Chronobiol Int. 1992;9:380–92.
81. Zaidan R, Geoffriau M, Brun J, et al. Melatonin in able to influence its secretion in humans: description of a phase-response curve. Neuroendocrinology. 1994;60:105–12.
82. Guerrero JM, Reiter RJ. Melatonin-immune system relationships. Curr Top Med Chem. 2002;2:167–79.
83. Withyachumnarnkul B, Nonaka KO, Santana C, et al. Interferon-gamma modulates melatonin production in rat pineal glands in organ culture. J Interferon Res. 1990;10:403–11.
84. Sutherland ER, Martin RJ, Ellison MC, Kraft M. Immunomodulatory effects of melatonin in asthma. Am J Respir Crit Care Med. 2002;166:1055–61.
85. Sulli A, Maestroni GJM, Villaggio B, et al. Melatonin serum levels in rheumatoid arthritis. Ann N Y Acad Sci. 2002;966:276–83.
86. Bartsch H, Bartsch C. Effect of melatonin on experimental tumors under different photoperiods and times of administration. J Neural Transm. 1981;52:269–79.
87. Lissoni P, Chilelli M, Villa S, et al. Five years survival in metastatic non-small cell lung cancer patients treated with chemotherapy alone or chemotherapy and melatonin: a randomized trial. J Pineal Res. 2003;35:12–5.
88. Ekmekcioglu C. Melatonin receptors in humans: biological role and clinical relevance. Biomed Pharmacother. 2006;60:97–108. Review.
89. Cardinali DP, Golombek DA, Rosenstein RE, et al. Melatonin site and mechanism of action: single or multiple? J Pineal Res. 1997;23:32–9.
90. Dubocovich ML, Delagrange P, Krause DN, Sugden D, Cardinali DP, Olcese J. International Union of Basic and Clinical pharmacology. LXXV. Nomenclature, classification, and pharmacology of G protein-coupled melatonin receptors. Pharmacol Rev. 2010;62:343–80.
91. Ebisawa T, Uchiyama M, Kajimura N, et al. Genetic polymorphisms of human melatonin 1b receptor gene in circadian rhythm sleep disorders and controls. Neurosci Lett. 2000;280:29–32.
92. Carrillo-Vico A, Garcia-Perganeda A, Naji L, et al. Expression of membrane and nuclear melatonin receptor mRNA and protein in the mouse immune system. Cell Mol Life Sci. 2003;60:2272–8.
93. Tan DX, Chen LD, Poegeller B, et al. Melatonin: a potent, endogenous hydroxyl radical scavenger. Endocr J. 1993;1:57–60.
94. Pandi-Perumal SR, Bahammam AS, Brown GM, Spence DW, Bharti VK, Kaur C, Hardeland R, Cardinali DP. Melatonin antioxidative defense: therapeutical implications for aging and neurodegenerative processes. Neurotox Res. 2013;23:267–300.

95. Manev H, Uz T, Kharlamov A, et al. In vivo protection against kainate-induced apoptosis by the pineal hormone melatonin: effect of exogenous melatonin and circadian rhythm. Restor Neurol Neurosci. 1996;9:251–6.
96. Benot S, Goberna R, Reiter RJ, Garcia-Mauriño S, Osuna C, Guerrero JM. Physiological levels of melatonin contribute to the antioxidant capacity of human serum. J Pineal Res. 1999;27:59–64.
97. Gitto E, Karbownik M, Reiter RJ, et al. Effects of melatonin treatment in septic newborns. Pediatr Res. 2001;50:756–60.
98. Fulia F, Gitto E, Cuzzocrea S, et al. Increased levels of malondialdehyde and nitrite/nitrate in the blood of asphyxiated newborns: reduction by melatonin. J Pineal Res. 2001;31:343–9.
99. Benes L, Claustrat B, Horriere F, Geoffriau M, Konsil J, Parrott KA, Degrande G, McQuinn RL, Ayres JW. Transmucosal, oral controlled release, and transdermal drug administration in human subjects: a cross-over study using melatonin. J Pharm Sci. 1997;86:1115–9.
100. Zhdanova IV, Wurtman RJ, Balcioglu A, Kartashov AI, Lynch HJ. Endogenous melatonin levels and the fate of exogenous melatonin: age effects. J Gerontol A Biol Sci Med Sci. 1998;53A:B293–8.

Melatonin and Pain: Therapeutic Applications

15

V. Srinivasan, Khek-Yu Ho, Dario Acuña-Castroviejo, Rahimah Zakaria, Amnon Brzezinski, and Edward C. Lauterbach

Abstract

Management and control of pain sensation is a matter of great clinical interest. Drugs like aspirin and nonsteroidal anti-inflammatory drugs (NSAIDS) exert their antinociceptive effects by inhibiting cyclooxygenases (COX), but their side effects such as gastrointestinal bleeding and ulceration make them unsafe for long-term clinical use. Thus, there is a need to find a safer antinociception. Melatonin's antinociceptive effects have been demonstrated in a number of experimental models of nociception. Its clinical roles in inflammatory pain, neuropathic pain, fibromyalgia, irritable bowel syndrome, and cluster headache are discussed in this chapter. The mechanism of melatonin's antinociceptive effects

V. Srinivasan, MSc, PhD, MAMS (✉)
Sri Sathya Sai Medical Educational and Research Foundation, An International Medical Sciences Research Study Center, Prasanthi Nilayam, 40-Kovai Thirunagar Extn, Goldwins, Coimbatore, TN 641014, India

National Health Service, Department of Mental Health, Psychiatric Service of Diagnosis and Treatment, Hospital "G. Mazzini", ASL 4, Teramo, Italy

Department of Neuroscience and Imaging, University "G.D' Annunzio", Chieti 66013, Italy
e-mail: sainivasan@yahoo.com, venkataramanujamsrinivasan6@gmail.com

K.-Y. Ho, MBBS (Syd Hons 1), MD (NUS)
Department of Gastroenterology and Hepatology, National University Hospital, 1E Kent Ridge Road, NUHS Tower Block, Level 10, Singapore, Singapore

Department of Medicine, National University of Singapore, 1E Kent Ridge Road, NUHS Tower Block, Level 10, Singapore, Singapore
e-mail: khek_yu_ho@nuhs.edu.sg

D. Acuña-Castroviejo, MD, PhD
Department of Physiology, Centro de Investigación Biomédica, Parque de Ciencias de la Salud, Avda. del Conocimiento s/n, Armilla, Granada 18100, Spain
e-mail: dacuna@ugr.es

R. Zakaria, MBBS, PhD (Physiology)
Department of Physiology, School of Medical Sciences, Universiti Sains Malaysia, Kubang Kerian, Kelantan 16150, Malaysia
e-mail: rahimah@kck.usm.my

A. Brzezinski, MD
Department of Obstetrics and Gynecology, Hadassah Hebrew-University Medical Center, Ein-Kerem, Jerusalem 91120, Israel
e-mail: amnonbrz@gmail.com

E.C. Lauterbach, MD
Department of Psychiatry and Behavioral Sciences, and the Department of Internal Medicine, Neurology Section, Mercer University School of Medicine, 655 First Street, Macon, GA 31201, USA
e-mail: eclbgnp@earthlink.net

V. Srinivasan et al. (eds.), *Melatonin and Melatonergic Drugs in Clinical Practice*, DOI 10.1007/978-81-322-0825-9_15, © Springer India 2014

via its interaction with a number receptor sites including opioidergic, benzodiazepinergic, muscarinic, nicotinic, serotonergic, α_1-adrenergic, α_2-adrenergic, and, most importantly, MT_1/MT_2 melatonergic receptors present in the dorsal horn of the spinal cord as well in the central nervous system is also highlighted in this chapter.

Keywords
Melatonin • Nociception • Allodynia • Inflammatory pain • Neuropathic pain

Introduction

By definition, "pain is an unpleasant sensory and emotional experience associated with actual or potential tissue damage or described in terms of such tissue" [1]. *Clinical pain* has been divided into two conditions, including *inflammatory pain* caused by inflammation and *neuropathic pain* caused by actual injury to the nervous system, and is characterized by persistent pain hypersensitivity [2]. In addition to hyperalgesia, neuropathic pain also manifests as allodynia (pain occurring in response to normally innocuous stimuli). Multiple nociceptive mechanisms underlie neuropathic pain [3]. As this type of pain can persist for years, it also causes psychiatric symptoms including anxiety, depression, and sleep disturbances [4, 5]. Pain also constitutes a symptom of major depressive disorder, suggesting pathophysiological similarities between clinical pain and certain psychiatric disorders, particularly major depression [6, 7]. The mechanism of pain perception is multifactorial, involving many biochemical, humoral, neurophysiological, and psychological factors [8]. Damage or inflammation to tissue releases a variety of inflammatory mediators such as prostaglandins (PGE_2), leukotrienes, bradykinin, substance P and inflammatory cytokines like tumor necrosis factor (TNF-α), ATP, and adenosine. Each of these substances either directly activates nociceptors or releases local allogeneic agents which sensitize nociceptors and enhance the neuronal excitability of pain transmission pathways [9]. The transmission of pain sensation involves nociceptors (the primary sensory nerve endings Aδ and C fibers) that have their central processes in the dorsal horn of the spinal cord.

The dorsal horn of the spinal cord is the first site of synaptic transfer in the nociceptive pathway, and it is the primary region where peripheral afferent signals are integrated and modulated. A number of neurotransmitter-receptor sites such as *N*-methyl-D-aspartic acid (NMDA), alpha-amino-3-hydroxy-5-methyl-4-isoxazolepropionic acid (AMPA), opioid (μ and δ), α_2-adrenoceptors, and adenosine are located in the dorsal horn projection neurons. The dorsal horn region of the spinal cord is the region of central sensitization and this is mediated by neurotransmitters including glutamate, substance P, and neurokinin that interact with the NMDA receptor system [10, 11]. In addition, the dorsal horn neuron is also subjected to the influences of interneurons of the dorsal horn itself and descending pathways that modulate pain perception [7, 12]. These spinal interneurons and descending neural tracts from the brain constitute endogenous pain modulatory systems that inhibit pain transmission signals. These pain modulatory systems are activated by opioid and GABAergic mechanisms located in and around the periaqueductal gray region (PAG). From the PAG, descending fibers project to the rostral ventrolateral medulla (RVM) and dorsolateral pontine structures that in turn send inhibitory projections to the spinal cord to induce antinociceptive effects. Inhibitory α_2-adrenergic, δ, μ, and k opioid and 5-HT_{1A} receptors are present in the postsynaptic dorsal horn neurons along with GABA-A/GABA-B receptors [7, 13]. Descending fibers synapse with primary afferent neurons and secondary neurons or interneurons to stimulate them to release opioid peptides.

Management and control of pain sensation is a matter of great clinical interest. Drugs like aspirin and nonsteroidal anti-inflammatory drugs (NSAIDS) exert their antinociceptive effects by inhibiting cyclooxygenases (COX) [14]. But the side effects of aspirin and NSAIDS including gastrointestinal bleeding and ulceration make them unsafe for long-term clinical use. Other classes of drugs like morphine or the anti-inflammatory drugs that act through the nitric oxide (NO)-cyclic GMP pathway exert their antinociceptive actions by blocking the ascending transmission of pain sensation [15]. The side effects associated with morphine including sedation, respiratory depression, and dependence complicate its use in controlling nociceptive mechanisms [16, 17]. Neuropathic pain is a frequent manifestation of neurodegenerative diseases. Although it is less appreciated in Parkinson's disease (PD), the prevalence of pain is nearly 40 % in PD. Pain presentations in PD include several categories such as musculoskeletal pain, radicular or neuropathic pain, and primary central parkinsonian pain [18]. Neurodegenerative mitochondrial and cytoskeletal cellular mechanisms producing painful hyperactivity in primary afferent nociceptors have been suggested as possible causative factors contributing to hyperalgesia [19]. Tricyclic antidepressants and gabapentin are often prescribed for the treatment of neuropathic pain with variable results of response, suggesting thereby the need for the development of novel analgesic drugs that can be used for effective treatment and management of inflammatory and neuropathic pain [20–22].

Melatonin and Nociception

Melatonin, the hormone secreted from the pineal gland and other areas in the body (see Chap. 2), plays important roles in antinociceptive mechanisms.

Diurnal variations in the perception of pain have been described both in rodents and humans [23–26]. It has been reported that patients suffer less pain during the dark phase of the photoperiod, and prolonged latencies in pain thresholds have been detected in healthy human subjects during nighttime. These observations were recorded by Laikin and his coworkers, and they attributed this phenomenon to high melatonin levels occurring at night and their possible analgesic effects [26]. Based upon this initial observation, a number of investigators have evaluated the antinociceptive effects of melatonin in animals by using a variety of experimental models and designs.

Melatonin's Role in Pain

Animal Models

Melatonin's antinociceptive effects have been demonstrated in animals like mice and rats in a number of experimental models of nociception as extensively discussed in an earlier review [27]. A brief analysis of this is presented in this paper with the aim of understanding the clinical significance of the antinociceptive and beneficial effects of melatonin. Using the hotplate test, it was shown that melatonin (20–40 mg/kg, i.p) exerted its maximal analgesic effect when given in the late afternoon. This analgesic effect was blunted by the administration of either the opiate antagonist naloxone or the central benzodiazepine antagonist flumazenil, showing thereby the involvement of central opioid and benzodiazepine (BZD) receptors [28]. Soon after, it was showed that β-endorphin, through μ-opioid receptors, is involved in melatonin-induced modulation of brain BZD receptors [29]. Dose-dependent antinociceptive effects of melatonin were evaluated by means of the hot-water tail-flick test in a group of rats in which melatonin, injected (i.p) at three different doses (30, 60, 120 mg/kg), produced dose-dependent antinociception [30]. The antinociceptive effect began within 15 min after injection and reached a peak in 30 min and with 60–120 mg/day doses lasted for 100 min. Melatonin's antinociceptive effect with 60–120 mg/kg (i.p) was antagonized by an i.c.v injection of naloxone within 10 min after injection and lasted for 45 min. As the i.c.v injection of naloxone blocked melatonin's antinociceptive effect, it was concluded that the CNS is the primary site for melatonin's antinociceptive effect. In another study, it was found that melatonin potentiated the antinociceptive effects of deltorphin-1a, a δ-opioid agonist, but not of the μ-opioid agonist endomorphin-1. In this study, melatonin was injected either i.p (1, 5, 25 mg/kg) or i.c.v (0.25, 0.5, 1 mg/kg), which produced significant tail withdrawal latencies, thereby confirming antinociceptive effects of melatonin [31]. A summary of the antinociceptive effects of melatonin in a variety of animal models is presented in Table 15.1.

Inflammatory Pain and Melatonin

Lipopolysaccharide (LPS) injection into the hind paws of mice (5 μg in 50 μl saline) significantly decreased the nociceptive threshold in the hotplate and tail-flick tests 6 and 10 h after injection. Prior injection of melatonin (5 or 10 mg/kg) significantly inhibited LPS-induced hyperalgesia at both time intervals. A noted finding of this study was that melatonin's effect on LPS-induced hyperalgesia was not reversed by the opiate antagonist naltrexone (4 mg/kg) [47]. In carrageenan-induced inflammation in rats, melatonin injection (0.5 and 1.0 mg/kg, i.p) increased nociceptive thresholds [48]. Melatonin also increased the antinociceptive effects of indomethacin and, further, reduced carrageenan-induced paw edema. Melatonin has been found to reduce the release of prostaglandins and recruitment of polymorphonuclear leukocytes at the inflammatory site in carrageenan-treated rats [49]. Prior injection of melatonin in 25–100 mg/kg doses attenuated the hyperalgesic responses to O_2^-. Melatonin has been suggested to inhibit inflammation and tissue damage by affecting COX-2 and inducible nitric oxide synthase expression (iNOS) [50]. Not only melatonin, but melatonin analogues such as the pyrrolol [1, 2α] indole derivatives 3, 5, 12, and 14 also exerted significant anti-inflammatory and analgesic effects in the carrageenan-induced paw edema study [51]. Melatonin also inhibited capsaicin-induced hyperalgesia, and naloxone pretreatment completely reversed melatonin's antinociceptive effects [52]. To evaluate the role of the spinal melatonin system in impeding the initiation or generation of capsaicin-induced secondary mechanical allodynia and hyperalgesia, melatonin or its antagonist 4-phenyl-2-propionamido-tetraline (4-P-PDOT) was administered intrathecally 30 min prior to capsaicin injection [53]. Intrathecal pre-administration of melatonin or its agonist significantly decreased or completely blocked the enhanced responses to von Frey filament stimulation following the injection of capsaicin. Melatonin also limited the intensity and duration of the secondary mechanical allodynia and hyperalgesia following capsaicin injection. It is concluded that the spinal melatonin system has the ability to impede the initiation and limit the development of "central sensitization" induced by capsaicin injection [53]. The effect of the melatonin agonist 6-chloromelatonin on capsaicin-induced mechanical allodynia and hyperalgesia was also evaluated. The increase in paw withdrawal frequency induced by capsaicin was significantly reduced by intrathecal injection of 6-chloromelatonin. This antinociceptive effect of 6-chloromelatonin was blocked by intrathecal administration of the MT_2 receptor selective antagonist 4-P-PDOT, suggesting thereby the involvement of spinal MT_2 receptors in the nociceptive transmission mechanism [53].

The formalin test is used as a model for assessing nociceptive behavior. Subcutaneous injection of 5 % formalin produces a licking response of the injected hindpaw in a biphasic pattern, involving rapid and brief withdrawal of the affected paw. The two phases of the licking/flinching response are phase 1 (0–9 min) and phase 2 (10–60 min). Melatonin administration decreased the licking/flinching responses in both phases [54–56]. In a recent study on formalin injection, intrathecal melatonin reduced the flinching response during phase 1 and phase 2, thereby attenuating both the facilitated state and acute pain evoked by formalin injection [32]. The antinociceptive effects of melatonin from some studies are also presented in Table 15.1 [57–59].

Table 15.1 Melatonin's antinociceptive actions: experimental animal studies

Animal model used	Melatonin or its agonist Dose and route	Effect of melatonin	Blocked by	Type of receptors involved	Reference
Hotplate	30 mg/kg i.p (melatonin)	Antinociception	Naloxone	Opioid	[26]
Inflammatory type of pain	25–100 mg/kg (melatonin)	Antinociception	–	–	[50]
Hotplate	20–40 mg/kg i.p (melatonin)	Antinociception	Naloxone and flumazenil	Opioid and BZD	[28]
Hot-water tail-flick test	30, 60, or 120 mg/kg i.p (melatonin)	Antinociception	Naloxone	Opioid	[30]
LPS model	5 and 10 mg i.p (melatonin)	Antinociception	–	–	[47]
Electrical stimulation of tail	0.5 and 1.0 mg i.p (melatonin)	Antinociception	–	–	[48]
Carrageenan-induced paw inflammation	5 and 10 mg i.p (melatonin)	Reduction of paw inflammation and antinociception	–	–	[49]
Hot-plate latency test	4 mg/kg s.c (melatonin) and equimolar 5.16, 5.13, 6.88, and 5.40 mg/kg s.c (melatonin analogue compounds 3, 5, 9a, and 12)	Antinociception	–	–	[51]
Capsaicin-induced hyperalgesia	Melatonin, 6-chloromelatonin	Antinociception	4-P-PDOT	MT_2 melatonin	[53]
Inflammatory pain model	150–600 μg/paw (melatonin)	Antinociception			[55]
Inflammatory pain	3, 10, and 30 μg intrathecal (melatonin)	Antinociception	Prazosin, yohimbine, atropine, mecamylamine	α_1- and α_2-adrenergic, nicotinic and muscarinic	[32]
Carrageenan-induced paw inflammation	5 and 10 mg i.p 0.25, 0.5, 1.0 mg i.c.v (melatonin)	Reduction of inflammation and antinociception	–	–	[57]
Paw withdrawal threshold	70 mg/kg i.v cumulative dose (210 mg/kg) (melatonin)	Antinociception	Naloxone or luzindole	Opioidergic and melatonergic	[58]
Tail-clamping response	38 mg/kg (35–41 mg/kg) (bromomelatonin)	Antinociception	–	–	[59]
Ligation of sciatic nerve (neuropathic pain)	120 mg/kg i.v 0.1 nmol i.c.v (melatonin)	Antinociception	Naloxone	Opioid peptides and L-arginine-NO pathway	[63]
Ligation of spinal nerves (neuropathic pain)	37.5–300 mg oral 3–100 μg intrathecal (melatonin)	Antinociception	Luzindole both oral and intrathecal and 4-P-PDOT	MT_1 and MT_2	[64]
Formalin injection model	150 mg/kg oral (melatonin)	Antinociception	4-P-PDOT	MT_2	[94]
Post-inflammatory visceral hyperalgesia to colorectal distension	60 mg/kg (melatonin)	Antinociception	Naltrexone or luzindole	Opioid or melatonin	[95]

Neuropathic Pain and Melatonin

Neuropathic pain due to nerve injury is associated with thermal hyperalgesia and mechanical allodynia. Partial tight ligation of the sciatic nerve in rats is a widely employed model, which produces spontaneous pain, allodynia, and hyperalgesia analogous to the clinical conditions of neuropathic pain [60–62]. In a study conducted in mice, ligation of the sciatic nerve produced pain-like behavior characterized by mechanical allodynia and thermal hyperalgesia [63]. Injection of melatonin at high doses (120 mg/kg, i.p) and 0.1 nmol i.c.v reduced paw withdrawal latencies in response to radiant heat stimulation of the injured hindpaw. Concomitant administrations of both L-arginine (200 mg/kg, i.p; 80 μg, i.c.v) and naloxone (1 mg/kg, i.p; 10 μg, i.c.v) reduced the effect of melatonin on thermal hyperalgesia. The findings of this study indicate that melatonin's effect on thermal hyperalgesia is mediated partially through the L-arginine-NO pathway [63]. In this study, concomitant administration of melatonin even at high doses (either through i.p or i.c.v) did not have any effect on mechanical allodynia. However, in another study of neuropathic pain using the L5/L6 spinal nerve ligation rat model, intrathecal (3–100 μg) or oral (37.5–300 mg/kg) administration of melatonin decreased tactile allodynia induced by spinal nerve ligation [64].

There is evidence that melatonin interacts with glutamatergic systems involving the NMDA receptor. In the study just mentioned, the concomitant administration of both melatonin (30 mg/kg) and dextromorphin (15 mg/kg) effectively reversed both thermal hyperalgesia and mechanical allodynia induced by ligation of spinal nerves, thereby suggesting the involvement of both melatonin MT_2 receptors and NMDA receptors in nociceptive mechanisms [64]. This antiallodynic effect of melatonin was diminished by intrathecal administration of luzindole (1–100 μg), a common MT_1/MT_2 receptor antagonist, and by oral (0.01–1.0 mg/kg) or intrathecal (0.1–10 μg) 4P-PDOT, a selective MT_2 receptor antagonist, suggesting the involvement of melatonin MT_2 receptors in the antiallodynic effects of melatonin [64]. Electrophysiological experiments showed that microiontophoretic injection of melatonin inhibits the activation of the NMDA receptor in rat striatum in a dose-dependent manner, involving the inhibition of the NMDA-dependent intracellular NO pathway [65]. Thus, NMDA receptors seem to be one of the targets for the antinociceptive actions of melatonin.

Dextromethomorphin is an NMDA receptor (NMDAR) antagonist and it is used for treating patients with neuropathic pain such as complex regional pain syndrome and painful diabetic neuropathy. Increased NMDAR activity contributes to central sensitization in certain types of neuropathic pain. Clinically used NMDAR antagonists such as ketamine and dextromethomorphin are effective in treating neuropathic pain [66].

Melatonin's Antinociceptive Role

Clinical Studies

Chronic pain is encountered in a number of clinical conditions such as fibromyalgia, pelvic pain conditions, irritable bowel syndrome, tension and cluster headaches, and migraine [67]. Similarly, a number of psychiatric conditions are associated with abnormal pain sensations. Pain thresholds in patients with post-traumatic stress disorder (PTSD) are significantly higher than controls or in patients with other conditions [33, 68]. Patients with depressive disorders suffer from painful symptoms like neck and back pain and abdominal pain, and painful symptoms in general are common in major depressive disorder [6, 69]. Conversely, chronic pain is suggested as a major risk factor for the development of major depressive disorder [34].

The link between pain and depressive disorders has been well studied, and it is suggested that a common pathophysiology may perhaps underlie these disorders [35, 70]. Serotonergic cell bodies located in the raphe nucleus and noradrenergic neurons located in the locus coeruleus project to various parts of the brain involved in the control of mood. The locus coeruleus and dorsal part of the raphe nucleus also project down to the spinal cord [36]. These descending pathways inhibit the transmission of pain sensations from sensory neurons of the dorsal horn of the spinal cord. Inhibitory α_2-adrenergic and 5-HT_{2A} receptors are also present on dorsal horn neurons [37]. A dysfunction of the descending neuronal pathways from the raphe nucleus and locus coeruleus can result in hypersensitivity of pain transmission systems, resulting in hyperalgesia and allodynia [7]. As pain and depression share common neuronal systems, drugs acting on serotonergic and noradrenergic systems are beneficial not only in treating depressive disorders but also in treating chronic clinical disorders of pain [7]. Perhaps this is best illustrated in conditions of neuropathic pain, where treatment with potent analgesics including opioids has been ineffective [22, 38]. Hence, tricyclic antidepressants are often prescribed in the clinical management of neuropathic pain [21, 22].

Melatonin and Fibromyalgia

Fibromyalgia is a clinical condition in which widespread debilitating musculoskeletal pain, hyperalgesia, allodynia, and stiffness of the body are found [71]. These patients suffer from sleep disturbances, depressive and anxiety symptoms, and impairment of memory and cognitive functions, collectively known as "fibro fog" [39, 40, 72]. The pathophysiology of fibromyalgia is thought to be due to abnormalities of the central pain processing mechanisms that cause central pain sensitization [41–43, 73]. Although few studies have carried out melatonin measurements in patients with fibromyalgia, a single study of 8 fibromyalgia patients showed significantly lower plasma and urinary melatonin (between 23:00 and 07:00 h) levels when compared to controls [44]. Treatment of fibromyalgia patients with melatonin has been carried out in two studies. In the first open label study carried out on 21 female patients, melatonin was administered in doses of 3 mg orally for 4 weeks 30 min before bed time [74]. Improvements with regard to pain, fatigue, and depressive symptoms were noted in these patients with melatonin therapy. In the second double-blind placebo-controlled study in 101 fibromyalgia patients, different doses of melatonin were used either alone or in combination with fluoxetine [75]. Patients were divided into four groups: group A patients ($n=24$) were treated with fluoxetine alone, group B patients ($n=27$) were treated with melatonin 5 mg/day, group C patients ($n=27$) were treated with fluoxetine (20 mg/day) and melatonin 3 mg/day, and group D patients ($n=23$) were treated with fluoxetine (20 mg/day) and melatonin 5 mg/day. Fluoxetine was given daily in the morning and melatonin was given each evening for 8 weeks. Treatment with fluoxetine alone improved symptoms including fatigue, anxiety, depression, and morning stiffness. Treatment with melatonin alone caused significant improvements in pain, fatigue, sleep/rest activity, depression, and morning stiffness. The combination of fluoxetine with melatonin caused even greater significant reductions in both anxiety and depressive symptoms, with reduction of fatigue symptoms in addition to each of the symptoms improved by each drug given individually. A noteworthy point emerging from this study is that, with all treatment modalities (fluoxetine, melatonin or a combination of both), there was a significant reduction of pain symptoms in fibromyalgia patients, showing the efficacy of the SSRI antidepressant fluoxetine and of melatonin in fibromyalgic pain [75]. Additional clinical studies in fibromyalgia patients also support that melatonin therapy is effective in treating pain associated with fibromyalgia [45, 76].

Melatonin and Irritable Bowel Syndrome

Another clinical condition in which melatonin has been found useful is irritable bowel syndrome (IBS). This condition is associated with abdominal pain, flatulence, constipation, diarrhea, and sleep disturbances. There are two randomized placebo-controlled clinical trials administering 3 mg/day of oral melatonin. In one study conducted in 40 patients, melatonin or placebo was given for 2 weeks [46]. Reductions in abdominal and rectal pain were noted. In another study in 24 women with IBS employing a cross-over design, patients received melatonin or placebo for 8 weeks followed by a 4-week washout period, after which they received the other treatment [77]. A reduction in pain symptoms with improvements in the IBS was noted in all 24 patients.

Melatonin and Migraine

In migraine, a clinical condition associated with attacks of severe headache and sleep disturbances, an association between nocturnal melatonin secretion and symptoms of migraine have been studied. Significantly lower urinary melatonin levels were found in ten migraine patients when compared to nine healthy controls [78]. Similarly, in a study in a large sample of 146 migraine sufferers with additional pain syndromes, significantly lower urinary 6-sulfatoxymelatonin was found in this group when compared to controls or migraine patients without additional pain syndromes [79]. In a study of migraine sufferers with disturbances in melatonin secretion (phase advance or phase delay), daily 5-h infusions of 4 μg melatonin/h relieved morning headache in four patients after the first infusion and two others obtained relief from morning headache after the third infusion, thereby showing a beneficial effect of melatonin in relieving the pain associated with migraine [80]. In a recent study, the melatonin agonist agomelatine has been used successfully for treating patients with migraine attacks. Agomelatine administered to patients suffering from migraine attacks (in doses of 25 mg/day for a duration of 6 months) decreased both the frequency and duration of migraine attacks and thus reduced the intensity of pain in migraine patients. Moreover, it also reduced significantly the severity of depression and normalized sleep disturbances [81]. This study, the first of its kind, demonstrates the beneficial effect of this melatonergic antidepressant in treating migraine attacks.

Melatonin and Cluster Headache

Melatonin is also involved in the pathogenesis of cluster headaches since its circadian rhythm is disrupted in this disorder [82]. A decrease in nocturnal melatonin secretion with a loss of melatonin rhythm has also been identified in cluster headache patients [83]. Based on these studies, melatonin was studied in the treatment of cluster headache patients in a double-blind placebo-controlled trial, in which melatonin caused a significant reduction in cluster headache attacks in the melatonin-treated group when compared to the control group [84]. In another study, a melatonin dose of 9 mg not only prevented the nocturnal cluster headaches but also prevented the daytime attacks as well [85]. These studies support the involvement of melatonin in the pathophysiology of cluster headaches. Pineal cysts, evident in 1.3–2.6 % of brain MRIs, have been commonly associated with headache. In a study by Peres et al., pineal cysts were found in five headache patients (four women and one man), two patients with migraine without aura, one patient with chronic migraine, one patient with aura, one with chronic migraine, and one with hemicrania continua [86]. Abnormal melatonin secretion and the presence of pineal cysts were found to be associated with headache in this group of patients. Several mechanisms, including free radicals scavenging, anti-inflammatory effects, inhibition of NOS activity, inhibition of dopamine release, GABA potentiation, and neurovascular regulation, have been proposed to explain beneficial treatment effects in cluster headaches and migraine attacks [86]. In an experimental animal model of headache induced by capsaicin, the c-fos expression response in the trigeminal nucleus caudalis (TNC) was studied in pinealectomized and control animals. Animals received capsaicin and melatonin in this study. Pinealectomized animals receiving capsaicin presented the highest number of c-fos-positive cells in the trigeminal nucleus caudalis, whereas animals injected with capsaicin and melatonin had a lower expression c-fos response similar to the control vehicle-treated group, showing melatonin's beneficial action in this experimental model [87].

Melatonin's Antinociceptive Actions

Possible Mechanisms

Early studies of melatonin's antinociceptive actions have shown that both opiate and BZD pathways are involved. The relationship of melatonin with the opioidergic system is complex. Recent studies suggest that melatonin can exert its antinociceptive effects by acting indirectly through a number of neurotransmitter systems and their related receptor sites, including benzodiazepinergic (BZD receptor), opioidergic (δ/κ/μ receptors), sigma system (sigma receptor), serotonergic ($5HT_{2A}$ receptor), dopaminergic (D_2 receptor), adrenergic (α_2 receptor), glutamatergic (NMDA receptor), and NO-cyclic GMP-PKG signalling pathway, and directly through melatonergic MT_1/MT_2 receptors [88]. Evidence for these interactions includes the reversal of melatonergic antinociceptive effects by the BZD antagonist flumazenil, δ/κ/μ opioid and sigma receptor antagonist naloxone, $5HT_{2A}$ receptor antagonist ketanserin, D_2 receptor antagonist sulpiride, the α_2-adrenoceptor antagonist yohimbine, and the NOS modulator L-arginine [28, 30, 63, 88, 89]. Evidence of direct melatonergic antinociception involves the MT_1/MT_2 antagonist luzindole and the MT_2 antagonist 4-P-PDOT [53, 59, 64]. Although modulation of these pathways play a role in melatonin's antinociceptive effects, the interaction of melatonin with both central and peripheral MT_1/MT_2 melatonin receptors seems crucial for melatonin's antinociceptive effects.

NMDA receptors in the spinal cord have been shown to be important in the transmission of pain sensation and potentiate spinal cord nociceptive synaptic transmission, an effect known as "wind-up," in which there is a repetitive increase in the intensity of C fiber stimulation [2, 90]. In a paradigm stimulating C fibers and inducing this "wind-up effect," melatonin's antinociceptive effect was evaluated. Different doses of melatonin (1.25, 2.5, 5.0, 10.0 mg/kg doses) produced dose-dependent decreases of "spinal wind-up," resulting in a complete suppression of wind-up at higher doses.

Melatonin's influence on spinal wind-up is attributed to its action on NMDA receptor-dependent intracellular NO generating pathways [91]. Nitric oxide has a diverse role in nociceptive transmission. It interacts with NMDA receptors and COX and induces a hyperalgesic effect, but by acting through cGMP-PKG-ATP-sensitive K^+ channels, NO also exerts an antinociceptive effect [13, 92]. Thus, melatonin interacts with a variety of systems, including benzodiazepine, opioidergic, serotonergic, dopaminergic, adrenergic, glutamatergic, the NO-cyclic GMP-PKG signalling pathway, and through diverse receptors including BZD, δ/κ/μ, sigma, 5-HT_{2A}, D_2, α_2, NMDA, NO, and MT_1/MT_2 receptors.

Role of Melatonin Receptors in Antinociceptive Mechanisms

Melatonin produces antinociception by inhibition of α_1-adrenergic, α_2-adrenergic, muscarinic, and nicotinic receptors in the spinal cord. One possible mechanism of action is suggested to be the activation of the cGMP system. Hence, it is possible that intrathecal melatonin, by increasing cGMP, may recapitulate the stimulation of α_1-adrenergic, α_2-adrenergic, muscarinic, and nicotinic receptors, thereby producing antinociception. Melatonin's exertion of direct antinociceptive effects through activation of MT_1 and MT_2 melatonin receptors has been demonstrated in a number of experimental studies on animals. This has been made possible by use of the common melatonin receptor (i.e., MT_1/MT_2) antagonist luzindole and specific MT_2 receptor antagonists like 4-P-PDOT or K185 (*N*-butanoyl-2-(5,6,7-trihydro-11-methoxybenzo[3, 4]cyclohept[2,1a]indole-13-yl)ethanamine). The antinociceptive effects of melatonin in neuropathic pain models and the localization of MT_1/MT_2 melatonin receptors in the thalamus, hypothalamus, dorsal horn of the spinal cord, spinal trigeminal tract, and trigeminal nucleus suggest that the antinociceptive actions of melatonin are mediated through melatonergic receptors. The

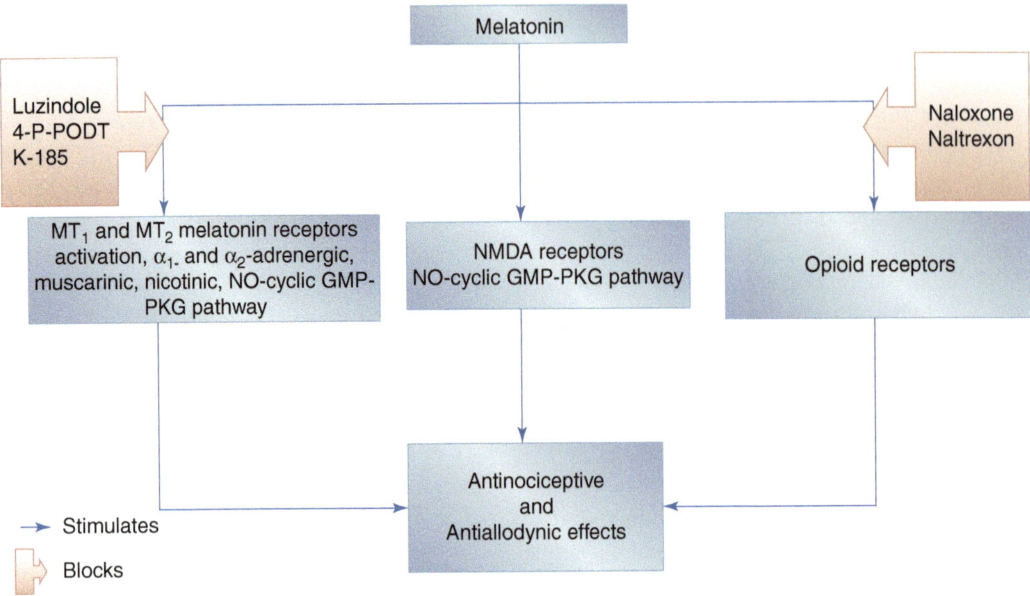

Fig. 15.1 Schematic diagram showing melatonin's antinociceptive actions

antinociceptive effects of melatonin and the melatonin agonist 2-bromomelatonin were each blocked by intrathecal administration of luzindole [93–95]. Similarly, the antinociceptive effect of intrathecal injection of 6-chloromelatonin was blocked by intrathecal administration of the melatonin MT_2 receptor blocking agent 4-P-PDOT [57]. The distribution of MT_1 and MT_2 melatonin receptors in lamina I–V and X of the spinal cord and their possible role in the mediation of antinociceptive actions of melatonin suggest that melatonin receptors do play a major role in the modulation of pain transmission pathways in the spinal cord as well as in the supraspinal region [47]. A schematic diagram showing the possible mechanisms of antinociceptive action is presented in Fig. 15.1.

Melatonin has been tried as premedication for surgical operating conditions including cataract surgery and also during tourniquet-related pain, and in both these conditions, melatonin reduced anxiety, improved preoperative analgesia, decreased tourniquet-related pain, and enhanced intraoperative and postoperative analgesia [96, 97].

Conclusion

Melatonin has exerted antinociceptive effects in a number of animal studies involving a diversity of models including acute pain, inflammatory pain, and neuropathic pain. While elucidating the mechanism of antinociceptive effects of melatonin, it has been noted that melatonin interacts with a number receptor sites including opioidergic, benzodiazepinergic, muscarinic, nicotinic, serotonergic, α_1-adrenergic, α_2-adrenergic, and, most importantly, MT_1/MT_2 melatonergic receptors present in the dorsal horn of the spinal cord as well in the central nervous system. Melatonin agonists such as 2-bromomelatonin, 6-chloromelatonin, and certain other pyrrolol indole derivatives of melatonin also exert significant anti-inflammatory and analgesic activity. In clinical disorders associated with chronic pain, e.g., fibromyalgia, depression, migraine and IBS, and cluster headaches, melatonin's use has been found beneficial in alleviating the pain that is associated with these disorders. In acute surgical conditions, melatonin's use reduced anxiety and enhanced both preoperative and postoperative analgesia.

Perhaps melatonin agonists with longer half-lives than melatonin (20–30 min) such as agomelatine (2 h) or even ramelteon (1–2 h) will also find clinical utility in the effective management and treatment of chronic pain and its associated clinical disorders.

References

1. Bonica JJ. The need of a taxonomy of pain. Pain. 1979;6:247–8.
2. Costigan M, Woolf CJ. Pain: molecular mechanisms. J Pain. 2000;1:35–44.
3. Jarvis MF, Boyce-Rustay JM. Neuropathic pain: models and mechanisms. Curr Pharm Des. 2009;15:1711–6.
4. Fishbain DA, Cutler R, Rossomoff HL, Rossomoff RS. Chronic-pain associated depression: antecedent or consequence of chronic pain. A review. Clin J Pain. 1997;13:116–37.
5. Blackburn-Munro G, Blackburn-Munro R. Chronic pain, chronic stress and depression: coincidence or consequence? Are hormones to blame? J Neuroendocrinol. 2001;13:1009–23.
6. Stahl SM. Does depression hurt? J Clin Psychiatry. 2002;63:273–4.
7. Stahl SM. Fibromyalgia-pathways and neurotransmitters. Hum Psychopharmacol. 2009;24:S11–7.
8. Shavali S, Ho B, Govitrpong P, Sawlom S, Ajjimaporn A, Klongpanichapak S, Ebadi M. Melatonin exerts its analgesic actions not by binding to opioid receptor subtypes but by increasing the release of β endorphin an endogenous opioid. Brain Res Bull. 2005;64:471–9.
9. Meyer RA, Ringkamp M, Campbell JN, Raja SN. Peripheral mechanisms of cutaneous nociception. In: McMahon S, Koltzenburg M, editors. Wall and Melzack's text book of pain. 5th ed. London: Elsevier; 2005. p. 3–34.
10. Riedel W, Neeck G. Nociception, pain, and antinociceptive mechanisms. J Rheumatol. 2001;60:404–15.
11. Pace MC, Mazzariello L, Passavanti MB, Sansone P, Barbarisi M, Aurillo C. Neurobiology of pain. J Cell Physiol. 2006;209:8–12.
12. Vanderah TW. Pathophysiology of pain. Med Clin North Am. 2007;91:1–12.
13. Cury Y, Picolo G, Guiterrez VP, Ferreira SH. Pain and analgesia: the dual effect of nitric oxide in the nociceptive system. Nitric Oxide. 2011;25(3):243–54.
14. Ferreira SH. Prostaglandins, aspirin like drugs, and analgesia. Nat New Biol. 1972;240:200–3.
15. Duarte LD, Lorenzetti BB, Ferreira SH. Peripheral analgesia and activation of the nitric-oxide-cyclic GMP pathway. Eur J Pharmacol. 1990;186:289–93.
16. Foley KM. Clinical tolerance to opioids. In: Bausmam AI, Besson JM, editors. Toward a new pharmacology of pain. Chichester: Wiley; 1991. p. 181–204.
17. Pasternak GW. When it comes to opiates, just say NO. J Clin Invest. 2007;117:3185–7.
18. Ford B. Pain in Parkinson's disease. Mov Disord. 2010;25 suppl 1:S98–103.
19. Reichling DB, Levine JD. Pain and death: neurodegenerative disease, mechanisms in the nociceptor. Ann Neurol. 2011;69(1):13–21.
20. MacFarlane BV, Wright A, O'Callaghan J, Benson HAE. Chronic neuropathic pain and its control by drugs. Pharmacol Ther. 1997;75:1–19.
21. Woolf CJ, Mannion RJ. Neuropathic pain: etiology, symptoms and mechanisms, and management. Lancet. 1999;353:1959–64.
22. Watson CP. The treatment of neuropathic pain: antidepressants and opioids. Clin J Pain. 2000;16:S49–55.
23. Crockett RS, Bornchein RL, Smith RP. Diurnal variations in response to thermal stimulation: mouse-hot plate test. Physiol Behav. 1977;18(2):193–6.
24. Davis GC, Buschbaum MS, Bunney Jr WE. Naloxone decreases diurnal variation in pain sensitivity and somatosensory evoked potentials. Life Sci. 1978;23:1449–60.
25. Pollmann L, Harris PH. Rhythmic changes in pain sensitivity in teeth. Int J Chronobiol. 1978;5(3):459–64.
26. Laikin MI, Miller CH, Stott ML, Winters WD. Involvement of the pineal gland and melatonin in murine analgesia. Life Sci. 1981;29:2543–51.
27. Srinivasan V, Pandi-Perumal SR, Spence DW, Moscovitch A, Trakht I, Brown GM, Cardinali DP. Potential use of melatonergic drugs in analgesia. Brain Res Bull. 2010;81:362–71.
28. Golombek DA, Escolar E, Burin LJ, Bristo-Sanchez MG, Cardinali DP. Time dependent melatonin analgesia in mice: inhibition by opiate or benzodiazepine antagonism. Eur J Pharmacol. 1991;194:25–30.
29. Gomar MD, Fernández B, Castillo JL, del Aguila CM, Acuña-Castroviejo D. Melatonin counteracts pinealectomy-dependent decreases in rat brain [3H] flunitrazepam binding through an opioid mechanism. Neurosci Lett. 1993;164(1–2):149–53.
30. Yu CX, Zhu CB, Xu SF, Cao XD, Wu GC. The analgesic effects of peripheral and central administration of melatonin in rats. Eur J Pharmacol. 2000;403:49–53.
31. Li SR, Wang T, Wang X, Dai X, Chen Q, Li RD. Melatonin enhances anti-nociceptive effects of δ but not μ opioid agonist in mice. Brain Res. 2005;1043(1–2):132–8.
32. Shin DJ, Jeong CW, Lee SH, Yoon MH. Receptors involved in antinociception of intrathecal melatonin in formalin test of rats. Neurosci Lett. 2011;494:207–10.
33. Schmahl C, Meinzer M, Zeuch A, Fichter M, Cebulla M, Kleindienst N, Ludäscher P, Steil R, Bohus M.

Pain sensitivity is reduced in borderline personality disorders, but not in post-traumatic stress disorder and bulimia nervosa. World J Biol Psychiatry. 2008;29:1–8.
34. Briley M. New hopes in the treatment of painful symptoms of depression. Curr Opin Investig Drugs. 2003;4:42–5.
35. Robinson MJ, Edwards SE, Iyengar S, Bymaster F, Clark M, Katon W. Depression and pain. Front Biosci. 2009;14:5031–51.
36. Wall PD, Melzack R. Text book of pain. 5th ed. New York: Churchill & Livingstone; 2005.
37. Stahl SM. Stahl's essential psychopharmacology. 3rd ed. Cambridge: Cambridge University Press; 2008.
38. Benedetti F, Vighetti S, Amanzio M, Casadio C, Oliaro A, Bergamasco B, Maggi G. Dose-response relationship of opioids in nociceptive and neuropathic postoperative pain. Pain. 1998;74(2–3):205–11.
39. Clauw DJ, Crofford LJ. Chronic widespread pain and fibromyalgia: what we know and what we do not know. Best Pract Res Clin Rheumatol. 2003;17: 685–701.
40. Arnold LM, Hudson JI, Keck Jr PE, Auchenbach MB, Javaras KN, Hess EV. Comorbidity of fibromyalgia and psychiatric disorders. J Clin Psychiatry. 2006;67:1219–25.
41. Bennett R. Fibromyalgia: present to future. Curr Rheumatol Rep. 2005;7:371–6.
42. Gracely RH, Petzke F, Wolf JM, Clauw DJ. Functional magnetic resonance imaging evidence of augmented pain processing in fibromyalgia. Arthritis Rheum. 2002;46:1333–43.
43. Staud R, Rodriguez ME. Mechanisms of disease: pain in fibromyalgia syndrome. Nat Clin Pract Rheumatol. 2006;2:90–8.
44. Wikner J, Hirsch U, Wetterberg L, Rojdmark S. Fibromyalgia – a syndrome associated with decreased nocturnal melatonin secretion. Clin Endocrinol (Oxf). 1998,49(2):179–83.
45. Reiter RJ, Acuna-Castroviejo D, Tan DX. Melatonin therapy for fibromyalgia. Curr Pain Headache Rep. 2007;11:339–42.
46. Song GH, Leng PH, Gwee KA, Moochhala SM, Ho KY. Melatonin improves abdominal pain in irritable bowel syndrome patients who have sleep disturbances: a randomized, double-blind, placebo controlled study. Gut. 2005;54:1402–7.
47. Raghavendra V, Agrewala JN, Kulkarni SK. Melatonin reversal of lipo-polysaccharides induced thermal and behavioural hyperalgesia in mice. Eur J Pharmacol. 2000;395(1):15–21.
48. El-Shenawy SM, Abdel-Salam OM, Baiuomy AR, EL-Batran S, Arbid MS. Studies on the inflammatory and anti-nociceptive effect of melatonin in the rat. Pharmacol Res. 2002;46(3):235–43.
49. Cuzzocrea S, Costantino G, Mazzon E, Caputi AP. Regulation of prostaglandin production in carrageenan-induced pleurisy by melatonin. J Pineal Res. 1999;27(12):9–14.
50. Esposito E, Paterniti I, Mazzon E, Bramant P, Cuzzocrea S. Melatonin reduces hyperalgesia associated with inflammation. J Pineal Res. 2010;49: 321–31.
51. Elmegeed GA, Baiuomy AR, Abdel-Salam OM. Evaluation of the anti- inflammatory and anti-nociceptive activities of the novel synthesized melatonin analogues. Eur J Med Chem. 2007;42(10):1285–92.
52. Mantovani M, Pertile R, Calixto JB, Santos AR, Rodriguez AL. Melatonin exerts its antidepressant like effect in the tail suspension test in mice: evidence for involvement of N-methyl-d-aspartate receptors and the L-arginine nitric oxide pathway. Neurosci Lett. 2003;1:1–4.
53. Tu Y, Sun RQ, Willis WD. Effects of intrathecal injections of melatonin analogs on capsaicin-induced secondary allodynia and hyperalgesia in rats. Pain. 2004;109:340–50.
54. Ray M, Mediratta PK, Mahajan P, Sharma KK. Evaluation of the role of melatonin in formalin induced pain response in pain. Indian J Med Sci. 2004;58(3):122–30.
55. Hernandez-Pacheo A, Araiza-Saldana CI, Granados-Soto V, Mixcoatlzecuati T. Possible participation of the nitric oxide-cyclic GMP protein kinase GK+ channels pathway in the peripheral antinociception of melatonin. Eur J Pharmacol. 2008;596:70–6.
56. Yoon MH, Park HC, Kim WM, Lee HG, Kim YO, Huang LJ. Evaluation for the interaction between intrathecal melatonin and clonidine or neostigmine on formalin-induced nociception. Life Sci. 2008;83: 845–50.
57. Billici D, Akpiner E, Kiziltuic A. Protective effective of melatonin in carrageenan induced acute local inflammation. Pharmacol Res. 2002;46:133–9.
58. Naguib MC, Hammond DL, Schmid III PG, Baker MT, Cutkomp J, Queral L, Smith T. Pharmacological effects of intravenous melatonin: comparative studies with thiopental and propofol. Br J Anaesth. 2003;90:504–7.
59. Naguib MC, Baker MT, Spadoni G, Gregerson M. The hypnotic and analgesic effects of bromomelatonin. Anesth Analg. 2003;97:763–8.
60. Seltzer Z, Dubner R, Shir Y. A novel behavioural model of neuropathic pain disorders produced in rats by partial sciatic nerve injury. Pain. 1990;43:205–18.
61. Seltzer Z. The relevance of animal neuropathy models of chronic pain in humans. Neurosciences. 1995;7:211–9.
62. Malmberg AB, Basbaum AI. Partial sciatic nerve injury in the mouse as a model of neuropathic pain: behavioural and neuroanatomical correlates. Pain. 1998;76:215–22.
63. Ulugol A, Dokmeci D, Guray G, Sapolyo N, Ozyigit F, Tamer M. Anti-hyperalgesic but not antiallodynic effect of melatonin in nerve injured neuropathic mice: possible involvements of the L-arginine-NO-pathway and opioid system. Life Sci. 2006;78: 1592–7.

64. Ambriz-Tututi M, Granados-Soto V. Oral and spinal melatonin reduces tactile allodynia in rats via activation of MT2 and opioid receptors. Pain. 2007;132(3):273–80.
65. Escames G, Macías M, León J, García JJ, Khaldy H, Martín M, Vives F, Acuña-Castroviejo D. Calcium-dependent effects of melatonin inhibition of glutamatergic response in rat striatum. J Neuroendocrinol. 2001;13(5):459–66.
66. Zhou HY, Chen SR, Pan HL. Treating N-methyl-D-aspartate receptors for treating neuropathic pain. Expert Rev Clin Pharmacol. 2011;4(3):379–88.
67. Woolf CJ. Pain: moving from symptom control toward mechanism-specific pharmacologic management. Ann Intern Med. 2004;140(6):441–51.
68. Defrin R, Ginzburg K, Solomon Z, Polad E, Block M, Covezensky M, Schreiber S. Quantitative testing of pain perception in subjects with PTSD-implications for the mechanism of the coexistence between PTSD and chronic pain. Pain. 2008;138: 450–9.
69. Lepin JP, Briley M. The epidemiology of pain in depression. Hum Psychopharmacol. 2004;19 Suppl 1:S3–7.
70. Delgado PL. Common pathways of depression and pain. J Clin Psychiatry. 2009;65:16–9.
71. Neumann L, Buskila D. Epidemiology of fibromyalgia. Curr Pain Headache Rep. 2003;7:362–8.
72. Mease PJ. Fibromyalgia syndrome: review of clinical presentation, pathogenesis, outcome measures, and treatment. J Rheumatol. 2005;75:6–21.
73. Bennett RM. Emerging concepts in the neurobiology of chronic pain: evidence of abnormal sensory processing in fibromyalgia. Mayo Clin Proc. 1999;74:385–98.
74. Citera G, Arias MA, Maldonado-Cocco JA, Lazaro MA, Rosemfett MG, Brusco LI, Scheines EJ, Cardinali DP. The effect of melatonin in patients with fibromyalgia: a pilot study. Clin Rheumatol. 2000;19:9–13.
75. Hussain SA, Al-Khalifa H, Jasim NA, Gorial FI. Adjuvant use of melatonin for treatment of fibromyalgia. J Pineal Res. 2011;50:267–71.
76. Acuña-Castroviejo D, Escames G, Reiter RJ. Melatonin therapy for fibromyalgia. J Pineal Res. 2006;40(1):98–9.
77. Lu WZ, Gwee KA, Moochhalla S, Ho YY. Melatonin improves bowel symptoms in female patients with irritable bowel syndrome: a double blind placebo controlled study. Aliment Pharmacol Ther. 2005;22: 927–34.
78. Brun J, Claustrat B, Saddier P, Chazot G. Nocturnal melatonin excretion is decreased in patients with migraine without aura attacks associated with means. Cephalalgia. 1995;15:136–9.
79. Masruha MR, de Souza Viera DS, Minett TS, Cipolla-Neto J, Zuckerman E, Vilanova LC, Peres MF. Low urinary 6-sulphatoxy-melatonin concentrations in acute migraine. J Headache Pain. 2008;9:221–34.
80. Claustrat B, Brun J, Geoffriau M, Zaidan R, Malloc C, Chazot G. Nocturnal plasma melatonin profile and melatonin kinetics during infusion in status migrainosus. Cephalalgia. 1997;17:511–7.
81. Tabeeva GR, Sergeev AV, Gromova SA. Possibilities of preventive treatment of migraine with MT1 and MT2 agonist and 5-HT2c receptor antagonist agomelatine (valdoxan). Zh Nevrol Psikhiatr Im S S Korsakova. 2011;111(9):32–6.
82. May A, Bahra A, Buchel C, Frackowiak RS, Goadsby PJ. Hypothalamic activation in cluster headache attacks. Lancet. 1998;352:275–8.
83. Chazot G, Claustrat B, Brun J, Jordon D, Sassolas G, Schott B. A chrono-biological study of melatonin, cortisol, growth hormone, and prolactin secretion in cluster headache attacks. Cephalalgia. 1984;4:213–20.
84. Leone M, D'Amico D, Moschiano F, Fraschini F, Bussone G. Melatonin versus placebo in the prophylaxis of cluster headache: a double blind pilot study with parallel groups. Cephalalgia. 1996;21:494–6.
85. Peres MFP, Rozen TD. Melatonin in the preventive treatment of chronic cluster headache. Cephalalgia. 2001;21:993–5.
86. Peres MFP. Melatonin, the pineal gland and their implications for headache. Cephalalgia. 2005;25:403–11.
87. Tanuri FC, de Lima E, Peres MF, Cabral FR, da grace Naffah-Mazzacoratti M, Cavalheiro EA, Cipolla-Neto J, Zukerman E, Amado D. Melatonin treatment decreases c-fos expression in a headache model induced by capsaicin. J Headache Pain. 2009;10: 105–10.
88. Mantovani M, Kaster MP, Pertile R, Calixto JB, Rodriguez AL, Santos AR. Mechanisms involved in the antinociception caused by melatonin in the mice. J Pineal Res. 2006;41:382–9.
89. Schmidtko A, Tegeder I, Geisslinger G. No NO, no pain? The role of nitric oxide and cGMP in spinal pain processing. Trends Neurosci. 2009;32:339–46.
90. Laurido C, Pelissie T, Soto-Mayono R, Valladares L, Flores F, Hernandez A. Effect of melatonin on rat spinal cord nociceptive transmission. Neuroreport. 2002;13:89–91.
91. Zhang Y, Quock LP, Chung E, Ohgami Y, Quock RM. Involvement of a NO-cyclic GMP-PKG signalling pathway in a nitrous oxide-induced antinociception in mice. Eur J Pharmacol. 2011;654:249–53.
92. Ambriz-Tututi M, Rocha-Gonzalez HI, Cruz SL, Granados-Soto V. Melatonin: a hormone that modulates pain. Life Sci. 2009;84:489–98.
93. Onal SA, Inalkac S, Kutlu S, Kelestimur H. Intrathecal melatonin increases the mechanical nociceptive threshold in the rat. Agriculture. 2004;16:35–40.
94. Espino R, Urquiza-Marín H, Ambriz-Tututi M, Araiza-Saldaña CI, Caram-Salas NL, Rocha-González HI, Mixcoatl-Zecuatl T, Granados-Soto V. Melatonin reduces formalin-induced nociception and tactile allodynia in diabetic rats. Eur J Pharmacol. 2007;577(1–3):203–10.

95. Mickle A, Sood M, Zhang Z, Shahmohammadi G, Sengupta JN, Miranda A. Antinociceptive effects of melatonin in a rat model of post-inflammatory visceral hyperalgesia: a centrally mediated process. Pain. 2010;149:555–64.
96. Ismail SA, Mowafii HA. Melatonin provides anxiolysis, enhances analgesia, decreases intra ocular pressure and promotes better operating conditions during cataract surgery under topical anesthesia. Anesth Analg. 2009;108:1146–51.
97. Mowafii HA, Ismail SA. Melatonin improves tourniquet tolerance and enhances postoperative analgesia in patients receiving intravenous regional anesthesia. Anesth Analg. 2008;107:1422–6.

Melatonin in Alzheimer's Disease: Focus on Neuroprotective Role

16

V. Srinivasan, Edward C. Lauterbach, Charanjit Kaur, Asma Hayati Ahmad, Mahaneem Mohamed, Atul Prasad, and Samuel D. Shillcutt

Abstract

Alzheimer's disease (AD) is characterized by a progressive loss of memory and cognitive function as well as behavioral and sleep disturbances including insomnia. The pathophysiology of AD has been attributed to oxidative stress-induced amyloid β-protein (Aβ) deposition. Abnormal tau protein, mitochondrial dysfunction, and protein hyperphosphorylation have been demonstrated in neural tissues of AD patients. AD patients exhibit severe sleep-wake disturbances associated with rapid cognitive decline and memory impairment. Optimally effective management of

V. Srinivasan, MSc, PhD, MAMS (✉)
Sri Sathya Sai Medical Educational and Research Foundation, An International Medical Sciences Research Study Center, Prasanthi Nilayam, 40-Kovai Thirunagar Extn, Goldwins, Coimbatore, TN 641014, India

National Health Service, Department of Mental Health, Psychiatric Service of Diagnosis and Treatment, Hospital "G. Mazzini", ASL 4, Teramo, Italy

Department of Neuroscience and Imaging, University "G.D' Annunzio", Chieti 66013, Italy
e-mail: sainivasan@yahoo.com, venkataramanujamsrinivasan6@gmail.com

E.C. Lauterbach, MD
Department of Psychiatry and Behavioral Sciences, and the Department of Internal Medicine, Neurology Section, Mercer University School of Medicine, 655 First Street, Macon, GA 31201, USA
e-mail: eclbgnp@earthlink.net

C. Kaur, MBBS, PhD
Department of Anatomy, Yong Loo Lin School of Medicine, National University of Singapore, BLK MD 10, 4 Medical Drive, Singapore 117597, Singapore
e-mail: antkaurc@nus.edu.sg

A.H. Ahmad, MBBS, MSc
M. Mohamed, MD, MSc, PhD
Department of Physiology, School of Medical Sciences, Universiti Sains Malaysia, Kubang Kerian, Kelantan 16150, Malaysia
e-mail: asma@kck.usm.my; mahaneem@kck.usm.my

A. Prasad, MBBS, MD, DM (Neurology)
Department of Neurology, Dr BL Kapur Superspeciality Hospital, Pusa Road, New Delhi, Delhi 110005, India
e-mail: prasad.atul@gmail.com

S.D. Shillcutt, PharmD, PhD
Department of Psychiatry and Behavioral Science, Mercer University School of Medicine, 655 First Street, Macon, GA 31201, USA
e-mail: shillcutt_s@mercer.edu

V. Srinivasan et al. (eds.), *Melatonin and Melatonergic Drugs in Clinical Practice*,
DOI 10.1007/978-81-322-0825-9_16,

AD patients requires a drug that can arrest Aβ-induced neurotoxic effects and restore the disturbed sleep-wake rhythm with improvement in sleep quality. In this context, the pineal hormone melatonin has been demonstrated to be an effective antioxidant that can prevent Aβ-induced neurotoxic effects through a variety of mechanisms. Sleep deprivation itself produces oxidative damage, impaired mitochondrial function, neurodegenerative inflammation, altered proteosomal processing, and abnormal activation of enzymes. Treating sleep disturbances is also necessary for preventing and arresting AD progression. Besides melatonin, use of melatonergic agonists such as ramelteon, agomelatine, and tasimelteon, which are now used clinically for treating insomnia and other sleep disorders, may also be beneficial in treating AD.

Keywords
Alzheimer's disease • Melatonin • Amyloid-β protein • Insomnia • Antioxidant • Sleep

Abbreviations

AD	Alzheimer's disease
apoE4	Apolipoprotein-E4
Aβ	Amyloid β-protein
ATP	Adenosine-5′-triphosphate
BDNF	Brain-derived neurotrophic factor
CSF	Cerebrospinal fluid
CypD	Cyclophilin D
ETC	Electron transport chain
H_2O_2	Hydrogen peroxide
MDA	Malondialdehyde
mtPTP	Mitochondrial permeability transition pore
O_2^-	Superoxide
PKA	Protein kinase
ROS	Reactive oxygen species

Introduction

Increased oxidative damage of the central nervous system has been suggested to cause age-associated neurodegenerative diseases like Alzheimer's disease (AD) and Parkinson's disease [1–5]. The brain is very susceptible to increased oxidative stress because of its high rate of oxygen consumption and high content of polyunsaturated fatty acids. Brain samples of AD patients have been shown to have increased protein, lipid, and DNA oxidation [6]. Protein carbonyl 3,3′-dityrosine and 3-nitrotyrosine levels in postmortem brain samples of AD patients produce increased oxidative and nitrosative protein modification in the hippocampal and neocortical regions [7].

Oxidative damage is related to other primary cytopathological features of AD including mitochondrial demise and amyloid-β (Aβ) protein accumulation. Other than age, one of the major risk factors for AD is gender. The higher incidence of AD in women than in men has been attributed to increased mitochondrial toxicity induced by Aβ proteins [8]. Increased Aβ levels trigger most important pathological features of AD such as tau hyperphosphorylation, formation of neurofibrillary tangles, synaptic dysfunction, and neuronal cell death [9]. Abnormal accumulation of Aβ protein results in the formation of toxic oligomers causing synaptic damage, alterations in signalling pathways related to synaptic plasticity, circuit hyperexcitability, and alterations in glutamate receptors [10]. Recent studies imply mitochondrial pathology as an important contributory factor in the late onset forms of AD [11].

Many of the current drugs used in treating patients with AD improve symptoms without any significant disease-modifying effects. It is estimated that the cost of care to the average AD patient family exceeds $90,000 per year [12] and the societal cost exceeds $100 billion per annum [13, 14]. These huge figures give evidence that there is an urgent need for speedy implementation of preventive treatment programs for arresting the progress of AD and other neurodegenerative diseases. In the last 15 years, studies have been done on the role of the pineal hormone melatonin in arresting the neurotoxic effects induced by Aβ in animal studies. Melatonin has been shown to antagonize Aβ-induced effects such as increased lipid peroxidation, increased oxidative stress, formation of protein carbonyl products, and mitochondrial pathological mechanisms [15]. Therefore, melatonin has substantial potential to prevent or delay AD progression which in turn reduces patient symptomatic burden, family expense, and societal cost. Moreover, its capacity to improve sleep disorders can improve AD symptoms and potentially reduces AD neuropathology as will be discussed below.

Molecular Pathophysiology of Alzheimer's Disease

There is a progressive loss of cognitive function in AD together with other neurobehavioral abnormalities including agitated behavior and profound sleep disturbances. Despite a lot of studies done on AD, its etiology remains unknown. Chronic inflammation associated with cytokine release, trace element neurotoxicity, and free radical generation have been suggested as possible contributory factors underlying the etiology of AD. The deposition of amyloid plaques in AD causes cell death by induction of oxidative stress, a primary pathogenic mechanism of AD. Aβ protein deposition initiates flavoenzyme-dependent increases in hydrogen peroxide (H_2O_2) and lipid peroxides that increase free radical generation [16]. Increased β-amyloid protein-induced oxidative stress together with decreased neurotrophic support [17] are major determinants of AD. Studies done in postmortem brain samples obtained from AD patients have shown extensive lipid, protein, and DNA oxidation [7]. Neural tissues of AD patients show increased levels of peroxidation end products such as malondialdehyde (MDA), 4-hydroxynonenal, carbonyls, and other species [18]. Although Aβ contributes to neuronal degeneration either directly or indirectly, its potential to cause AD depends on an individual's susceptibility to Aβ-mediated toxicity.

Mitochondrial Involvement in Alzheimer's Disease

Mitochondria are the major source of reactive oxygen species (ROS) and also the primary target of attack by ROS and reactive nitrogen species [19]. Damage to the mitochondrial respiratory chain can cause breakdown of the mitochondrial membrane proton potential, opening of the mitochondrial permeability transition pore (mtPTP), and consequent induction of apoptosis, leading to further generation of free radicals. These free radicals produce a vicious cycle that ultimately results in cell death by apoptotic or necrotic processes [20]. Studies have shown the involvement of mitochondrial ROS production and subsequent mitochondrial abnormalities in the pathophysiology of AD [21]. Mitochondrial superoxide (O_2^-) production plays a critical role in the pathological events following the elevation of Aβ peptide levels. The histopathological changes of AD such as extracellular accumulation of oligomeric and fibrillar Aβ peptides and intracellular neurofibrillary tangles induce functional deficits of the mitochondrial respiratory chain complexes which in turn results in mitochondrial dysfunction and enhanced oxidative stress [22].

Amyloid β-Peptide and Mitochondrial Interaction as Triggering Event for the Pathogenesis of Alzheimer's Disease

The faulty metabolism of amyloid precursor protein as the initiating event in the pathogenesis of AD has been suggested by the amyloid cascade hypothesis proposed by Hardy and Selkoe (2002) [23]. There is a subject of debate whether extracellular Aβ-induced mitochondrial damage is the initial triggering event in AD as Aβ appears within the mitochondria long before the appearance of extracellular Aβ deposits. The enzymes that transfer Aβ to mitochondria have been identified as a complex of translocases of both the inner membrane and outer membrane [24]. The presence of intracellular Aβ is one of the major reasons for the reduced oxygen consumption caused by the electron transport chain since Aβ diminishes the enzymatic activity of respiratory chain complexes III and IV [23]. Other neurotoxic mechanisms, such as the formation of ionic channels that allows increased calcium uptake by mitochondria and mtPTP opening with subsequent inhibition of respiratory complexes [25], have been suggested for Aβ-induced neurotoxicity that is mediated via intramitochondrial interactions. Rosales-Corral et al. (2012) has demonstrated that Aβ can accumulate both intracellularly and intramitochondrially [26], in which intracerebral injection of fibrillar Aβ caused accumulation of Aβ both intracellularly and intramitochondrially, deep within the cristae. This finding supports other investigators' views on intramitochondrial accumulation of Aβ. Other than inhibiting mitochondrial respiratory complex activities, disturbances in mitochondrial dynamics have also been demonstrated in AD patients. This includes disturbances in mitochondrial structure, impairment of dynamin-related peptide, and imbalances in fission and fusion, with consequent neuronal damage and synaptic loss [27]. Significant disturbances of mitochondrial proteins and lipids also occur following intramitochondrial accumulation of Aβ, which in turn causes functional impairment of mitochondria in AD [26]. Translocation of cyclophilin D (CypD), a Ca^{2+}-associated protein found in the mtPTP, from the matrix to the inner membrane caused by an interaction of Aβ with CypD, results in opening of the mtPTP and consequent mitochondrial swelling, with ensuing cellular and synaptic alterations [28]. Deficiency of CypD has been shown to attenuate Aβ-induced mitochondrial oxidative stress, thereby reducing Aβ-related synaptic dysfunction and cognitive impairment [29]. From this finding it is evident that the interaction of Aβ and CypD is one of the major causes for mitochondrial pathology in AD. Therefore, the mitochondrial aspect of AD with regard to Aβ-induced free radical formation, excitation-dependent calcium overload, and its consequences for the mitochondrial membrane potential and mtPTP must be taken into account to effectively treating AD with suitable drug therapy. Prevention or reduction of increased oxidative stress seen in AD patients should be the primary goal of effective treatment for AD.

Melatonin in the Treatment of Alzheimer's Disease

Melatonin is an interesting neuroprotective agent as it shows multiple properties antagonizing oxidative stress. The proposed mechanisms on the neuroprotective effects of melatonin include its (1) antioxidant, including influences on mitochondrial metabolism; (2) antifibrillogenic; and (3) cytoskeletal, including the suppression of protein hyperphosphorylation. Although these actions are observed at pharmacological concentrations, the relevance of these findings can be appreciated if one considers the relatively high rates of melatonin secretion into the cerebrospinal fluid (CSF), uptake into the brain tissue, and metabolization of melatonin into other neuroprotective compounds such as the kynuramines N^1-acetyl-N2-formyl-5-methoxykynuramine and N^1-acetyl-5-methoxykynuramine [30]. Melatonin has been shown to prevent the death of neuroblastoma cells exposed to Aβ. Pappolla et al. (1997) [31] first demonstrated that co-incubation of murine neuroblastoma cells (N2a) with Aβ and melatonin significantly reduced several features of apoptosis including cellular shrinkage and formation of membrane blebs.

Recent studies on astrocytes show that astrocytic apoptosis contributes to the pathogenesis of AD. Astrocytes exhibit tau phosphorylation and activation of stress kinases, as seen in AD neuronal pathology. They also produce apolipoprotein-E4 (apoE4) which aggravates Aβ effects [32]. The Aβ protein and astrocyte-neuron interaction potentiates the neurodegeneration of AD. During interaction with Aβ, astrocytes lose control over glial nitric oxide production, thereby forming neurotoxic peroxynitrate. Treatment of C6 astroglioma cells with melatonin effectively prevents the increase in nitric oxide production induced by Aβ [33].

Studies on the possible antioxidative and anti-apoptotic actions of melatonin in arresting neuronal lesions have been done using animal models of AD. Okadaic acid induces physiological and biochemical changes similar to those seen in AD. Following administration of okadaic acid, increased levels of 4-hydroxynonenal (a product of lipid peroxidation) in cultured neuronal cells (SY5Y cells) has been found [34]. In another study, the effect of okadaic acid on NIE 115 neuronal cells was effectively prevented with administration of antioxidants like vitamin C or melatonin [35]. In this study, melatonin was found superior to vitamin C as it prevented free radical-induced damage with greater efficiency and increased the activities of enzymes glutathione-S transferase and glutathione reductase, which were not found with vitamin C [35]. In a model of APP 695 Tg mice, senile plaques appear in the cerebral cortex as early as the age of 8 months. These mice have behavioral manifestations and memory impairments as seen in AD patients. Administration of melatonin (10 mg/kg) ameliorated learning and memory deficits and reduced the number of apoptotic neurons in these mice [36].

Anti-amyloid Actions of Melatonin: Molecular Mechanisms

Melatonin exerts its anti-amyloid actions through several mechanisms. Aβ by inducing oxidative stress damages mitochondrial DNA, forms protein carbonyl, induces lipid peroxidation, impairs mitochondrial membrane structure and respiration, and breaks down the mitochondrial membrane potential. All these actions that produce mitochondrial dysfunction are prevented by melatonin administration. Melatonin also inhibits the formation of amyloid fibrils, as demonstrated by different techniques. Both $A\beta_{1-40}$ and $A\beta_{1-42}$ peptides are effectively inhibited by melatonin [37, 38]. A structural analog of melatonin, namely, indole-3-propionic acid, not only shares melatonin's radical scavenging activity [39] but also exhibits similar or even higher antifibrillogenic activity. Melatonin reverses the pro-fibrillogenic activity of apoE4 and antagonizes neurotoxicity induced by combinations of Aβ and apoE4 or apoE3 [40]. Melatonin also reverses glycogen synthase kinase-3 activation which shows that melatonin not only acts as an antioxidant but also interferes with the phosphorylation system, especially stress kinases [41]. Melatonin has attenuated tau hyperphosphorylation induced by wortmannin [42]. Tyrosine kinase receptors [43], important elements of the phosphorylation system, and neurotrophins are adversely affected by Aβ and other oxidotoxins. In neuroblastoma cells, melatonin normalized tyrosine kinase receptor and neurotrophin expression [43]. A schematic diagram showing the neuroprotective actions of melatonin are presented in Fig. 16.1 and additional information is provided in Table 16.1.

Melatonin's Neuroprotective Role for Mitochondrial Homeostasis in Alzheimer's Disease

The neuroprotective role of melatonin in AD not only depends upon its radical scavenging action but also on its additional actions such as protecting the mitochondrial membranes and mitochondrial DNA from oxidative insults, stimulation of glutathione synthesis, reduction of oxidized glutathione levels, and maintenance of mitochondrial electron flux. The electron transport chain (ETC) represents a major source of ROS within the cell [44]. Complex I and III of the ETC have been identified as the two principal sites of superoxide anion (O_2^-) generation [45]. The O_2^- formed is disposed of by several pathways. A portion of it re-donates electrons to the ETC at cytochrome c [46]. Another fraction is converted into H_2O_2 and O_2 by the mitochondrial manganese-containing subform of superoxide dismutase [47]. Melatonin's mitochondrial actions take place within the organelle. Melatonin, which

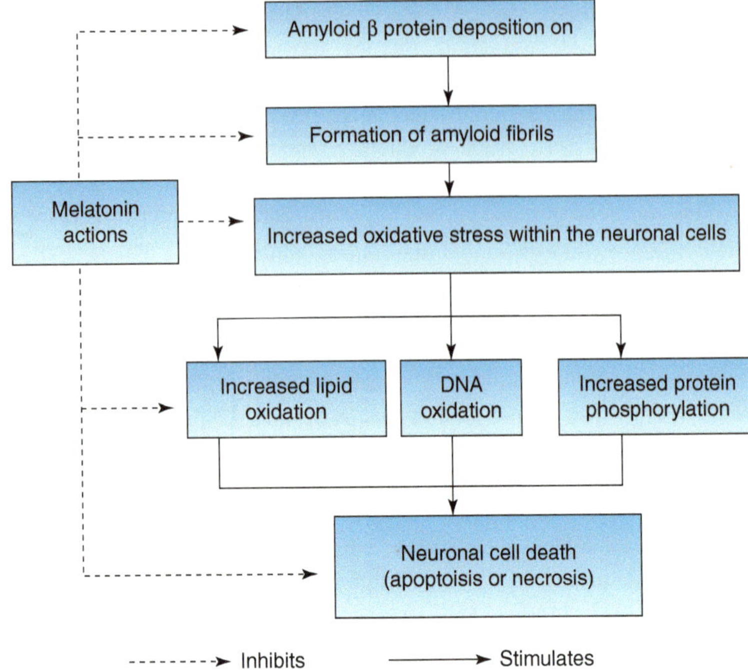

Fig. 16.1 Pathophysiology of Alzheimer's disease and melatonin's neuroprotective actions

Table 16.1 Summary of melatonin's neuroprotective effects in Alzheimer's disease Mechanisms

1. Inhibition of amyloid β-protein deposition
2. Inhibits the formation of amyloid fibrils
3. Scavenges free radicals induced by amyloid β-protein
4. Inhibits lipid peroxidation reactions in neural tissue
5. Suppresses protein hyperphosphorylation
6. Activates GSK3 (glycogen synthase kinase)
7. Prevents cytoskeletal disorganization
8. Improves sleep quality in Alzheimer's disease patients and thereby arrests neurodegenerative development

Table 16.2 Summary of melatonin's beneficial actions on mitochondrial physiology and metabolism in amyloid-β-induced neural tissues

1. Prevents intramitochondrial effects of amyloid β effects
2. Prevents opening of mitochondrial transition pores
3. Increases mitochondrial respiratory enzyme complex activities
4. Safeguards electron flow through transport chain
5. Increases intramitochondrial glutathione pool
6. Prevents intramitochondrial lipid peroxidation
7. Prevents mitochondrial DNA oxidation
8. Increases ATP synthesis
9. Prevents cell death by necrotic effects or apoptotic effects

possesses a balanced amphiphilicity, crosses the cell membranes with ease and is concentrated within subcellular compartments [48]. Melatonin's effects on electron flux have two aspects. Firstly, it increases the activities of mitochondrial respiratory complexes I and IV in a time-dependent manner [49]. This effect of melatonin, namely, the improvement of electron transport capacity in mitochondria, is remarkable as these effects are observed in senescence-accelerated mice [50]. Secondly, melatonin antagonizes calcium overload which can perturb the mitochondrial membrane potential. Melatonin has been shown to prevent calcium overload and counteract the collapse of the mitochondrial membrane potential induced by H_2O_2 [51], and it also inhibited the opening of the mtPTP, thereby preventing the occurrence of apoptosis. A summary of melatonin's neuroprotective actions on mitochondrial physiology and metabolism are presented in Table 16.2 and Fig. 16.2. Melatonin also activates signalling pathways, namely, the Bcl-2 pathway that stabilizes mitochondrial

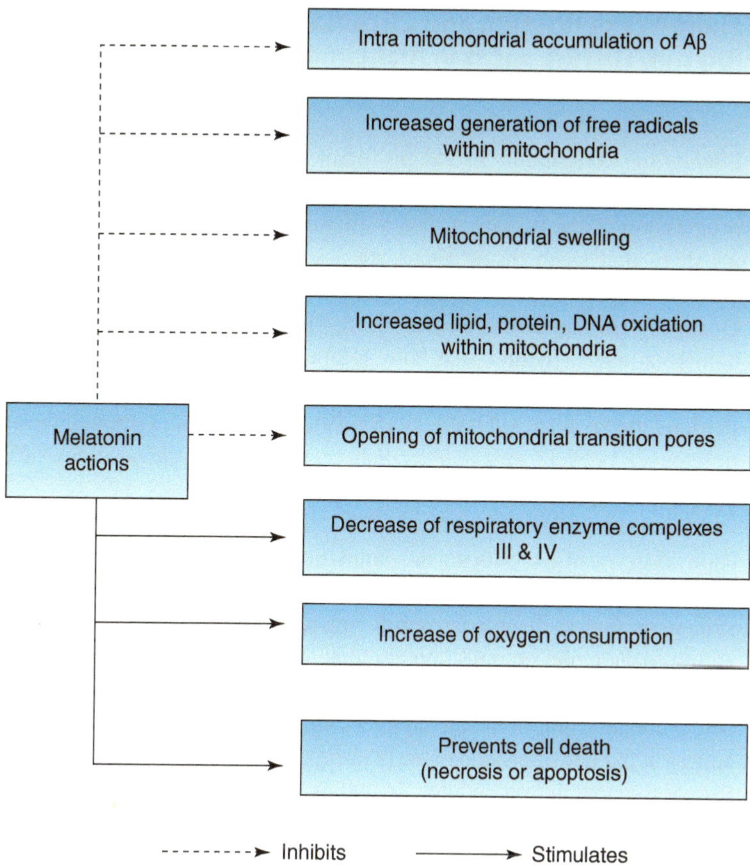

Fig. 16.2 Melatonin's effects on mitochondrial pathophysiology in Alzheimer's disease

function by antiapoptotic Bcl-2 family modulators. Melatonin enhances Bcl-2 expression with consequent inhibition of Aβ-induced cell death [52]. Caspase-3 is known to be directly linked to cytochrome c release and is related to cell death in AD [53], and this is downregulated by melatonin. Thus, the apoptosis-inducing factors liberated during mitochondrial damage are effectively inhibited by melatonin through a variety of mechanisms, which in turn prevents the neuronal cell death seen in AD.

Melatonin's Neuroprotective Actions in Alzheimer's Disease

Glutamate receptors, specifically *N*-Methyl-D-aspartate receptors, are involved in the pathophysiology of AD [54]. Excessive glutamate activity causing excessive calcium influx activates a number of enzymes including phospholipases, endonucleases, neuronal nitric oxide synthase, and proteases that can result in neuronal toxicity leading to several neurodegenerative diseases including AD [54]. Melatonin shows a neuroprotective effect by reducing the NMDA-induced high Ca^{2+} influx. The regulation of intracellular Ca^{2+} by melatonin is explained through its action on melatonin MT2 receptors, and cAMP-dependent protein kinase (PKA) is involved in the activation of calcium channels. Melatonin, by acting through MT2 receptors, decreases cAMP formation and thereby blocks PKA activation [55]. Both MT1 and MT2 receptors are found to be decreased in the cortical regions of AD patients [56].

Sleep-Wake Rhythm and Circadian Rhythm Disturbances in Alzheimer's Disease

Studies in AD patients reveal profound disturbances in sleep-wake cycles that correlate with progression of the disease. Cross-sectional studies show that sleep disturbances are associated with memory and cognitive impairments. Disruption of the circadian timing system and numerous overt rhythms like body temperature, glucocorticoid, melatonin, and other hormonal rhythms are seen in AD patients [57–59]. Phase differences between rest-activity and core body temperature cycles are also significantly delayed in AD patients [60]. A chronobiological phenomenon observed in AD patients in conjunction with sleep-wake disturbances is *sundowning*, in which symptoms such as disorganized thinking, reduced ability to maintain attention on external stimuli, and motor disturbances like agitation, wandering, perceptual, and emotional disturbances all tend to appear in the late afternoon or early evening [61]. Chronotherapeutic procedures including exposure to bright light in selected circadian phases alleviated sundowning symptoms including wandering, agitation, and delirium and also improved sleep-wake patterns in AD patients [62].

Melatonin Levels in Alzheimer's Disease

Studies have shown that melatonin levels are lower in AD patients compared to age-matched controls [63–66]. Decreased CSF melatonin levels in AD patients were attributed to reduced melatonin production rather than to the diluting effects of CSF. CSF melatonin levels decreased even in preclinical stages (Braak stage 1) when patients did not yet manifest cognitive impairment, suggesting that a reduction in CSF melatonin may be an early marker for the first stages of AD [66, 67]. The decreased melatonin level in AD has also been attributed to defective retinohypothalamic tract or suprachiasmatic nucleus-pineal connections. However, decreased nocturnal melatonin levels correlate with the severity of mental impairment of patients with dementia [68]. Recently, it has been suggested that the choroid plexus portal theory of CSF circulation gives an explanation for the neuropathology of AD. Contrary to earlier views expressed in medical text books that the CSF absorption occurs through the arachnoid granules into the superior sagittal sinus, present evidence indicates that CSF is moved from the choroid fissure into the ventricular system. Understanding of the consequences of deficient CSF melatonin together with the understanding of the CSF circulation through these portals may provide answers to the puzzles of AD pathophysiology [69].

Melatonin's Potential Therapeutic Value in Alzheimer's Disease

Replacement of physiological levels of melatonin in the brain as AD patients have a profound deficiency in endogenous melatonin production may represent a treatment for arresting the progress of AD. Melatonin's vasoprotective properties could conceivably help in maintaining cerebral blood flow and might therefore help to reduce clinical deterioration of AD patients. In addition, AD patients show a greater breakdown of the circadian sleep-wake cycle when compared to similarly aged non-demented controls. Amelioration of sleep disturbances is of paramount importance in treating AD patients as sleep disturbances exacerbate memory and cognitive impairment [70]. In a study conducted in 14 AD patients with 6–9 mg of melatonin/day and follow-up over a 2–3 year period, it was noted that melatonin improved sleep quality in most of the patients [71, 72]. Sundowning, diagnosed clinically, was no longer detectable in 12 out of 14 patients, and reductions in cognitive impairment and amnesia were noted [71, 72]. This should be contrasted with significant deterioration of the clinical conditions of the disease expected in patients after a 1–3 year evolution of AD [72]. A number of other studies support the efficacy of melatonin in treating AD patients. Administration of melatonin (6 mg/day) for 4 weeks to 7 AD patients reduced aberrant night-time activity compared to placebo [73]. Alleviation of sundowning and sleep improvement was reported in 11 elderly AD patients treated with melatonin (3 mg/day at bedtime) [62]. In this study, a significant decrease in agitated behavior and daytime sleepiness were also noted. Reduction of sundowning with the administration of 3 mg of melatonin was reported using actigraphy in 7 AD patients [74]. In a double-blind study conducted in AD patients, it was noted that 3 mg/day of melatonin significantly prolonged actigraphically evaluated sleep time, decreased activity at night-time, and improved cognitive functions [75]. In a multicenter, randomized, placebo-controlled clinical trial in a large sample of 157 AD patients with sleep disturbances, patients were randomly assigned to one of three treatment groups (placebo, 2.5 mg slow release melatonin or 10 mg melatonin). Melatonin or placebo was administered for a period of 2 months with actigraphic monitoring, and an increased nocturnal total sleep time and decreased waking after sleep onset was noted in the melatonin group. A significant improvement in sleep quality on subjective measures using caregiver ratings was noted in the 2.5 mg sustained-release melatonin group as compared to the placebo group [76]. Nevertheless, in a recent study, melatonin 8.5 mg immediate release and 1.5 mg sustained release was administered at 10.00 PM for ten consecutive nights to patients with AD. There was no significant difference between placebo and melatonin on sleep, circadian rhythms, or agitation [77]. Supraphysiological dose of melatonin has been attributed to the lack of beneficial effect of melatonin on sleep. Melatonin can also act at multiple different levels besides tackling the sleep and circadian rhythm disturbances seen in AD. The antioxidant, mitochondrial, and antiamyloidogenic effects of melatonin can be viewed as potentially interfering with the onset of AD. As such, melatonin has several obvious advantages over other comparable compounds, including most other antioxidants. The question of whether melatonin has therapeutic value in preventing or treating AD, affecting disease initiation, or progression of the neuropathology and its driving mechanisms, remains to be answered by future multicenter double-blind clinical trials. In the meantime, it is suggested that improvement of insomnia in neurodegenerative conditions specifically in AD with melatonin represents a clinically effective option that potentially may also help in arresting the progression of the disease as well as offering neuroprotection against the development of AD.

Melatonin-Lithium Combination and Ramelteon for Treatment of Alzheimer's Disease

In a recent review of psychopharmacological approaches to neuroprotection, Lauterbach et al. (2010) suggested a trial of lithium (a mood stabilizer) with melatonin since this combination can potentially synergize neuroprotective effects on Aβ, hyperphosphorylated tau, ROS, mtPTP, and apoptosis, with lithium also potentially improving ubiquitylation [78]. It is suggested that treatments lowering plasma Aβ will be beneficial for reducing the risk of developing AD.

Ramelteon, the newly developed melatonergic agonist, exhibits greater affinity for MT1/MT2 melatonin receptors than melatonin itself. It has been suggested that melatonin's neuroprotective effects might be enhanced by the rapid onset of action of ramelteon when applied in the treatment of AD [79]. A neuroprotective neurotrophic effect of ramelteon in AD is suggested by the recent finding in which ramelteon increased the neural content of brain-derived neurotrophic factor (BDNF) in cultured mouse cerebellar granule cells [80]. Both melatonin and ramelteon may have important roles in treating AD given melatonin's involvement in the possible etiology of AD as well as the hypnotic and chronobiotic properties of both drugs. As melatonin and its receptors are involved in the regulation of neurotrophic factors as well as in neurodevelopment, and if ramelteon treatment is efficient in regulating brain BDNF levels, these melatoninergic compounds will have promising roles as therapeutic agents in treating AD and other neurodegenerative diseases [81]. Since melatonin also exerts its neuroprotective actions by modulating intramitochondrial energy regulating complexes, ramelteon also may exert intramitochondrial actions and may prove to be beneficial in arresting AD progression [82].

Conclusion

Melatonin has established clinical effects on sleep disturbances and other clinical features of AD. Deposition of Aβ protein, oxidative stress, and their neurotoxic effects are suggested as the major contributing factors for the pathogenesis of AD. Intramitochondrial accumulation of Aβ protein, inhibition of respiratory complexes, increased electron leakage, decreased oxygen consumption, and decline of adenosine-5′-triphosphate (ATP) levels caused by increased oxidative stress are the major reasons for the neuronal cell death seen in AD. As melatonin has significant antioxidant properties, it can be of therapeutic value in arresting the progression of AD. Since ramelteon has greater potency in activating MT1 and MT2 melatonin receptors, it may increase the antioxidative capacity of AD patients by increasing the synthesis of antioxidative enzymes and, thereby, has potential therapeutic value in treating AD patients. Moreover, its action of regulating BDNF levels also suggests neuroprotective potential in treating AD. Multicenter clinical trials of ramelteon and melatonin are now required for proving the efficacy of the melatonergic drug ramelteon in the treatment of AD.

References

1. Vollicer L, Crino B. Involvement of free radicals in dementia of Alzheimer's type hypothesis. Neurobiol Aging. 1990;11:567–71.
2. Markesbery W. Oxidative stress hypothesis in Alzheimer's disease. Free Radic Biol Med. 1997;23: 134–47.
3. Christen Y. Oxidative stress and Alzheimer's disease. Am J Clin Nutr. 2000;71:621S–9.
4. Smith MA, Rottkamp CA, Nunomura A, Raina AK, Perry G. Oxidative stress in Alzheimer's disease. Biochim Biophys Acta. 2000;1502:139–44.
5. Srinivasan V. Melatonin oxidative stress and neurodegenerative diseases. Indian J Exp Biol. 2002;40: 668–79.
6. Subbarao KV, Richardson JS, Ang LS. Autopsy samples of Alzheimer's cortex show increased peroxidation in vitro. Neurochem Res. 1990;55:342–5.
7. Pamplona R, Dalfo E, Ayala V, Bellmunt MJ, Prat J, Ferrer I, et al. Proteins in human brain cortex are modified by oxidation, glyco-oxidation and lipoxidation. Effects of Alzheimer's disease and identification of lipoxidation targets. J Biol Chem. 2005;280:21522–30.
8. Vina J, lloret A. Why women have more Alzheimer's disease than men: gender and mitochondrial toxicity of amyloid-beta peptide. J Alzheimers Dis. 2010;20(S2):527–33.
9. Simon AM, Frechilla D, del Rio J. Perspectives on the amyloid cascade hypothesis of Alzheimer's disease. Rev Neurol. 2010;50(11):667–75.
10. Crews L, Masliah E. Molecular mechanisms of neurodegeneration in Alzheimer's disease. Hum Mol Genet. 2010;19(R1):R12–20.
11. Swerdlow RH, Burns JM, Khan SM. The Alzheimer's disease: mitochondrial cascade hypothesis. J Alzheimers Dis. 2010;20(S2):265–79.
12. Aarsland D, Sharp S, Ballard C. Psychiatric and behavioural symptoms in Alzheimer's disease and other dementias: etiology and management. Curr Neurol Neurosci Rep. 2005;5:345–54.
13. Alzheimer's Association. Alzheimer's disease facts and figures. Chicago: Alzheimer's Association; 2007.
14. Rice DP, Fillit HM, Max W, Knopman DS, Lloyd JR, Dasgupta S. Prevalence, cost and treatment of Alzheimer's disease and related dementia: a managed care perspective. Am J Manag Care. 2001;7(8):809–18.
15. Pappolla MA, Chyan Y-J, Bozner P, Soto C, Reiter RJ, Brewer G, et al. Dual anti-amyloidogenic and anti-oxidant properties of melatonin. A new therapy for Alzheimer's disease. In: Iqbal K, Mortimer JA, Winblad B, Wisniewski HM, editors. Research advance in Alzheimer's disease. New York: Wiley; 1999. p. 661–9.
16. Hensley K, Carney JM, Mattson MP, Aksenova M, Harris M, Wu JF, Floyd RA, Butterfield DA. A model for beta amyloid aggregation and neurotoxicity based on free radical generation by the peptide relevance to Alzheimer's disease. Proc Natl Acad Sci U S A. 1994;91:3270–4.
17. Hock C, Heese K, Muller-Spahn F, Hulette C, Rosenberg C, Otten U. Decreased trkA neurotrophin receptor expression in the parietal cortex of patients with Alzheimer's disease. Neurosci Lett. 1998;241:151–4.
18. Markesbery WR, Carney JM. Oxidative alterations in Alzheimer's disease. Brain Pathol. 1999;9:133–46.
19. Raha S, Robinson BH. Mitochondria, oxygen free radicals, disease and aging. Trends Biochem Sci. 2000;25:502–8.
20. Lenaz G. The mitochondrial production of reactive oxygen species: mechanisms and implications in human pathology. IUBMB Life. 2001;52:159–64.
21. Kim JS, He L, Lemasters JJ. Mitochondrial permeability transition pore: a common pathway to necrosis

and apoptosis. Biochem Biophys Res Commun. 2003;304:463–70.

22. Muller WE, Eckert A, Kurz G, Eckert GP, Leuner K. Mitochondrial dysfunction: common final pathway in brain aging and Alzheimer' disease – therapeutic aspects. Mol Neurobiol. 2010;41(2–3):159–71.
23. Reddy PH, Manczak M, Mao P, Calkins MJ, Reddy AP, Shirendeb U. Amyloid β and mitochondria in aging and Alzheimer's disease: implications for synaptic damage and cognitive decline. J Alzheimers Dis. 2010;20(S2):S499–512.
24. Hardy J, Selkoe DJ. The amyloid hypothesis of Alzheimer's disease: progress and problems on the road to therapeutics. Science. 2002;297:353–6.
25. Petersen CA, Alikhani N, Behbahani H, Wiehager B, Pavlov PF, Alafuzoff I, et al. The amyloid beta – peptide is imported into mitochondria via the TOM import machinery and localized to mitochondrial cristae. Proc Natl Acad Sci U S A. 2008;105:13145–50.
26. Rosales-Corral SA, Acuña-Castroviejo D, Coto-Montes A, Boga JA, Manchester LC, Fuentes-Broto L, Korkmaz A, Ma S, et al. Alzheimer's disease: pathological mechanisms and the beneficial effects of melatonin. J Pineal Res. 2012;52(2):167–202.
27. Mattson MP, Liu D. Energetics and oxidative stress in synaptic plasticity and neurodegenerative disorders. Neuromolecular Med. 2002;2:215–31.
28. Connern CP, Halestrap AP. Recruitment of mitochondrial cyclophilin to the mitochondrial inner membrane under conditions of oxidative stress that enhance the opening of a calcium–sensitive non-specific channel. Biochem J. 1994;302(S2):321–4.
29. Du H, Guo L, Fang F, Yon SS. Cyclophilin D deficiency attenuates mitochondrial and neuronal perturbations and ameliorates learning and memory in Alzheimer's disease. Nat Med. 2008;14:1097–105.
30. Reiter RJ, Tan DX. Role of CSF in the transport of melatonin. J Pineal Res. 2002;33:61.
31. Pappolla MA, Sos M, Omar RA, Bick RJ, Hickson-Bick DL, Reiter RJ. Melatonin prevents death of neuro-blastoma cells exposed to the Alzheimer amyloid peptide. J Neurosci. 1997;17:1683 90.
32. Malchiodi-Albedi F, Domenici MR, Paradisi S, Bernardo A, Ajmone-Cat MA, Minghetti L. Astrocytes contribute to neuronal impairment in βA toxicity increasing apoptosis in rat hippocampal neurons. Glia. 2001;34:68–72.
33. Feng Z, Zhang JT. Protective effect of melatonin on β–amyloid induced apoptosis in rat astroglioma C6 cells and its mechanism. Free Radic Biol Med. 2004;37:1790–801.
34. Wang J, Tung YC, Li XT, Iqbal K, Grundke-Iqbal I. Hyperphosphorylation and accumulation of neurofilament proteins in Alzheimer's disease brain and in okadaic acid treated SY5Y cells. FEBS Lett. 2001;507:81–7.
35. Montilla-Lopez P, Munoz-Agueda MC, Feijoo Lopez M, Munoz-Castaneda JR, Bujalance-Arenas I, Tunez-Finana I. Comparison of melatonin versus vitamin on oxidative stress and antioxidant enzyme activity in Alzheimer's disease induced by okadaic acid in neuroblastoma cells. Eur J Pharmacol. 2002;451:237–43.
36. Kawarabayashi T, Younkin LH, Saido TC, Shoji M, Ashe KH, Younkin SG. Age-dependent changes in brain, CSF, and plasma amyloid β protein in the Tg 2576 transgenic mouse model of Alzheimer's disease. J Neurosci. 2001;21:372–81.
37. Matsubara E, Bryant-Thomas T, Quinto JP, Hendry TL, Poeggeler B, Herbert D, et al. Melatonin increases survival and inhibits oxidative and amyloid pathology in a transgenic mouse model of Alzheimer's disease. J Neurochem. 2003;85:1101–8.
38. Cheng X, Breemen RB. Mass spectrometry – based screening for inhibitors of β-amyloid protein aggregation. Anal Chem. 2005;77:7012–5.
39. Poeggeler B, Pappolla MA, Hardeland R, Rassoulpour A, Hodgkins PS, Guidetti P, et al. Indole-3-propionic acid: a potent hydroxyl radical scavenger in rat brain. Brain Res. 2001;815:322–8.
40. Matsubara E, Sekijima Y, Tokuda T, Urakami K, Amari M, Shizuka-Ikeda M, Tomidokoro Y, et al. Soluble Aβ homeostasis in AD and DS: impairment of anti amyloidogenic protection by lipoproteins. Neurobiol Aging. 2004;25:833–41.
41. Li XC, Wang XF, Zhang JX, Wang Q, Wang JZ. Effect of melatonin on calyculin A-induced tau phosphorylation. Eur J Pharmacol. 2005;510:25–30.
42. Liu SJ, Wang JZ. Alzheimer-like tau phosphorylation induced by wortmannin in vivo and its attenuation by melatonin. Acta Pharmacol Sin. 2002;23:183–7.
43. Reyes-Toso CF, Ricci CR, de Mignone IR, Reyes PR, Linares LM, Albornoz LE, et al. In vitro effect of melatonin on oxygen consumption in liver mitochondria of rats. Neuro Endrocrinol Lett. 2003;24:341–4.
44. Barja G, Herrero A. Localization at complex I and mechanism of higher free radical production of brain nonsynaptic mitochondria in the short-lived rat than in longevous pigeon. J Bioeneg Biomembr. 1998;30: 235–43.
45. Genova ML, Merlo-Pich M, Bernacchia A, Bianchi C, Biondi A, Bovina C, et al. The mitochondrial production of reactive oxygen species in relation to aging and pathology. Ann N Y Acad Sci. 2004;1011: 86–100.
46. Fridovich I. Superoxide radical and superoxide dismutases. Annu Rev Biochem. 1995;64:97–112.
47. Menendez-Pelaez A, Poeggeler B, Reiter RJ, Barlow-Walden L, Pablos ML, Tan DX. Nuclear localization of melatonin in different mammalian species: immuno cytochemical and radioimmunoassay evidence. J Cell Biochem. 1993;53:373–82.
48. Martin M, Macias M, Leon J, Escames G, Khaldy H, Acuna-Castroviejo D. Melatonin increases the activity of the oxidative phosphorylation enzymes and the production of ATP in rat brain and liver mitochondria. Int J Biochem Cell Biol. 2002;34:348–57.
49. Okatani Y, Wakatsuki A, Reiter RJ, Miyahara Y. Acutely administered melatonin restores hepatic mitochondrial physiology in old mice. Int J Biochem Cell Biol. 2003;35:367–75.

50. Jou M-J, Peng T-I, Reiter RJ, Jou SB, Wu HY, Wen ST. Visualization of anti oxidative effects of melatonin at the mitochondrial level during oxidative stress-induced apoptosis of rat brain astrocytes. J Pineal Res. 2004;37:55–70.
51. Jang MH, Jung SB, Lee MH, Kim CJ, Oh YT, Kang I, et al. Melatonin attenuates amyloid beta- induced apoptosis in mouse microglial BV2 cells. Neurosci Lett. 2005;380(1–2):26–31.
52. Aliev G, Palacious HH, Walrafen B, Lipsitt AE, Obrenovich ME, Morales L. Brain mitochondria as a primary target in the development of treatment strategies for Alzheimer's disease. Int J Biochem Cell Biol. 2009;41:1989–2004.
53. Louneva N, Cohen JW, Han LY, Talbot K, Wilson RS, Bennelt DA, et al. Caspase-3, is enriched in postsynaptic densities and increased in Alzheimer's disease. Am J Pathol. 2008;173:1488–95.
54. Lau A, Tymianski M. Glutamate receptors, neurotoxicity and neuro-degeneration. Pflugers Arch. 2010;460:525–42.
55. Slaner O, Pelisek V, Vanecek J. Melatonin inhibits pituitary adenylyl cyclase-activating polypeptide–induced increase of cyclic AMP accumulation and [Ca2+] in cultured cells of neonatal rat pituitary. Neurochem Int. 2000;36:213–9.
56. Brunner P, Sozer-Topcular N, Jockers R, Ravid R, Fraschini F, Eckert A, et al. Pineal and cortical melatonin receptors MT1 and MT2 are decreased in Alzheimer's disease. Eur J Histochem. 2006;50: 311–6.
57. Harper DG, Stopa EG, McKee AC, Satlin A, Harlan PC, Goldstein R, et al. Differential circadian rhythm disturbances in men with Alzheimer's disease and frontotemporal degeneration. Arch Gen Psychiatry. 2001;58:353–60.
58. Giubilei F, Patacchioli FR, Antonini G, Sepe MM, Tisei P, Bastianello S, et al. Altered circadian cortisol secretion in Alzheimer's disease: clinical and neuroradiological aspects. J Neurosci Res. 2001;66:262–5.
59. Mishima K, Tozawa T, Satoh K, Matsumoto Y, Hishikawa Y, Okawa M. Melatonin secretion rhythm disorders in patients with senile dementia of Alzheimer's type with disturbed sleep-waking. Biol Psychiatry. 1999;45:417–21.
60. van Someren EJW. Circadian rhythms and sleep in human aging. Chronobiol Int. 2000;17:233–43.
61. Cohen-Mansfield J, Garfinekel D, Lipson S. Melatonin for treatment of sundowning in elderly persons with dementia – a preliminary study. Arch Gerontol Geriatr. 2000;31:65–76.
62. Yamadera H, Ito T, Susuki H, Asayama K, Ito R, Endo S. Effects of bright light on cognitive and sleep-wake (circadian) rhythm disturbances in Alzheimer type of dementia. Psychiatry Clin Neurosci. 2000;54:352–3.
63. Uchida K, Okamoto N, Ohara K, Morita Y. Daily rhythm of serum melatonin in patients with dementia of the degenerative type. Brain Res. 1996;717:154–9.
64. Ohashi Y, Okamoto K, Uchida K, Iyo M, Mori N, Morita Y. Daily rhythm of serum melatonin levels and effect of light exposure in patients with dementia of the Alzheimer's disease. Biol Psychiatry. 1999;145:1646–52.
65. Wu YH, Matthijis GP, Feenstra MG, Zhou JN, SastrTorano J, Van Kan HJ, et al. Molecular changes underlying reduced pineal melatonin levels in Alzheimer's disease: alterations in preclinical and clinical stages. J Clin Endocrinol Metab. 2003;88:5898–906.
66. Zhou JN, Liu RY, Kamphorst W, Hofman MA, Swaab DF. Early neuro-pathological Alzheimer's changes in aged individuals are accompanied by decreased cerebrospinal fluid melatonin levels. J Pineal Res. 2003;35:125–30.
67. Skene DJ, Swaab DF. Melatonin rhythmicity: effect of age and Alzheimer's disease. Exp Gerontol. 2003;38:199–206.
68. Magri F, Locatelli M, Balza G, Molla G, Cuzzoni G, Fioravanti M, et al. Changes in endocrine circadian rhythms as markers of physiological and pathological brain ageing. Chronobiol Int. 1997;14:385–96.
69. Maurizi CP. Choroid plexus portals and a deficiency of melatonin can explain the neuropathology of Alzheimer's disease. Med Hypotheses. 2010;74: 1059–66.
70. McCurry SM, Reynolds CF, Ancoli-Israel S, Teri L, Vitiello MV. Treatment of sleep disturbance in Alzheimer's disease. Sleep Med Rev. 2000;4:603–28.
71. Brusco LJ, Marquez M, Cardinali DP. Melatonin treatment stabilizes chronobiological and cognitive symptoms in Alzheimer's disease. Neuro Endocrinol Lett. 1998;19:111–5.
72. Brusco LI, Marquez M, Cardinali DP. Monozygotic twins with Alzheimer's disease treated with melatonin. Case report. J Pineal Res. 1998;25:260–8.
73. Mishima K, Okawa M, Hozumi S, Hishikawa Y. Supplementary administration of artificial bright light and melatonin as potent treatment for disorganized circadian rest activity and dysfunctional autonomic and neuroendocrine systems in institutionalized demented elderly patients. Chronobiol Int. 2000;17:419–32.
74. Mahlberg R, Kunz D, Sutej I, Kuhl KP, Hellweg R. Melatonin treatment of day-night rhythm disturbances and sundowning in Alzheimer's disease an open-label pilot study using actigraphy. J Clin Psychopharmacol. 2004;24:456–9.
75. Asayama K, Yamadera H, Ito T, Suzuki H, Kudo Y, Endo S. Double blind study of melatonin effects on the sleep-wake rhythm; cognitive and non-cognitive functions in Alzheimer type dementia. J Nippon Med Sch. 2003;70:334–41.
76. Singer C, Tractenberg RE, Kaye J, Schafer K, Gamst A, Grundtman M, et al. A multicenter, placebo controlled trial of melatonin for sleep disturbances in Alzheimer's disease. Sleep. 2003;26:893–901.

77. Gehrman PR, Connor DJ, Martin JL, Shochat T, Corey-Bloom J, Ancoli-Israel S. Melatonin fails to improve sleep or agitation in double-blind randomized placebo-controlled trial of institutionalized patients with Alzheimer's disease. Am J Geriatr Psychiatry. 2010;17:166–9.
78. Lauterbach EC, Victoroff J, Coburn KL, Shillcutt SD, Doonan SM, Mendez MF. Psychopharmacological neuroprotection in neurodegenerative disease: assessing the preclinical data. J Neuropsychiatry Clin Neurosci. 2010;22(1):8–18.
79. Lauterbach EC, Shillcutt SD, Victoroff J, Coburn KL, Mendez MF. Psychopharmacological neuroprotection in neurodegenerative disease: heuristic clinical applications. J Neuropsychiatry Clin Neurosci. 2010;22(2):130–54.
80. Imbesi M, Uz T, Dzitoyeva S, Manev H. Stimulatory effects of melatonin receptor agonist, ramelteon, on BDNF in mouse cerebellar granule cells. Neurosci Lett. 2008;439(1):34–6.
81. Srinivasan V, Kaur C, Pandi-Perumal S, Brown GM, Cardinali DP. Melatonin and its agonist ramelteon in Alzheimer's disease: possible therapeutic value. Int J Alzheimers Dis. 2011. doi:10.4061/2011/741974.
82. Srinivasan V, Lauterbach EC, Ahmed AH, Prasad A. Alzheimer's disease: focus on the neuroprotective role of melatonin. J Neurol Res. 2012. doi:10.402/jnr93w.

Melatonin in Parkinson's Disease and Its Therapeutic Potential

17

V. Srinivasan, U.S. Srinivasan, Charanjit Kaur, Rahimah Zakaria, Zahiruddin Othman, Edward C. Lauterbach, and Dario Acuña-Castroviejo

Abstract

Although the etiology of Parkinson's disease (PD) is not known, most patients with PD experience sleep-related problems like difficulty in initiating and maintaining sleep, excessive daytime sleepiness, sleep fragmentation, and reductions in non-REM or REM sleep. Since melatonin and its analogues have sleep promoting and sleep-wake rhythm-regulating actions, interest has been focused on the role of melatonin in PD. Interestingly use of melatonin in animal models of PD has shown that melatonin has been useful in improving the neurotoxic effects of administration of 1-methyl-4-phenyl-1,2,3,6-tetrahydropyridine (MPTP), rotenone,

V. Srinivasan, MSc, PhD, MAMS (✉)
Sri Sathya Sai Medical Educational and Research Foundation, An International Medical Sciences Research Study Center, Prasanthi Nilayam, 40-Kovai Thirunagar Extn, Goldwins, Coimbatore, TN 641014, India

National Health Service, Department of Mental Health, Psychiatric Service of Diagnosis and Treatment, Hospital "G. Mazzini", ASL 4, Teramo, Italy

Department of Neuroscience and Imaging, University "G.D' Annunzio", Chieti 66013, Italy
e-mail: sainivasan@yahoo.com, venkataramanujamsrinivasan6@gmail.com

U.S. Srinivasan, MBBS, MCh
Department of Neurosurgery, Fortis Malar Hospital, Gandhi Nagar Main Road, Adyar, Chennai, TN 600020, India
e-mail: sanjoosmruthi@yahoo.com

C. Kaur, MBBS, PhD
Department of Anatomy, Yong Loo Lin School of Medicine, National University of Singapore, BLK MD 10, 4 Medical Drive, Singapore 117597, Singapore
e-mail: antkaurc@nus.edu.sg

R. Zakaria, MBBS, PhD (Physiology)
Department of Physiology, School of Medical Sciences, Universiti Sains Malaysia, Kubang Kerian, Kelantan 16150, Malaysia
e-mail: rahimah@kck.usm.my

Z. Othman, MD, MMed (Psychiatry)
Department of Psychiatry, School of Medical Sciences, Hospital Universiti Sains Malaysia, Kubang Kerian, Kelantan 16150, Malaysia
e-mail: zahir@kb.usm.my

E.C. Lauterbach, MD
Department of Psychiatry and Behavioral Sciences and the Department of Internal Medicine, Neurology Section, Mercer University School of Medicine, 655 First Street, Macon, GA 31201, USA
e-mail: eclbgnp@earthlink.net

D. Acuña-Castroviejo, MD, PhD
Department of Physiology, Centro de Investigación Biomédica, Parque de Ciencias de la Salud, Avda. del Conocimiento s/n, Armilla, Granada 18100, Spain
e-mail: dacuna@ugr.es

V. Srinivasan et al. (eds.), *Melatonin and Melatonergic Drugs in Clinical Practice*, DOI 10.1007/978-81-322-0825-9_17, © Springer India 2014

or maneb and paraquat. Being an antioxidant melatonin counteracted the MPTP-induced lipid per oxidation. The finding of reduced expression of MT_1 and MT_2 melatonin receptors in amygdale and substantia nigra of patients with PD supports the involvement of melatonergic system in the possible etiology of PD. Use of melatonin or its analogues may be beneficial in treating patients with PD for improving the sleep quality and also for enhancing the neuroprotection against oxidative stress seen in PD.

Keywords
Parkinson's disease • Melatonin • Oxidative stress • Sleep quality • Neuroprotection

Introduction

The development of age-related diseases like Alzheimer disease, Parkinson's disease (PD), and other neurodegenerative diseases has been attributed in part to an increased generation of free radicals and associated enhanced oxidative stress seen in these patients [1, 2]. The central nervous system exhibits a high susceptibility to oxidative stress because of its high oxygen consumption rate. Moreover the brain is enriched with polyunsaturated fatty acids that render it easily susceptible to oxidative attack [3]. The neuronal death or damage that occurs following the oxidative attack leads to disruption and loss of certain physiological functions and behaviors crucial for normal living. In this chapter, attention is focused on the possible etiology of PD and primary features of PD including sleep disturbances. This chapter considers how melatonin deficiency is involved in the etiology of PD and how it can be helpful both as an effective antioxidant and as a sleep regulator in controlling PD sleep disturbances. Free radicals are an initiating factor in PD [4]. Indeed enhanced oxidative stress has been demonstrated in the brain of PD patients [5]. Studies reveal that the prevalence of sleep disturbances is nearly 100 % in PD [6, 7]. As melatonin has been demonstrated to be an effective antioxidant and free radical scavenger, and as it is also involved in sleep regulation, it plays a potentially important role in both the etiology and treatment of PD [8].

Pathophysiology of PD

PD is a neurodegenerative disorder with a multifactorial etiology, but mainly due to a loss of dopaminergic nigrostriatal function. Research studies by Braak and colleagues reveal that Lewy body pathology is pronounced not only in the substantia nigra but also in many other CNS regions like the lower brainstem and autonomic nervous system, as has been evidenced in recent studies [9–11]. It is thought that other neurological and psychiatric manifestations may precede the traditional motor manifestations of PD [12]. Insomnia and depression form integral features of PD and are considered to be *primary manifestations* in PD [13]. Case–control and cohort studies suggest that depressive and anxiety disorders may be one of the earliest manifestations of PD [14, 15]. Since sleep disturbances seen in PD are associated with cognitive decline and psychiatric symptoms, attention should be focused on the development of targeted interventions in sleep [16]. A diagram showing multiple factors involved in the etiology of Parkinson's disease is presented in Figs. 17.1 and 17.2.

There is also much evidence for the possible involvement of the retino-hypothalamic system in the etiology of PD since circadian rhythm disturbances are common in this disease [17]. Parkinsonian symptoms themselves undergo circadian fluctuations. Patients with PD often experience worsening of symptoms in the afternoon and evening. Patients with PD experience

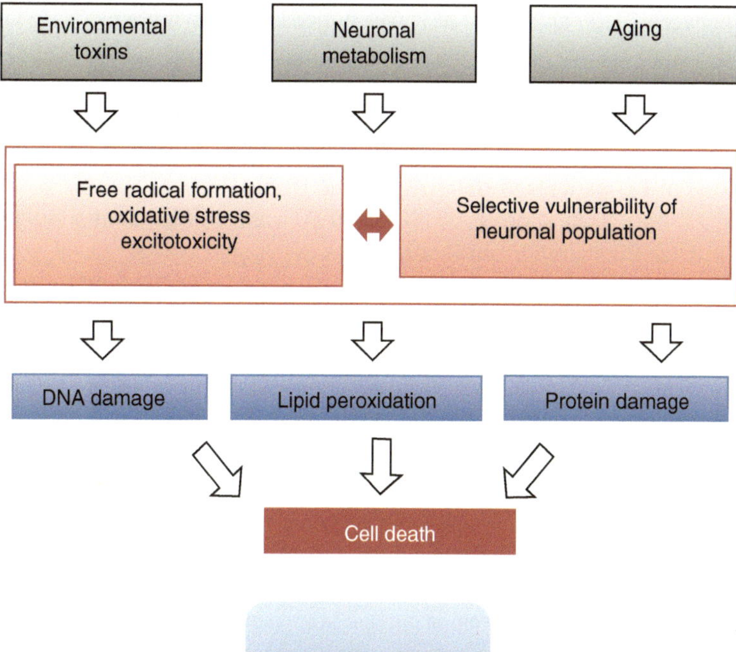

Fig. 17.1 Parkinson's disease: diagram showing various factors that trigger Parkinson's disease

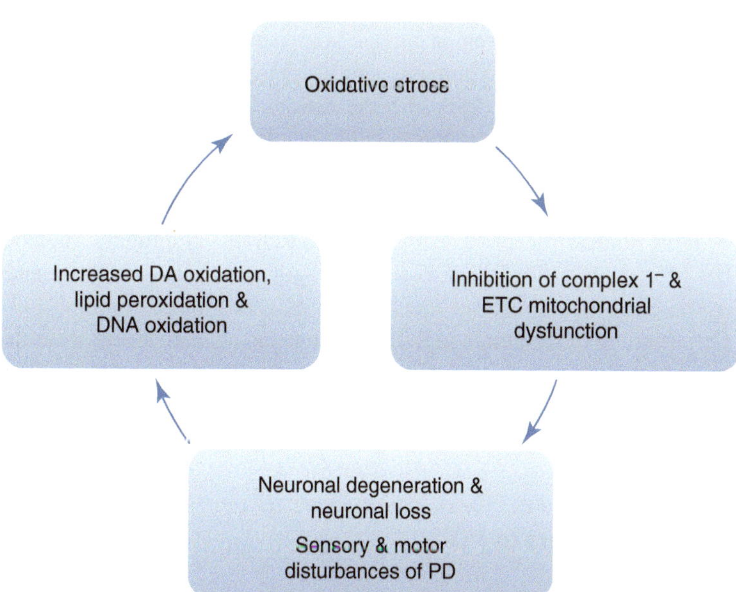

Fig. 17.2 Role of oxidative stress in the pathogenesis of Parkinson's disease

time-dependent responsiveness to dopaminergic stimulation [18]. Recently, many studies of molecular clock mechanisms regulating circadian physiology and behavior in mammals have been undertaken in both the central circadian pacemaker, the suprachiasmatic nucleus (SCN), and various peripheral tissues and cells [19]. Several circadian genes known as key "clock genes" have been identified. Of these, *Per1* and *Bmal1* are regarded as the best markers of the molecular clock. Disruptions of *Bmal1* and *Per1* in mice have been shown to cause altered circadian behavior and dysregulation of circadian patterns in gene expression [20, 21]. Circadian clock genes *Per1* and *Bmal1* have been located in leukocytes of healthy humans, and hence, study of these genes in patients with PD has been recently undertaken [22, 23]. *Per1* and *Bmal1* expression in leukocytes of patients with PD and normal controls were investigated between 21:00 and 09:00 h. It was noticed that the expression of *Bmal1* but not *Per1* was greatly reduced in PD during this dark phase, suggesting thereby that a peripheral molecular clock is altered in PD patients. Moreover *Bmal1* expression in PD patients correlated with the Unified PD Rating Scale score at 06:00 and 09:00 h and with the Pittsburgh Sleep Quality Index Score at 06:00 h [24].

Melatonin, the major neurohormone secreted by the pineal gland, is a *chronobiotic* that has significant circadian rhythm regulatory function, and it exerts its action through MT_1 and MT_2 melatonin receptors expressed in the central circadian clock, namely, the SCN of the ventral hypothalamus [25]. Melatonin receptors also have been located in other regions of the brain [26, 27]. Melatonin MT_1 and MT_2 receptors are found expressed in the human amygdala and substantia nigra of healthy humans, and decreased expression of MT_1 and MT_2 in these regions in patients with PD suggests the possible involvement of "melatonin in the pathophysiology of PD" [28]. Clock genes are also under the control of ROR nuclear receptors. Among them, RORγ has been recently identified as a direct regulator of the circadian control of clock genes in vivo [29]. Binding of melatonin to ROR receptors may be also another pathway explaining the beneficial effects of melatonin on the circadian alterations in PD patients.

Sleep Disorders in PD

Sleep disorders constitute one of the major non-motor features of PD and even serve as "preclinical marker" of the disease. Between 42 and 98 % of patients with PD experience sleep-related symptoms [6, 30, 31]. Sleep disturbances in PD encompass insomnia, excessive daytime sleepiness, and REM sleep behavior disorder (RSBD) [32]. There is difficulty in initiating and maintaining sleep [31]. These sleep disorders in PD are classified as primary sleep disorders that are intrinsic to PD and those that are secondary due to medication, etc. [33]. Among the non-motor symptoms (NMS) of PD, sleep disturbances and particularly RSBD are very important and even predict the diagnosis of PD as ascertained by motor symptoms [34, 35].

REM Sleep Behavior Disorder in PD

RSBD in PD is poorly understood and may occur as a prodromal feature predating motor symptoms by several years. Its prevalence is suggested to be 60 % in PD patients and it has been suggested to be predictive of dementia in longitudinal studies [34, 35]. RBSD is characterized by a loss of skeletal muscle atonia with prominent motor activity and dreaming [36]. Numerous cases of RBD have been found in clinically diagnosed PD [37–40]. Loss of REM sleep atonia and/or increased locomotor drive is suggested as the likely mechanism for the clinical expression of human RSBD [41]. It is a dream disorder similar to REM motor disorder and there is a tendency for the dream content to involve an aggressive, attacking, or chasing theme. Nightmare behaviors like screaming, kicking, punching, and injuring the bed partner are quite common [41, 42]. Nocturnal disturbances and sleep arousals as measured by actigraphy are specific to RSBD seen in PD [16]. Loss of hypocretin neurons and cells secreting melanin-concentrating hormone (MCH) in the hypothalamus of PD patients is said to be responsible for nocturnal insomnia, RSBD, and hallucinations. In a study conducted on the hypothalamus of 11 PD patients and five control subjects, a loss of hypothalamic hypocretin and MCH neurons has been found in PD [43]. However, a recent study undertaken in regard to these issues indicates that changes in orexin/hypocretin do not necessarily underpin RSBD sleep disturbances [44]. It is suggested that probing into the components of the circadian system that mediates the onset and timing of REM sleep, including the pattern and timing of melatonin secretion, combined with clinic pathological studies may prove to be vital for defining the neuroanatomical correlates of RSBD in PD [16].

Excessive Daytime Sleepiness

Excessive daytime sleepiness (EDS) occurs in PD patients and its prevalence ranges from 15 to 50 % [45, 46]. However, in another study, the prevalence of EDS was found to be 41 % in PD patients compared to 24 % in a control population [47]. Although it is suggested that intake of both dopamine (DA) and levodopa are contributory factors for the development of EDS, EDS also could be due to the underlying pathology of PD [46, 48].

Depression in PD

Parkinson's disease is complicated by depression, and a number of studies have used antidepressants including nortriptyline and paroxetine for controlling depressive features of PD [49, 50].

Melatonin Receptors and PD

Melatonin exerts its physiological actions through G-protein-coupled MT_1 and MT_2 melatonin receptors expressed both singly and together in various cells and tissues of the body [51, 52]. Functional melatonin receptors have been localized in the in different areas of the brain such as the SCN, cerebellum, hippocampus, and central dopaminergic pathways like the substantia nigra, caudate-putamen, ventral tegmental areas, and nucleus accumbens [53–56]. In this context it is significant to note that the expression of both MT_1 and MT_2 receptors are decreased in the substantia nigra of patients with PD. Melatonin exerts many of its physiological actions by binding with these membrane-bound MT_1 and MT_2 receptors only. A frequently observed primary effect is a reduction in cyclic AMP. A third melatonin-binding site known as MT_3 has been described and it appears to be quinine reductase [57]. Melatonin exerts some of its actions by binding with calmodulin, reticulin, as well as to nuclear receptors of the retinoic acid receptor family RZR β, RORα-1, RORα-2 [58–60]. Melatonin's much pronounced antioxidant actions are receptor independent. Melatonin is involved in the control of various physiological functions of the body including the control of reproductive processes, sleep regulation, immune mechanisms of the body, and regulation of circadian and sleep-wake rhythms [61–70]. In addition to these abovementioned physiological actions, melatonin in pharmacological doses inhibits tumor growth and has shown to be of potential therapeutic value in treating breast cancer, prostate cancer, melanoma, and cancer of the GI tract [71–73]. Melatonin also exerts antinociceptive and antiallodynic actions and this has been demonstrated in several experimental models of animal studies [74].

Melatonin's Neuroprotective Role in Animal Models of PD

Animal models employing altered brain DA function after injecting 6-hydroxydopamine (6-OHDA) into the nigrostriatal pathway of the rat, or by injecting the neurotoxin 1-methyl-4-phenyl-1,2,3,6-tetrahydropyridine (MPTP), that produce behavioral deficits are commonly employed for studying the efficacy of various therapeutic agents used for the treatment of PD [75]. The loss of DA neurons occurring in these animal models causes severe sensory and motor impairments that give rise to tremor, rigidity, and kinesis similar to those seen in PD patients [76]. In a study using the MPTP model of PD, melatonin was able to counteract MPTP-induced lipid peroxidation in striatal, hippocampal, and midbrain regions [77]. Using the same MPTP model, melatonin's ability to prevent mitochondrial damage was also demonstrated. These authors also reported that melatonin administration was able to prevent the motor disturbances induced by MPTP in a synergistic manner with deprenyl. Moreover, neuronal cell death in the nigrostriatal pathway was again demonstrated [78]. MPTP elicits its neurotoxic effects by an increase in nitric oxide (NO) radicals derived from inducible

NO synthase (iNOS) which act primarily on DA neurons, while NO radicals derived from neuronal NOS (nNOS) damage dopaminergic fibers and terminals in the striatum. Hence, it is suggested that therapies for treating PD require agents that inhibit the degenerative effects of iNOS in the substantia nigra pars compacta [79]. As melatonin can effectively downregulate iNOS and prevent NO radical formation in the brain [80], it can be considered as a potential therapeutic agent for treating PD [81, 82]. In this regard, melatonin and some melatonin derivatives have been tested as iNOS antagonists in the MPTP model of PD. In these studies, cytosolic and mitochondrial iNOS, induced by MPTP administration, were blunted after the administration of melatonin and structural analogues [83, 84].

The neuroprotective action of melatonin in experimental animal models has been found in other studies [85, 86]. In a recent study that explored melatonin's neuroprotective effect, the effects of rotenone (a specific inhibitor of the mitochondrial complex I,) were studied in rats. Rotenone produced behavioral, pathological, and biochemical manifestations that resemble those seen in PD [87, 88]. Rotenone induces neurodegeneration of the substantia nigra by releasing hydroxyl (OH) radicals that cause oxidative stress, resulting from complex I inhibition [89]. Rotenone has been shown to cause glutathione (GSH) depletion in the cell body region of the substantia nigra. Administration of melatonin at various doses (10, 20, 30 mg/kg) independently attenuated rotenone-induced GSH depletion. Moreover, a significant reduction in rotenone-induced ·OH formation and increases in the activity of mitochondrial superoxide dismutase (SOD) and catalase were also observed within the rotenone-damaged substantia nigra [90]. The results of this study support the potential beneficial effects of melatonin in treating PD.

It is suggested that 6-OHDA could be generated per se from excessive DA in the brain, and increased production of this neurotoxin could be the reason for selective degeneration of the DA-containing substantia nigra as seen in PD. Following L-dopa administration, dopaminergic nuclei and serotonergic nuclei in the brain are overloaded with DA, and this increased DA can cause production of 6-OHDA in the brain [91]. Using this concept, an in vitro study involving generation of 6-OHDA and evaluating melatonin's ability to prevent the formation of 6-OHDA. Employing a ferrous-ascorbate dopamine (FAD) hydroxyl radical generating system, the addition of DA (1 mM) caused 6-OHDA production. The DA-dependent production of 6-OHDA was decreased by melatonin in a dose-dependent manner. Similarly, an in vivo study was carried out in mice involving the daily administration of melatonin (30 mg/kg) along with L-DOPA for 7 days. Melatonin significantly reduced the L-DOPA or L-DOPA+MPTP-induced generation of striatal 6-OHDA by 21 and 32 %, respectively, when compared with the same groups not treated with melatonin. This study demonstrates that melatonin has the potential to inhibit 6-OHDA generation as demonstrated in both in vitro and in vivo studies in the brain [92]. Melatonin's neuroprotective effects in animal models of PD are summarized in Table 17.1.

Mitochondrial Dysfunction in PD and the Neuroprotective Effects of Melatonin and AMK

The MPTP model of PD is a valuable tool for studying not only the participation of various factors like oxidative/nitrosative stress, excitotoxicity, and inflammation in the pathogenesis of PD but also in studying the role of mitochondrial dysfunction in the pathogenesis of PD. MPTP is metabolized into 1-methyl-4-phenylpyridinium (MPP^+) that is taken up into the dopaminergic neurons through dopamine transporters and accumulates in the mitochondria of the substantia nigra pars compacta [93]. MPP^+, by binding with complex I of electron transport chain (ETC) and inhibiting it [94], thereby causes increased generation of reactive oxygen species (ROS). These results in oxidative damage to the ETC, reduced ATP production and nigral cell death [95–97]. MPP^+, by inducing microglial activation and iNOS expression in the substantia nigra, has been shown to produce large amounts of NO and

Table 17.1 Melatonin's neuroprotective effects in animal models of PD

Model used for PD phenotype	Effects seen	Melatonin's beneficial neuroprotective effects against PD	Reference
6-OHDA injection model	Loss of DA neurons and severe sensory and motor impairments with tremor, rigidity, and akinesia as seen in PD patients	Melatonin counteracted the neurotoxic effects of 6-OH DA injection and prevented the occurrence of sensory and motor impairments	[85, 86]
Ferrous-ascorbate DA generating system (in vitro model)	Increased 6-OHDA generation	Melatonin administration decreased 6-OHDA generation in dose-dependent manner	[92]
Maneb- or paraquat-induced nigrostriatal degeneration	Striatal DA tyrosine hydroxylase activity, decreased Increased lipid peroxidation and degenerative changes seen in nigrostriatal pathway – loss of locomotor activity	Melatonin administration delayed degenerative changes by reducing oxidative stress and improved locomotor activity	[116]
MPTP injection	Generates peroxy nitrate inhibits ETS and mitochondrial function and consequent neuronal cell death	Both melatonin and AMP counteracted the effects of MPTP, increased complex I, and reduced lipid peroxidation; nitrate prevented the neuronal cell loss	[84]

neuronal cell death [97, 98]. NO, by reacting with O_2^-, generates highly toxic peroxynitrite ($ONOO^-$) that impairs mitochondrial function by causing irreversible inhibition of all ETC complexes [99], producing neuronal cell death [100, 101]. Recently, the participation of mitochondrial iNOS (i-mtNOS) in the mitochondrial dysfunction and nigrostriatal degeneration in PD was studied in the MPTP mouse model. In this study, it was found that MPTP administration induced i-mtNOS in the mitochondria of the substantia nigra leading to marked production of NO. Moreover, complex I inhibition, NO production, and lipid peroxidation levels were significantly higher in the substantia nigra than in the striatum after treatment with MPTP. Treatment with the melatonin agonists (aMT) and N1-acetyl-5-methoxykynuramine (AMK) counteracted the effects of MPTP in both brain nuclei, increasing complex I activity above control values in substantia nigra ($P<0.001$), and striatum ($P<0.05$) mitochondria. Both aMT and AMK counteracted the effects of MPTP on lipid peroxidation levels in the cytosol ($P<0.05$) and in the mitochondria of the substantia nigra ($P<0.001$). Similarly, both aMT and AMK reduced nitrites to control values in the cytosol ($P<0.05$) and mitochondria ($P<0.001$). An emerging feature of this study is that AMK, the brain metabolite of aMT, was as efficient as aMT treatment in counteracting i-mtNOS production, oxidative stress, and mitochondrial dysfunction induced by MPTP [84]. These data indicate that the development of i-mtNOS antagonists, primarily aMT, AMT, or any other melatonin agonist, may hold promise as therapeutic strategies for treating PD [84].

Melatonin as a Therapeutic Agent in the Treatment of PD

Experimental animal studies pointed out that melatonin as an effective antioxidant has the potential for offering neuroprotection in patients with PD and for treating cognitive disorders in PD [102, 103]. Clinical studies in this direction are rather nil. However, melatonin has been used for treating sleep problems, insomnia, and daytime sleepiness. In a study undertaken in 40 patients with PD (11 women, 29 men; mean age 61.7 ± 8.4 years; range 43–76 years) for a treatment period of 2 weeks, melatonin was administered in doses ranging from 5 mg to 50 mg/day [104]. Melatonin was administered (5 or 50 mg) 30 min before bedtime to avoid any possible circadian phase shift; as such shifts can occur if melatonin is administered at any other time. All subjects were taking stable doses of antiparkinsonian medications during the course of the study. Treatment with 50 mg of melatonin significantly increased nighttime sleep ($P<0.05$) compared to placebo as revealed by actigraphy. Subjective reports of overall sleep disturbance improved significantly on 5 mg of melatonin when compared to 50 mg or placebo. It was found that high doses of melatonin (50 mg) were well tolerated in this study [104]. With the finding of reduced expression of melatonin MT_1 and MT_2 receptors in patients with PD, there is a possibility that the melatonergic system is involved in the abnormal sleep mechanisms seen in PD and in the pathophysiology of PD as well. Hence, therapeutic strategies should aim at targeting the use of melatonin and its agonists like ramelteon to treating not only the non-motor symptoms of the PD but also for preventing the progression of the disease itself. However, the use of melatonin as an adjunct therapy to either halt the progression or provide symptomatic relief in PD has been questioned [13].

Bright Light Treatment, Melatonin, and PD

Exposure to light of 1,000–1,500 lx for 1–1.5 h, 1 h prior to bedtime at 22.00 h for 2–5 weeks in 12 patients has improved the bradykinesia and rigidity observed in PD [105]. A reduction in agitation and psychiatric side effects were also reported in this study. The authors suggest that activation of the circadian system by antagonizing melatonin secretion with bright light has a therapeutic value in treating the symptoms of PD [17]. Bright light has been employed in treating depressive symptoms. But suppression of melatonin secretion is not the likely mechanism by which artificial light exerts its therapeutic effect [106]. Two possible mechanisms have been proposed for the possible therapeutic effects of bright light. First, bright light could reset the phase of abnormal circadian rhythms seen in depressed patients [106]. Secondly, evening bright light exposure, although it produces momentary melatonin suppression, actually causes a rebound increase of melatonin secretion in the late night period [107]. Bright light exposure ultimately facilitates melatonin secretion rather than suppressing it, and this is said to be responsible for the therapeutic efficacy of bright light in affective disorders. Hence, in the case of PD, bright light might also improve the symptoms of PD, but certainly not by antagonizing melatonin secretion but by instead inducing the rebound effect of enhancing melatonin secretion.

Potential Use of Melatonin Agonists in the Treatment of PD

Available evidences indicate that both sleep induction as well as maintenance of sleep at appropriate circadian phases are substantially affected in PD patients. Moreover, the onset and timing of REM sleep also is very much impaired in PD patients [16]. REM sleep behavior disorder, seen commonly in PD patients, occurs much earlier and is predictive of dementia [34, 35]. Treatment of sleep disturbances seen in PD patients with appropriate drugs may help not only in solving sleep problems but may also help to prevent the progression of PD as well. As the conventional drugs like benzodiazepines that aroused for the treatment of insomnia may worsen the cognitive and memory impairment associated with PD, a hypnotic drug lacking these side effects would be preferred. Melatonin is a likely candidate as it exerts its hypnotic and chronobiotic effects by acting through MT_1 and MT_2 receptors located in the SCN. Although melatonin significantly improves the subjective quality of sleep, sleep abnormalities persist in PD [105]. Since melatonin has a short half-life (less than 30 min), a melatonin agonist with a longer duration of action and enhanced bioavailability might be of greater benefit than melatonin in promoting sleep initiation and efficiency [108]. Recently, the melatonin agonist ramelteon, a chronohypnotic agent, has been introduced for treating patients with insomnia. Ramelteon is a novel melatonin receptor agonist at $MT_1$and MT_2 receptors and has a longer duration of action than melatonin [109]. The efficacy and safety of ramelteon in treating insomnia has been established in a number of clinical studies [110]. Ramelteon may have great therapeutic potential in treating the sleep problems seen in PD, including RSBD. Apart from treating sleep disturbances, ramelteon can alter the sleep-wake rhythm as well and, hence, can be beneficial in correcting the REM rhythm abnormality seen in PD patients. Use of the novel melatonergic antidepressant agomelatine may also be potentially quite advantageous in treating PD as it may be helpful for treating both depression and sleep disorders seen in patients with PD.

Additional Symptomatic and Neuroprotective Considerations Regarding Melatonin and Its Agonists in PD

Melatonin and the MT_1/MT_2 receptor agonist ramelteon have been considered from the standpoint of their symptomatic and neuroprotective potential in PD. In addition to the considerations detailed above, the data indicate that improved sleep by itself can engender improvements in PD motor symptoms, dementia, and behavioral and cognitive features that are quite prevalent in PD and related conditions. Indeed, melatonin itself has been reported to improve anxiety, delirium, disturbances in attention, and some aspects of memory and dementia, prominent disorders in PD [104]. Dementia in PD and the closely related dementia with Lewy bodies, delirial, attentional, and mnestic features are especially common. It is interesting to note that sleep deprivation alone promotes pathogenic protein proliferation, proteasomal dysfunction, oxidative stress, mitochondrial impairment, and neuroinflammation [111, 112]. The hypnotic advantages of these drugs have the potential to intervene therapeutically in these processes. Moreover, treatment studies of melatonin demonstrate the inhibition of pathological alpha-synuclein oligomerization and aggregation (critical to Lewy body formation in PD), dopamine autoxidation, ETC complex I and IV loss, mitochondrial degeneration, and apoptotic cascades, resulting in the preservation of nigral and striatal neurons [111, 112]. Furthermore, melatonin stimulates neurotrophins including BDNF and GDNF and promotes stem cell viability and neuritogenesis [113]. Ramelteon has been documented to stimulate BDNF production [113]. Melatonin and, its agonist, ramelteon therefore appear to have potential as symptomatic and neuroprotective treatment agents for treating patients with PD. As PD patients also manifest many psychiatric symptoms [114, 115], the use of the first melatonergic antidepressant, namely, agomelatine will be also beneficial in treating both sleep disturbances and for treating psychiatric symptoms as well.

Conclusions

Animal models of PD employing MPTP and 6-hydroxydopamine indicate that free radical generation in the nigrostriatal system is involved in the pathogenesis of PD. Since non-motor symptoms of PD like sleep disorders, particularly REM sleep disorder, occur in majority of PD patients and can present long before PD motor symptom manifestations, treating the sleep disorders of PD may be essential both for preventing and delaying the progression of this disease. Current evidence points to melatonin and melatonin receptors in PD pathophysiology. Therapeutic strategies for the control of PD should consider the therapeutic application of melatonin or its receptor agonists like ramelteon and the melatonergic antidepressant agomelatine. However, only clinical trials can prove the efficacy of melatonin and its agonists in the treatment of PD.

References

1. Olanow CW. An introduction to the free radical hypothesis in Parkinson's disease. Ann Neurol. 1992;32:S2–9.
2. Fahn S, Cohen G. The oxidant stress hypothesis in Parkinson's disease: evidence supporting it. Ann Neurol. 1992;32:804–12.
3. Reiter RJ, Tan DX, Burkhardt S. Reactive oxygen and nitrogen species and cellular and organismal decline: amelioration with melatonin. Mech Ageing Dev. 2002;123:1007–19.

4. Adams JD, Odunze IN. Oxygen free radicals and Parkinson's disease. Free Radic Biol Med. 1991;10:161–9.
5. Dexter DT, Carter CJ, Wells FR, Javoy-Agid F, Agid Y, Lees AJ, Jenner P, Marsden CD. Basal lipid peroxidation in substantia nigra is increased in Parkinson's disease. J Neurochem. 1989;52:381–9.
6. Lees AJ, Blackburn NA, Campell VL. The night time problems of Parkinson's disease. Clin Neuropharmacol. 1988;11:512–9.
7. Pal PK, Clane S, Samii A, Fleming JA. A review of normal sleep and its disturbances in Parkinson's disease. Parkinsonism Relat Disord. 1999;5:1–17.
8. Srinivasan V. Melatonin, oxidative stress and neurodegenerative diseases. Indian J Exp Biol. 2002;40: 668–79.
9. Braak H, Del Tredici K, Rub U, de Vas RAI, Jansen Steur ENH, Braak E. Staging of brain pathology related to sporadic Parkinson's disease. Neurobiol Aging. 2003;24:197–211.
10. Braak H, Sastre M, Bohl JRE, de Vos RAI, Del Tradici K. Parkinson's disease: lesions in dorsal horn layer 1, involvement of parasympathetic and sympathetic pre and post ganglionic neurons. Acta Neuropathol. 2007;113:421–9.
11. Beach TG, Adler CH, Lue L, Sue LI, Bachalakuri J, Henry-Watson J, et al. Arizona Parkinson's disease Consortium. Unified staging system for Lewy body disorders: correlation with nigrostriatal degeneration, cognitive impairment and motor dysfunction. Acta Neuropathol. 2009;117:613–34.
12. Savica R, Rocca WA, Ahlskog E. When does Parkinson disease start? Arch Neurol. 2010;67:798–801.
13. Willis GL, Armstrong SM. A therapeutic role for melatonin antagonism in experimental models of Parkinson's disease. Physiol Behav. 1999;66:785–95.
14. Shiba M, Bower JH, Maraganore DM, McDonnell SK, Peterson BJ, Ahlskog JE, et al. Anxiety disorders and depression disorders preceding Parkinson's disease: a case controlled study. Mov Disord. 2000;159:669–77.
15. Weisskopf MG, Chen H, Schwarzschild MA, Kawachi I, Ascherio A. Prospective study of phobic anxiety and risk of Parkinson's disease. Mov Disord. 2003;18:646–51.
16. Naismith SL, Rogers NL, Mackenzie J, Hickie IB, Lewis SJ. The relationship between actigraphically defined sleep disturbance and REM sleep behaviour disorder in Parkinson's disease. Clin Neurol Neurosurg. 2010;112:420–3.
17. Willis GL. Parkinson's disease as a neuroendocrine disorder of circadian function: dopamine-melatonin imbalance and the visual system in the genesis and progression of the degenerative process. Rev Neurosci. 2008;19:245–316.
18. Bruguerolle B, Simon N. Biologic rhythms and Parkinson's disease: a chrono-pharmacologic approach to considering fluctuations in function. Clin Neuropharmacol. 2002;25:194–201.
19. Liu S, Cai Y, Sothern RB, Guan Y, Chan P. Chronobiological analysis of circadian patterns in transcription of seven clock genes in six peripheral tissues in mice. Chronobiol Int. 2007;24:793–820.
20. Cermakian N, Monaco L, Pando MP, Dierich A, Sasone-Corsi P. Altered behavioural rhythms and clock gene expression in mice with a targeted mutation in the period 1 gene. EMBO J. 2001;20:3967–74.
21. Kondratov RV, Kondratova AA, Gorbacheva VY, Vykhovanets OV, Antoch MP. Early age related pathologies in mice deficient in BMAL1, the core components of the circadian clock. Genes Dev. 2006;20:1868–73.
22. Boivin DB, James FO, Wu A, Cho-Park PF, Xiong H, Sun ZS. Circadian clock genes oscillate in human peripheral blood mononuclear cells. Blood. 2003;102:4143–5.
23. Fukuya H, Emoto N, Nonaka H, Yagita K, Okamura H, Yokoyama M. Circadian expression of clock genes in human peripheral leukocytes. Biochem Biophys Res Commun. 2007;354:924–8.
24. Cai Y, Liu S, Sothern RB, Xu S, Chan P. Expression of clock genes Per1 and Bmal1 in total leukocytes in health and Parkinson's disease. Eur J Neurol. 2010;17:550–4.
25. Srinivasan V. The pineal gland: its physiological and pharmacological role. Indian J Physiol Pharmacol. 1989;33:263–72.
26. Reppert SM, Weaver DR, Ebisawa T. Cloning and characterization of a mammalian melatonin receptor that mediates reproductive and circadian responses. Neuron. 1994;13:1177–85.
27. Reppert SM, Godson C, Mahle CD, Weaver DR, Slaugenhaupt SA, Gusella JF. Molecular characterization of a second melatonin receptor expressed in human retina and brain: the Melib melatonin receptor. Proc Natl Acad Sci U S A. 1995;92:8734–8.
28. Adi N, Mash DC, Ali Y, Singer C, Shehadeh L, Papapetropoulos S. Melatonin MT1 and MT2 receptor expression in Parkinson's disease. Med Sci Monit. 2010;16:BR61–7.
29. Takeda Y, Jothi R, Jetter AM. ROR γ directly regulates the circadian expression of clock genes and downstream targets in vivo. Nucleic Acids Res. 2012;40(17):8519–35.
30. Kumar S, Bhatia M, Behari M. Sleep disorders in Parkinson's disease. Mov Disord. 2002;17:775–81.
31. Brotini S, Gigli GL. Epidemiology and clinical features of sleep disorders in extra-pyramidal disease. Sleep Med. 2004;5:169–79.
32. Garcia-Borreguero D, Larrosa O, Bravo M. Parkinson's disease and sleep. Sleep Med Rev. 2003;7:115–29.
33. Friedman JH, Chou KL. Sleep and fatigue in Parkinson's disease. Parkinsonism Relat Disord. 2004;10:S27–35.
34. Vendette M, Gagnon JF, Decary A, Massicotte-Marquez J, Postuma RB, Doyan J, et al. REM sleep

behaviour disorder predicts cognitive impairment in Parkinson's disease without dementia. Neurology. 2007;69:1843–9.
35. Marion MH, Qurashi M, Marshall G, Foster O. Is REM sleep behaviour disorder (RBD) a risk factor of dementia in idiopathic Parkinson's disease? J Neurol. 2008;255:192–6.
36. Olson EJ, Boeve BF, Silber MH. Rapid eye movement sleep behaviour disorder: demographic, clinical and laboratory findings in 93 cases. Brain. 2000;123:331–9.
37. Schenck CH, Bundlie SR, Mahowald MW. Delayed emergence of a Parkinsonian disorder in 38 % of 29 older women initially diagnosed with idiopathic rapid eye movement sleep behaviour disorder. Neurology. 1996;46:388–93.
38. Silber MH, Ahlskog JE. REM sleep behaviour disorder in Parkinsonian syndromes. Sleep Res (abstract). 1992;21:313.
39. Boeve B, Silber M, Ferman T. REM sleep behaviour disorder in Parkinsonn's disease and dementia with Lewy bodies. J Geriatr Psychiatry Neurol. 2004;17:146–57.
40. Boeve BF, Silber MH, Saper CB, Ferman TJ, Dickson DW, Parisi JE, et al. Pathophysiology of REM sleep behaviour disorder and relevance to neurodegenerative disease. Brain. 2007;130:2770–88.
41. Fantini ML, Corona A, Clerisi S, Ferini-Strambi L. Aggressive dream content without daytime aggressiveness in REM sleep behaviour disorder. Neurology. 2005;65:1010–5.
42. Jahan I, Hauser RA, Sullivan KL, Miller A, Zesiewicz TA. Sleep disorders in Parkinson's disease. Neuropsychiatr Dis Treat. 2009;5:535–40.
43. Thannickal TC, Lai YY, Siegel JM. Hypocretin (orexin) cell loss in Parkinson's disease. Brain. 2007;130:1586–95.
44. Compta Y, Santamaria J, Ratti L, Tolosa E, Iranzo A, Munoz E, et al. Cerebrospinal hypocretin, daytime sleepiness and sleep architecture in Parkinson's disease dementia. Brain. 2009;132:3308–17.
45. Tandberg E, Larsen JP, Karlsen NK. Excessive daytime sleepiness and sleep benefit in Parkinson's disease. A community based study. Mov Disord. 1999;14:922–7.
46. Arnulf I, Konofal E, Merino-Andreu M, Houeto JL, Mesnage V, Welter ML, et al. Parkinson's disease and sleepiness: an integral part of PD. Neurology. 2002;58:1019–24.
47. Brodsky MA, Godbold J, Roth T, Olanow CW. Sleepiness in Parkinson's disease: a controlled study. Mov Disord. 2003;18:668–72.
48. Mehta SH, Morgan JC, Sethi KD. Sleep disorders associated with Parkinson's disease: role of dopamine, epidemiology, and clinical scales of assessment. CNS Spectr. 2008;13:6–11.
49. Dobkin RD, Menza M, Bienfait KL, Gara M, Marin H, Mark MH, et al. Depression in Parkinson's disease: symptom improvement and residual symptoms after acute pharmacologic management. Am J Geriatr Psychiatry. 2010;19:222–9.
50. Weintraub D, Mavandadi S, Mamikonyan E, Siderowf AD, Duda JE, Hurtig HI, et al. Atomoxetine for depression and other neuropsychiatric symptoms in Parkinson's disease. Neurology. 2010;75:448–55.
51. Dubocovich ML, Cardinali DP, Delagrange P, Krause DN, Strosberg D, Sugden D, et al. Melatonin receptors. In: The IUPHAR compendium of receptor characterization and classification. 2nd ed. London: IUPHAR Media; 2000. p. 271–7.
52. Dubocovich ML, Markowska M. Functional MT_1 and MT_2 melatonin receptor in mammals. Endocrine. 2005;27:101–10.
53. Liu C, Weaver DR, Jin X, Shearman LP, Pieschl RL, Gribkoff VK, et al. Molecular dissection two distinct actions of melatonin on the suprachiasmatic circadian clock. Neuron. 1997;19:91–102.
54. Al Ghoul WM, Herman MD, Dubocovich ML. Melatonin receptor subtype expression in human cerebellum. Neuroreport. 1998;9:4063–8.
55. Savaskan E, Olivieri G, Meier F, Brydon L, Jockers R, Ravid R, et al. Increased melatonin 1a-receptor immunoreactivity in the hippocampus of Alzheimer's disease patients. J Pineal Res. 2002;32:59–62.
56. Uz T, Arsian AD, Kurtuncu M, Imbesi M, Akhisaroglu M, Dwivedi Y, et al. The regional and cellular expression profile of the melatonin receptor MT_1 in the central dopaminergic system. Brain Res Mol Brain Res. 2005;136:45–53.
57. Nosjean O, Ferro M, Coge F, Beauverger P, Henlin JM, Lefoulon F, et al. Identification of the melatonin binding site MT3 as the quinine reductase2. J Biol Chem. 2000;275:31311–7.
58. Benitez-King G. Melatonin as a cytoskeletal modulator: implications for cell physiology and disease. J Pineal Res. 2006;49:1–9.
59. Macias M, Escames G, Leon J, Coto-Montes A, Sbihi Y, Osuna A, et al. Calrcticulin melatonin: an unexpected relationship. Eur J Biochem. 2003;270: 832–40.
60. Wiesenberg I, Missbach M, Kahlen JP, Schrader M, Carlberg C. Transcriptional activation of the nuclear RZR α by the pineal gland hormone melatonin and identification of CGP 52608 as a synthetic ligand. Nucleic Acids Res. 1995;23:327–33.
61. Reiter RJ. The pineal and its hormones in the control of reproduction in mammals. Endocr Rev. 1980;1:109–31.
62. Srinivasan V, Spence DW, Pandi-Perumal SR, Zakaria R, Bhatnagar KP, Brzezinski A. Melatonin and human reproduction. Gynecol Endocrinol. 2009;25:779–85.
63. Wurtman RJ, Zhdanova I. Improvement of sleep quality by melatonin. Lancet. 1995;346:1491.
64. Guerrero JM, Reiter RJ. Melatonin-immune system relationships. Curr Top Med Chem. 2002;2:167–79.
65. Srinivasan V, Maestroni GJM, Cardinali DP, Esquifino AI, Pandi-Perumal SR, Miller SC.

Melatonin, immune function and aging. Immun Ageing. 2005;2:17.
66. Srinivasan V, Spence DW, Trakt I, Pandi-Perumal SR, Cardinali DP, Maestroni GJ. Immunomodulation by melatonin: its significance for seasonally occurring diseases. Neuroimmunomodulation. 2008;15:93–101.
67. Armstrong SM. Melatonin: the internal zeitgeber of mammals? Pineal Res Rev. 1989;7:157–202.
68. Deacon S, Arendt J. Melatonin-induced temperature suppression and its acute phase shifting effects correlate in a dose dependent manner in humans. Brain Res. 1995;688:77–85.
69. Arendt J, Skene DJ. Melatonin as a chronobiotic. Sleep Med Rev. 2005;9:25–39.
70. Rajaratnam SM, Middleton B, Stone BM, Arendt J, Dijk DJ. Melatonin advances the circadian timing of EEG sleep and directly facilitates sleep without altering its duration in extended sleep opportunities in humans. J Physiol. 2004;561:339–51.
71. Blask DE, Sauer LA, Dauchey RT. Melatonin as a chronobiotic/anticancer agent: cellular, biochemical, and molecular mechanisms of action and their implications for circadian based cancer therapy. Curr Top Med Chem. 2002;2:113–32.
72. Srinivasan V, Spence DW, Pandi-Perumal SR, Trakht I, Esquifino AI, Cardinali DP, et al. Melatonin, environmental light and breast cancer. Breast Cancer Res Treat. 2008;108:339–50.
73. Srinivasan V, Spence DW, Pandi-Perumal SR, Trakht I, Cardinali DP. Therapeutic actions of melatonin in cancer: possible mechanisms. Integr Cancer Ther. 2008;7:189–203.
74. Srinivasan V, Pandi-Perumal SR, Spence DW, Moscovitch A, Trakht I, Brown GM, et al. Potential use of melatonergic drugs in analgesia: mechanisms of action. Brain Res Bull. 2010;81:362–71.
75. Chieuh CC, Burns RS, Markey DM, Jacobowitz DM, Kopin IJ. Primate model of parkinsonism: selective lesion of nigrostriatal neurons by 1-methyl-4-phenyl-1,2,3,6 tetrahydropyridine produces an extrapyramidal syndrome in rhesus monkeys. Life Sci. 1985;36:213–8.
76. Terzioglu M, Galter D. Parkinson's disease: genetic versus toxic induced rodent models. FEBS J. 2008;275:1384–91.
77. Acuña-Castroviejo D, Coto-Montes A, Gaia MM, Ortiz GG, Reiter RJ. Melatonin is protective against MPTP-induced striatal and hippocampal lesions. Life Sci. 1997;60:L23–9.
78. Khaldy H, Leon J, Escames G, Bikjdaouene L, Acuña-Castroviejo D. Synergistic effects f melatonin and deprenyl protect against MPTP-induced mitochondrial damage and DA depletion. Neurobiol Aging. 2003;24:491–500.
79. Antolin I, Mayo JC, Sainz RM, del Brio ML, Herrera F, Martin V, et al. Protective effect of melatonin in chronic experimental model of Parkinson's disease. Brain Res. 2002;943:163–73.
80. Zhang Y, Dawson VL, Dawson TM. Oxidative stress and genetics in the pathogenesis of Parkinson's disease. Neurobiol Dis. 2000;7:240–50.
81. Cuzzocrea S, Zingarelli B, Gilad E, Hake P, Salzman AL, Szabo C. Protective effect of melatonin in carrageenan-induced models of local inflammation: relationship to its inhibitory effect on nitric oxide production and its peroxynitrite scavenging activity. J Pineal Res. 1997;23:106–16.
82. Srinivasan V, Pandi-Perumal SR, Maestroni GJM, Esquifino AI, Hardeland R, Cardinali DP. Role of melatonin in neurodegenerative diseases. Neurotox Res. 2005;7:293–318.
83. Entrena A, Camacho ME, Carrion MD, Lopez-Cara LC, Velasco G, Leon J, et al. Kynurenamines as neural nitric oxide synthase inhibitors. J Med Chem. 2005;48:8174–81.
84. Tapias V, Escames G, Lopez LC, Entrena A, Camacho E, Espinosa A, et al. Melatonin and its brain metabolite N^1-acetyl-5-methoxy-kynuramine prevent mitochondrial nitric oxide synthase induction in Parkinsonian mice. J Neurosci Res. 2009;87:3002–10.
85. Dabbeni-Sala F, Di Santo S, Franceschini D, Skaper SD, Giusti P. Melatonin protects against 6-OHDA-induced neurotoxicity in rats: a role for mitochondrial complex I activity. FASEB J. 2001;15:164–70.
86. Thomas B, Mohankumar KP. Melatonin protects against oxidative stress caused by 1-methyl-4-phenyl-1,2,3,6- tetra hydropyridine in the mouse nigrostriatum. J Pineal Res. 2004;36:25–32.
87. Saravanan KS, Sindhu KM, Mohankumar KP. Acute intranigral infusion of rotenone in rats causes progressive biochemical lesions in the striatum similar to Parkinson's disease. Brain Res. 2005;1049: 147–55.
88. Sindhu KM, Saravanan KS, Mohankumar KP. Behavioural differences in a rotenone-induced hemiparkinsonian rat model developed following intranigral or median forebrain bundle infusion. Brain Res. 2005;1051:25–34.
89. Saravanan KS, Sindhu KM, Senthilkumar KS, Mohanakumar KP. L-Deprenyl protects against rotenone-induced oxidative stress mediated dopaminergic neurodegeneration in rats. Neurochem Int. 2006;49:28–40.
90. Saravanan KS, Sindhu KM, Mohankumar KP. Melatonin protects against rotenone-induced oxidative-stress in a hemiparkinsonian model. J Pineal Res. 2007;42:247–53.
91. Maharaj H, Sukhdev Maharaj D, Scheepers M, Mokokong R, Daya S. L-DOPA administration enhances 6-hydroxydopamine generation. Brain Res. 2005;1063:180–6.
92. Borah A, Mohankumar KP. Melatonin inhibits 6-hydroxydopamine production in the brain to protect against experimental parkinsonism in rodents. J Pineal Res. 2009;47:293–300.

93. Przedborski S, Tieu K, Perier C, Vila M. MPTP as a mitochondrial neurotoxic model of Parkinson's disease. J Bioenerg Biomembr. 2004;36:375–9.
94. Greenmyre JT, Sherer TB, Betarbet R, Panov AV. Complex 1 and Parkinson's disease. IUBMB Life. 2001;52:135–41.
95. Rego AC, Oliveira CR. Mitochondrial dysfunction and reactive oxygen species in excitotoxicity and apoptosis: implications for the pathogenesis of neurodegenerative diseases. Neurochem Res. 2003;28: 1563–74.
96. Tretter L, Sipos I, Adam-Vizi V. Inhibition of neuronal damage by complex I deficiency and oxidative stress in Parkinson's disease. Neurochem Res. 2004; 29:569–77.
97. Liberatore GT, Jackson-Lewis V, Vukosavic S, Mandir AS, Vila M, McAuliffe WG, et al. Inducible nitric oxide synthase stimulates dopaminergic neurodegeneration in the MPTP model of Parkinson's disease. Nat Med. 1999;5:1403–9.
98. Brown GC, Bal-Price A. Inflammatory neurodegeneration mediated by nitric oxide, glutamate, and mitochondria. Mol Neurobiol. 2003;27:325–55.
99. Brown GC, Borutaite V. Inhibition of mitochondrial respiratory complex I by nitric oxide, peroxynitrite, and S-nitrosothiols. Biochim Biophys Acta. 2004; 1658:44–9.
100. Muravchick S, Levy RJ. Clinical implications of mitochondrial dysfunction. Anesthesiology. 2006; 105:819–37.
101. Zhang I, Dawson VL, Dawson TM. Role of nitric oxide in Parkinson's disease. Pharmacol Ther. 2006; 109:33–41.
102. Arushanian EB. A hormonal drug melatonin in the treatment of cognitive function disorders in parkinsonism. Eksp Klin Farmakol. 2010;73:35–9.
103. Dowling GA, Mastick J, Colling E, Carter JH, Singer CM, Aminoff MJ. Melatonin for sleep disturbances in Parkinson's disease. Sleep Med. 2005;6:459–66.
104. Medeiros CA, Carvalhedo de Bruin PF, Lopes LA, Magalhaes MC, de Lourdes Seabra M, de Bruin VM. Effect of exogenous melatonin on sleep and motor dysfunction in Parkinson's disease: a randomized, double blind, placebo–controlled study. J Neurol. 2007;254:459–64.
105. Willis GL, Turner EJ. Primary and secondary features of Parkinson's disease improve with strategic exposure to bright light: a case series study. Chronobiol Int. 2007;24:521–37.
106. Beck-Friis J, Borg G, Wetterberg L. Rebound increase of nocturnal serum melatonin levels following evening suppression of bright light exposure in healthy men. Ann N Y Acad Sci. 1985;453:371–5.
107. Srinivasan V. Psychoactive drugs, pineal gland and affective disorders. Prog Neuropsychopharmacol Biol Psychiatry. 1989;13:653–64.
108. Turek FW, Gillette MU. Melatonin, sleep and circadian rhythms: rationale for development of specific melatonin agonists. Sleep Med. 2004;5:523–32.
109. Kato K, Hirai K, Nishiyama K, Uchikawa O, Fukatsu K, Ohkawa S, et al. Neurochemical properties of ramelteon (TAK 375), a selective MT1/MT2 receptor agonist. Neuropharmacology. 2005;48:301–10.
110. Srinivasan V, Zakaria R, Othman Z, Brzezinski A, Prasad A, Brown GM. Melatonergic drugs for therapeutic use in insomnia and sleep disturbances of mood disorders. CNS Neurol Disord Drug Targets. 2012;11:180–9.
111. Lauterbach EC, Victoroff J, Coburn KL, Shillcutt SD, Doonan SM, Mendez MF. Psychopharmacological neuroprotection in neurodegenerative disease: assessing the preclinical data. J Neuropsychiatry Clin Neurosci. 2010;22:8–18.
112. Lauterbach EC, Shillcutt SD, Victoroff J, Coburn KL, Mendez MF. Psychopharmacological neuroprotection in neurodegenerative disease: heuristic clinical applications. J Neuropsychiatry Clin Neurosci. 2010;22:130–54.
113. Imbesi M, Uz T, Dzitoyeva S, Manev H. Stimulatory effects of melatonin receptor agonist, ramelteon on BDNF in mouse cerebellar granule cells. Neurosci Lett. 2008;439:34–6.
114. Lauterbach EC. The neuropsychiatry of Parkinson's disease. Minerva Med. 2005;96:155–73.
115. Lauterbach EC. The neuropsychiatry of Parkinson's disease and related disorders. Psychiatr Clin North Am. 2004;27:801–25.
116. Singhal NK, Srivastava G, Patel DK, Jain SK, Singh MP. Melatonin or silymarin reduces maneb- and paraquat-induced Parkinson's disease phenotype in the mouse. J. Pineal Res. 2011;50:97–109.

Melatonin and Its Agonists in Sleep Disorders

18

Amnon Brzezinski

Abstract

Exogenous melatonin reportedly induces drowsiness and sleep and may ameliorate sleep disturbances, including the nocturnal awakenings associated with old age. Daytime administration of exogenous melatonin (when it is not present endogenously) promotes sleep in humans and results in sleeplike brain activity patterns at specific areas such as the precuneus and hippocampus. However, existing studies on the hypnotic efficacy of melatonin have been highly heterogeneous in regard to inclusion and exclusion criteria, measures to evaluate insomnia, doses of the medication, and routes of administration.

The inconsistent reports about the effectiveness of exogenous melatonin in the treatment of insomnia brought about the development of more potent melatonin analogs with prolonged effects and the design of slow-release melatonin preparations. The melatonergic receptor ramelteon is a selective melatonin-1 (MT1) and melatonin-2 (MT2) receptor agonist with negligible affinity for other neuronal receptors, including gamma-aminobutyric acid and benzodiazepine receptors. It was found effective in increasing total sleep time and sleep efficiency as well as in reducing sleep latency, in insomnia patients. The melatonergic antidepressant agomelatine, displaying potent MT1 and MT2 melatonergic agonism and relatively weak serotonin 5-HT2C receptor antagonism, reportedly is effective in the treatment of depression-associated insomnia. A review of the currently available evidence regarding the effects of these compounds on sleep quality is presented in this chapter.

Keywords

Melatonin • Melatonin agonists • Sleep • Insomnia • Ramelteon • Agomelatine

A. Brzezinski, MD
Department of Obstetrics and Gynecology,
Hadassah Hebrew-University Medical Center,
Ein-Kerem, Jerusalem, 91120, Israel
e-mail: amnonbrz@gmail.com

V. Srinivasan et al. (eds.), *Melatonin and Melatonergic Drugs in Clinical Practice*,
DOI 10.1007/978-81-322-0825-9_18, © Springer India 2014

Introduction

In humans, the circadian rhythm of melatonin release from the pineal gland is highly synchronized with the habitual hours of sleep, and the daily onset of melatonin secretion is well correlated with the onset of the steepest increase in nocturnal sleepiness ("sleep gate") [1, 2]. Serum melatonin levels were reported to be significantly lower (and the time of peak melatonin values was delayed) in elderly subjects with insomnia compared with age-matched subjects with no insomnia [3]. Exogenous melatonin reportedly induces drowsiness and sleep and may ameliorate sleep disturbances, including the nocturnal awakenings associated with old age [4, 5]. However, existing studies on the hypnotic efficacy of melatonin have been highly heterogeneous in regard to inclusion and exclusion criteria, measures to evaluate insomnia, doses of the medication, and routes of administration. Adding to this complexity, there continues to be considerable controversy over the meaning of the discrepancies that sometimes exist between subjective and objective (polysomnographic) measures of good and bad sleep [6].

Thus, attention has been focused either on the development of more potent melatonin analogs with prolonged effects or on the design of prolonged-release melatonin preparations [7]. The MT1 and MT2 melatonergic receptor ramelteon was effective in increasing total sleep time and sleep efficiency, as well as in reducing sleep latency, in insomnia patients [8–10]. The melatonergic antidepressant agomelatine, displaying potent MT1 and MT2 melatonergic agonism and relatively weak serotonin 5-HT2C receptor antagonism, was found effective in the treatment of depression-associated insomnia [11–15]. Other melatonergic compounds are currently developed [16, 17].

Exogenous Melatonin

Melatonin's two well-established physiological effects—promotion of sleep and entrainment of circadian rhythms—are both mediated by two specific receptor proteins in the brain, and not by the gamma-aminobutyric acid (GABA) receptors through which most hypnotic agents act. This difference probably explains why, unlike the GABA-agonist drugs, which are true "sleeping pills," exogenous melatonin does not suppress rapid eye movement (REM) sleep nor, in general, affect the distribution of sleep stages [18].

Measurements of melatonin in body fluids in elderly subjects have convincingly demonstrated an age-related impairment of nocturnal pineal melatonin synthesis [19–21]. Several studies have shown the importance of melatonin both for the initiation and for maintenance of sleep [22]. In all diurnal animals and in human beings, the onset of melatonin secretion coincides with the timing of increase in nocturnal sleep propensity [23].

In 2005 a meta-analysis of 17 studies, involving 284 subjects that satisfied inclusion criteria, demonstrated that melatonin treatment significantly decreased sleep latency and increased sleep efficiency and total sleep duration [24]. The inclusion criteria were that a study includes at least six subjects, all adults, be randomized and double blinded, involves placebo-controlled clinical trials, and uses objective measures of sleep evaluation. Studies could utilize crossover or parallel group designs; however, case reports were excluded. Statistical significance was obtained in spite of considerable variations among the studies in melatonin doses and routes of administration, the general health of the subjects, and the measures used to evaluate sleep. The effects of exogenous melatonin on sleep have been examined under three types of experimental conditions in relation to the onset or offset of endogenous melatonin secretion.

In some studies, the hormone was administered during the daily light period, such that blood melatonin levels would be transiently elevated but would then return to baseline before the initiation of nocturnal melatonin secretion. Such experiments were used to demonstrate that melatonin decreases sleep latency at any time in the afternoon or evening and that this effect is independent of an action on sleep rhythms (since no treatment can immediately shift the phase of a circadian rhythm by 8–10 h).

In others, the hormone was given close enough to the onset of darkness for blood melatonin levels to still be elevated when nocturnal melatonin secretion started. The period during which plasma melatonin levels were continuously elevated would thus be prolonged. Such experiments reflected the use of melatonin to decrease sleep latency and maintain continuous sleep in, for example, a shift worker or eastbound world traveler who needed to start sleeping earlier.

In yet others, the hormone was given at the end of the light period to older insomniacs with low nighttime plasma melatonin levels. The intent was to prolong the portion of the night during which their plasma melatonin concentrations would be in the same range as those of noninsomniac young adults.

In all these situations, oral melatonin decreased sleep latency and, when tested, increased sleep duration and sleep efficiency. A 0.3 mg dose was either as effective as or more effective than higher doses, particularly when the hormone was administered for several days [18]. This dose had no effect on body temperature, affirming that, while pharmacologic doses can cause hypothermia, melatonin's ability to promote sleep is not mediated by such a change, as had been suggested. The hormone had no consistent effect on sleep architecture (e.g., REM time). Its effects differed from those of most hypnotic drugs, since after receiving melatonin, subjects could readily keep from falling asleep if they chose so, and their cognitive abilities the next morning were unchanged or improved.

In a study of 30 people who were 50 years old or older and did or did not suffer from clinically significant insomnia (i.e., sleep efficiencies of 70–80 % in the insomniacs versus 92 % in controls), melatonin was found to produce statistically and clinically significant improvements in sleep efficiency among insomniacs [18].

In yet another meta-analysis published on the same year (2005), the authors found that melatonin decreased sleep onset latency (−11.7 min; 95 % confidence interval [CI]: −18.2, −5.2); it was decreased to a greater extent in people with delayed sleep phase syndrome (−38.8 min; 95 % CI: −50.3, −27.3; $n=2$) compared with people with insomnia (−7.2 min; 95 % CI: −12.0, −2.4; $n=12$) [25]. The former result appears to be clinically important. However, they conclude that melatonin is not effective in treating most primary sleep disorders with short-term use (4 weeks or less) but that there was evidence to suggest that melatonin was effective in treating delayed sleep phase syndrome with short-term use.

A meta-analysis published in 2009 focused on exogenous melatonin for sleep problems in individuals with intellectual disability [26]. Nine studies (including a total of 183 individuals with intellectual disabilities) showed that melatonin treatment decreased sleep latency by a mean of 34 min ($P<0.001$), increased total sleep time by a mean of 50 min ($P<0.001$), and significantly decreased the number of wakes per night ($P<0.05$). The authors concluded that melatonin decreases sleep latency and number of wakes per night and increases total sleep time in individuals with intellectual disabilities.

It should be noted that very recently, an official regulatory—the European Food Safety Authority (EFSA)—has evaluated the available evidence that melatonin can reduce the time it takes for normal sleepers and patients with insomnia to fall asleep [27]. It concluded that there is evidence that "a cause and effect relationship exist…between the consumption of melatonin and reduction of sleep onset latency…" and that "… 1 mg of melatonin should be consumed close to bedtime…"

Also, a recent consensus of the British Association for Psychopharmacology on evidence-based treatment of insomnia, parasomnia, and circadian rhythm sleep disorders concluded that melatonin is the first-choice treatment when a hypnotic is indicated in patients over 55 years [28].

Melatonin Receptors Agonists

Because melatonin has a short half-life (<30 min), its efficacy in promoting and maintaining sleep has not been uniform in the studies undertaken so far. Thus, the need for the development of prolonged-release preparations of melatonin or of melatonin agonists with a longer duration of action on sleep regulatory structures in the brain arose [29]. In accordance with this idea, slow-release forms of melatonin were developed (e.g., Circadin[R], a 2-mg preparation developed by Neurim, Tel Aviv, Israel, and approved by the European Medicines Agency in 2007) [7]. Their efficacy in treatment of sleep disorders in various populations was recently reported [7, 30].

A "sleep-switch" model to describe the regulation of sleep wakefulness was originally proposed by Saper and his colleagues [31, 32]. It consists of "flip-flop" reciprocal inhibitions among sleep-associated activities in the ventrolateral preoptic nucleus and wakefulness-associated activities in the locus coeruleus, dorsal raphe, and tuberomammillary nuclei. The SCN has an active role both in promoting wakefulness and in promoting sleep, and this depends upon a complex neuronal network and a number of neurotransmitters released (GABA, glutamate, arginine vasopressin, somatostatin, etc.) [33, 34].

The high density of melatonin receptors in the hypothalamic suprachiasmatic nuclei (SCN) may suggest that melatonin affects sleep and the sleep-wakefulness cycle by acting on these receptors [35, 36]. Thus, the need arose for the development of melatonin receptors agonists with a longer duration of action, and hopefully more potent in affecting sleep quality. The melatonin analogs ramelteon, agomelatine, tasimelteon, and TK-301 are examples of this strategy.

Ramelteon

Ramelteon (Rozerem[R]; Takeda Pharmaceuticals, Osaka, Japan) is a melatonergic hypnotic analog that has been demonstrated to be effective in clinical trials. It is a tricyclic synthetic analog of melatonin with the chemical name of (*S*)-*N*-[2-(1,6,7,8-tetrahydro-2*H*-indeno[5,4-b] furan-8-yl)-ethyl]propionamide (Fig. 18.1). In 2005, ramelteon was approved by the US Food and Drug Administration (FDA) for treatment of insomnia. It is a selective agonist for MT1/MT2 receptors without significant affinity for other receptor sites [9, 36]. In vitro binding studies have shown that ramelteon affinity for MT1 and MT2 receptors is 3–16 times higher than that of melatonin. The selectivity of ramelteon for MT1 has been found to be greater than that of MT2 receptors. The selectivity of MT1 receptors by ramelteon may suggest that it targets sleep onset more specifically than melatonin itself [37].

Ramelteon is administered usually by the oral route and is absorbed rapidly by the gastrointestinal tract [38]. The half-life of circulating ramelteon is in the range of 1–2 h which is much longer than that of melatonin. The influence of

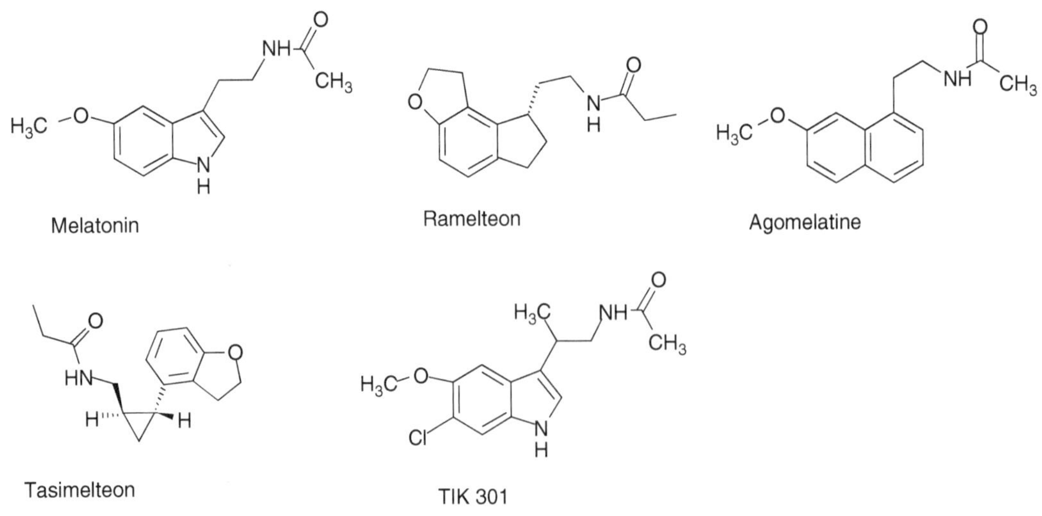

Melatonin

Ramelteon

Agomelatine

Tasimelteon

TIK 301

Fig. 18.1 The chemical structure of melatonin and melatonin agonists

age and gender on the pharmacokinetics and the pharmacodynamics of ramelteon was evaluated in healthy volunteers (young, 18–34 years; elderly 63–79 years) after administration of a single dose of ramelteon. Compared with young individuals, the clearance of ramelteon was significantly reduced in elderly individuals. No significant effect of gender was observed [38].

Ramelteon is metabolized mainly in the liver via oxidation to hydroxyl and carbonyl groups and then conjugated with glucuronide [39]. Cytochrome P450 (CPY) 1A2 is the major hepatic enzyme involved in ramelteon metabolism. Four principal metabolites of ramelteon (M-I, M-II, M-III, M-IV) have been identified [39]. Among these, M-II has been found to occur in a much higher concentration with systemic levels of 20- to 100-fold greater than those of ramelteon itself.

Although the activity of M-II is 30-fold lower than that of ramelteon, its exposure exceeds that of ramelteon by a factor of 30. Hence, it is suggested that M-II may contribute significantly to the net clinical effect of ramelteon intake. Although MT1 and MT2 receptors are widely distributed in the brain outside of the SCN [40–44], the high density of melatonin receptors in the SCN and their relationship to the circadian pacemaker function are highly suggestive of an SCN melatonin receptor role in sleep regulation. Ramelteon specificity for MT1 and MT2 melatonin receptors indicates that its probable sleep-related site of action is in the SCN.

Ramelteon may accelerate sleep onset by influencing the hypothalamic sleep switch downstream from the SCN in the same way as melatonin [10, 45]. Ramelteon promotes sleep onset through the inhibition of SCN electrical activity and the consequent inhibition of circadian wake signal, thereby activating the specific sleep-circuit pathway.

Ramelteon's efficacy as hypnotic drug was evaluated in a group of freely moving monkeys (Macaca fascicularis) in comparison with that of melatonin and zolpidem [45]. Ramelteon and melatonin were administered in doses of 0.003, 0.03, and 0.3 mg/kg and 0.3, 1, and 3 mg/kg, respectively, to independent groups of animals. Zolpidem was administered in doses 1, 3, 10, or 30 mg/kg to a third group of monkeys. All drugs were administered orally at18:00 h, and the polysomnographic (PSG) recording of sleep was continuously taken from 17:00 to 7:00 h. Ramelteon at a dose of 0.03 or 0.3 mg/kg significantly reduced sleep onset latency (SOL) for both light sleep and NREM sleep as melatonin and its analogs in insomnia and depression compared to controls. Both doses of ramelteon increased total sleep time (TST), whereas the lowest dose employed (0.003 mg/kg) was ineffective. Melatonin administration at a 0.3 mg/kg dose significantly reduced latency to SOL for light sleep but not for NREM sleep [46]. At a dose of 1 mg and 3 mg/kg, melatonin tended to shorten SOL and increased TST, but these changes were marginally significant. The administration of zolpidem (1–30 mg/kg) did not produce any significant effect on SOL or TST at any of the doses tested. From these results, it was concluded that ramelteon has a potent sleep-inducing effect not shared by either melatonin or zolpidem [46]. In another study conducted in rhesus monkeys, ramelteon did not induce either abuse or dependence after administering daily at a dose of 10 mg/kg for 1 year [47].

In a double-blind study including 829 insomniac patients (mean age, 72.4 years), ramelteon, at a dose of 4–8 mg/day, brought about a significant 16–35 % reduction in SOL [48]. TST was increased by both doses of ramelteon. In another randomized, multicenter double-blind, placebo-controlled crossover study including 107 patients followed by PSG, ramelteon was administered in doses of 4–32 mg/day [49]. The treatment decreased latency to first sleep (LFS) and increased TST significantly.

A short-term evaluation of the efficacy of ramelteon was performed in 100 elderly subjects by administering 4 and 8 mg doses in a two-night/three-day period crossover design [50]. LPS decreased, and TST and SE augmented as compared to placebo. Likewise, the efficacy of ramelteon in reducing SOL and in increasing TST and SE was evaluated in 405 patients administered with 8 or 16 mg of ramelteon for 5 weeks in a double-blind placebo-controlled study [51].

The results confirmed the effect of ramelteon to reduce SOL and to increase SE and TST[51].

Ramelteon's hypnotic action (at an 8 mg dose) was so rapid that it caused significant reductions in SOL within a week (63 % for ramelteon versus 39.7 % for placebo, $P<0.001$) [52]. This reduction in LPS was sustained throughout the 5 weeks of study (63 and 65.9 % ramelteon versus 41.2 and 48.9 % placebo at the end of the third and fifth weeks, respectively) [52]. Reduction in LPS after ramelteon was also noted in healthy human subjects in a 6-week-long study using an 8 mg dose; in this study on healthy human subjects, ramelteon also increased TST [53].

In yet another 6-month-long study performed in 451 adults suffering from chronic insomnia drawn from different centers across the globe (mainly the USA, Europe, Russia, and Australia), ramelteon consistently reduced LPS when compared with placebo [54]. The baseline LPS decreased from 70.7 to 32.0 min at week 1 (with ramelteon), and this reduction in LPS was maintained at months 1, 3, 5, and 6. No adverse effects, like next-morning residual effects, rebound insomnia, or withdrawal effects, were noted [54].

In a double-blind placebo-controlled study involving a large number of Japanese patients with chronic insomnia ($N=1,130$), the efficacy and safety of 4 and 8 mg ramelteon were evaluated [55]. At a 4 mg dose of ramelteon, no statistically significant differences were found in subjective SOL as compared to the placebo group, while with 8 mg of ramelteon, a significant increase in TST and a decrease in SOL were observed. The same investigators evaluated the efficacy and safety of ramelteon in 190 Japanese adults with chronic insomnia treated for a period of 24 weeks [56]. TST significantly increased with an 8 mg/day dose of ramelteon, and this was maintained for 20 weeks. In this study, ramelteon was well tolerated and did not cause residual effects, rebound insomnia, withdrawal symptoms, or dependence after 24 weeks of continuous treatment [56].

Summarizing Ramelteon's studies, it seems that in all clinical studies undertaken so (in various doses ranging from 4 to 32 mg/day) in patients with chronic insomnia, the drug reduced SOL and increased sleep duration [10, 57] without significant adverse effects.

Agomelatine

Disturbances in sleep are prominent features of depression. Antidepressant drugs that are also effective in alleviating sleep disturbances can be of better therapeutic value in treating depressive disorders [58]. It is suggested that an ideal antidepressant should not only decrease sleep onset difficulties and wakefulness after sleep onset but should also promote the feelings of freshness and alertness during daytime [59].

The newly introduced melatonergic antidepressant agomelatine (Valdoxan; Servier, Neuilly-sur-Seine, France) is endowed with these properties. Agomelatine, a naphthalenic compound chemically designated as *N*-(2-[7-methoxy-1-naphthalenyl]ethyl) acetamide, acts on both MT1and MT2 melatonergic receptors and also acts as an antagonist to 5-HT_{2C} receptors at a three orders of magnitude greater concentration [11]. It does not show any significant affinities for muscarinic, histaminergic, adrenergic, and dopaminergic receptor subtypes [60] (Fig. 18.1).

Agomelatine has been licensed by European Medicines Agency (EMEA) for the treatment of major depressive disorder (MDD). In several animal models of depression like the forced swimming test, the learned helplessness model [61], and the social stress model [62], agomelatine displayed antidepressant activity. It has been hypothesized that agomelatine has a unique mechanism of action because its effects are mediated through MT1/MT2 melatonergic receptors and 5-HT_{2C} serotonergic receptors, acting differently at different circadian phases of the day/night cycle [63]. Through this dual action, agomelatine may promote and maintain sleep at night and helps to maintain alertness during daytime.

Agomelatine given before sleep would have an immediate sleep-promoting melatonergic effect that would prevail over its potentially antihypnotic 5-HT_{2C} antagonism [63]. In contrast, during the day, the drug's 5-HT_{2C} antagonism would predominate over the melatonergic action, thus having an alerting action. 5-HT_{2C} receptors are concentrated in the frontal cortex, amygdala, hippocampus, and cortico-limbic structures that are involved in the regulation of mood and cognition [64]. They are also present in the SCN [65], and antidepressants, while exerting their therapeutic effects, decrease the number of SCN 5-HT_{2C} receptors in those structures [66].

One criticism of this dual interpretation of agomelatine action is the large differences in affinity for the putative action on serotonergic receptors as compared to the melatonergic one (about three orders of magnitude greater concentration are needed to exert 5-HT_{2C} antagonism) [11]. Moreover, both melatonin and ramelteon have been shown to display antidepressant-like effects even though they are not reportedly known to affect serotonergic activity significantly [67–69].

As agomelatine addresses sleep disturbances as well as depressive symptoms and has early onset of action even in a severely depressed population, it stands unique among the antidepressants for effective management of MDD [12]. Because sleep disturbances constitute one of the prominent features of depressive illness and are among the diagnostic criteria of DSM-IV [70], it is not strange that the melatonergic activity of agomelatine (or ramelteon) could be beneficial for this symptom. Patients suffering from MDD or bipolar disorder exhibit marked difficulties in initiation and maintenance of sleep, poor quality of sleep, and frequent nocturnal and early morning wakening [58].

The American National Institute of Mental Health (NIMH) Epidemiological Catchment Area (ECA) study of sleep disturbances and psychiatric disorders identified sleep disturbances as a highly significant risk factor for subsequent development of depression [13].

The effectiveness of agomelatine in reducing the sleep complaints of depressed patients has been evaluated. Altered intra-night temporal distribution of REM sleep with increased amounts of early REM sleep and reduction in SOL to REM sleep is the specific EEG sleep pattern that is associated with depression [71]. Hence, prevention of persistent sleep disturbances would help to reduce the risk of relapse or recurrence of depressive disorders. The treatment of depressive patients with agomelatine for 6 weeks increased the duration of NREM sleep without affecting REM sleep, thereby causing improvements in both sleep quality and continuity [14]. In the study that compared the effect of agomelatine (25 mg) with the antidepressant venlafaxine, agomelatine promoted sleep earlier and scored higher on the criteria of getting into sleep as assessed by the Leeds Sleep Evaluation Questionnaire [72]. The improvement in sleep quality was evident from first week of treatment with agomelatine, whereas venlafaxine did not produce any beneficial effect. This can be important clinically in as much as improvement in sleep disturbances often precede that of depressive symptoms [73–75]. Agomelatine has also been shown effective in reducing circadian rhythm disturbances seen in MDD [76].

Other Melatonin Agonists

Tasimelteon, [VES-162] *N*-([(1R,2R)-2-(2,3-dihydro-1-benzofuran-4-yl)cyclopropyl]methyl) propanamide, is a MT1/MT2 agonist developed by Vanda Pharmaceuticals that completed phase III trial in 2010 (Fig. 18.1). In animal studies, tasimelteon exhibited the circadian phase shifting properties of melatonin [77]. In clinical studies on 39 healthy human subjects with transient insomnia after a 5-h phase advance, tasimelteon was administered randomly at doses of 10, 20, 50, or 100 mg against placebo [16]. A decrease in SOL, an increased in SE, and a shift in melatonin rhythm were noticed. In a further extended study involving 411 healthy human subjects after a 5-h phase advance, the administration of tasimelteon improved SE and reduced SOL and wake after sleep onset [16]. In both these phase II and phase III clinical trials, the side effects of tasimelteon did not differ from that of placebo. Long-term studies are needed to establish the effectiveness and safety of tasimelteon in treating insomnia [78]. The FDA granted tasimelteon orphan drug designation status for blind individuals without light perception with a non-24-h sleep-wake disorder in 2010.

TIK-301 (formerly LY-156,735) has been in a phase II clinical trial in the USA since 2002. Originally, it was developed by Eli Lilly and Company and called LY-156,735. In 2007, Tikvah Pharmaceuticals took over the development and named it TIK-301. It is a chlorinated derivative of melatonin with MT1/MT2 agonist activity and 5-HT2C antagonist activity. Its formula is *N*-[2-(6-chloro-5-methoxy-1*H*-indol-3-yl)propyl] acetamide (Fig. 18.1). TIK-301 pharmacokinetics, pharmacodynamics, and safety have been examined in a placebo-controlled study using 20, 35, 50, and 100 mg/day doses in healthy volunteers [79]. Unlike melatonin, TIK-301 induced sleepiness at all doses studied and did not cause unwanted effects like hypothermia, hypotension, or bradycardia.

In another double-blind study on 40 patients with chronic insomnia, TIK-301 was administered at doses of 20, 40, and 100 mg with placebo on two nights with 5 days washout period between treatments [17]. TIK-301 produced significant improvement in subjective and objective measures of SOL at higher doses with a trend of improvement at 20 mg doses. The FDA granted TIK-301 orphan drug designation in 2004, to use as a treatment for circadian rhythm sleep disorder in blind individuals without light perception and individuals with tardive dyskinesia.

Summary

The data presented above clearly indicate that exogenous melatonin and its various analogs promote and maintain sleep. However, there is inconsistency and discrepancy among the large number of reports regarding the degree of efficacy and the clinical significance of these effects. The results of endogenous melatonin's action in insomnia have not been consistent probably because the studies described in existing publications on melatonin's efficacy have utilized different inclusion and exclusion criteria, different outcome measures to evaluate insomnia, different doses of the hormone, and different routes and timing of its administration. There also continues to be considerable controversy over the meaning of the discrepancies that sometimes exist between subjective and objective (polysomnographic) measures of good and bad sleep. Adding to this complexity is melatonin's short half-life and ready metabolism after oral administration of fast-release preparations. Hence, prolonged-release melatonin preparations and melatonin agonists were introduced and have shown good results in treating insomnia.

It is noteworthy that most of the trials that examined the efficacy of melatonin in people with primary sleep disorders were of relatively short trial duration (4–6 weeks or less), as were the trials examining the safety of melatonin in this population (3 months or less). Therefore, the reported efficacy and safety of melatonin may reflect only the short-term effects of melatonin. Long-term safety and efficacy studies are needed for melatonin and especially for melatonin's agonists, particularly considering the pharmacological activity of their metabolites.

References

1. Brzezinski A. Melatonin in humans. N Engl J Med. 1997;336:186–95.
2. Shochat T, Haimov I, Lavie P. Melatonin: the key to the gate of sleep. Ann Med. 1998;30(1):109–14.
3. Haimov I, Lavie P, Laudon M, Herer P, Vigder C, Zisapel N. Melatonin replacement therapy of elderly insomniacs. Sleep. 1995;18(7):598–603.
4. Zhdanova IV, Lynch HJ, Wurtman RJ. Melatonin – a sleep-promoting hormone. Sleep. 1997;20:899–907.
5. Zhdanova IV, Friedman L. Melatonin for treatment of sleep and mood disorders. In: Mischolon D, Rosenbaum J, editors. Natural medications for psychiatric disorders: considering the alternatives. Philadelphia: Williams & Wilkins; 2002. p. 147–74.
6. Nowell PD, Mazumdar S, Buysse DJ, Dew MA, Reynolds 3rd CF, Kupfer D. Benzodiazepines and zolpidem for chronic insomnia: a meta-analysis of treatment efficacy. JAMA. 1997;278(24):2170–7.
7. Lemoine P, Nir T, Laudon M, Zisapel N. Prolonged-release melatonin improves sleep quality and morning alertness in insomnia patients aged 55 years and older and has no withdrawal effects. J Sleep Res. 2007;16:372–80.
8. Kato K, Hirai K, Nishiyama K, et al. Neurochemical properties of ramelteon (TAK-375), a selective

MT1/MT2 receptor agonist. Neuropharmacology. 2005;48:301–10.
9. Miyamoto M. Pharmacology of ramelteon, a selective MT1/MT2 receptor agonist: a novel therapeutic drug for sleep disorders. CNS Neurosci Ther. 2009;15:32–51.
10. Pandi-Perumal SR, Srinivasan V, Spence DW, et al. Ramelteon: a review of its therapeutic potential in sleep disorders. Adv Ther. 2009;26:613–26.
11. Millan MJ, Gobert A, Lejeune F, et al. The novel melatonin agonist agomelatine (S20098) is an antagonist at5-hydroxytryptamine2C receptors, blockade of which enhances the activity of frontocortical dopaminergic and adrenergic pathways. J Pharmacol Exp Ther. 2003;306:954–64.
12. Srinivasan V, Cardinali DP, Pandi-Perumal SR, Brown GM. Melatonin agonists for treatment of sleep and depressive disorders. J Exptl Integ Med. 2011;1:149–58.
13. Kennedy SH, Emsley R. Placebo-controlled trial of agomelatine in the treatment of major depressive disorder. Eur Neuropsychopharmacol. 2006;16:93–100.
14. Llorca PM. The antidepressant agomelatine improves the quality of life of depressed patients: implications for remission. J Psychopharmacol. 2010;24:21–6.
15. Srinivasan V, Brzezinski A, Spence DW, et al. Sleep, mood disorders and antidepressants: the melatonergic antidepressant agomelatine offers a new strategy for treatment. Psychiatrica Fennica. 2010;41:168–87.
16. Rajaratnam SM, Polymeropoulos MH, Fisher DM, et al. Melatonin agonist tasimelteon (VEC-162) for transient insomnia after sleep-time shift: two randomised controlled multicentre trials. Lancet. 2009;373:482–91.
17. Zemlan FP, Mulchahey JJ, Scharf MB, et al. The efficacy and safety of the melatonin agonist beta-methyl-6-chloromelatonin in primary insomnia: a randomized, placebo-controlled, crossover clinical trial. J Clin Psychiatry. 2005;66:384–90.
18. Zhdanova IV, Wurtman RJ, Regan MM, et al. Melatonin treatment for age-related insomnia. J Clin Endocrinol Metab. 2001;86(10):4727–30.
19. Haimov I, Laudon M, Zisapel N, et al. Sleep disorders and melatonin rhythms in elderly people. BMJ. 1994;309:167.
20. Hughes RJ, Badia P. Sleep-promoting and hypothermic effects of daytime melatonin administration in humans. Sleep. 1997;20:124–31.
21. Leger D, Laudon M, Zisapel N. Nocturnal 6-sulfatoxymelatonin excretion in insomnia and its relation to the response to melatonin replacement therapy. Am J Med. 2004;116:91–5.
22. Cajochen C, Jewett ME, Dijk DJ. Human circadian melatonin rhythm phase delay during a fixed sleep-wake schedule interspersed with nights of sleep deprivation. J Pineal Res. 2003;35:149–57.
23. Lavie P. Melatonin: role in gating nocturnal rise in sleep propensity. J Biol Rhythms. 1997;12:657–65.
24. Brzezinski A, Vangel MG, Wurtman RJ, et al. Effects of exogenous melatonin on sleep: a meta-analysis. Sleep Med Rev. 2005;9:41–50.
25. Buscemi N, Vandermeer B, Hooten N, et al. The efficacy and safety off exogenous melatonin for primary sleep disorders: a meta-analysis. J Gen Int Med. 2005;20:1151–8.
26. Braam W, Smits MG, Didden R, Korzilius H, Van Geijlswijk IM, Curfs LM. Exogenous melatonin for sleep problems in individuals with intellectual disability: a meta-analysis. Dev Med Child Neurol. 2009;51(5):340–9.
27. European Food Safety Authority. Scientific Opinion on the substantiation of a health claim related to melatonin and reduction of sleep onset latency (ID 1698, 1790, 4080) pursuant to Article 13(1) of Regulation (EC) No 1924/2006. EFSA J. 2011;9(6):2241.
28. Wilson SJ, Nutt DJ, Alford C, et al. British Association for Psychopharmacology consensus statement on evidence-based treatment of insomnia, parasomnias and circadian rhythm disorders. J Psychopharmacol. 2010;24:1577–601.
29. Turek FW, Gillette MU. Melatonin, sleep, and circadian rhythms: rationale for development of specific melatonin agonists. Sleep Med. 2004;5:523–32.
30. Garfinkel D, Zorin M, Wainstein J, Matas Z, Laudon M, Zisapel N. Efficacy and safety of prolonged-release melatonin in insomnia patients with diabetes: a randomized, double-blind, crossover study. Diabetes Metab Syndr Obes. 2011;4:307–13.
31. Saper CB, Lu J, Chou TC, Gooley J. The hypothalamic integrator for circadian rhythms. Trends Neurosci. 2005;28:152–7.
32. Saper CB, Scammell TE, Lu J. Hypothalamic regulation of sleep and circadian rhythms. Nature. 2005;437:1257–63.
33. Kalsbeek A, Perreau-Lenz S, Buijs RM. A network of (autonomic) clock outputs. Chronobiol Int. 2006;23:521–35.
34. Reghunandanan V, Reghunandanan R. Neurotransmitters of the suprachiasmatic nuclei. J Circadian Rhythms. 2006;4:2.
35. Reppert SM, Weaver DR, Ebisawa T. Cloning and characterization of a mammalian melatonin receptor that mediates reproductive and circadian responses. Neuron. 1994;13:1177–85.
36. Dubocovich ML, Delagrange P, Krause DN, et al. International union of basic and clinical pharmacology. LXXV. Nomenclature, classification, and pharmacology of G protein coupled melatonin receptors. Pharmacol Rev. 2010;62:343–80.
37. Cajochen C. TAK-375 Takeda. Curr Opin Investig Drugs. 2005;6:114–21.
38. Greenblatt DJ, Harmatz JS, Karim A. Age and gender effects on the pharmacokinetics and pharmacodynamics of ramelteon, a hypnotic agent acting via melatonin receptorsMT1 and MT2. J Clin Pharmacol. 2007;47:485–96.
39. Stevenson S, Bryson S, Amayke D, Hibberd M. Study to investigate the absolute bioavailability of a single oral dose of ramelteon (TAK-375) in healthy male subjects. Clin Pharmacol Ther. 2004;75:P22.

40. Wu YH, Zhou JN, Balesar R, et al. Distribution of MT1melatonin receptor immunoreactivity in the human hypothalamus and pituitary gland: colocalization of MT1 with vasopressin, oxytocin, and corticotropin-releasing hormone. J Comp Neurol. 2006;499:897–910.
41. Savaskan E, Olivieri G, Meier F, et al. Increased melatonin1a-receptor immunoreactivity in the hippocampus of Alzheimer's disease patients. J Pineal Res. 2002;32:59–62.
42. Savaskan E, Ayoub MA, Ravid R, et al. Reduced hippocampalMT2 melatonin receptor expression in Alzheimer's disease. J Pineal Res. 2005;38:10–6.
43. Savaskan E, Jockers R, Ayoub M, et al. The MT2 melatonin receptor subtype is present in human retina and decreases in Alzheimer's disease. Curr Alzheimer Res. 2007;4:47–51.
44. Brunner P, Sozer-Topcular N, Jockers R, et al. Pineal and cortical melatonin receptors MT1 and MT2 are decreased in Alzheimer's disease. Eur J Histochem. 2006;50:311–6.
45. Srinivasan V, Pandi-Perumal SR, Trahkt I, et al. Melatonin and melatonergic drugs on sleep: possible mechanisms of action. Int J Neurosci. 2009;119:821–46.
46. Yukuhiro N, Kimura H, Nishikawa H, et al. Effects of ramelteon (TAK-375) on nocturnal sleep in freely moving monkeys. Brain Res. 2004;1027:59–66.
47. France CP, Weltman RH, Koek W, Cruz CM, Mcmahon LR. Acute and chronic effects of ramelteon in rhesus monkeys (Macaca mulatta): dependence liability studies. Behav Neurosci. 2006;120:535–41.
48. Roth T, Seiden D, Sainati S, et al. Effects of ramelteon on patient-reported sleep latency in older adults with chronic insomnia. Sleep Med. 2006;7:312–8.
49. Erman M, Seiden D, Zammit G, Sainati S, Zhang J. An efficacy, safety, and dose–response study of Ramelteon in patients with chronic primary insomnia. Sleep Med. 2006;7:17–24.
50. Roth T, Seiden D, Wang-Weigand S, Zhang J. A 2-night,3-period, crossover study of ramelteon's efficacy and safety in older adults with chronic insomnia. Curr Med Res Opin. 2007;23:1005–14.
51. Zammit G, Erman M, Wang-Weigand S, et al. Evaluation of the efficacy and safety of ramelteon in subjects with chronic insomnia. J Clin Sleep Med. 2007;3:495–504.
52. Mini L, Wang-Weigand S, Zhang J. Ramelteon 8 mg/d versus placebo in patients with chronic insomnia: post hoc analysis of a 5-week trial using 50% or greater reduction in latency to persistent sleep as a measure of treatment effect. Clin Ther. 2008;30:1316–23.
53. Dobkin RD, Menza M, Bienfait KL, et al. Ramelteon for the treatment of insomnia in menopausal women. Menopause Int. 2009;15:13–8.
54. Mayer G, Wang-Weigand S, Roth-Schechter B, et al. Efficacy and safety of 6-month nightly ramelteon administration in adults with chronic primary insomnia. Sleep. 2009;32:351–60.
55. Uchimura N, Ogawa A, Hamamura M, et al. Efficacy and safety of ramelteon in Japanese adults with chronic insomnia: a randomized, double-blind, placebo-controlled study. Expert Rev Neurother. 2011;11:215–24.
56. Uchiyama M, Hamamura M, Kuwano T, et al. Long-term safety and efficacy of ramelteon in Japanese patients with chronic insomnia. Sleep Med. 2011;12:127–33.
57. Pandi-Perumal SR, Srinivasan V, Poeggeler B, Hardeland R, Cardinali DP. Drug insight: the use of melatonergic agonists for the treatment of insomnia-focus on ramelteon. Nat Clin Pract Neurol. 2007;3:221–8.
58. Lam RW. Sleep disturbances and depression: a challenge for antidepressants. Int Clin Psychopharmacol. 2006;21(Suppl1):S25–9.
59. Kupfer DJ. Depression and associated sleep disturbances: patient benefits with agomelatine. Eur Neuropsychopharmacol. 2006;16 Suppl 5:S639–43.
60. Bourin M, Mocaer E, Porsolt R. Antidepressant-like activity of S 20098 (agomelatine) in the forced swimming test in rodents: involvement of melatonin and serotonin receptors. J Psychiatry Neurosci. 2004;29:126–33.
61. Bertaina-Anglade V, La Rochelle CD, Boyer PA, Mocaer E. Antidepressant-like effects of agomelatine(S 20098) in the learned helplessness model. Behav Pharmacol. 2006;17:703–13.
62. Fuchs E, Simon M, Schmelting B. Pharmacology of a new antidepressant: benefit of the implication of the melatonergic system. Int Clin Psychopharmacol. 2006;21 Suppl 1:S17–20.
63. Millan MJ. Multi-target strategies for the improved treatment of depressive states: conceptual foundations and neuronal substrates, drug discovery and therapeutic application. Pharmacol Ther. 2006;110:135–370.
64. Landolt HP, Wehrle R. Antagonism of serotonergic5-HT2A/2C receptors: mutual improvement of sleep, cognition and mood? Eur J Neurosci. 2009;29:1795–809.
65. Varcoe TJ, Kennaway DJ. Activation of 5-HT2C receptors acutely induces Per1 gene expression in the rat SCN in vitro. Brain Res. 2008;1209:19–28.
66. Martin JR, Bos M, Jenck F, et al. 5-HT2C receptor agonists: pharmacological characteristics and therapeutic potential. J Pharmacol Exp Ther. 1998;286:913–24.
67. Detanico BC, Piato AL, Freitas JJ, et al. Antidepressant like effects of melatonin in the mouse chronic mild stress model. Eur J Pharmacol. 2009;607:121–5.
68. Mcelroy SL, Winstanley EL, Martens B, et al. A randomized, placebo-controlled study of adjunctive ramelteon in ambulatory bipolar I disorder with manic symptoms and sleep disturbance. Int Clin Psychopharmacol. 2010;26:48–53.
69. Crupi R, Mazzon E, Marino A, et al. Melatonin treatment mimics the antidepressant action in chronic corticosterone treated mice. J Pineal Res. 2010;49:123–9.
70. Loo H, Hale A, Dhaenen H. Determination of the dose of agomelatine, a melatoninergic agonist and selective 5-HT2Cantagonist, in the treatment of major depressive disorder: a placebo-controlled dose range study. Int Clin Psychopharmacol. 2002;17:239–47.
71. Calabrese JR, Guelfi JD, Perdrizet-Chevallier C. Agomelatine adjunctive therapy for acute bipolar

depression: preliminary open data. Bipolar Disord. 2007;9:628–35.

72. Di Giannantonio M, Di Iorio G, Guglielmo R, et al. Major depressive disorder, anhedonia and agomelatine: an open-label study. J Biol Regul Homeost Agents. 2011;25:109–14.
73. Lopes MC, Quera-Salva MA, Guilleminault C. Cycling alternating pattern in the NREM sleep of patients within major depressive disorder: baseline results and change overtime with a new antidepressant. Sleep Med. 2005;6(Suppl2):87–8.
74. Lopes MC, Quera-Salva MA, Guilleminault C. Non-REM sleep instability in patients with major depressive disorder: subjective improvement and improvement of non-REM sleep instability with treatment (Agomelatine). Sleep Med. 2007;9:33–41.
75. Hardeland R, Poeggeler B, Srinivasan V, et al. Melatonergic drugs in clinical practice. Arzneimittelforschung. 2008;58:1–10.
76. Kasper S, Hajak G, Wulff K, et al. Efficacy of the novel antidepressant agomelatine on the circadian rest-activity cycle and depressive and anxiety symptoms in patients with major depressive disorder: a randomized, double-blind comparison with sertraline. J Clin Psychiatry. 2010;71:109–20.
77. Vachharajani NN, Yeleswaram K, Boulton DW. Preclinical pharmacokinetics and metabolism of BMS-214778, a novel melatonin receptor agonist. J Pharm Sci. 2003;92:760–72.
78. Lankford DA. Tasimelteon for insomnia. Expert Opin Investig Drugs. 2011;20:987–93.
79. Mulchahey JJ, Goldwater DR, Zemlan FP. A single blind, placebo controlled, across groups dose escalation study of the safety, tolerability, pharmacokinetics and pharmacodynamics of the melatonin analog beta-methyl-6-chloromelatonin. Life Sci. 2004;75:1843–56.

Agomelatine in Depressive Disorders

19

Sidney H. Kennedy and Franca M. Placenza

Abstract

Major depressive disorder (MDD) is a debilitating disease with significant personal, social, and economic burden and continues to be the leading cause of disability worldwide. Disappointing rates of remission following treatment with first-line antidepressants primarily targeting the serotonin and norepinephrine systems have provided the impetus for developing alternative treatments targeting novel mechanisms. There is a strong association between MDD and disturbances in circadian rhythm. Agomelatine is a novel antidepressant with actions on the melatonergic system which play a fundamental role in synchronizing circadian rhythms. Its actions as a melatonin receptor (M1 and M2) agonist and as a serotonin receptor (5-HT2c) antagonist also trigger increased dopamine activation in the frontal cortex and decreased glutamatergic actions elsewhere in the brain. Compared to other first-line antidepressants, agomelatine has favorable efficacy and tolerability. In particular, it demonstrates superior effects on sleep and alertness and an absence of sexual dysfunction, making it a useful alternative for the treatment of MDD.

Keywords

Agomelatine • Major depressive disorder • Antidepressant • Melatonin • Efficacy • Tolerability • Neurobiology

Introduction

Major depressive disorder (MDD) is a leading cause of disability worldwide and is also associated with increased morbidity and mortality [1]. Despite the emergence of numerous antidepressants primarily acting on the serotonin and/or norepinephrine transporter, the rate of remission following antidepressant treatment remains disappointing [2]. Central monoamine function

S.H. Kennedy, MD, FRCPC (✉)
Department of Psychiatry,
University Health Network, University of Toronto,
EN8-222, 200 Elizabeth Street, Toronto,
ON M5G2C4, Canada
e-mail: sidney.kennedy@uhn.ca

F.M. Placenza, PhD
Department of Psychiatry, University Health Network,
EN8-222, 200 Elizabeth Street, Toronto,
ON M5G2C4, Canada
e-mail: franca.placenza@uhn.ca

V. Srinivasan et al. (eds.), *Melatonin and Melatonergic Drugs in Clinical Practice*,
DOI 10.1007/978-81-322-0825-9_19, © Springer India 2014

continues to be an important avenue for research into the etiopathology and treatment of depression; however, other neurobiological pathways have been identified as targets for antidepressant treatment [3].

Preclinical Evidence to Support the Antidepressant Effects of Agomelatine

With evidence to support a strong association between MDD and disturbances in circadian rhythm [4], drugs that restore circadian rhythm have potential as antidepressants. Since melatonin plays a fundamental role in synchronizing circadian rhythms, through actions on melatonin receptors (MT1 and MT2) situated on suprachiasmatic nucleus neurons [5], it was reasonable to evaluate the role of agomelatine – an MT1 and MT2 agonist and 5-HT2c antagonist – as a putative antidepressant [6].

Agomelatine has no effect on serotonin release but dose-dependently enhances release of extracellular frontocortical dopamine (DA) and norepinephrine (NE) [7]. There is also evidence that agomelatine increases dopamine firing rates [8] and prevents stress-induced glutamate release in rats [9]. In each of these studies, neither melatonin nor a 5-HT2c antagonist alone increased dopamine or norepinephrine; nor did they demonstrate antidepressant effects [8, 9]. Agomelatine has also displayed neurogenic properties via increased cell proliferation and survival of newly formed cells in the dentate gyrus of the hippocampus with agomelatine treatment in rats [10].

Pharmacology

Agomelatine undergoes rapid metabolism and has a half-life of 1–2 h with peak plasma concentration at 1–2 h. Approximately 90 % of the drug is metabolized by CYP1A2, with CYP2C9 and CYP2C19 contributing to a lesser extent. Agomelatine itself does not inhibit or induce cytochrome p450 enzymes, and the propensity for drug interactions is generally low. While many enzyme inhibitors (e.g., paroxetine, valproic acid, lorazepam) have no significant interaction with agomelatine, both fluvoxamine and ciprofloxacin (potent CYP1A2 inhibitors) prevent agomelatine metabolism and should not be co-prescribed. Enzyme inducers such as nicotine may decrease serum levels of agomelatine and require administration of the 50 mg dose.

Antidepressant Efficacy in Middle Life and Late Life Depression

The original dose finding study identified agomelatine 25 mg as the most effective starting dose [11]. Subsequent studies supported an increase to 50 mg in patients who had failed to show minimal improvement after 2–4 weeks [12, 13]. A further dose finding study compared agomelatine 10, 25, and 25–50 mg to placebo and confirmed that 25 mg is the minimal effective dose [14]. Results from placebo-controlled trials demonstrated a broad spectrum of action across depressive symptoms, including the core "mood" and "loss of interest" items as well as anxiety, sleep, and other somatic symptoms [15]. Two additional placebo-controlled trials performed in the United States using different protocols yielded positive but contradictory results: in one trial the 25 mg but not the 50 mg agomelatine dose was superior to placebo and in the other, 50 mg but not 25 mg was superior to placebo [16, 17]. There is also clear evidence that agomelatine has significant efficacy in preventing relapse [18].

The influence of severity and anxiety has also been examined in agomelatine studies. Greater severity of depression was associated with increased antidepressant efficacy in both middle life [19] and elderly [20] depressed patients. Similarly, in anxious depressed patients, there was a significantly greater effect on anxiety and depressive symptoms compared to SSRI and SNRI antidepressants [21] (see also Chap. 20).

Comparison of Agomelatine to SSRI and SNRI Antidepressants

Venlafaxine, fluoxetine, sertraline, and escitalopram are among the most frequently prescribed first-line antidepressants [22] and have all been evaluated in active comparison trials with agomelatine. In two of these active comparator studies, agomelatine had a statistically significant advantage when compared to fluoxetine in severely depressed patients (1.49 points, $p<0.05$) [23] and when compared to sertraline (1.68 points $p<0.05$) [24], while equivalent rates of efficacy were reported in the venlafaxine and escitalopram comparisons. In a meta-analysis of these comparative trials, there was a significant advantage to agomelatine on both HAMD-17 (1.37 points; $p<0.001$) and the Clinical Global Impression of Improvement Scale (0.24 points; $p<0.001$) [25]. These differences in favor of agomelatine remained statistically significant in an analysis of the 6-month double-blind extension phases of these trials [26]. It is likely that the higher retention rate by patients on agomelatine compared to active comparator drugs contributed to these favorable rates of sustained responses [27].

Specific Attributes of Agomelatine Compared to Other Antidepressants

A number of the active comparator trials had a primary end point designed to evaluate unique aspects of agomelatine. For example, the early effects of agomelatine on sleep and alertness were superior to venlafaxine [28], and, in comparison to sertraline, patients receiving agomelatine reported significantly better "ease of getting to sleep" and "quality of sleep" [24]. The ability of agomelatine to provide antidepressant efficacy in the absence of sexual dysfunction has also been evaluated in two trials. The first involved healthy volunteer students who received agomelatine 25 or 50 mg, paroxetine 20 mg or placebo for 8 weeks. The incidence of sexual dysfunction in the group who received paroxetine was 62 %, while the two agomelatine groups did not differ from placebo in the incidence of sexual dysfunction and both were under 5 % [29]. Similar findings were reported in a study designed to evaluate the rate of sexual dysfunction in remitted depressed patients who were sexually active following 12 weeks of either agomelatine 50 mg or venlafaxine 150 mg. At the end of this trial, 80 % of remitted patients on agomelatine were free of sexual dysfunction compared to 50 % of those taking venlafaxine [30]. This ability to avoid sexual dysfunction is thought to be related to the antagonism of 5-HT2c receptors and facilitation of dopamine release particularly in the frontal cortex [31]. It is also likely that the advantage of agomelatine compared to venlafaxine in a clinical trial designed to explore effects on anhedonia [32] using a specifically developed anhedonia scale [33] may also relate to the indirect effects of agomelatine on release of dopamine and norepinephrine in the frontal cortex [7].

In addition to depression, there is also an emerging literature on the efficacy of agomelatine in the treatment of generalized anxiety disorder in acute [34] and relapse prevention trials [35] as well as in comparison to other antidepressants including escitalopram [36]. To date there are limited data on the efficacy of agomelatine in bipolar depression, in other anxiety disorders including obsessive-compulsive disorder and panic disorder, and also in the treatment of depression in children and youth.

Tolerability and Safety

In general, agomelatine has a favorable side effect profile, with pooled data from the pivotal trials indicating that only dizziness occurred significantly more frequently with agomelatine than with placebo [25]. Agomelatine is also devoid of weight gain, cardiac conduction alterations, or effects on blood pressure. Based on preliminary monitoring of liver function, the European Medicines Agency requires evaluation of hepatic enzymes prior to and during the initial phases of antidepressant treatment with agomelatine. The reported rates of enzyme elevation at or above three times upper limit of normal are in 1.4 % of patients on 25 mg daily and 2.5 % of patients at 50 mg daily [37]; in the majority of cases, these elevations appeared early in treatment and returned to normal levels after drug discontinuation. It remains unknown how these rates compare to elevations in hepatic enzymes with other antidepressants or psychotropic medications.

Finally a number of naturalistic studies have been carried out in European countries, involving several thousand patients who received treatment with agomelatine. Data from these "real-world" trials confirm the efficacy, tolerability, and safety as previously reported and provide additional information on drug safety when agomelatine is used in combination with other antidepressants. In general, these naturalistic studies have confirmed both effectiveness and safety [38] and provide additional evidence of good functional outcomes [39].

In summary, agomelatine is a "first in class" antidepressant with favorable efficacy and tolerability compared to other first-line antidepressants. Given the heterogeneity of MDD, based on clinical presentations and underlying neurobiological disturbances, agomelatine represents a useful alternative for the treatment of MDD.

References

1. Collins PY, Patel V, Joestl SS, March D, Insel TR, Daar AS, Scientific Advisory Board and the Executive Committee of the Grand Challenges on Global Mental Health, Anderson W, Dhansay MA, Phillips A, Shurin S, Walport M, Ewart W, Savill SJ, Bordin IA, Costello EJ, Durkin M, Fairburn C, Glass RI, Hall W, Huang Y, Hyman SE, Jamison K, Kaaya S, Kapur S, Kleinman A, Ogunniyi A, Otero-Ojeda A, Poo MM, Ravindranath V, Sahakian BJ, Saxena S, Singer PA, Stein DJ. Grand challenges in global mental health. Nature. 2011;475(7354):27–30.
2. Warden D, Rush AJ, Trivedi MH, Fava M, Wisniewski SR. The STAR*D project results: a comprehensive review of findings. Curr Psychiatry Rep. 2007;9(6):449–59.
3. Rizvi SJ, Kennedy SH. Emerging drugs for major depressive disorder: an update. Expert Opin Emerg Drugs. 2012;17(3):285–94.
4. Germain A, Kupfer DJ. Circadian rhythm disturbances in depression. Hum Psychopharmacol. 2008;23(7):571–85.
5. Schulz P, Steimer T. Neurobiology of circadian systems. CNS Drugs. 2009;23 Suppl 2:3–13.
6. de Bodinat C, Guardiola-Lemaitre B, Mocaër E, Renard P, Muñoz C, Millan MJ. Agomelatine, the first melatonergic antidepressant: discovery, characterization and development. Nat Rev Drug Discov. 2010;9(8):628–42.
7. Millan MJ, Gobert A, Lejeune F, Dekeyne A, Newman-Tancredi A, Pasteau V, Rivet JM, Cussac D. The novel melatonin agonist agomelatine (S20098) is an antagonist at 5-hydroxytryptamine2C receptors, blockade of which enhances the activity of frontocortical dopaminergic and adrenergic pathways. J Pharmacol Exp Ther. 2003;306(3):954–64.
8. Chenu F, El Mansari M, Blier P. Electrophysiological effects of repeated administration of agomelatine on the dopamine, norepinephrine, and serotonin systems in the rat brain. Neuropsychopharmacology. 2013;38:275–84.
9. Tardito D, Milanese M, Bonifacino T, Musazzi L, Grilli M, Mallei A, Mocaer E, Gabriel-Gracia C, Racagni G, Popoli M, Bonanno G. Blockade of stress-induced increase of glutamate release in the rat prefrontal/frontal cortex by agomelatine involves synergy between melatonergic and 5-HT2c receptor-dependent pathways. BMC Neurosci. 2010;11:68.
10. Banasr M, Soumier A, Hery M, Mocaër E, Daszuta A. Agomelatine, a new antidepressant, induces regional changes in hippocampal neurogenesis. Biol Psychiatry. 2006;59(11):1087–96.
11. Lôo H, Daléry J, Macher JP, Payen A. Pilot study comparing in blind the therapeutic effect of two doses of agomelatine, melatonin- agonist and selective 5HT2c receptors antagonist, in the treatment of major depressive disorders. Encéphale. 2003;29(2):165–71.
12. Kennedy SH, Emsley R. Placebo-controlled trial of agomelatine in the treatment of major depressive disorder. Eur Neuropsychopharmacol. 2006;16:93–100.
13. Olié JP, Kasper S. Efficacy of agomelatine, a MT1/MT2 receptor agonist with 5-HT2c antagonistic properties, in major depressive disorder. Int J Neuropsychopharmacol. 2007;10(5):661–73.
14. Kennedy SH, Avedisova A. Efficacy and safety of 3 agomelatine dose regimens (10, 25, 25–50 mg) versus placebo in out-patients suffering from moderate to severe Major Depressive Disorder. EPA April 08, 2013. Nice.
15. Demyttenaere K. Agomelatine: a narrative review. Eur Neuropsychopharmacol. 2011;21 Suppl 4:S703–9.
16. Stahl SM, Fava M, Trivedi MH, Caputo A, Shah A, Post A. Agomelatine in the treatment of major depressive disorder: an 8-week, multicenter, randomized, placebo-controlled trial. J Clin Psychiatry. 2010; 71(5):616–26.
17. Zajecka J, Schatzberg A, Stahl S, Shah A, Caputo A, Post A. Efficacy and safety of agomelatine in the treatment of major depressive disorder: a multicenter, randomized, double-blind, placebo-controlled trial. J Clin Psychopharmacol. 2010;30(2):135–44.
18. Goodwin GM, Emsley R, Rembry S, Rouillon F, Agomelatine Study Group. Agomelatine prevents relapse in patients with major depressive disorder without evidence of a discontinuation syndrome: a 24-week randomized, double-blind, placebo-controlled trial. J Clin Psychiatry. 2009;70(8):1128–37.
19. Montgomery SA, Kasper S. Severe depression and antidepressants: focus on a pooled analysis of placebo-controlled studies on agomelatine. Int Clin Psychopharmacol. 2007;22(5):283–91.
20. Heun R, Ahokas A, Boyer P, Gimenez-Montesinos N, Pontes-Soares F, Olivier V. The efficacy of agomelatine

in elderly patients with major recurrent depressive disorder: a placebo controlled study. J Clin Psychiatry. 2013;74(6):587–94.
21. Stein DJ, Picarel-Blanchot F, Kennedy SH. Efficacy of the novel antidepressant agomelatine for anxiety symptoms in major depression. Hum Psychopharmacol. 2013;28(2):151–9.
22. Lam RW, Kennedy SH, Grigoriadis S, McIntyre RS, Milev R, Ramasubbu R, Parikh SV, Patten SB, Ravindran AV, Canadian Network for Mood and Anxiety Treatments (CANMAT). Canadian Network for Mood and Anxiety Treatments (CANMAT) clinical guidelines for the management of major depressive disorder in adults. III. Pharmacotherapy. J Affect Disord. 2009;117 Suppl 1:S26–43.
23. Hale A, Corral RM, Mencacci C, Ruiz JS, Severo CA, Gentil V. Superior antidepressant efficacy results of agomelatine versus fluoxetine in severe MDD patients: a randomized, double-blind study. Int Clin Psychopharmacol. 2010;25(6):305–14.
24. Kasper S, Hajak G, Wulff K, Hoogendijk WJ, Montejo AL, Smeraldi E, Rybakowski JK, Quera-Salva MA, Wirz-Justice AM, Picarel-Blanchot F, Baylé FJ. Efficacy of the novel antidepressant agomelatine on the circadian rest-activity cycle and depressive and anxiety symptoms in patients with major depressive disorder: a randomized, double-blind comparison with sertraline. J Clin Psychiatry. 2010;71(2):109–20.
25. Kasper S, Corruble E, Hale A, Lemoine P, Montgomery SA, Quera-Salva MA. Antidepressant efficacy of agomelatine versus SSRI/SNRI: results from a pooled analysis of head-to-head studies without a placebo control. Int Clin Psychopharmacol. 2013;28(1):12–9.
26. Demyttenaere K, Corruble E, Hale A, Quera-Salva MA, Picarel-Blanchot F, Kasper S. A pooled analysis of six month comparative efficacy and tolerability in four randomized clinical trials: agomelatine versus escitalopram, fluoxetine, and sertraline. CNS Spectr. 2013;11:1–8.
27. Kennedy SH, Rizvi SJ. Agomelatine in the treatment of major depressive disorder: potential for clinical effectiveness. CNS Drugs. 2010;24(6):479–99.
28. Lemoine P, Guilleminault C, Alvarez E. Improvement in subjective sleep in major depressive disorder with a novel antidepressant, agomelatine: randomized, double-blind comparison with venlafaxine. J Clin Psychiatry. 2007;68:1723–32.
29. Montejo AL, Prieto N, Terleira A, Matias J, Alonso S, Paniagua G, Naval S, Parra DG, Gabriel C, Mocaër E, Portolés A. Better sexual acceptability of agomelatine (25 and 50 mg) compared with paroxetine (20 mg) in healthy male volunteers. An 8-week, placebo-controlled study using the PRSEXDQ-SALSEX scale. J Psychopharmacol. 2010;24(1):111–20.
30. Kennedy SH, Rizvi S, Fulton K, Rasmussen J. A double-blind comparison of sexual functioning, antidepressant efficacy, and tolerability between agomelatine and venlafaxine XR. J Clin Psychopharmacol. 2008;28(3):329–33.
31. Montejo A, Majadas S, Rizvi SJ, Kennedy SH. The effects of agomelatine on sexual function in depressed patients and healthy volunteers. Hum Psychopharmacol. 2011;26(8):537–42.
32. Martinotti G, Sepede G, Gambi F, Di Iorio G, De Berardis D, Di Nicola M, Onofrj M, Janiri L, Di Giannantonio M. Agomelatine versus venlafaxine XR in the treatment of anhedonia in major depressive disorder: a pilot study. J Clin Psychopharmacol. 2012;32(4):487–91.
33. Snaith RP, Hamilton M, Morley S, Humayan A, Hargreaves D, Trigwell P. A scale for the assessment of hedonic tone the Snaith-Hamilton Pleasure Scale. Br J Psychiatry. 1995;167(1):99–103.
34. Stein DJ, Ahokas AA, de Bodinat C. Efficacy of agomelatine in generalized anxiety disorder: a randomized, double-blind, placebo-controlled study. J Clin Psychopharmacol. 2008;28(5):561–6.
35. Stein DJ, Ahokas A, Albarran C, Olivier V, Allgulander C. Agomelatine prevents relapse in generalized anxiety disorder: a 6-month randomized, double-blind, placebo-controlled discontinuation study. J Clin Psychiatry. 2012;73(7):1002–8.
36. Stein D, Marquez MS, Höschl C, et al. Efficacy and tolerability of agomelatine in generalized anxiety disorder (GAD): a randomised double-blind, placebo-controlled trial with escitalopram as validator. Int J Neuropsychopharmacol. 2012;15(S1).P-04-019.
37. European Medicines Agency. Evaluation of Medicines for Human Use. CHMP Assessment Report for Valdoxan. Doc. Ref.: EMEA/655251/2008, London, 20 Nov 2008.
38. Laux G, VIVALDI Study Group. The antidepressant agomelatine in daily practice: results of the non-interventional study VIVALDI. Pharmacopsychiatry. 2012;45(7):284–91.
39. Novotny V, Pecenak J. Agomelatine in depression treatment, multicenter study in Slovakia. Int J Psych Clin Pract. 2011;15 Suppl 2:33–4.

Melatonin in Mood Disorders and Agomelatine's Antidepressant Efficacy

20

V. Srinivasan, Edward C. Lauterbach, Samuel D. Shillcutt, Domenico De Berardis, Preetha Sharone Kuppuswamy, Rahimah Zakaria, Zahiruddin Othman, Dario Acuña-Castroviejo, and Timo Partonen

V. Srinivasan, MSc, PhD, MAMS (✉)
Sri Sathya Sai Medical Educational and Research Foundation, An International Medical Sciences Research Study Center, Prasanthi Nilayam, 40-Kovai Thirunagar Extn, Goldwins, Coimbatore, TN 641014, India

National Health Sevice, Department of Mental Health, Psychiatric Service of Diagnosis and Treatment, Hospital "G. Mazzini", ASL 4, Teramo, Italy

Department of Neuroscience and Imaging, University "G.D' Annunzio", Chieti 66013, Italy
e-mail: sainivasan@yahoo.com, venkataramanujamsrinivasan6@gmail.com

E.C. Lauterbach, MD
Department of Psychiatry and Behavioral Sciences, and the Department of Internal Medicine, Neurology Section, Mercer University School of Medicine, 655 First Street, Macon, GA 31201, USA
e-mail: eclbgnp@earthlink.net

S.D. Shillcutt, PharmD, PhD
Department of Psychiatry and Behavioral Science, Mercer University School of Medicine, 655 First Street, Macon, GA 31201, USA
e-mail: shillcutt_s@mercer.edu

D. De Berardis, MD, PhD
Department of Mental Health, Psychiatric Service of Diagnosis and Treatment, Hospital "G. Mazzini", Piazza Italia 1, Teramo 64100, Italy
e-mail: dodebera@aliceposta.it

P.S. Kuppuswamy, MD
Department of Psychiatry and Psychology, Mayo Clinic College of Medicine, 200 First Street SW, Rochester, MN 55905, USA
e-mail: preethasharone@gmail.com

R. Zakaria, MBBS, MSc, PhD (Physiology)
Department of Physiology, School of Medical Sciences, Universiti Sains Malaysia, Kubang Kerian, Kelantan 16150, Malaysia
e-mail: rahimah@kck.usm.my

Z. Othman, MD, MMed (Psychiatry)
Department of Psychiatry, School of Medical Sciences, Hospital Universiti Sains Malaysia, Kubang Kerian, Kelantan 16150, Malaysia
e-mail: zahir@kb.usm.my

D. Acuña-Castroviejo, MD, PhD
Department of Physiology, Centro de Investigación Biomédica, Parque de Ciencias de la Salud, Avda. del Conocimiento s/n, Armilla, Granada 18100, Spain
e-mail: dacuna@ugr.es

T. Partonen, MD, PhD
Department of Mental Health and Substance Abuse Services, National Institute for Health and Welfare, Mannerheimintie 166, FI-00300 Helsinki, Finland
e-mail: timo.partonen@thl.fi

V. Srinivasan et al. (eds.), *Melatonin and Melatonergic Drugs in Clinical Practice*,
DOI 10.1007/978-81-322-0825-9_20, © Springer India 2014

Abstract

Numerous clinical studies have shown that melatonin is involved in the pathogenesis of mood disorders like major depressive disorder, bipolar disorder, and seasonal affective disorder or winter depression. Many clinical symptoms seen in depressive patients suggest that disturbances of sleep and circadian rhythms play an important role in the pathophysiology of mood disorders. Disturbances of sleep-wake rhythms and circadian rhythms are linked to malfunctioning of SCN-pineal-melatonin axis. As a rhythm regulating factor and as a hormone involved in the physiological regulation of sleep-wake rhythm, melatonin plays an important role in regulating sleep and circadian rhythm disturbances of mood disorders. Melatonin receptors, namely, MT_1 and MT_2, are found expressed in the suprachiasmatic nucleus of the hypothalamic region, an area concerned with the regulation of various circadian rhythms and sleep-wake rhythm. Although pharmacotherapy of mood disorders has long been associated with the modulation of monoaminergic systems of neuronal circuits in different regions of the brain that are involved in the regulation of mood, attention has been paid in recent years for the development of drugs that can shift, reset, and stabilize the circadian rhythms and improve the quality of sleep. In this context agomelatine, a novel antidepressant with MT_1/MT_2 agonistic and 5-HT_{2c} antagonistic properties, has been introduced. Having proved its efficacy as an effective antidepressant in various animal models of depression, agomelatine has been introduced as an antidepressant for treating patients with major depressive disorders in many European countries and also in the USA. Agomelatine has also been used for treating patients with bipolar disorder, winter depression, and anxiety disorder and has demonstrated its clinical efficacy with rapid onset of action, comparable to other antidepressants like SSRIs and SNRIs. But unlike these drugs, agomelatine does not exhibit adverse side effects like worsening of insomnia or sexual problems, and hence, it is considered as an antidepressant of choice for effective treatment of mood disorders.

Keywords

Melatonin • Agomelatine • Mood disorders • Antidepressant • Sleep-wake rhythms

Introduction

Major depressive disorder (MDD) is a heterogeneous syndrome that comprises a variety of physiological, neuroendocrine, behavioral, and psychological symptoms [1]. The common sleep disturbances reported by patients with depression include delayed sleep onset, early morning wakefulness, reversal of the normal morning peaks in subjective mood, energy, and alertness, and day time fatigue. Several studies point out that there are profound disturbances in sleep and circadian rhythms in depressive disorder [2, 3]. Although unipolar and bipolar depressive patients can be differentiated on the basis of symptoms they manifest, the sleep disturbances exhibited by manic patients, unipolar depressed patients, and bipolar depressed patients are almost similar [4–7]. Polysomnographic studies of sleep disturbances in patients with major depressive disorder show reduced rapid eye movement (REM) latency, elevated REM density, and decreased slow-wave sleep and increased stage 1 and stage 2 sleep [8]. REM sleep is regulated by circadian timekeeping system, while NREM sleep is regulated by homeostatic sleep system [9]. The presence of sleep abnormalities is seen not only in depressive patients but also in the first-degree relatives of depressed patients, suggesting thereby that sleep changes can be viewed as "markers" of depression [10]. As sleep and circadian rhythm disturbances constitute primary symptoms in affective disorders including major depressive disorder (MDD), bipolar disorder (BD), and seasonal affective disorder, the study of a common underlying sleep pathophysiology in these disorders has become a necessity for using appropriate pharmacological agents to normalize the sleep issues in order to achieve complete remission of symptoms. As the key endogenous neurohormone involved in the physiological regulation of circadian rhythms and sleep-wake cycles, melatonin plays an important role in the etiology of mood disorders like major depressive disorder, bipolar disorder, and seasonal affective disorder [11–13]. It is suggested that drugs that cause shifts, resetting, and stabilization of rhythms are considered as the most important for treatment of mood disorders.

Role of Melatonin in Mood Disorders: Studies in Major Depressive Disorder

The interest of melatonin in mood disorders dates back to 1979, when three research groups independently reported lower nocturnal melatonin levels in a group of depressed patients [14–16]. The clinical finding of a subgroup of patients with low nocturnal melatonin levels led to the formulation of "low-melatonin syndrome" in depressed patients in 1983 [17]. Further studies revealed that only depressed patients who had abnormal response to DST (dexamethasone suppression test) had lower nocturnal melatonin levels when compared to healthy control subjects [18–21]. Dexamethasone suppression test (DST) has been used as a possible biological marker for melancholic depression in adults [22]. Increased melatonin levels in patients with major depression have been documented by some other studies. It was suggested that discordant results on melatonin levels in depressed patients may be due to different clinical entities. Phase advances and phase delay of melatonin rhythm have been noted in a number of studies on patients with major depressive disorder [23–25]. Phase shift of melatonin rhythm is considered as a prominent feature of major depressive disorder, suggesting thereby circadian rhythm abnormality in MDD. The duration of 6-sulfatoxymelatonin excretion was also found to be longer in these patients. Treatment of patients with major depressive disorder with imipramine, desipramine, or monoamine oxidase inhibitor caused significant increase in the amplitude of melatonin secretion or urinary 6-sulfatoxymelatonin secretion [26]. The changes in melatonin levels combined with clinical findings seen in depressed patients before and after antidepressant therapy points to the possible involvement of melatonin in the pathophysiology of mood disorders [3, 27].

Melatonin in Bipolar Affective Disorders

Sleep disturbances are a significant aspect of bipolar affective disorders, especially decreased need for sleep which is considered as one of the diagnostic criteria for both BD types I and II. Patients with BD exhibit several abnormalities in circadian rhythms and a circadian preference for evening [28–30]. Patients with BD experience marked reduction in sleep in the night before they switch from depression to mania [31].

A recent study analyzed abnormalities in melatonin biosynthesis pathway in patients with bipolar disorder, and results showed mutations in acetylserotonin O-methyltransferase (ASMT) (a key enzyme in the synthesis of melatonin) genes associated with low ASMT activity were observed in BD, thereby suggesting a role of melatonin as a "susceptibility factor" in BD [32].

Reduction in the amplitude of melatonin secretion was reported in bipolar depressed patients during their depressed phase which was restored back to normal with remission of symptoms [33]. A longitudinal study on a single patient showed an increase of melatonin secretion noted during manic phase as compared to euthymic or depressed phase [34]. However in a study on a group of nine patients with mood disorders, lower melatonin levels were noted during manic, euthymic, and depressed phases as compared to healthy controls. Melatonin levels in bipolar depressed patients can therefore be considered as a *trait marker* of bipolar disorder rather than a state marker [35].

The phase position of melatonin also varies in bipolar disorders. Phase advance in melatonin levels was noted in bipolar patients when compared to normal healthy controls. Phase advance of nocturnal melatonin peak by one hour was noted during manic phase which preceded euthymic or depressed phase [36]. In a study on bipolar I patients, delayed peak melatonin secretion and melatonin levels lower than 60 pg/ml also have been reported. In a pilot clinical study on eleven manic patients who had treatment-resistant insomnia, Bersani used melatonin as an add-on for 30 days with no change made to their antimanic drug regimen. A significant improvement in sleep duration was observed concurrent with a marked decrease in the severity of mania [37]. These studies suggest abnormalities in both the phase and amplitude of melatonin secretion in patients with bipolar depression.

Melatonin in Seasonal Affective Disorder

In seasonal affective disorder (SAD), recurrent episodes of depression occur during winter months and euthymia during summer season. These patients have delayed circadian rhythms. Lewy and his co-workers suggested that relative phase shifting of the circadian rhythms in relation to the timing of sleep-wake rhythm is responsible for the pathogenesis of seasonal affective disorder [38]. Seasonal alteration of melatonin rhythms has been found in some studies on patients with SAD and also elevated daytime melatonin levels in SAD patients during winter season, but healthy control subjects did not manifest any such alterations of seasonal melatonin rhythms in this study [39, 40].

Some studies reported seasonal variations in melatonin rhythms in healthy control subjects also [41–44]. Patients with SAD exhibit phase delay of circadian rhythms, and this has been suggested to be due to later dawn of the winter months that result in disruption of molecular rhythms of SCN and the sleep-wake cycle of SAD patients. Application of bright light in the morning by phase advancing circadian rhythms corrects the phase angle between circadian and sleep-wake schedules and corrects the underlying abnormality in SAD [45, 46].

In SAD patients the most prominent marker of seasonal variations was the change in the melatonin offset [40]. A study by Wehr et al. reported that patients with SAD generate a biological signal of a change in season in a manner similar to that of photoperiodic animals [40].

Pharmacotherapy of Mood Disorders

Most antidepressant medications including selective reuptake inhibitors (SSRIs), serotonin and norepinephrine reuptake inhibitors (SNRIs), tricyclic antidepressants (TCAs), and monoamine oxidase inhibitors (MAOIs) work by targeting the monoamines like serotonin, norepinephrine, and dopamine [47]. There is increasing evidence that suggests that mood disorders are caused by several other hormonal and neurotransmitter systems like brain-derived neurotrophic factor (BDNF), amino acid neurotransmitters, GABA, corticotrophin-releasing factor (CRF), and substance P [48]. As monoaminergic antidepressants were identified primarily through serendipity, a need to develop drugs that could act through circadian system and sleep mechanisms was felt, and thus, melatonergic antidepressants were developed [3].

Moreover, most of the antidepressants that are currently used have varying effects on sleep, while some antidepressants like TCAs and 5-HT receptor antagonists promote sleep initiation and maintenance, and many other antidepressants like SSRIs such as fluoxetine and SNRI (venlafaxine) exert adverse effects on sleep [49]. Most pharmacoepidemiologic surveys indicate that at least one third of patients taking SSRIs receive concomitant sedative-hypnotic medications [50]. Hence clinicians consider antidepressant effects on sleep as potentially important determining factor in selecting the therapeutic option to treat patients with depressive symptoms [51, 52]. The possibility that insomnia does not primarily reflect a consequence or accompanying phenomenon of affective disorders but rather represent a *major triggering factor for the development of depressive disorders* is a new concept. Hence there is a need for development of novel antidepressants that can ameliorate symptoms of insomnia and circadian rhythm dysfunction [53, 54].

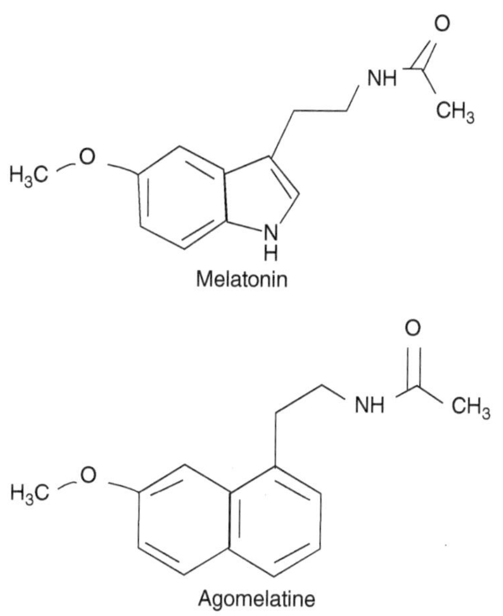

Agomelatine: Chemistry and Pharmacodynamics

Agomelatine, a naphthalenic compound chemically designated as *N*-[2-(7-methoxynaphth-1-yl)ethyl] acetamide or S-20098, is a newly developed selective agonist for MT_1 and MT_2 receptors with antagonism to $5\text{-}HT_{2c}$ receptors [55]. Agomelatine displays overall selectivity (>100 fold) for MT_1 and MT_2 melatonin receptors sites. Agomelatine's half-life is longer than that of melatonin (~2 h) in humans and is metabolized in the liver by three CYP isoenzymes CYPA1, CYPA2, and CYP2C9. The main metabolites of agomelatine are 3-hydroxy S20098, 3-hydoxy, 7-methoxy S20098, 7-desmethyl S20098, and dihydrodiol S20098. Agomelatine has no significant affinity to histaminergic, muscarinic, dopaminergic, and adrenergic receptors. The mean terminal elimination half-life is 2.3 h [55]. Agomelatine's structure is shown in Fig. 20.1.

Fig. 20.1 Melatonin is *N*-acetyl methoxytryptamine and is a hormone synthesized by the pineal gland and also in many other tissues in the body like the retina, gut, lymphocytes, and thymus where it plays an autocrine or paracrine role. Agomelatine is a synthetic analog of melatonin, and it is a naphthalenic compound chemically designated as *N*-[2-(7-methoxynapth-1-yl] acetamide that acts both on MT_1 and MT_2 melatonergic receptors and on $5\text{-}HT_{2c}$ receptors and is a novel antidepressant

Agomelatine's Mechanism of Antidepressant Effects

Agomelatine (Valdoxan[R]) was developed by Servier and Novartis in the USA. In February 2009, Valdoxan was approved by the Europe, the Middle East, and Africa (EU-EMEA) for the treatment of MDD in European countries and is available in all European countries. Although phase III clinical trials have been conducted in the USA, the drug is yet to be approved by the US Food and Drug Administration (FDA). Agomelatine acts synergistically on both melatonergic (MT_1/MT_2) and $5\text{-}HT_{2c}$ receptors [56]. It is an interesting finding that both melatonergic receptors MT_1 and MT_2 and $5\text{-}HT_{2c}$ receptors are expressed in the SCN and other brain areas involved in the pathophysiology of depression, namely, the cerebral cortex, hippocampus,

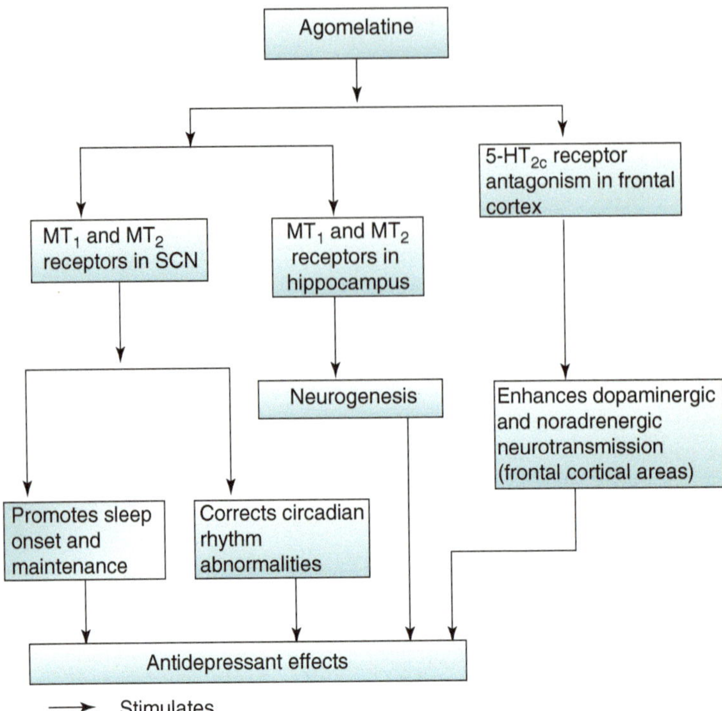

Fig. 20.2 This diagram shows various mechanisms through which agomelatine exerts antidepressant actions. Being a melatonergic agonist, it acts on both MT_1 and MT_2 melatonergic receptors present in SCN and corrects both sleep-wake rhythm and circadian rhythm abnormalities, both of which are essential for its antidepressant actions [2]. Secondly, agomelatine's 5-HT 2c antagonism in the frontal cortex enhances dopaminergic and noradrenergic neurotransmission to areas in the CNS involved in mood regulation and thereby enhances mood [3]. Agomelatine also promotes neurogenesis in hippocampal regions of the brain that are essential for regulation of mood. By acting through all these different mechanisms, agomelatine exerts its antidepressant actions more than any other conventional antidepressants that are in clinical use today

amygdala, and thalamus [57]. Both receptors (MT_1/MT_2 and 5-HT_{2c}) exhibit circadian fluctuations and are regulated by light and biological clock [57]. The combined actions of agomelatine on melatonergic and 5-HT_{2c} receptors help to resynchronize disturbed circadian rhythms and abnormal sleep patterns and will be effective in treating the mood spectrum disorders including MDD, BPD, and SAD [54].

Agomelatine's antidepressant actions are attributed to its sleep-promoting and chronobiotic actions mediated by MT_1 and MT_2 melatonergic receptors present in the SCN as well as due to its effects on the blockade of 5-HT_{2c} receptors. Blockade of 5-HT_{2c} receptors causes release of both norepinephrine (NE) and dopamine (DA) at the frontocortical dopaminergic and noradrenergic pathways. It is well known that dopaminergic and adrenergic mechanisms in the frontal cortex modulate mood and cognitive functions, and antidepressants improve mood and cognition by enhancing the release of NE and DA [58]. The probable mechanism by which agomelatine exerts its antidepressant actions is shown in Fig. 20.2.

Agomelatine exhibits similar actions to that of melatonin in synchronization of circadian rhythms following brief exposure, and this has been demonstrated in various animal models [59–61]. Agomelatine influences daily patterns of locomotor activity, running wheel activity, and body temperature rhythm [59]. The circadian rhythm regulating effect of agomelatine has been demonstrated in young healthy subjects in a double-blind crossover design study in which administration of agomelatine 5–100 mg in the early evening induced phase advance of various rhythms like dim-light saliva melatonin onset, core body temperature minimum, and proximal skin temperature [62]. In another double-blind crossover study, prolonged administration of agomelatine (50 mg/50 days) significantly advanced the circadian rhythm of body temperature by an average of 2 h and cortisol by an average of 1.5–2.0 h in healthy older men (51–76 years old) [63]. These studies demonstrate agomelatine's circadian entrainment and phase-shifting effects in humans.

The antidepressant mechanism of action of agomelatine has been studied in animals by its neurogenic effects on the ventral hippocampus. The ventral hippocampus is implicated in mood and anxiety regulation [64]. Agomelatine reversed the decreased neurogenesis in the glucocorticoid receptor-impaired mice, an animal model of depression, and in corticosterone-treated mice, thereby demonstrating that the hippocampus is also one of its target areas through which agomelatine exerts its antidepressant effects [65, 66].

Agomelatine has demonstrated its antidepressant effects in several animal models of depression like forced swimming test, learned helplessness model, chronic mild stress, and psychosocial stress which have been discussed in an earlier review paper [67].

Clinical Studies with Agomelatine

Clinical efficacy assessment of agomelatine is based on symptomatic relief as measured by Hamilton Depression Rating Scale, HAM-D [68]. A 50 % reduction in the HAM-D baseline score is defined as the *response* to antidepressant therapy, whereas the absence of depressive symptoms and return back to premorbid level of functioning is considered as *remission* [69]. Agomelatine's efficacy as an antidepressant has been assessed in both acute-phase trials and relapse prevention trials as compared to placebo.

In three acute-phase studies conducted with agomelatine, the superiority of agomelatine over placebo was found in 25 mg/day and with increased dose of 50 mg/day [70–72]. The primary outcome for *efficacy* in these studies was the change in the 17-item HDRS score from baseline. Remission rates were found to be significantly higher for agomelatine in the study of Loo et al. (15 % higher), whereas in another study the remission rate was only 7.5 % higher in the total population and 9.1 % higher in the subgroup with severe depression [70, 71]. In the randomized double-blind placebo-controlled trial study of Loo et al. consisting of 711 patients (MDD = 698; BD = 13) diagnosed as per DSM-IV, patients were randomized to receive agomelatine 1, 5, or 25 mg once daily in the evening or placebo during the 8-week study period [70]. Paroxetine 20 mg/day was also used in the study but as a validator of the study methodology and study population. One third of these patients had severe depression (HAM-D 17 score >25). Agomelatine at a dose of 25 mg/day showed a statistically significant efficacy compared to placebo based on the mean final HAM-D score in this study. The time to respond was significantly shorter in the agomelatine 25 mg/day group in comparison to placebo and also was shorter with reference to paroxetine group which showed significant improvement after 4 weeks of treatment, whereas agomelatine 25 mg/day was significantly superior to placebo after 2 weeks of treatment [70].

Similarly the clinical efficacy of agomelatine in MDD was confirmed in another double-blind, placebo-controlled study [71]. In this study (n = 212 patients), agomelatine was administered in 25 and 50 mg doses. On completion of 6 weeks of treatment period, agomelatine was found to be significantly more effective than the placebo group. Significant improvement in the severity of disease as measured with Clinical Global Impression of Severity (CGI-S) was noted with agomelatine compared to placebo. Among the agomelatine 50 mg-treated group (34 % of patients), the HAM-D score decreased from 26.1 ± 2.6 at baseline to 17.5 ± 7.4 at week 6 compared to the placebo group which showed a decrease from 26.7 ± 2.8 to 20.4 ± 6.0. Also, agomelatine at a dose of 50 mg/day was observed to be effective in patients who failed to show improvement after 2 weeks on a dose of 25 mg/day [71].

In another study on 238 patients with moderate to severe major depression, treatment with agomelatine (25–50 mg) resulted in significant decrease of the HAM-D final scores with reference to baseline scores. The severity of the disease as measured with CGI-S also significantly improved with agomelatine [72]. The clinical efficacy of agomelatine was also proved in another double-blind randomized study on 332 patients treated either with agomelatine 25–50 mg/day or with venlafaxine (75–150 mg/day). After 6 weeks of treatment, the antidepressant efficacy of agomelatine was similar to that of venlafaxine as measured by CGI severity. However agomelatine showed greater efficacy in improving subjective sleep than venlafaxine as measured with Leeds Sleep Evaluation Questionnaire (LSEQ) [73].

Agomelatine's efficacy was studied in patients with seasonal affective disorder [74]. Thirty-seven acutely depressed patients with SAD diagnosed as per DSM-IV-TR criteria were selected in an open study, and agomelatine was administered at a dose of 25 mg/day for over 14 weeks. Clinical efficacy was assessed by Structured Interview Guide for the Hamilton Rating Scale (SIGH-SAD) and CGI-S and improvement by circa screen, a self-rating scale for the assessment of sleep and circadian rhythm disorders, and hypomania scale. Response and remission rates were computed from SIGH-SAD score. Response was defined as a reduction of SIGH-SAD total score of more than 50 % from baseline score. Remission was defined as SIGH-SAD total score of less than 8 points. Significant reduction of SIGH-SAD total score was noted from the second week onwards with agomelatine ($p<0.001$). Treatment effects were progressive and sustained throughout the course of trial (baseline score 29.8 ± 4.6, final score at 14 weeks 8.4 ± 10.1). CGI-S score was 4.5 ± 1.0 at baseline, at 14 weeks 1.9 ± 1.3. The reduction in CGI-S score with agomelatine was significant ($p<0.001$). From this study it was noted that 75.7 % of patients had responded to agomelatine treatment. This study being the first of its kind on agomelatine effect in SAD shows that agomelatine exerts its antidepressant action from the second week onwards. The antidepressant efficacy of agomelatine was sustained in a large number of patients revealing sustained remission during the entire period of the study [74].

Clinical efficacy of agomelatine (50 mg) was compared with venlafaxine (target dose of 150 mg) in a total population of 276 (male and female patients). Both treatments resulted in equivalently high rates of remission (agomelatine 73 %, venlafaxine XR 66.9 %), but treatment-emergent sexual dysfunction was significantly less prevalent among patients who received agomelatine, whereas venlafaxine XR was associated with significantly greater deterioration on the sex effects scale domain of desire and orgasm. From this study it is evident that agomelatine is endowed with efficacious antidepressant effect with a superior sexual side effect profile compared with venlafaxine XR [75].

Antidepressant efficacy of agomelatine was also evaluated in patients with BD type I. BD patients on lithium ($n=14$) or valpromide ($n=7$) were given adjunctive open-label agomelatine at 25 mg/day for a minimum of 6 weeks, followed by an additional optional extension up to 46 weeks. Marked improvement (>50 % from baseline HAM-D score) was noted. Among the severely depressed patients (HAM-D score >25.2), 47.6 % responded as early as 1 week of initiating treatment. Of the 19 patients who entered the optional extension period for a mean of 211 days, 11 completed the 1-year extension on agomelatine. During the optional extension period, three lithium-treated patients experienced manic or hypomanic episodes, one of which was treatment related. Otherwise agomelatine 25 mg/day has been found effective for treating BD type I patients (experiencing a major depressive episode), when co-medicated with lithium or valpromide [76].

In a 24-week randomized double-blind treatment study, patients were randomly assigned to receive agomelatine ($n=133$) or placebo ($n=174$); *the time to relapse* was evaluated by using the Kaplan-Meier method of survival analysis. During the 6-month evaluation period, the incidence of relapse was significantly lower in patients who continued to receive agomelatine than those switched to placebo ($p = 0.0001$). The cumulative relapse rate at 6 months for agomelatine-treated patients was 21.7 %, and for placebo-treated patients, it was 46.6 %. From this *long-term study*, it was concluded that *agomelatine is an effective and safe antidepressant* and that the incidence of relapse was significantly lower in patients who continued agomelatine compared to those who switched to placebo [77].

In an 8-week double-blind trial, the *efficacy and safety* of two fixed doses of agomelatine were evaluated in patients with moderate to severe major depressive disorder [78]. Primary efficacy variable was assessed by using HAM-D 17-item scale on 511 MDD patients. Secondary efficacy was assessed by using Clinical Global Impression-Improvement Scale (CGI-I), CGI-S, sleep disability by LSEQ, and disability by Sheehan Disability Scale. Patients were randomized (1:1:1) to once-daily agomelatine 25 mg, agomelatine 50 mg, and placebo. Patients who received agomelatine 50 mg showed statistically significant improvement in HAM-D 17 score from the first baseline visit through the 8-week period. At week 8, the statistical significance was $p = 0.004$ with agomelatine 50 mg, whereas with 25 mg it was $p = 0.505$. Also agomelatine 50 mg was found to be superior than placebo in all other secondary efficacy variables in this study CGI-1 ($p = 0.012$), CGI-S ($p = 0.003$), patients ability to get to sleep ($p < 0.001$), and quality of sleep ($p = 0.002$). These results confirm the significant antidepressant efficacy of agomelatine 50 mg/day with positive effects on sleep. Transient aminotransferase elevations were noted in 4.5 % of the patients in the agomelatine 50 mg group [78].

The efficacy, safety, and tolerability of fixed doses of agomelatine 25 and 50 mg/day were evaluated during an 8-week, multicenter double-blind parallel group trial on outpatients with moderate to severe major depressive disorder as compared to placebo [79]. In this study patients were randomly assigned (1:1:1) to receive once-daily dose of agomelatine 25 mg, agomelatine 50 mg, or placebo. Agomelatine 50 mg/day caused statistically significant reduction in HDRS (17) total score from 2 to 6 weeks but not at week 8 ($p = 0.144$). But higher proportion of patients receiving agomelatine 25 mg/day showed clinical response ($p = 0.013$), clinical remission ($p = 0.07$), and improvement according to the CGI-I ($p = 0.065$) compared to those receiving placebo. However no statistically significant difference between patients receiving agomelatine 50 mg/day and placebo was noted. From this study, agomelatine 25 mg/day was found effective in the treatment of patients with moderate to severe intensity and was safe and well tolerated throughout the 8-week period, whereas agomelatine 50 mg/day provided evidence for its antidepressant efficacy until week 6 of treatment [79].

In a group of severely depressed patients ($n = 252$) with HAM-D score of more than 25 and CGI-S score of 4 and above, an 8-week randomized, double-blind study was carried out with agomelatine and fluoxetine (agomelatine 25–50 mg/day; fluoxetine 20–40 mg/day). The mean decrease in HAM-D 17 total score over 8 weeks was significantly greater with agomelatine than with fluoxetine with a group difference of 1.49. The percentage of responders at last post-baseline assessment was higher with agomelatine on both HAM-D 17, decrease in total score by 50 % from baseline (71.7 % agomelatine vs. 68.8 % fluoxetine; $p = 0.060$), and CGI-improvement score (77.7 % vs. 68.8 %; $p = 0.023$). Although both the treatments were safe and well tolerated, agomelatine showed superior antidepressant efficacy over fluoxetine [80].

The efficacy of agomelatine over sertraline was evaluated in a randomized, double-blind study carried out for 6 weeks. Outpatients with DSM-IV-TR diagnosis of major depressive disorder received either agomelatine 25–50 mg/day ($n = 154$) or sertraline 50–100 mg/day ($n = 159$) for 6 weeks, and efficacy on depression symptoms was evaluated using HAM-D 17 scale and CGI-S; sleep efficiency, sleep latency, and circadian-rest activity were evaluated. Over the 6-week treatment period, depressive symptoms improved significantly more with agomelatine than with sertraline ($p < 0.05$) and also anxiety symptoms ($p<0.05$). A significant improvement in sleep latency ($p<0.001$) and sleep efficiency from week 1 to 6 was observed with agomelatine as compared to sertraline. The relative amplitude of the circadian rest-activity cycle was also in favor of agomelatine as compared to sertraline. All these findings indicate that agomelatine has more beneficial effects on depressed patients [81].

Di Giannantonio and his co-investigators carried out an 8-week open-label study to prove the efficacy of agomelatine (25–50 mg/day) on depressive symptoms in 32 patients with major depressive disorder. Secondary endpoints were the effect of agomelatine on anhedonia assessed by the Hamilton Rating Scale. Of the 24 patients who completed 8 weeks of treatment, significant improvements were noted at all visits on the HAM-D ($p<0.05$), HAM-A (anxiety scale) ($p<0.01$), SHAPS ($p<0.05$), and LESQ-sleep scale ($p<0.05$). Five subjects were remitters (17 %) at week 1. At the end of the trial period, 18 subjects were remitters (60 %). No serious adverse effects or aminotransferase elevations were noted. Not only the evidence for early response to agomelatine treatment and clinical improvements were obtained from this study, but this study is the first of its kind where agomelatine was found to be effective in the treatment of anhedonia [82].

In addition to mood disorders, obsessive-compulsive disorder has also been successfully treated with agomelatine [83]. In this single-case study, agomelatine was administered (25 mg/day) and symptoms of OCD were evaluated at 2 weeks, at 3 weeks, and at the end of 6 weeks. After 2 weeks of treatment, the dose was titrated to 50 mg/day resulting in a gradual improvement of symptoms, and full clinical remission was maintained after 6 weeks of treatment with agomelatine 50 mg/day. In a case series report on six patients with SSRI-refractory OCD, agomelatine 50 mg/day was initiated and patients were followed up for 12 weeks. Three out of six patients showed a Yale-Brown Obsessive Compulsive Scale (Y-BOCS) score reduction of ≥35 %, indicating a possible role of agomelatine in SSRI-refractory OCD patients [84] (Table 20.1).

Safety and Tolerability of Agomelatine

Agomelatine has exhibited a good tolerability and safety in all the clinical studies that have been undertaken so far. The frequency of adverse effects reported (with both 25 and 50 mg/day) such as headache, anxiety, abdominal pain, and diarrhea are similar to that reported for placebo [70]. The cardiovascular profile of agomelatine is also the same as that of placebo with the mean heart rate and blood pressure of patients unchanged [85]. The side effect profile of agomelatine has shown to be good in individual trials as well as pooled analyses. The specific side effects like increases in body weight or sexual dysfunction which are common with some other antidepressants are not seen with agomelatine [86, 87]. Agomelatine's ability to improve sleep-related complaints is not associated with daytime sedation [86].

Impaired sexual function that often occurs with other antidepressants is a major cause of noncompliance [88]. Specific trials were conducted on the effects of agomelatine on sexual function [75]. Agomelatine's effect on sexual dysfunction was compared with venlafaxine ER (by sexual function questionnaire). Desire, arousal, orgasm scores, and the total sexual dysfunction were significantly greater in venlafaxine-treated patients. By the analysis of medication-induced side effects and sexual symptoms associated with intake of antidepressants (either agomelatine or venlafaxine), it was shown that 7.3 % of agomelatine-treated patients and 15.7 % of venlafaxine-treated patients reported deterioration of sexual function [75].

With regard to discontinuation symptoms, only fewer patients discontinued treatment with agomelatine compared to fluoxetine (11.9 % vs. 18.6 %); agomelatine vs. venlafaxine (2.2 % vs. 8.6 %); and agomelatine vs. sertraline (13.6 % vs. 18.9 %) [75, 78, 80]. A double-blind placebo-controlled study on 192 patients was undertaken to assess for any discontinuation symptoms with agomelatine using Discontinuation-Emergent Signs and Symptoms (DESS) checklist [89]. These patients were randomized to receive either

Table 20.1 Agomelatine's antidepressant effects: clinical studies

Agomelatine dosage	Type of patient	Number of patients	Type of study	Duration of study (weeks)	Antidepressant response	Reference
1, 5, 25 mg/day	MDD	711	Double-blind, placebo-controlled	8	25 mg/day was more effective than placebo	[70]
25 and 50 mg/day	MDD	212	Double-blind, placebo-controlled	6	Effective in depressed and severely depressed patients	[71]
25 and 50 mg/day	MDD	238	Double-blind, placebo-controlled	6	Improved depressive symptoms and sleep	[72]
25 mg/day	MDD	332 agomelatine ($n=165$); venlafaxine ($n=167$)	Double-blind randomization	6	Agomelatine showed superior antidepressant and sleep quality	[73]
25 mg/day	SAD	37	Open study	14	Remission was sustained	[74]
25 mg/day	BD type I	21 lithium ($n=14$); valpromide ($n=7$)	Open label	6	Improved depression	[76]
50 mg/day	MDD	276 agomelatine ($n=137$); venlafaxine XR ($n=139$).	Double-blind	12	Agomelatine showed superior antidepressant efficacy	[75]
25 and 50 mg/day	MDD	339	Double-blind, placebo-controlled	24	Very effective antidepressant effect	[77]
25 and 50 mg/day	MDD	511	Double-blind, placebo-controlled	8	50 mg/day has significant antidepressant efficacy with positive effects on sleep	[78]
25 and 50 mg/day	MDD	403	Double-blind, placebo-controlled	8	25 mg/day was effective for moderate to severe intensity	[79]
25–50 mg/day	MDD (severe)	515 agomelatine ($n=252$); fluoxetine ($n=263$)	Double-blind randomization	8	Agomelatine showed superior antidepressant efficacy	[80]
25–50 mg/day	MDD	313 agomelatine ($n=154$); sertraline ($n=159$)	Double-blind randomization	6	Agomelatine showed superior antidepressant and sleep quality	[81]
25–50 mg/day	MDD	30	Open-label study	8	Significant response	[82]

agomelatine 25 mg/day or paroxetine 20 mg/day for 12 weeks followed by an abrupt discontinuation of treatment for 2 weeks during which they were randomized to placebo or their initial antidepressant. Compared to paroxetine, no discontinuation symptoms were noted in patients who discontinued agomelatine [89].

In terms of parameters, mild elevations in serum aminotransferases were reported in 1.1 % of the patients treated with agomelatine, and these increases were isolated and reversible and occurred without any clinical signs of liver damage [86]. In other recent studies, aminotransferase elevations were noted in 2.4 % of the patients in one study and 4.5 % of the patients treated with agomelatine 50 mg/day [78]. These elevations in aminotransferases seen with 50 mg/day of agomelatine are not accompanied by any clinical signs of liver damage but only reflected the higher prevalence of hepatobiliary disorders at baseline, according to medical history, in the agomelatine 50 mg/day group than in agomelatine 25 mg or placebo group (both at 0.6 %).

Conclusion

The role of melatonin in mood disorders like MDD, BD, and SAD has been supported by a number of clinical, physiological, and chronobiological studies. The altered levels of melatonin seen in different groups of mood disorders and circadian rhythm changes in various bodily functions have suggested abnormalities in the functioning of the biological clock located in the SCN of the hypothalamus which are implicated in the pathogenesis of various types of mood disorders. Hence treatment interventions based on the use of antidepressant medications that can shift, reset, and stabilize the functioning of the circadian clock and its rhythms will be greatly helpful in ameliorating symptoms of depressive illness. Agomelatine, a novel melatonergic antidepressant with dual mechanism of action of stimulating MT_1 and MT_2 melatonergic receptors of SCN and 5-HT_{2c} antagonism in the frontal cortex, amygdala, hippocampus, and cortico-limbic structures involved in the regulation of mood and cognition, has been shown to be beneficial in treatment of MDD, SAD, and BD. Agomelatine's 5-HT_{2c} antagonism also enhances frontocortical dopaminergic and noradrenergic transmission which is essential for modulation of mood and antidepressant effect [54, 58]. In addition to its therapeutic efficacy, agomelatine does not manifest any of the adverse effects like sexual dysfunction, sleep disturbances, and discontinuation effects commonly seen with the use of other antidepressants. Its clinical efficacy in major depressive disorder combined with its early onset of action and its good tolerability and safety has been supported by a number of clinicians and research workers and reviewed in recent times [52, 53, 57, 67, 69, 85, 86, 90, 91].

References

1. Nestler EJ, Barrot M, DeLeone RJ, Eisch AJ, Gold SJ, Monteggia LM. Neurobiology of depression. Neuron. 2002;34:13–25.
2. Germain A, Kupfer DJ. Circadian rhythm disturbances in depression. Hum Psychopharmacol. 2008; 23:571–85.
3. Srinivasan V, Pandi-Perumal SR, Trakht I, Spence DW, Hardeland R, Poeggeler B, Cardinali DP. Pathophysiology of depression: role of sleep and the melatonergic system. Psychiatry Res. 2009;165(3):201–14.
4. Riemann D, Berger M, Voderholzer U. Sleep and depression: results from psycho-biological studies. Biol Psychol. 2001;57:67–103.
5. Hudson JI, Lipinski JF, Keck Jr PE, Aizley HG, Lukas SE, Rothschild AJ, Waternaux CM, Kupfer DJ. Polysomnographic characteristics of young manic patients. Comparison with unipolar depressed patients and normal control subjects. Arch Gen Psychiatry. 1992;49(5):378–83.
6. Plante DT, Winkelman JW. Sleep disturbance in bipolar disorder: therapeutic implications. Am J Psychiatry. 2008;165(7):830–43.
7. Hudson JI, Lipinski JF, Frankenburg FR, Grochocinski VJ, Kupfer DJ. Electroencephalographic sleep in mania. Arch Gen Psychiatry. 1988;45(3):267–73.
8. Steiger A, Kimura M. Wake and sleep EEG provide biomarkers in depression. J Psychiatr Res. 2010;44(4):242–52.
9. Dijk DJ, Czeisler CA. Contribution of the circadian pacemaker and the sleep haemostat to sleep propensity, sleep structure, electroencephalographic slow waves and sleep spindle activity in humans. J Neurosci. 1995;15:3526–38.

10. Lustberg L, Reynolds CE. Depression and insomnia: questions of cause and effect. Sleep Med Rev. 2000;4:253–62.
11. Wetterberg L. Melatonin in adult depression. In: Shafii M, Shafii SL, editors. Melatonin in psychiatric and neoplastic disorders. Washington, DC: American Psychiatry Press; 1998. p. 43–79.
12. Lewy AJ, Sack RL, Cutler NL. Melatonin in circadian phase sleep and mood disorders. In: Shafii M, Shafii SL, editors. Melatonin in psychiatric and neoplastic disorders. Washington, DC: American Psychiatry Press; 1998. p. 81–104.
13. Mayeda A, Nurnberger JI. Melatonin and circadian rhythms in bipolar mood disorder. In: Shafii M, Shafii SL, editors. Melatonin in psychiatric and neoplastic disorders. Washington, DC: American Psychiatry Press; 1998. p. 105–23.
14. Beck-Friis J, Ljunggren JG, Thoren M, von Rosen D, Kjellman BF, Wetterberg L. Melatonin, cortisol and ACTH in patients with major depressive disorders and healthy humans with special reference to the outcome of the dexamethasone suppression test. Psychoneuroendocrinology. 1985;10:173–86.
15. Kennedy SH, Garfinkel PE, Parienti V, Costa D, Brown GM. Changes in melatonin levels but not cortisol levels are associated with depression in patients with eating disorders. Arch Gen Psychiatry. 1989;46:73–8.
16. Sack RL, Lewy AJ. Melatonin and major affective disorders. In: Miles A, Philbrick DRS, Thompson C, editors. Melatonin: clinical perspectives. New York: Oxford University Press; 1988. p. 205–27.
17. Wetterberg L, Beck-Friis J, Aperia B, Petterson U. Melatonin/cortisol ratio in depression (letter). Lancet. 1979;2:1361.
18. Wetterberg L. Clinical importance of melatonin. Prog Brain Res. 1979;52:539–47.
19. Mendlewicz J, Linkowski P, Branchey L, Weinberg U, Weitzman ED, Branchey M. Abnormal 24 hour pattern of melatonin secretion in depression. Lancet. 1979;2:1362.
20. Beck-Friis J, Hanssen T, Kjellman BF, Ljunggren J-G, Unden F, Wetterberg L. Serum melatonin and cortisol in human subjects after the administration of dexamethasone and propranolol. Psychopharmacol Bull. 1979;19:646–8.
21. Beck-Friis J, Kjellman BF, Aperia B, Undén F, von Rosen D, Ljunggren JG, Wetterberg L. Serum melatonin in relation to clinical variables in patients with major depressive disorder and a hypothesis of low melatonin syndrome. Acta Psychiatr Scand. 1985;71:319–30.
22. Carrol BJ. The dexamethasone suppression test for melancholia. Br J Psychiatry. 1982;140:292–304.
23. Nair NP, Hariharasubramanian N, Pilapil C. Circadian rhythm of plasma melatonin in endogenous depression. Prog Neuropsychopharmacol Biol Psychiatry. 1984;8:715–8.
24. Wehr TA, Sack DA, Duncan WC, Mendelson WB, Rosenthal NE, Gillin JC, Goodwin FK. Sleep and circadian rhythms in affective patients isolated from external time cues. Psychiatry Res. 1985;15:327–39.
25. Tuunainen A, Kripke DF, Elliott JA, Assmus JD, Rex KM, Klauber MR, Langer RD. Depression and endogenous melatonin in postmenopausal women. J Affect Disord. 2002;69:149–58.
26. Golden RN, Markey SP, Risby ED, Rudorfer MV, Cowdry RW, Potter WZ. Antidepressants reduce whole-body norepinephrine turnover while enhancing 6-hydroxymelatonin output. Arch Gen Psychiatry. 1988;45:150–4.
27. Srinivasan V, Smits M, Spence W, Lowe AD, Kayumov L, Pandi-Perumal SR, Parry B, Cardinali DP. Melatonin mood disorders. World J Biol Psychiatry. 2006;7:138–51.
28. Harvey AG. Sleep and circadian rhythms in bipolar disorder: seeking synchrony, harmony, and regulation. Am J Psychiatry. 2008;165:820–9.
29. Ahn YM, Chang J, Joo YH, Kim SC, Lee KY, Kim YS. Chronotype distribution in bipolar I disorder and schizophrenia in a Korean sample. Bipolar Disord. 2008;10:271–5.
30. Mansour HA, Wood J, Chowdari KV, Dayal M, Thase ME, Kupfer DJ, Monk TH, Devlin B, Nimgaonkar VL. Circadian phase variation in bipolar I disorder. Chronobiol Int. 2005;22:571–84.
31. Sitaram N, Gillin JC, Bunney Jr WE. The switch process in manic-depressive illness. Circadian variations in time of switch and sleep and manic ratings before and after switch. Acta Psychiatr Scand. 1978;58:267–78.
32. Etain B, Dumaine A, Bellivier F, Pagan C, Francelle L, Goubran-Botros H, Moreno S, Deshommes J, Moustafa K, Le Dudal K, Mathieu F, Henry C, Kahn JP, Launay JM, Mühleisen TW, Cichon S, Bourgeron T, Leboyer M, Jamain S. Genetic and functional abnormalities of the melatonin biosynthesis pathway in patients with bipolar disorder. Hum Mol Genet. 2012;21(18):4030–7.
33. Souetre E, Salvati E, Belugou JL, Pringuey D, Candito M, Krebs B, Ardisson JL, Darcourt G. Circadian rhythms in depression and recovery: evidence for blunted amplitude in the main chronobiological abnormality. Psychiatry Res. 1989;28:263–78.
34. Kennedy SH, Tighe S, McVey G, Brown GM. Melatonin and cortisol "switches" during mania, depression and euthymia in a drug free bipolar patient. J Nerv Ment Dis. 1989;177:300–3.
35. Kennedy SH, Kutcher SP, Ralevski E, Brown GM. Nocturnal melatonin and 24 hr 6-sulfatoxymelatonin levels in various phases of bipolar disorder. Psychiatry Res. 1996;63:219–22.
36. Lewy AJ, Wehr T, Gold PW. Plasma melatonin in manic depressive illness. In: Usdin E, Kopin IJ, Barchas JD, editors. Catecholamines: basic and clinical frontiers. Oxford: Pergamon Press; 1979. p. 1173–5.
37. Bersani G, Garavini A. Melatonin add-on in manic patients with treatment resistant insomnia. Prog Neuropsychopharmacol Biol Psychiatry. 2000;24: 185–91.

38. Lewy AJ, Sack RL, Singer CM, White DM, Hoban TM. Winter depression and phase shift hypothesis for bright light's therapeutic effects: history, theory and experimental evidence. J Biol Rhythms. 1988;3: 121–34.
39. Danilenko KV, Putilov AA, Russkikh GS, Duffy LK, Ebbesson SO. Diurnal and seasonal variations of melatonin and serotonin in women with seasonal affective disorder. Arctic Med Res. 1994;53:137–45.
40. Wehr TA, Duncan Jr WC, Sher L, Aeschbach D, Schwartz PJ, Turner EH, Postolache TT, Rosenthal NE. A circadian signal of change of season in patients with seasonal affective disorders. Arch Gen Psychiatry. 2001;58:1108–14.
41. Touitou Y, Fevre M, Bogden A, Reinberg A, De Prins J, Beck H, Touitou C. Patterns of plasma melatonin with ageing and mental condition: stability of nyctohemeral rhythms and differences in seasonal variations. Acta Endocrinol (Copenh). 1984;106:145–51.
42. Kivela A, Kauppila A, Ylöstalo P, Vakkuri O, Leppäluoto J. Seasonal, menstrual and circadian secretions of melatonin, gonadotropins and prolactin in women. Acta Physiol Scand. 1988;132:321–7.
43. Honma K, Honma S, Kohsaka M, Fukuda N. Seasonal variation in the human circadian rhythm: dissociation between sleep and temperature rhythms. Am J Physiol. 1992;262:R885–91.
44. Morera AL, Abreu P. Seasonality of psychopathology and circannual melatonin rhythms. J Pineal Res. 2006;41:279–83.
45. Lewy AJ, Bauer VK, Cutler NL, Sack RL, Ahmed S, Thomas KH, Blood ML, Jackson JM. Morning vs evening light treatment of patients with winter depression. Arch Gen Psychiatry. 1988;55:890–6.
46. Terman JS, Terman JS. Light therapy for seasonal and non seasonal depression: protocol, safety and side effects. CNS Spectr. 2005;10:647–63.
47. Ruhe HG, Mason NS, Schene AH. Mood is indirectly related to serotonin, norepinephrine and dopamine levels in humans: a meta-analysis of mono amine depletion studies. Mol Psychiatry. 2007;12:331–59.
48. Rakofsky JJ, Holtzheimer PE, Nemeroff CB. Emerging targets for antidepressant therapies. Curr Opin Chem Biol. 2009;13:291–302.
49. Pandi-Perumal SR, Trakht I, Srinivasan V, Spence DW, Poeggeler B, Hardeland R, Cardinali DP. The effect of melatonergic and non-melatonergic antidepressants on sleep: weighing the alternatives. World J Biol Psychiatry. 2008;4:1–13.
50. Thase ME. Pharmacotherapy of bipolar depression: an update. Curr Psychiatry Rep. 2006;8:478–88.
51. Winokur A, Gary KA, Rodner S, Rae-Red C, Fernando AT, Szuba MP. Depression, sleep physiology and antidepressant drugs. Depress Anxiety. 2001;14:19–28.
52. De Martinis NA, Winokur A. Effects of psychiatric medications on sleep and sleep disorders. CNS Neurol Disord Drug Targets. 2007;6:17–29.
53. Srinivasan V, Brzezinski A, Spence DW, Pandi-Perumal SR, Hardeland R, Brown GM, Cardinali DP. Sleep, mood disorders and anti depressants the melatonergic antidepressant agomelatine offers a new strategy for treatment. Psychiatrica Fennica. 2010;41:168–80.
54. Kennedy SH, Young AH, Blier P. Strategies to achieve clinical effectiveness: refining existent therapies and pursuing emerging targets. J Affect Disord. 2011;132 Suppl 1:S21–8.
55. Papp M, Gruca P, Boyer PA, Mocaër E. Effect of agomelatine in the chronic mild stress model of depression in the rat. Neuropsychopharmacology. 2003;28:604–703.
56. San L, Arranz B. A novel mechanism of antidepressant action involving melatonergic serotonergic system. Eur Psychiatry. 2008;23:396–402.
57. Masana MJ, Benlousif S, Dubocovich ML. Circadian rhythm of MT_1 melatonin receptor expression in the suprachiasmatic nucleus of the C3H/HeN mouse. J Pineal Res. 2000;28:185–92.
58. Millan MJ, Gobert A, Rivet JM, Adhumeau-Auclair A, Cussac D, Newman-Tancredi A, Dekeyne A, Nicolas JP, Lejeune F. Mirtazapine enhances frontocortical dopaminergic and corticolimbic adrenergic but not serotonergic transmission by blockade of alpha-2 adrenergic and serotonergic 2c receptors; a comparison with citalopram. Eur J Neurosci. 2000;12:1079–95.
59. Redman JR, Guardiola-Lemaitre B, Brown M, Delagrange P, Armstrong SM. Dose dependent effects of S-20098 a melatonin agonist on direction of re-entrainment of rat circadian activity rhythms. Psychopharmacology (Berl). 1995;118:385–90.
60. Pitrosky B, Kirsch R, Malan A, Mocaer E, Pevet P. Organization of rat circadian rhythms during daily infusions or melatonin or S20098, a melatonin agonist. Am J Physiol. 1999;277:812–28.
61. Van Reeth O, Weibel L, Olivares E, Maccari S, Mocaer E, Turek FW. Melatonin or a melatonin agonist corrects age-related changes in circadian response to environmental stimulus. Am J Physiol Regul Integr Comp Physiol. 2001;80:1582–91.
62. Krauchi K, Cajochen C, Mori D, Graw P, Wirz-Justice A. Early evening melatonin and S-20098 advance circadian phase and nocturnal regulation of core body temperature. Am J Physiol. 1997;272:R1178–88.
63. Leproult R, Van Onderbergen A, L'Hermite-Baleriaux M, Van Cauter E, Copinschi G. Phase-shifts of 24-h rhythms of hormonal release and body temperature following early evening administration of the melatonin agonist agomelatine in healthy older men. Clin Endocrinol (Oxf). 2005;63:298–304.
64. Bannerman DM, Deacon RM, Brady S, Bruce A, Sprengel R, Seeburg PH, Rawlins JN. A comparison of GluR-A deficient and wild type mice on a test battery assessing sensorimotor, affective and cognitive behaviours. Behav Neurosci. 2004;118:643–7.
65. Paizanis E, Renoir T, Lelievre V, Saurini F, Melfort M, Gabriel C, Barden N, Mocaër E, Hamon M, Lanfumey L. Behavioural and neoplastic effects of the new-generation antidepressant agomelatine compared to fluoxetine in glucocorticoid receptor impaired mice. Int J Neuropsychopharmacol. 2010;13:759–74.

66. Rainer Q, Xia L, Guilloux JP, Gabriel C, Mocaër E, Hen R, Enhamre E, Gardier AM, David DJ. Beneficial behavioural and neurogenic effects of agomelatine in a model of depression/anxiety. Int J Neuropsychopharmacol. 2012;15:321–35.
67. Pandi-Perumal SR, Srinivasan V, Cardinali DP, Monti MJ. Could agomelatine be the ideal antidepressant? Exp Rev Neurother. 2006;6(11):1595–608.
68. Hamilton M. Development of a rating scale for primary depressive illness. Br J Soc Clin Psychol. 1967;6:278–96.
69. Eser D, Baghai TC, Moller HJ. Agomelatine: the evidence for its place in the treatment of depression. Core Evid. 2009;3:171–9.
70. Loo H, Hale A, D'haenen H. Determination of the dose of agomelatine, a melatonergic agonist and selective 5-HT(2C) antagonist in the treatment of major depressive disorder. Int Clin Psychopharmacol. 2002;17:239–47.
71. Kennedy SH, Emsley RA. Placebo-controlled trial of agomelatine in the treatment of major depressive disorder. Eur Neuropsychopharmacol. 2006;16(2):93–100.
72. Olie JP, Kasper S. Efficacy of agomelatine, a MT1/MT2 receptor agonist with 5-HT2c antagonistic properties in major depressive disorder. Int J Neuropsychopharmacol. 2007;10(5):661–73.
73. Lemoine R, Guilleminault C, Alvarez E. Improvement in subjective sleep in major depressive disorder with a novel antidepressant agomelatine: randomized, double-blind comparison with venlafaxine. J Clin Psychiatry. 2007;68:1723–32.
74. Pjrek E, Winkler D, Konstantinidis A, Willeit M, Praschak-Rieder N, Kasper S. Agomelatine in the treatment of seasonal affective disorder. Psychopharmacology (Berl). 2007;190:575–9.
75. Kennedy SH, Rizvi S, Fulton K, Rasmussen J. A double blind comparison of sexual functioning, antidepressant efficacy, and tolerability between agomelatine and venlafaxine XR. J Clin Psychopharmacol. 2008;28(3):329–33.
76. Calabrese JR, Guelfi JD, Perdrizet-Chevallier C, Agomelatine Bipolar study group. Agomelatine adjunctive therapy for acute bipolar depression: preliminary open data. Bipolar Disord. 2007;6:628–35.
77. Goodwin GM, Emsley R, Rembry S, Rouillon F, Agomelatine Study Group. Agomelatine prevents relapse in patients with major depressive disorder without evidence of a discontinuation syndrome: a 24-week randomized, double-blind, placebo controlled trial. J Clin Psychiatry. 2009;70(8):1128–37.
78. Zajecka J, Schatzberg A, Stahl S, Shah A, Caputo A, Post A. Efficacy and safety of agomelatine in treatment of major depressive disorder: a multicenter, randomized double-blind, placebo controlled trial. J Clin Psychopharmacol. 2010;30(2):135–44.
79. Stahl SM, Fava M, Trivedi MH, Caputo A, Shah A, Post A. Agomelatine in the treatment of major depressive disorder: an 8 week, multicenter, randomized, placebo controlled trial. J Clin Psychiatry. 2010;71(5):616–26.
80. Hale A, Corral RM, Mencacci C, Ruiz JS, Severo CA, Gentil V. Superior antidepressant efficacy results of agomelatine versus fluoxetine in severe MDD patients: a randomized double-blind study. Int Clin Psychopharmacol. 2010;25(6):305–14.
81. Kasper S, Hajak G, Wulff K, Hoogendijk WJ, Montejo AL, Smeraldi E, Rybakowski JK, Quera-Salva MA, Wirz-Justice AM, Picarel-Blanchot F, Baylé FJ. Efficacy of the novel antidepressant agomelatine on the circadian rest-activity cycle and depressive and anxiety symptoms in patients with major depressive disorder: a randomized, double blind comparison with sertraline. J Clin Psychiatry. 2010;71(2):109–20.
82. Di Giannantonio M, Di Iorio G, Guglielmo R, De Berardis D, Conti CM, Acciavatti T, Cornelio M, Martinotti G. Major depressive disorder, anhedonia and agomelatine: an open-label study. J Biol Regul Homeost Agents. 2011;25(1):109–14.
83. De Berardis D, Serroni N, Campanella D, Olivieri L, Moschetta FS, Conti CM, Conti P, Di Giannantonio M. A case of obsessive-compulsive disorder successfully treated with agomelatine monotherapy. J Clin Psychopharmacol. 2012;32(2):289–90.
84. Fornaro M. Switching from serotonin reuptake inhibitors to agomelatine in patients with refractory obsessive-compulsive disorder: a 3 month follow-up case series. Ann Gen Psychiatry. 2011;10(1):5.
85. Rouillon F. Efficacy and tolerance profile of agomelatine and practical use in depressed patients. Int Clin Psychopharmacol. 2006;21 Suppl 1:531–5.
86. Kennedy SH, Rizvi SJ. Agomelatine in the treatment of major depressive disorder: potential for clinical effectiveness. CNS Drugs. 2010;24(6):479–99.
87. Montejo AL, Prieto N, Terleira A, Matias J, Alonso S, Paniagua G, Naval S, Parra DG, Gabriel C, Mocaër E, Portolés A. Better sexual acceptability of agomelatine (25 mg-50 mg) compared with paroxetine (20 mg) in healthy male volunteers. An 8 week, placebo controlled study using the PRSEXDQ-SALSEX scale. J Psychopharmacol. 2010;24:111–20.
88. Rosen RC, Lane RM, Menza M. Effects of SSRIs on sexual function: a critical review. J Clin Psychopharmacol. 1999;19:67–85.
89. Montgomery SA, Kennedy SH, Burrows GD, Lejoyeux M, Hindmarch I. Absence of discontinuation symptoms with agomelatine and occurrence of discontinuation with paroxetine. A randomized double-blind placebo controlled discontinuation study. Int Clin Psychopharmacol. 2004;19:271–80.
90. Fornaro M, Prestia Colicchio S, Perugi G. A systematic, updated review on the antidepressant agomelatine focussing on its melatonergic modulation. Curr Neuropharmacol. 2010;8:287–304.
91. De Berardis D, Di Lorio G, Acciavatti T, Conti C, Serroni N, Olivieri L, Cavuto M, Martinotti G, Janiri L, Moschetta FS, Conti P, Di Giannantonio M. The emerging role of melatonin agonists in the treatment of major depression: focus on agomelatine. CNS Neurol Disord Drug Targets. 2011;10(1):119–32.

The Role of Agomelatine in the Treatment of Anxiety Disorders

21

Domenico De Berardis, Nicola Serroni, Marilde Cavuto, Michele Fornaro, Giovanni Martinotti, Francesco Saverio Moschetta, and Massimo Di Giannantonio

Abstract

Anxiety disorders (ADs) are the most common type of psychiatric disorders. Pharmacological options studied for treating ADs may include several compounds such as benzodiazepines, tricyclic antidepressants (TCAs), noradrenergic and specific serotonergic drug (NaSSA), and dual-reuptake inhibitors of serotonin and noradrenaline (SNRIs). However, the selective serotonin reuptake inhibitors (SSRIs) are the gold standard of the treatment of ADs, but some patients do not respond or withdraw the treatment due to adverse effects. Agomelatine, a new antidepressant, acts synergistically on both the melatonergic and the 5-HT2c receptors and has been shown effective in the treatment of major depression. Moreover, there is evidence that suggests efficacy of agomelatine in the treatment of ADs. Therefore, the aim of this chapter is to review the current literature about agomelatine in the treatment of ADs. The clinical trials evaluating agomelatine in the treatment of generalized anxiety disorder are few but, overall, encouraging on establishing its efficacy. Apart from some interesting case reports, to date, no large studies are present in literature about agomelatine and other ADs such as panic disorder, social anxiety disorder, obsessive-compulsive disorder, and post-traumatic stress

D. De Berardis, MD, PhD (✉) • N. Serroni, MD
F. Saverio Moschetta, MD
Department of Mental Health,
Psychiatric Service of Diagnosis and Treatment,
Hospital "G. Mazzini", Piazza Italia 1,
Teramo 64100, Italy
e-mail: dodebera@aliceposta.it;
serroni.nicola@virgilio.it;
saverio.moschetta@aslteramo.it

M. Cavuto, MD, BA
IASM, L'Aquila 64100, Italy
e-mail: marilde_cavuto@virgilio.it

M. Fornaro, MD, PhD
Department of Education Science,
University of Catania, Via Ofelia N.1,
Catania 95125, Italy
e-mail: dott.fornaro@gmail.com

G. Martinotti, MD, PhD
M. Di Giannantonio, MD, PhD
Department of Neuroscience and Imaging,
"G.D'Annunzio", University of Chieti,
Via dei Vestini 33, Chieti 66013, Italy
e-mail: giovanni.martinotti@gmail.com;
digiannantonio@unich.it

V. Srinivasan et al. (eds.), *Melatonin and Melatonergic Drugs in Clinical Practice*,
DOI 10.1007/978-81-322-0825-9_21, © Springer India 2014

disorder. Therefore, the clinical efficacy and the relative good tolerability of agomelatine may be further investigated to widen the therapeutic spectrum of ADs.

Keywords
Anxiety disorders • Agomelatine • Melatonin • Serotonin • Noradrenaline • Dopamine • Efficacy • Tolerability

Introduction

Anxiety disorders (ADs) are among the most common mental disorders, with lifetime prevalence rates for experiencing any AD ranging from 10.4 to 28.8 % and 12-month prevalence rates of about 18 % [1]. ADs can adversely affect quality of life, mobility, education, employment, social functioning, health care, and physical well-being [2]. The ADs are a group of psychiatric disorders whose key features include excessive anxiety, fear, worry, avoidance, and compulsive rituals. The most prevalent anxiety disorders listed in the *Diagnostic and Statistical Manual of Mental Disorders*, Fifth Edition (DSM-V) include panic disorder with and without agoraphobia, obsessive-compulsive and related disorders, social phobia, generalized anxiety disorder, specific phobia, and trauma- and stressor-related disorders (post-traumatic stress disorder). ADs are often associated with other psychiatric disorders, including major depression (MD), substance abuse, and bipolar disorder (BD) [3].

Several antidepressants have demonstrated some degree of efficacy in the treatment of ADs [4, 5]. Of these, selective serotonin reuptake inhibitors (SSRIs), serotonin-norepinephrine reuptake inhibitors (SNRIs), and noradrenergic and specific serotonergic antidepressant (NaSSA) are currently preferred, being generally safer and better tolerated than tricyclic antidepressants (TCAs) or monoamine oxidase inhibitors (MAOIs) [6].

Recently, because ADs are often associated with desynchronization of internal rhythms, it has been suggested that resetting normal circadian rhythms may have anxiolytic potential [7, 8]. The circadian pacemaker or biological clock, located in the suprachiasmatic nuclei (SCN) of the anterior hypothalamus, on top of the optic chiasma, is the site of generation of circadian rhythms and prepares the organism to anticipate the daily changes in the environment [9]. The activation of melatonergic MT1 receptors directly inhibits firing of neurons in the SCN, thus regulating the amplitude of circadian rhythmicity and facilitating sleep promotion, whereas melatonin-mediated activation of MT2 receptors is responsible for inducing phase shifts and therefore is involved in the entrainment of circadian rhythmicity [5, 7].

Agomelatine, a melatonergic antidepressant with a rapid onset of action, has been shown effective in various types of mood disorders [10, 11]. Moreover, there is evidence that suggests efficacy of agomelatine in the treatment of ADs, and, therefore, the aim of this chapter is to review the current literature about agomelatine in the treatment of ADs.

Clinical Pharmacology of Agomelatine

Agomelatine (Valdoxan®/Thymanax®) (S20098, *N*-[2-(7-methoxynaphth-1-yl)ethyl]acetamide) was first reported in the literature in 1992, among a series of synthetic naphthalene melatonin analogs [11]. Agomelatine was synthesized with the intention of developing a drug that would easily cross the blood–brain barrier and synchronize the circadian rhythm [12]. Investigations of the action of agomelatine on over 80 receptors and enzymes revealed a high affinity for MT1 (K_i=0.1 nM) and MT2 (K_i=0.12 nM), where it exerts an agonistic activity [13], and a moderate affinity for 5-HT2c ($pK_i=6.2$ μM), where it acts as an antagonist [14]. Although it also interacted with 5HT2b receptors, they are poorly represented in the central nervous system and have uncertain functional significance [15]. Agomelatine does not show significant affinity for any of the monoamine transporters or for adrenergic, noradrenergic, dopaminergic, muscarinic, and histaminic receptors [16]. Agomelatine's half-life is longer than that of melatonin (~2 h) in humans and is metabolized in the liver by three CYP isoenzymes, CYPA1, CYPA2, and CYP2C9 [11]. The main metabolites of agomelatine are 3-hydroxy S20098, 3-hydroxy, 7-methoxy S20098, 7-desmethyl S20098, and dihydrodiol S20098. A major oxidative metabolite in humans is 3-hydroxy-7 desmethyl agomelatine, which has low affinity for MT1/MT2 and 5-HT2c receptors [17]. The mean terminal elimination half-life is 2.3 h.

Agomelatine, is administered once daily at a dose of between 25 and 50 mg/day at bedtime [12]. In February 2009, agomelatine was approved by the European Medicines Agency for the treatment of major depression (MD) and is available in several European countries [18].

The major hypothesis to explain the antidepressant action of agomelatine is that this compound could act synergistically on both the melatonergic and the 5-HT2c receptors [19]. This synergy could be implemented at the level of circadian rhythms, with the melatonergic action prevailing during the night and the serotoninergic action prevailing during the day [20]. In vivo data indicate that agomelatine enhances the levels of dopamine (DA) and norepinephrine (NE) in the frontal cortex, but not in the nucleus accumbens or striatum, likely secondary to the blockade of the inhibitory input of 5-HT2c receptors to cortical dopaminergic and adrenergic pathways [21]. In addition, 5-HT outflow in the frontal cortex remained unchanged, and chronic treatment with agomelatine did not cause any adaptive changes in the activity of pre- and postsynaptic 5-HT1a receptors [22]. This finding is notable because the absence of any effect on 5-HT outflow and the absence of functional changes of 5-HT1a receptors allow inference that agomelatine's antidepressant action is not mediated through the mechanisms known for tricyclics, SSRIs, and monoamine oxidase inhibitors [23]. In depressed patients, agomelatine was also found to be effective in reducing sleep complaints, as well as in increasing the duration of slow-wave sleep (SWS), and normalizing sleep structure [18]. Agomelatine normalizes non-rapid eye movement sleep (NREM) in depressed patients [24].

The combined actions of agomelatine on MT1/MT2 and 5-HT2c receptors facilitate the resynchronization of altered circadian rhythms and abnormal sleep patterns and are effective in treating mood disorders of all kinds with a well-recognized specific action on anhedonia dimension [25].

Why Agomelatine May Be Useful in the Treatment of ADs?

Initially, the anxiolytic properties of agomelatine were evaluated in animal models of anxiety [26]. It was demonstrated that morning and evening agomelatine (10–75 mg/kg) administration in rats increased responses in the elevated plus maze and Vogel tests, suggesting the involvement of both the melatonin and the 5-HT2c receptors in the mechanism of anxiolytic-like action of agomelatine [27].

Moreover, in rats, social defeat by an aggressive male conspecific is a natural stressor which is known to induce a state of stress and anxiety as expressed by reduction in behavioral activity, an increase in immobility, and an increase in exploring the enclosed aggressive dominant [28]. Tuma et al. [7] tested the hypothesis whether acute or sub-chronic agomelatine would antagonize the negative consequences of a social defeat in male Wistar rats. They found that social defeat-induced changes were clearly reduced by sub-chronic administration of agomelatine and to a lesser extent by its acute intraperitoneal administration, whereas the acute melatonin did not significantly affect the social defeat-induced behavioral changes.

Unlike agomelatine, the anxiolytic effects were seen independently of the time of day of its administration [29]. As the pretreatment with a selective melatonergic antagonist (prazocine) prevented the anxiolytic effect of agomelatine in the evening but not in the morning, it was suggested that the anxiolytic effect may be related to the 5-HT2c antagonistic property of such drug [30].

In fact, it was demonstrated that mice genetically lacking 5-HT2c receptors showed reduced anxiety, whereas, in other experimental models, 5-HT2c receptor agonists show anxiogenic properties [31]. In fact, while acute administration of SSRIs increases anxiety in rodents through the indirect activation of 5-HT2c receptors, their chronic administration reduces anxiety due to a downregulation of the same receptors [32, 33]. Translating the evidence in humans, it is well known that the antidepressant mirtazapine, a potent antagonist of 5-HT2c receptors, showed anxiolytic properties in patients with MD and GAD [34, 35]. Agomelatine has antagonist properties at native, rat and cloned, human 5-HT2c receptors in vitro [36]. The antagonism of 5-HT2c receptors induced by agomelatine especially in the amygdala and hippocampus may be associated with anxiolytic properties [37]. Moreover, through the blockade of 5-HT2c receptors, agomelatine may also enhance extracellular levels of NA in hippocampus, therefore increasing anxiolytic response [9].

In addition to its 5-HT2c antagonistic properties, it is also possible that anxiolytic effect of agomelatine may also involve the activation of melatonergic receptors in response to anxious states [38]. It is well known that melatonin secretion is under the facilitatory control of pineal β-adrenoceptors (ARs) which are innervated by stress-sensitive adrenergic neurons and several stressful and anxiogenic stimuli may enhance pineal release of melatonin [39]. In a prospective, randomized, double-blind study on 200 adults, Naguib and Samarkandi [40] demonstrated that treatment with melatonin reduced preoperative anxiety. Moreover, melatonin premedication significantly decreased the doses of both propofol and thiopental required to induce anesthesia. It was also demonstrated that melatonin showed anxiolytic properties in mice [41]. To summarize these observations, it was proposed that such actions may be exerted through enhancement of γ-amino butyric acid (GABA)-related pathways: however, this hypothesis needs further confirmation [42].

Review of Current Literature on Agomelatine Treatment of ADs

Generalized Anxiety Disorder (GAD)

Efficacy of agomelatine on anxiety symptoms, especially in the treatment of GAD, has become the object of investigation starting from the observation that agomelatine was effective in reducing anxiety symptoms associated with MD [43].

To date, there are two published randomized, placebo-controlled trials (RCTs) that evaluated agomelatine efficacy and tolerability in GAD. Stein et al. [44] evaluated 121 patients diagnosed with GAD but no comorbid disorders, randomized to agomelatine (25–50 mg/day) or placebo for 12 weeks. Only nine patients failed to complete the trial (92.6 % completers), and there were no differences in rates of withdrawal between agomelatine and placebo. Study results demonstrated significant superiority of agomelatine 25–50 mg as compared with placebo, and the difference between groups was statistically significant in favor of agomelatine from week 6 onward. Moreover, secondary outcome measures, including improvement in associated disability, were consistent with the efficacy of agomelatine. In particular, improvement in sleep symptoms on the self-rated Leeds Sleep Evaluation Questionnaire was more marked on agomelatine than on placebo, including the items for sleep initiation, quality of sleep, and sleep awakening. In this trial, agomelatine was as well tolerated as placebo without development of discontinuation symptoms. The most common emergent adverse events reported more frequently in the agomelatine than in the placebo groups were dizziness (7.9 % vs. 3.4 %) and nausea (4.8 % vs. 1.7 %). However, it should be considered that this clinical trial was for short-term (12 weeks) acute treatment, and therefore, longer trials were necessary to determine the extended response and maintenance of effect from agomelatine treatment in GAD.

In fact, more recently, Stein et al. [45] evaluated the efficacy and tolerability of agomelatine in the prevention of relapse in patients with GAD. Patients who responded to a 16-week course of agomelatine 25–50 mg/day treatment were randomly assigned to receive continuation treatment with agomelatine ($n=113$) or placebo ($n=114$) for 26 weeks, and the main outcome measure was the time to relapse during the maintenance period. These authors reported that, during the 6-month maintenance period, in the intention-to-treat population, the proportion of patients who relapsed during the double-blind period in the agomelatine group (22 patients, 19.5 %) was lower than in the placebo group (35 patients, 30.7 %). The risk of relapse over 6 months was significantly lower with agomelatine than placebo, and the risk of relapse over time was reduced by 41.8 % for agomelatine-treated patients. Moreover, agomelatine was well tolerated throughout the study, and there were no differences in discontinuation symptoms after withdrawal of agomelatine in comparison to maintenance on agomelatine. The most frequent emergent adverse events with agomelatine were similar to those reported during the double-blind treatment period and included headache (11.3 %), nasopharyngitis (9.9 %), dizziness (8 %), nausea (6.5 %), dry mouth (5.7 %), somnolence (5.0 %), and fatigue (4.4 %). Fourteen patients treated with agomelatine had at least one emergent potentially clinically significant abnormal liver enzyme value, but were not discontinued from the study and monitored for liver enzymes.

However, despite these positive observations, it should be noted that patients with GAD frequently have comorbid psychiatric and medical illnesses and such trials excluded significant psychiatric and medical comorbidity: therefore, future studies should be extended to, for example, primary-care settings to substantiate generalizability of these result to the general patient population.

Obsessive-Compulsive Disorder (OCD)

It has been demonstrated that OCD may be associated with disruption of circadian rhythms [46]. Healthy subjects with delayed bedtimes have been reported to have increased rates of obsessive-compulsive symptoms, as compared with non-delayed bedtime subjects [47]. This observation on healthy subjects seems also to apply to patients with clinically diagnosed OCD as they may show hypervigilance and problems falling asleep [48]. As reported by Mukhopadhyay et al. [49], a substantial number of patients with severe, enduring OCD also suffer with delayed sleep phase, which seems to be specifically linked to OCD as opposed to comorbid depression. Moreover, alterations in hormone concentrations, including adrenocorticotropin, corticotropin-releasing hormone, and cortisol, all biomarkers of circadian rhythms, have been reported in patients with OCD [50]. Overall, OCD patients may suffer hyperactivity of the hypothalamic-pituitary-adrenal axis, resulting in increased secretion of adrenocorticotropic hormone and cortisol and a reduced secretion of melatonin [51–53]. Also dehydroepiandrosterone secretion may be substantially higher in the OCD subject than healthy controls [36].

Taken together, these findings support the notion that agomelatine, on the basis of its capability of restoring circadian rhythms, may be useful in the treatment of OCD, but data present in literature are mainly case reports and case series. However, as expected, encouraging evidence emerged when agomelatine was used in the treatment of this disorder. Fornaro et al. [54] reported the outcome of six treatment-refractory OCD patients with or without comorbid mood and/or other anxiety disorders who were switched from SSRIs to agomelatine 50 mg/day and followed up for 12 weeks. Three out of six patients, in particular those with relevant circadian rhythm subjective impairment, showed a Yale-Brown Obsessive Compulsive Scale (Y-BOCS) score reduction of ≥35 %, suggesting a potential role of agomelatine in some SSRI-refractory cases. Da Rocha and Correa [55] described the case of a 17-year-old black male patient with a 3-year history of OCD (mainly contamination obsessions with cleaning and washing compulsions) who did not respond to sertraline (200 mg daily) for 7 months, clomipramine (225 mg daily) for 5 months, augmentation with risperidone (2 mg daily) for 6 months, and aripiprazole (10 mg daily) for 35 days. When agomelatine 25 mg/day was added to his treatment, an improvement in the depressive as well as OCD symptoms was observed and persisted over time.

Recently, De Berardis et al. [56] reported on a 25-year-old female OCD patient with ritual washing of hands and genitals in response to contamination obsessions as well as checking compulsions. She had been treated first with fluvoxamine up to 300 mg/day for approximately 1 year and then with sertraline 200 mg/day and alprazolam 1.5 mg/day for approximately 10 months. Quetiapine up to 450 mg/day was added for almost 6 months to sertraline but was discontinued due to adverse effects. A subsequent trial with clomipramine 150 mg/day was stopped after 3 months due to drowsiness and severe constipation, without observed improvement. At the time of observation, she was taking escitalopram 30 mg/day at the morning for approximately 5 months without improvement but without reported severe adverse effects. Agomelatine 25 mg/day at bedtime was prescribed in addition to escitalopram, and this combination led first to a significant improvement of symptoms and then to complete remission.

Panic Disorder (PD)

To date, there is only one published case report on agomelatine in the treatment of PD. Fornaro [57] described the case of a 24-year-old man who was previously treated with paroxetine (15 mg/day) and clonazepam (2 mg/day) in conjunction with 40 mg/day propranolol for sweating at the age of 21 years, with substantial remission. However, the patient refused to continue maintenance treatment due to loss of libido and ejaculation delay. After a 3-year-long absence, he again required medical assistance because of recurrent panic attacks. The patient decided to start a trial treatment with agomelatine 25 mg/day, and 2 months after beginning the new therapy, his fear of having panic attacks disappeared due to successful therapeutic effects and the absence of reoccurring panic attacks. No significant side effects were observed during the 5-month trial of agomelatine monotherapy 25 mg/day.

Social Anxiety Disorder (SAD)

To date, there is only one published case report on agomelatine in the treatment of SAD. Crippa et al. [58] evaluated a 25-year-old single man with generalized SAD refractory to several pharmacological trials. In fact, he was treated at different times with several singular medications for SAD, including sertraline, citalopram, escitalopram, duloxetine, clonazepam, and venlafaxine, without effects on symptoms and distressing adverse effects such as sexual dysfunction (sertraline and citalopram), nausea and insomnia (duloxetine), sedation (clonazepam), or paradoxical dysphoria (sertraline and citalopram). Agomelatine (25 mg/day) was prescribed, and a partial reduction of social anxiety and physical symptoms within 4 weeks was observed. The dosage was then increased to 50 mg/day, with a striking reduction in anticipatory/performance anxiety and improvements in interpersonal relationships/social functioning within 10 weeks. A 6-month follow-up observation showed no relapse of SAD symptoms and no adverse effects were reported during the treatment period.

Post-traumatic Stress Disorder (PTSD)

To date, there is only one published case report on agomelatine in the treatment of PTSD. De Berardis et al. [59] studied a 44-year-old female housewife with no history of psychiatric disorders who showed a clinical PTSD 5 months after a traffic accident. On the basis of patient's request and refusal to take medications because of fear of weight gain and sexual side effects, they prescribed agomelatine 25 mg/day at bedtime, considering that insomnia and nightmares were her most disturbing symptoms. After 2 weeks, an improvement in PTSD symptoms and sleep quality was observed and medication titrated to 50 mg/day. At the end of the fourth week, further improvement was observed, and after another 5 weeks of continuous improvement, the patient achieved full remission. No adverse effects related to agomelatine were reported.

Conclusions

The analysis of current literature suggests that agomelatine may be a promising treatment for ADs. Agomelatine seems to be efficacious especially in treatment-resistant patients who have failed therapy with other agents such as SSRIs and SNRIs. Moreover, agomelatine seems useful to obtain patient' full recovery without residual symptoms than merely response but without complete recovery and with persistence of subclinical anxiety symptoms. In the majority of the studies and case reports, agomelatine has shown good tolerability, in most cases superior to conventional treatments (such as SSRIs and SNRIs), and this may have led to a favorable response, considering that AD subjects are more distressed by adverse effects (even if these are in the mild-to-moderate range) than patients with other psychiatric disorders. However, the clinical efficacy of this drug will be more evident once more widely prescribed by physicians. The results of the clinical trials evaluating agomelatine in the treatment of GAD are supportive of its efficacy on ADs without severe adverse effects. However, to date, the long-term efficacy of agomelatine (>6 months) has not been yet investigated deeply, and therefore, further long-term studies are needed.

Apart from some interesting and encouraging case reports (especially in OCD), no RCTs are, to date, present in literature about agomelatine and other ADs. Therefore, the clinical efficacy and the relative good tolerability of such drug in other ADs than GAD must be further investigated with randomized, double-blind placebo-controlled studies in order to widen the therapeutic spectrum of ADs and confirm the positive results drawn from case reports.

Disclosure This manuscript was entirely funded by the authors, and no pharmaceutical companies were informed of or were involved in the paper. All authors contributed to this chapter with equal efforts. The authors have no potential conflict of interest directly relevant to the contents of the paper.

References

1. Wittchen HU, Jacobi F. Size and burden of mental disorders in Europe – a critical review and appraisal of 27 studies. Eur Neuropsychopharmacol. 2005;15(4):357–76.
2. De Berardis D, Campanella D, Serroni N, Sepede G, Carano A, Conti C, et al. The impact of alexithymia on anxiety disorders: a review of the literature. Curr Psychiatry Rev. 2008;4(2):80–6.
3. Conway KP, Compton W, Stinson FS, Grant BF. Lifetime comorbidity of DSM-IV mood and anxiety disorders and specific drug use disorders: results from the National Epidemiologic Survey on Alcohol and Related Conditions. J Clin Psychiatry. 2006;67(2):247–57.
4. De Berardis D, Conti CM, Serroni N, Moschetta FS, Olivieri L, Carano A, et al. The effect of newer serotonin-noradrenalin antidepressants on cytokine production: a review of the current literature. Int J Immunopathol Pharmacol. 2010;23(2):417–22.
5. De Berardis D, Serroni N, Carano A, Scali M, Valchera A, Campanella D, et al. The role of duloxetine in the treatment of anxiety disorders. Neuropsychiatr Dis Treat. 2008;4(5):929–35.
6. Pasquini M, Berardelli I. Anxiety levels and related pharmacological drug treatment: a memorandum for the third millennium. Ann Ist Super Sanita. 2009;45:193–204.
7. Tuma J, Strubbe JH, Mocaër E, Koolhaas JM. Anxiolytic-like action of the antidepressant agomelatine (S 20098) after a social defeat requires the integrity of the SCN. Eur Neuropsychopharmacol. 2005;15(5):545–55.
8. André C. Anxiety and circadian rhythms. Encéphale. 2009;35 Suppl 2:S76–9.
9. Srinivasan V, Pandi-Perumal SR, Trahkt I, Spence DW, Poeggeler B, Hardeland R, et al. Melatonin and melatonergic drugs on sleep: possible mechanisms of action. Int J Neurosci. 2009;119(6):821–46.
10. Di Giannantonio M, Di Iorio G, Guglielmo R, De Berardis D, Conti CM, Acciavatti T, et al. Major depressive disorder, anhedonia and agomelatine: an open-label study. J Biol Regul Homeost Agents. 2011;25(1):109–14.

11. Martinotti G, Sepede G, Gambi F, Di Iorio G, De Berardis D, Di Nicola M, Onofrj M, Janiri L, Di Giannantonio M. Agomelatine versus venlafaxine XR in the treatment of anhedonia in major depressive disorder: a pilot study. J Clin Psychopharmacol. 2012;32(4):487–91.
12. De Berardis D, Di Iorio G, Acciavatti T, Conti C, Serroni N, Olivieri L, Cavuto M, Martinotti G, Janiri L, Moschetta FS, Conti P, Di Giannantonio M. The emerging role of melatonin agonists in the treatment of major depression: focus on agomelatine. CNS Neurol Disord Drug Targets. 2011;10(1):119–32.
13. Kasper S, Hamon M. Beyond the monoaminergic hypothesis: agomelatine, a new antidepressant with an innovative mechanism of action. World J Biol Psychiatry. 2009;10(2):117–26.
14. San L, Arranz B. Agomelatine: a novel mechanism of antidepressant action involving the melatonergic and the serotonergic system. Eur Psychiatry. 2008;23(6):396–402.
15. de Bodinat C, Guardiola-Lemaitre B, Mocaër E, Renard P, Muñoz C, Millan MJ. Agomelatine, the first melatonergic antidepressant: discovery, characterization and development. Nat Rev Drug Discov. 2010;9(8):628–42.
16. Olié JP, Kasper S. Efficacy of agomelatine, a MT1/MT2 receptor agonist with 5-HT2c antagonistic properties, in major depressive disorder. Int J Neuropsychopharmacol. 2007;10(5):661–73.
17. Pandi-Perumal SR, Trakht I, Srinivasan V, Spence DW, Poeggeler B, Hardeland R, et al. The effect of melatonergic and non-melatonergic antidepressants on sleep: weighing the alternatives. World J Biol Psychiatry. 2009;10(2):342–54.
18. European public assessment report (EPAR) – Valdoxan. Accessed via http://www.ema.europa.eu/docs/en_GB/document_library/EPAR_-_Summary_for_the_public/human/000915/WC500046224.pdf on 20 Oct 2013.
19. Racagni G, Riva MA, Molteni R, Musazzi L, Calabrese F, Popoli M, Tardito D. Mode of action of agomelatine: synergy between melatonergic and 5-HT2c receptors. World J Biol Psychiatry. 2011;12(8):574–87.
20. Quera-Salva MA, Vanier B, Laredo J, Hartley S, Chapopot F, Moulin C, et al. Major depressive disorder, sleep EEG and agomelatine: an open-label study. Int J Neuropsychopharmacol. 2007;10(5):691–6.
21. Srinivasan V, De Berardis D, Shillcutt SD, Brzezinski A. Role of melatonin in mood disorders and the antidepressant effects of agomelatine. Expert Opin Investig Drugs. 2012;21(10):1503–22.
22. Zupancic M, Guilleminault C. Agomelatine: a preliminary review of a new antidepressant. CNS Drugs. 2006;20(12):981–92.
23. Demyttenaere K. Agomelatine: a narrative review. Eur Neuropsychopharmacol. 2011;21 Suppl 4:S703–9.
24. Quera Salva MA, Hartley S, Barbot F, Alvarez JC, Lofaso F, Guilleminault C. Circadian rhythms, melatonin and depression. Curr Pharm Des. 2011;17(15):1459–70.
25. Di Giannantonio M, Martinotti G. Anhedonia and major depression: the role of agomelatine. Eur Neuropsychopharmacol. 2012;22 Suppl 3:S505–10.
26. Pandi-Perumal SR, Srinivasan V, Maestroni GJM, Cardinali DP, Poeggeler B, Hardeland R. Melatonin: nature's most versatile biological signal? FEBS J. 2006;273:2813–38.
27. Papp M, Litwa E, Gruca P, Mocaer E. Anxiolytic-like activity of agomelatine and melatonin in three animal models of anxiety. Behav Pharmacol. 2006;17(8):9–18.
28. Paul ED, Hale MW, Lukkes JL, Valentine MJ, Sarchet DM, Lowry CA. Repeated social defeat increases reactive emotional coping behavior and alters functional responses in serotonergic neurons in the rat dorsal raphe nucleus. Physiol Behav. 2011;104(2):272–82.
29. Gruca P, Przegalinski E, Mrowiec S, Lason M, Papp M. Evidence for antidepressant and anxiolytic-like activities of melatonin and agomelatine in animal models. Eur Neuropsychopharmacol. 2004;14:S230.
30. De Berardis D, Acciavatti T, Di Iorio G, Corbo M, Serroni N, Campanella D, et al. The melatonergic system: effects on sleep and implications for the treatment of psychiatric disorders. Chronophysiol Ther. 2011;1:59–67.
31. Heisler LK, Zhou L, Bajwa P, Hsu J, Tecott LH. Serotonin 5-HT(2C) receptors regulate anxiety-like behavior. Genes Brain Behav. 2007;6:491–6.
32. Jenck F, Moreau JL, Berendsen HH, Boes M, Broekkamp CL, Martin JR, et al. Antiaversive effects of 5HT2C receptor agonists and fluoxetine in a model of panic-like anxiety in rats. Eur Neuropsychopharmacol. 1998;8(3):161–8.
33. Nunes-de-Souza V, Nunes-de-Souza RL, Rodgers RJ, Canto-de-Souza A. 5-HT2 receptor activation in the midbrain periaqueductal grey (PAG) reduces anxiety-like behaviour in mice. Behav Brain Res. 2008;187(1):72–9.
34. Gambi F, De Berardis D, Sepede G, Campanella D, Galliani N, Carano A, et al. Effect of mirtazapine on thyroid hormones in adult patients with major depression. Int J Immunopathol Pharmacol. 2005;18(4):737–44.
35. Gambi F, De Berardis D, Campanella D, Carano A, Sepede G, Salini G, et al. Mirtazapine treatment of generalized anxiety disorder: a fixed dose, open label study. J Psychopharmacol. 2005;19(5):483–7.
36. Millan MJ, Brocco M, Gobert A, Dekeyne A. Anxiolytic properties of agomelatine, an antidepressant with melatoninergic and serotonergic properties: role of 5-HT2c receptor blockade. Psychopharmacology (Berl). 2005;177(4):448–58.
37. Tardito D, Milanese M, Bonifacino T, Musazzi L, Grilli M, Mallei A, et al. Blockade of stress-induced increase of glutamate release in the rat prefrontal/frontal cortex by agomelatine involves synergy between melatonergic and 5-HT2c receptor-dependent pathways. BMC Neurosci. 2010;11:68.
38. Fornaro M, Prestia D, Colicchio S, Perugi G. A systematic, updated review on the antidepressant

agomelatine focusing on its melatonergic modulation. Curr Neuropharmacol. 2010;8(3):287–304.
39. Li X, Borjigin J, Snyder SH. Molecular rhythms in the pineal gland. Curr Opin Neurobiol. 1998;8(5):648–51.
40. Naguib M, Samarkandi AH. The comparative dose–response effects of melatonin and midazolam for premedication of adult patients: a double-blinded, placebo-controlled study. Anesth Analg. 2000;91(2):473–9.
41. Karakaş A, Coşkun H, Kaya A, Kücük A, Gündüz B. The effects of the intraamygdalar melatonin injections on the anxiety like behavior and the spatial memory performance in male Wistar rats. Behav Brain Res. 2011;222(1):141–50.
42. Cheng XP, Sun H, Ye ZY, Zhou JN. Melatonin modulates the GABAergic response in cultured rat hippocampal neurons. J Pharmacol Sci. 2012;119(2):177–85.
43. Lôo H, Hale A, D'haenen H. Determination of the dose of agomelatine, a melatoninergic agonist and selective 5-HT(2C) antagonist, in the treatment of major depressive disorder: a placebo-controlled dose range study. Int Clin Psychopharmacol. 2002;17(5):239–47.
44. Stein DJ, Ahokas AA, de Bodinat C. Efficacy of agomelatine in generalized anxiety disorder: a randomized, double-blind, placebo-controlled study. J Clin Psychopharmacol. 2008;28(5):561–6.
45. Stein DJ, Ahokas A, Albarran C, Olivier V, Allgulander C. Agomelatine prevents relapse in generalized anxiety disorder: a 6-month randomized, double-blind, placebo-controlled discontinuation study. J Clin Psychiatry. 2012;73(7):1002–8.
46. Lange KW, Lange KM, Hauser J, Tucha L, Tucha O. Circadian rhythms in obsessive-compulsive disorder. J Neural Transm. 2012;119(10):1077–83.
47. Coles ME, Schubert JR, Sharkey KM. Delayed bedtimes and obsessive-compulsive symptoms. Behav Sleep Med. 2012;10(4):258–65.
48. Wulff K, Gatti S, Wettstein JG, Foster RG. Sleep and circadian rhythm disruption in psychiatric and neurodegenerative disease. Nat Rev Neurosci. 2010;11(8):589–99.
49. Mukhopadhyay S, Fineberg NA, Drummond LM, Turner J, White S, Wulff K, et al. Delayed sleep phase in severe obsessive-compulsive disorder: a systematic case-report survey. CNS Spectr. 2008;13(5):406–13.
50. Bigos KL, Folan MM, Jones MR, Haas GL, Kroboth FJ, Kroboth PD. Dysregulation of neurosteroids in obsessive compulsive disorder. J Psychiatr Res. 2009;43(4):442–5.
51. Monteleone P, Catapano F, Tortorella A, Di Martino S, Maj M. Plasma melatonin and cortisol circadian patterns in patients with obsessive-compulsive disorder before and after fluoxetine treatment. Psychoneuroendocrinology. 1995;20(7):763–70.
52. Millet B, Touitou Y, Poirier MF, Bourdel MC, Hantouche E, Bogdan A, et al. Plasma melatonin and cortisol in patients with obsessive-compulsive disorder: relationship with axillary temperature, physical activity, and clinical symptoms. Biol Psychiatry. 1998;44(9):874–81.
53. Gustafsson PE, Gustafsson PA, Ivarsson T, Nelson N. Diurnal cortisol levels and cortisol response in youths with obsessive-compulsive disorder. Neuropsychobiology. 2008;57(1–2):14–21.
54. Fornaro M. Switching from serotonin reuptake inhibitors to agomelatine in patients with refractory obsessive-compulsive disorder: a 3 month follow-up case series. Ann Gen Psychiatry. 2011;10:5.
55. da Rocha FF, Correa H. Is circadian rhythm disruption important in obsessive-compulsive disorder (OCD)? A case of successful augmentation with agomelatine for the treatment of OCD. Clin Neuropharmacol. 2011;34(4):139–40.
56. De Berardis D, Serroni N, Campanella D, Olivieri L, Moschetta FS, Conti CM, et al. A case of obsessive-compulsive disorder successfully treated with agomelatine monotherapy. J Clin Psychopharmacol. 2012;32(2):289–90.
57. Fornaro M. Agomelatine in the treatment of panic disorder. Prog Neuropsychopharmacol Biol Psychiatry. 2011;35(1):286–7.
58. Crippa JA, Hallak JE, Zuardi AW, Chagas MH, Quevedo J, Nardi AE. Agomelatine in the treatment of social anxiety disorder. Prog Neuropsychopharmacol Biol Psychiatry. 2010;34(7):1357–8.
59. De Berardis D, Serroni N, Marini S, Moschetta FS, Martinotti G, Di Giannantonio M. Agomelatine for the treatment of posttraumatic stress disorder: a case report. Ann Clin Psychiatry. 2012;24(3):241–2.

22 Melatonin in the Etiology, Pathophysiology, and Management of Schizophrenia

George Anderson and Michael Maes

Abstract

Emerging data suggests that melatonin has been overlooked in the developmental etiology, course, and treatment of schizophrenia. The neuroimmune and oxidative stress factors in the pathophysiology of schizophrenia and the nature of specific symptoms including circadian dysregulation, sleep disturbance, and metabolic disturbances suggest a significant role for melatonin in course and treatment. Importantly side effects of antipsychotics including tardive dyskinesia, weight gain, and metabolic dysregulation highlight an important therapeutic role for the adjunctive use of melatonin. It is proposed that melatonin interacts with the tryptophan catabolite pathway, known to be altered in schizophrenia. The decrease in melatonin in schizophrenia is mediated by increased activation of the tryptophan catabolite pathway driving tryptophan away from serotonin and melatonin production. This impacts cognition, affect, and motivational processing via changes in the cortex, amygdala, and striatum, respectively. Importantly melatonin may improve not only the quality of life but also the drastic decrease in life expectancy in schizophrenia patients.

Keywords

Melatonin • Schizophrenia • Antipsychotics • Metabolism • Inflammation • Stress • Neuroprogression • Leptin • Agomelatine • Ramelteon

G. Anderson, BSc (Hons), MPhil (Cl. Psych) (✉)
CRC, Rm 30, 57 Laurel St, Glasgow
G11 7QT, Scotland, UK
e-mail: anderson.george@rocketmaiil.com

M. Maes, MD, PhD
Department of Psychiatry,
Chulalongkorn University Hospital, 1873 Rama IV
Road, Bangkok 10330, Thailand
e-mail: dr.michaelmaes@hotmail.com

V. Srinivasan et al. (eds.), *Melatonin and Melatonergic Drugs in Clinical Practice*,
DOI 10.1007/978-81-322-0825-9_22, © Springer India 2014

Introduction

Schizophrenia is a chronic and debilitating disorder affecting around 1 % of people worldwide and is poorly understood and treated [1]. Schizophrenia is also associated with a 25-year decrease in life expectancy, which is not explained by increased levels of suicide [2]. The induction of metabolic syndrome by antipsychotics is generally recognized as a significant contributing factor to decreased life expectancy. For clinical psychiatrists this poses a moral dilemma: antipsychotic medication is the only treatment available for containing psychotic symptoms, but concurrently such treatment contributes to decreased life expectancy and associated longer-term health problems. Given that schizophrenia is being increasingly recognized as an immuno-inflammatory disorder, the changes associated with medication-induced obesity will interact with the course and management of schizophrenia [3]. This is arguably the major ethical and practical issue faced in the management of schizophrenia today.

As well as a role in sleep induction and the regulation of the circadian rhythm [4], melatonin's role in the etiology, course, and management of schizophrenia has received scant attention. Melatonin has a potential role in all three of these aspects of schizophrenia. Any contribution of melatonin to the inhibition of antipsychotic side effects, especially metabolic dysregulation [5, 6], would be of major clinical significance.

This chapter aims to spotlight the under-investigated role of melatonin in schizophrenia, proposing that its adjunctive use will contribute to the alleviation of many of the side effects of both typical and atypical antipsychotics, concurrently contributing to an increase in life expectancy and quality of life. The possible utility of melatonergic drugs, including ramelteon and agomelatine, is also discussed.

Etiology of Schizophrenia

Recent conceptualizations of schizophrenia suggest a powerful role for maternal infection in increasing the risk of schizophrenia in the offspring [7], with epidemiological studies showing that between 38 and 46 % of schizophrenia cases are due to maternal infection, both viral and bacterial [8]. Not every case of maternal infection is associated with the induction of schizophrenia in the offspring, leading to the idea of a "second hit," which can take many forms including childhood trauma and stress [9]. A consequence of maternal infection is an altered offspring immuno-inflammatory response, giving subsequent immune challenges a different character contributing to a second hit but also triggering symptom exacerbations in adulthood. A major mediator of altered neuronal activity is immuno-inflammatory-driven changes in the levels of specific tryptophan catabolites (TRYCATs), including kynurenic acid (KYNA) and quinolinic acid (QUIN), which can have inhibitory and excitatory/excitotoxic effects on neurons, respectively. The induction of the TRYCAT pathways is mediated by the activation of indoleamine 2,3-dioxygenase (IDO) and tryptophan 2,3-dioxygenase (TDO). TDO is a curtailed pathway leading to only kynurenine or KYNA production, whereas IDO is associated with the induction of a wider range of TRYCATs, including QUIN and 3-hydroxy-kynurenine (3-OHK), the latter also being neurotoxic. Normally over 95 % of tryptophan is used in the production of TRYCATs, with any further induction of IDO or TDO depriving the availability of tryptophan for serotonin and melatonin production. Thus levels of melatonin production, by the pineal gland as well as immune cells, are intimately associated with the immuno-inflammatory processes that are proposed to drive the etiology and course of schizophrenia.

Melatonin and Schizophrenia: Etiology

Given the powerful role of prenatal maternal infection in mediating an increased risk of schizophrenia in the offspring, it is of note that pregnancy is a period of significant oxidative stress for the mother. In normal pregnancy the placenta produces gradually increasing levels of melatonin over the course of gestation in a non-circadian manner [10]. This has significant consequences for the mother, placenta, and fetus. Melatonin in the placenta seems to make the placenta more efficient at nutrient uptake [11]. During viral infection, increased levels of antioxidants are known to inhibit the extent of infection, with melatonin modulating both viral and bacterial infections [12]. In macrophages, melatonin inhibits the levels of proinflammatory cytokine production to viral infection via the inhibition of the NF-κB transcription factor [13]. This would suggest that variations in maternal, and especially placental melatonin, would have a significant impact on the course of pregnancy as well as the consequences arising from maternal infection.

Many of the schizophrenia susceptibility genes are regulated by oxidative stress, suggesting that melatonin's antioxidative and anti-inflammatory effects would inhibit the influence of these predominantly early developmentally expressed susceptibility genes. The oxidative stress increase in preeclampsia is associated with an increased risk of schizophrenia in the offspring [14]. Recent data shows that melatonin levels, melatonin receptors, and the conversion of serotonin to *N*-acetylserotonin (NAS) and melatonin by arylalkylamine *N*-acetyltransferase (AANAT) are significantly reduced in preeclamptic pregnancies [15]. Preeclampsia is associated with decreased levels of IDO at the maternal-fetal interface, so decreased melatonin is not a consequence of tryptophan being driven down the IDO pathways and away from melatonin and serotonin production. Any increase in placental TDO, highly expressed only in early pregnancy in the rodent, is still to be investigated in preeclampsia. However, it seems that preeclampsia results in increased levels of placental serotonin [15], suggesting that levels of AANAT are rate limiting for NAS and melatonin production. An increase in placental serotonin may be of particular relevance to fetal outcomes. The placenta is a significant source of serotonin for the early-stage fetus, modulating the development of axons and neuronal connectivity [16]. Any significant increase or decrease in serotonin results in altered neuronal development, concurrently increasing anxiety levels in the offspring.

Maternal obesity increases preeclampsia risk three to tenfold [17, 18]. Maternal obesity is linked to increased levels of leptin and associated increased leptin resistance. Leptin is highly produced by the placenta in normal pregnancy but is dramatically increased in preeclamptic pregnancies [19]. In women increased levels of leptin and leptin resistance are associated with decreased melatonin production, and in animals leptin increases levels of AANAT [20], increasing NAS and melatonin production from serotonin. Although requiring experimental validation, this seems to suggest that increased levels of leptin resistance would be associated with decreased placental melatonin production, with negative consequences for the mother, placenta, and fetus, as well as concurrently altering leptin and melatonin's powerful regulation of the immune and cortisol systems. As such decreased melatonin may be a significant modulator, if not mediator, of conditions of pregnancy associated with heightened schizophrenia risk in the offspring.

Another significant innate [21] and adaptive [22] immune regulator is vitamin D (vit D). Decreased vit D increases the risk of schizophrenia in the offspring, at least in part mediated by increased risk of infection as well as preeclampsia [23, 24]. In other human conditions, a synergistic interaction of melatonin and vit D has been shown to occur, including in the inhibition of breast cancer cell proliferation [25]. As to whether melatonin and vit D interact at the maternal-fetal interface in the regulation of preeclampsia and offspring schizophrenia risk remains to be determined. The melatonin-1 receptor (MT1r) is a susceptibility gene for schizophrenia [26]. The above would suggest that some of the influence of MT1r variants on schizophrenia risk might be in the placenta and early-stage fetus.

A corollary of both maternal stress/infection and preeclampsia is decreased placental 11b-hydroxysteroid-dehydrogenase type 2 (11b HSD2), leading to increased cortisol to the placenta and the fetus [27, 28]. Increased transfer of cortisol modulates fetal development including decreasing neurogenesis and increasing the renin-angiotensin system (RAS) both peripherally and centrally. Melatonin is known to prevent the long-term glucocorticoid inhibition of neurogenesis [29]. Melatonin significantly inhibits cortisol's glucocorticoid receptor (Gcr) nuclear translocation [30], likely mediated via increased Bcl-2-associated athanogene-1 (BAG-1). Any increase in BAG-1 by melatonin would also potentiate the effects of vitamin D3, which is chaperoned by BAG-1 to the nuclear vit D receptor [31]. BAG-1 induction could therefore contribute to the melatonin interactions with the effects of vit D, as suggested above [25].

The impact of the prenatal increase in placental cortisol transfer on the RAS will increase childhood and adult blood pressure, as well as increasing adult hypertension susceptibility [32]. Melatonin, in part via increased peripheral vasodilation, decreases hypertension as well as increasing neurogenesis. As such variations in melatonin, as with leptin, will act to inhibit cortisol's prenatal effects, as well as regulating later factors that constitute a "second hit" [33].

It is important to emphasize that not all women who experience infection or preeclampsia in pregnancy have offspring that go on to develop schizophrenia. A "second hit" is necessary, which may take many forms, including trauma and social stress, but which may ultimately be an immune response, acting on a prenatally altered immune system [7]. Variations in melatonin and the susceptibility allele of the MT1r may then be impacting on the nature and consequences of the "second hit." Melatonin is safe and efficacious for many conditions in neonates and older children [34], suggesting its safe use in the modulation of the early developmental factors in the etiology of schizophrenia.

A further corollary of the above is that schizophrenia should be associated with increased levels of anxiety and depression, and indeed this is the case. One study of schizophrenic patients found that 61 % met criteria for a diagnosis of depression, previously undiagnosed [35]. This has led to the proposal that the early developmental etiology of schizophrenia acts to prime people for a heightened susceptibility to comorbid depression [36], which is suggested to be mediated by an immune-/inflammatory-induced increase in IDO and TDO activity, driving tryptophan away from serotonin and melatonin production and to the production of TRYCATs, including KYNA and QUIN. As well as having relevance to the prenatal etiology and to stress-induced exacerbations in adult manifestations of the disorder, such changes may also enhance the likelihood of a "second hit."

The mechanisms through which this is mediated may have parallels to the animal literature on the nature of chronic unpredictable mild stress (CUMS), which increases depression via the central enhancement of QUIN in the amygdala and striatum, and a trend KYNA increase in the frontal cortex [37, 38]. Stress-induced cortisol transiently increases interleukin-18 (IL-18) [39]. IL-18 levels positively correlate with increased cortisol in human medical conditions [40]. IL-18 levels are increased in schizophrenia [41], with IL-18 being a schizophrenia susceptibility gene [42]. IL-18, predominantly via the induction of interferon-gamma (IFNy) but also independently, increases IDO including in microglia. A resultant increase in QUIN activates the *N*-methyl-D-ASPARTATE receptor (NMDAr), increasing neuronal activity in specific CNS regions, with excitotoxicity occurring at higher concentrations. This would suggest that prenatal infection primes not only an increase in the comorbid expression of depression, but also may act to prime the "second hit" effects of stress.

It remains to be determined as to whether prenatal stress-/infection- or preeclampsia-induced increases in placental cortisol transfer also increase IL-18 and the TRYCAT pathway, with consequences not only in the developing fetus but also for the childhood "second hit" and adult exacerbations. The prefrontal cortex, amygdala, and striatum are significant sites for changes in schizophrenia. These same areas show TRYCAT changes induced by CUMS leading to a proposed occluded role for the relatively early developing amygdala in the coordination of wider CNS changes [43]. This remains to be fully examined, but melatonin and vit D are likely to inhibit and protect against such putative consequences of dysregulated cortisol. Such enhancement of the TRYCAT pathway will contribute to the low melatonin levels commonly found in schizophrenia.

Melatonin and the Course of Schizophrenia

The immuno-inflammatory changes crucial to the etiology of schizophrenia are also relevant to the immuno-pathophysiological changes occurring during the course of the disorder. Two recent meta-analyses have highlighted the role of monocytic activation in schizophrenia, including enhanced production of proinflammatory cytokines (PICs). Concurrently T cell activation driving a Th1-like pattern of PICs is also evident [44, 45]. However, a mixed immune response with increased Th2-like, as well as TH1-like, cytokines has also been found [46]. An increase in neuroinflammation is also evident in schizophrenic patients, suggesting that developmental neuroinflammation caused by maternal prenatal infections is pathophysiologically relevant in driving the course of adult manifestations, contributing to progressive brain changes and to the progression of the disorder itself [7]. This is, in part, mediated by increased oxidative damage, leading to lipid peroxidation, DNA damage, and oxidatively modified proteins [47]. Schizophrenia as well as bipolar disorder has been conceptualized as both a circadian and metabolic disorder, with increased oxidative stress-induced damage contributing to mitochondrial dysfunction and vice versa [48].

As a regulator of the immune and circadian systems as well as being a powerful antioxidant, anti-inflammatory [49, 50], and inducer of mitochondrial oxidative phosphorylation [51], variation in levels of endogenous melatonin is likely to modulate such factors relevant to the course of schizophrenia. In addition to being an antioxidant, melatonin also increases the production of nuclear factor erythroid-derived-2 (NF-E2)-related factor (Nrf-2)-induced endogenous antioxidants [52] via the phosphorylation and inhibition of glycogen synthase kinase-3b (GSK-3b).

As an inhibitor of cortisol's Gcr nuclear translocation [30], melatonin will modulate the stress, immune, and atrophy effects of cortisol. Melatonin also increases neuronal levels of the longevity protein sirtuin-1 [53], suggesting its impact on the significant decrease in longevity in schizophrenia [2]. Diminished daily amplitude in melatonin has been shown in women with metabolic syndrome [54], suggesting that metabolic dysregulation, including as induced by antipsychotics, may contribute to melatonin changes in schizophrenia.

An accumulating body of evidence in the past two decades suggests that alterations in melatonin play a role in the course and pathophysiology of schizophrenia. A decrease in nocturnal melatonin has been shown in paranoid schizophrenic patients under medication, as well as in a drug-free sample [55, 56]. The typical diurnal variation in melatonin is also frequently lost in schizophrenia [57] including in a medicated sample [58], which is generally associated with decreased levels of melatonin production, but not always [59]. This suggests that antipsychotic medication does not normalize melatonin dysregulation. Changes in the circadian rhythm of melatonin have also been shown, including phase advance [60]. Monozygotic twins discordant for schizophrenia also show significant melatonin differences [61]. In fact CT measurements of cortex atrophy are correlated with levels of pineal gland loss from calcification [62].

Neuroprogression, Schizophrenia, and Melatonin

Data in recent decades has highlighted a slow neurodegeneration in schizophrenia, especially in the left temporal lobe and prefrontal cortex [63]. This is often coupled with decreased neurogenesis as well as increased apoptosis, inflammation, and decreased antioxidant status. In fact many of the susceptibility genes for schizophrenia are also susceptibility genes for, or significantly altered in, Alzheimer's [3, 64], suggesting overlaps with processes associated with neuronal loss. This is also likely to make a contribution to changes in symptom presentation over the course of schizophrenia. Melatonin, via its anti-inflammatory, antioxidant effects [65] as well increasing neurogenesis, is likely to have inhibitory impacts on neuroprogression and neurodegeneration. Substantiating this, melatonin shows significant benefits in many models of neurodegenerative disorders and is currently being trialed for efficacy in human disorders, including Alzheimer's [66].

More specific cognitive deficits in schizophrenia are thought to be mediated by increased levels of KYNA in the prefrontal cortex [67], inhibiting the alpha7 nicotinic acetylcholine receptor (a7nAChr) and decreasing levels of glutamate, noradrenalin, and acetylcholine in the frontal cortex, in turn contributing to suboptimal arousal associated cognitive deficits [67]. Concurrently the inhibition of the a7nAChr on GABAergic interneurons decreases GABAergic activity, dysregulating cortex pyramidal neurons synchronization by the GABAergic network [68]. Astrocyte TDO is a significant inducer of KYNA, with TDO2 being a susceptibility gene for schizophrenia [69]. Cortisol and the cAMP pathway are the main inducers of TDO [70], and both are inhibited by melatonin, suggesting melatonin benefits to this aspect of cognition. Melatonin positively regulates cognitive processing in some stress paradigms [71], suggesting efficacy against the stress effects on cognition in the course, as well as the etiology, of schizophrenia. Interestingly nicotinic receptors in rodents have been shown to have a circadian rhythm driven by melatonin [72]. As to how relevant this would be in the regulation of optimized human cognition requires further investigation.

Sleep, Schizophrenia, and Melatonin

Sleep disturbance is relevant to the course of many psychiatric disorders, occurring in over 80 % of people with schizophrenia. This can occur despite relative stability of presenting symptoms and mental state, with many showing significant circadian and melatonin misalignment [48]. Sleep disturbance, as one would expect, is linked to poor quality of life and may be particularly exacerbated when positive symptoms are prominent [73]. The adjunctive use of melatonin has been shown to not only enhance sleep quality, but also to improve mood and daytime functioning [74]. A study by Bromundt and colleagues showed that a regular circadian sleep rhythm is associated with improved prefrontal cortex functioning, but with no significant impact on wider symptom presentations [75]. There is currently great interest in melatonin compounds as anxiolytics and antidepressants, and given the high levels of undiagnosed depression comorbid with schizophrenia, some of the efficacy of melatonergic compounds may be mediated by decreased levels of anxiety and depression, contributing to improved sleep. Certainly any sleep-promoting effects of melatonin will enhance quality of life. However, it should be noted that the melatonin sleep-promoting effects might be subject to alteration in some people with schizophrenia [76].

Wider Aspects of Schizophrenia and Melatonin

Schizophrenia is associated with very high levels of drug and alcohol abuse/addiction, which will contribute to increased levels of depression and wider medical problems, in turn contributing to peripheral organ dysregulation and immuno-inflammatory activation. Melatonin has protective effects in most organs, and melatonin and melatonergic drugs are proposed as having efficacy in the treatment and management of alcohol addiction and associated problems [77].

As well as significantly modulating the immune response, both melatonin and vit D would inhibit the raised levels of osteoporosis, evident over the course of schizophrenia [78]. Melatonin increases mesenchymal stem cell differentiation into osteoblasts, decreasing their differentiation into adipocytes [79].

An increase in somatization is evident in schizophrenia and is often included in measures of depression. Recent data shows that somatization, and not depression, is associated with increased ratios of kynurenine/KYNA and kynurenine/tryptophan, suggesting that increased levels of TRYCAT pathway activation may be more associated with somatization than depression per se [80]. As to how relevant these changed ratios would be to the high comorbidity of somatization and depression in schizophrenia is unknown. Recent data suggests that alterations in melatonin rhythm are particularly evident in people with psychosomatic complaints [81] and that melatonin has some analgesic properties [82]. This could suggest that a disrupted melatonin rhythm is more strongly associated with increased somatization in schizophrenia.

Much cutting-edge research has focussed on changes in microRNAs (miRNA) and epigenetic changes, including in schizophrenia [83]. Recent work in cancer cells shows that melatonin has significant impacts on levels of miRNAs and levels of methylation of a number of genes [84]. This is likely to be a promising area for future research in schizophrenia, contributing to an understanding of the heterogeneity in the disorder and to more targeted treatments.

Melatonin Adjunctive to Antipsychotics

The moral question posed by antipsychotic-induced metabolic syndrome and the 25-year decrease in life expectancy in schizophrenia [85] may in part find an answer in melatonin [86]. Melatonin is a peripheral vasodilator and decreases blood pressure. In maintaining neuronal sirtuin-1 levels under challenge [87], it is readily linked to pathways that are classically associated with increased longevity [88]. Melatonin decreases or prevents diet-induced obesity in animal models [89] and increases mitochondria oxidative phosphorylation [51], in turn attenuating metabolic syndrome. Most antipsychotics, as well as mood stabilizers lithium and valproate, have metabolic side effects, resulting in weight gain, raised leptin, and glucose dysregulation [5, 6]. Melatonin provides protection against such side effects [90, 91].

The antipsychotic-induced increase in leptin, and subsequent increased leptin resistance, may be of particular importance. In a nonpsychiatric sample of men with metabolic syndrome, nighttime levels of melatonin are negatively correlated with levels of leptin [92], suggesting that leptin resistance decreases nocturnal melatonin production. Decreased nighttime melatonin is associated with non-dipping nighttime blood pressure, a forerunner to hypertension [93]. Normally leptin, produced predominantly by adipocytes, feeds back to the hypothalamus to decrease appetite. However, under conditions of leptin resistance, there is an increased peripheral level of leptin but decreased leptin transport over the blood–brain barrier (BBB). Increases in triglycerides decrease leptin transport over the BBB [94]. Melatonin is known to decrease levels of circulating triglycerides [95]. As a powerful immune regulator, an increase in peripheral leptin modulates immuno-inflammatory responses and as such is likely to interact with the altered immuno-inflammatory activity that is intimately associated with driving the course of schizophrenia. Leptin has also been shown to decrease levels of CUMS-induced depression [96], suggesting that changes in levels of leptin may have relevance to stress-induced exacerbations as well as comorbid depression. This suggests that antipsychotic-induced weight gain is not simply a side effect but is interactive with the disorder itself. This is relevant to the proposal that the increased efficacy of olanzapine is related to its relatively enhanced ability to increase weight, although this may be via the coordinated changes in cholesterol and lipid raft regulation [97].

Leptin has a number of similar effects as melatonin, including increasing TH1-like cytokines, natural killer cell activity, and neurogenesis, as well as inhibiting the cAMP pathways and the effects of cortisol [98]. Also like melatonin, leptin increases the phosphorylation and inhibition of GSK-3b [96] and is therefore likely to increase Nrf-2 and endogenous antioxidants. It is unknown if leptin increases BAG-1, although its induction of bcl-2 and cortisol inhibition would suggest that this not unlikely. Leptin has recently been shown to have antidepressant effects [96] and to be protective in Alzheimer's [99, 100]. As such a loss of leptin effects in the CNS would be likely to increase levels of cortisol and cAMP induction of TDO, with resulting increases in

KYNA, a7nAChr inhibition, and associated cognitive inhibition, concurrently also impacting on levels of neuroprogression and neurodegeneration. The loss of leptin receptor activity in the rodent forebrain mediates the association of leptin to depression, including via increased levels of synaptic long-term depression (LTD) [101]. It requires investigation as to whether this is mediated by increased levels of astrocyte TDO and KYNA activation.

In a variety of animal models of diet-induced obesity, melatonin has been shown to not only decrease weight but also to decrease levels of peripheral leptin and leptin resistance. As well as providing protection against metabolic syndrome, melatonin, via the inhibition of antipsychotic-induced leptin resistance, would inhibit the dysregulation of the immuno-inflammatory pathways that are relevant to the course and etiology of schizophrenia. Such a perspective would suggest that leptin, if targeted to the CNS, would be beneficial in the treatment of schizophrenia and that melatonin may have some efficacy via the regulation of leptin resistance. Interestingly the antidepressant fluvoxamine has been suggested to decrease levels of leptin resistance, putatively via decreased endoplasmic reticulum stress [102].

The atypical antipsychotic olanzapine decreases melatonin by 55 % in rodents [103], and preliminary data suggests that similar effects may occur in treated schizophrenic patients, correlating with aspects of metabolic dysregulation, which the adjunctive use of low-dose melatonin helped to prevent [104]. The dose of melatonin in this trial was low, and far higher levels need testing given the lack of any significant side effects at higher dosage. However, in another study over a very short treatment period, olanzapine had no significant impact on melatonin levels in a sample of schizophrenic patients [105]. This work requires replication over a longer time frame and with varying levels of adjunctive melatonin. Given the long-standing data on the efficacy of melatonin in animal models of obesity and metabolic dysregulation, it seems surprising that there is a relative paucity of human trials. This would seem a system error, in so much that melatonin is very cheap and available over the counter in the USA, meaning that pharmaceutical companies have little interest in financing clinical trials, postponing interest until the development of melatonergic drugs such as ramelteon and agomelatine.

In an 8-week trial, ramelteon significantly decreased cholesterol levels and showed a trend decrease in abdominal and trunk fat [106]. However, in rodent models of Alzheimer's, ramelteon had no protective effects, unlike melatonin [107], suggesting that melatonin may have additional qualities not replicated by the MTr effects of ramelteon. Also longer-term ramelteon treatment resulted in fragmentation of aspects of the circadian rhythm, unlike the effects of melatonin [66]. This may be of particular relevance to processes of neuroprogression in schizophrenia.

Agomelatine is a MT1 and 2r agonist and serotonin 5-HT2Cr antagonist, being marketed as an anxiolytic and antidepressant. Given the high levels of often-unrecognized depression that is comorbid with schizophrenia, it would seem likely that trials of agomelatine in schizophrenia will occur. Data in rodents shows that agomelatine directly and indirectly increases the levels of dopamine, noradrenalin, and serotonin, with the effects on dopamine and serotonin being mediated by the melatonin effects of the drug [108]. Agomelatine also decreases levels of acute stress-induced excitatory glutamate efflux from the amygdala and hippocampus, possibly indicating an impact on stress-induced depression and wider symptom exacerbations in schizophrenia [109]. Interestingly agomelatine reverses the effects of prenatal restraint stress in the induction of later anxiety and depression features [110], indicating a possible impact on the early developmental etiology of schizophrenia and its priming for comorbid depression [36]. However, there is no data on how agomelatine would modulate the immuno-inflammatory and TRYCAT pathways. Like other antidepressants agomelatine increases levels of neurogenesis, cell survival, and BDNF [111]. As to whether agomelatine would have any additional utility, including in metabolic dysregulation, requires investigation.

Melatonin, adjunctive to antipsychotics, may augment the drug utility, including via the targeting of immuno-inflammation and oxidative stress, simultaneously decreasing symptom relapses that contribute to neuroprogression and treatment resistance [49, 50, 112]. The importance of the TRYCAT pathways is exemplified by the data showing altered 3-OHK in schizophrenia and its correlation with both clinical symptom presentations and response to treatment [113, 114]. As to how melatonin would modulate basal and antipsychotic-induced expression of specific TRYCATs requires investigation.

Of the antipsychotics an increased risk of pneumonia is particularly linked to clozapine, especially around the time of initial prescription [115]. Vit D levels and the vit D induction of the endogenous antimicrobial cathelicidin [116] are likely to be a significant modulator of pneumonia as a side effect, given that the risk of and mortality from pneumonia are regulated by vit D and cathelicidin. As to whether melatonin would interact with vit D, including via increased BAG-1, to modulate pneumonia susceptibility requires experimental investigation. Used on its own, melatonin in animal models attenuates bacteria-induced lung inflammation [117] and has shown efficacy in the management of pneumonia and COPD [118]. The use of melatonin in patients with lung disorders, which often has associated sleep disturbance, may result primarily in better regulation of sleep. Given the relevance of the immuno-inflammatory model to the course of schizophrenia and the known immuno-inflammatory effects of clozapine [119], the optimization of melatonin and vit D at the time of the initial prescribing of clozapine, and other antipsychotics, may attenuate the emergence of pneumonia, as well as metabolic dysregulation.

First-generation antipsychotic medications are associated with the side effect of tardive dyskinesia (TD). There are a number of risk factors for TD, including genetic [120] and pro-inflammatory [121]. In a small sample study, melatonin, at a low dose (2 mg/day), did not modulate the emergence of TD [122]. However, when given at 10 mg/day, melatonin significantly decreases TD [123]. Genetic variations in the MT1r have been shown to interact with antipsychotic medication in the susceptibility to TD [124]. Most recent work on the prevention of TD has focussed on the efficacy of antioxidants, including melatonin [125].

Conclusions

In summary, melatonin has a role in the developmental etiology, course, and management of schizophrenia. Its optimization, including in conjunction with vit D3 at initial presentation, could inhibit the development of schizophrenia as well as the extent and progression of symptoms. Minimally, it would limit antipsychotic side effects, contributing to the alleviation of metabolic dysregulation, sleep disorders, leptin resistance, neuroprogression, and tardive dyskinesia, concurrently increasing the dreadful decrease in life expectancy and quality of life of a still devalued population of people.

References

1. Tandon R, Keshavan MS, Nasrallah HA. Schizophrenia, "just the facts": what we know in 2008. 2. Epidemiology and etiology. Schizophr Res. 2008;102:1–18.
2. Flaum M. Strategies to close the "mortality gap". Am J Psychiatry. 2010;167(2):120–1.
3. Anderson G, Maes M. Schizophrenia: linking prenatal infection to hypoNMDAr, immune-inflammation, demyelination, susceptibility genes, IDO, neuroprogression and treatment. Prog Neuropsychopharmacol Biol Psychiatry. 2013;42:5–19.
4. Marczynski TJ, Yamaguchi N, Ling GM, Grodzinska L. Sleep induced by the administration of melatonin (5-methoxyn-acetyltrptamine) to the hypothalamus in unrestrained cats. Experientia. 1964;20(8):435–7.
5. Bushe CJ, Leonard BE. Blood glucose and schizophrenia: a systematic review of prospective randomized clinical trials. J Clin Psychiatry. 2007;68(11):1682–90.
6. Tardieu S, Micallef J, Gentile S, Blin O. Weight gain profiles of new anti-psychotics: public health consequences. Obes Rev. 2003;4(3):129–38.
7. Meyer U, Feldon J, Dammann O. Schizophrenia and autism: both shared and disorder-specific pathogenesis via perinatal inflammation? Pediatr Res. 2011;69(5 Pt 2):26R–33.
8. Brown AS, Derkitis EJ. Prenatal infection and schizophrenia: a review of epidemiologic and translational studies. Am J Psychiatry. 2010;167(3):261–80.

9. Read J, Perry BD, Moskowitz A, Connolly J. The contribution of early traumatic events to schizophrenia in some patients: a traumagenic neurodevelopmental model. Psychiatry. 2001;64:319–45.
10. Parry BL, Meliska CJ, Sorenson DL, Lopez AM, Martinez LF, Nowakowski S, et al. Plasma melatonin circadian rhythm disturbances during pregnancy and postpartum in depressed women and women with personal or family histories of depression. Am J Psychiatry. 2008;165(12):1551–8.
11. Richter HG, Hansell JA, Raut S, Giussani DA. Melatonin improves placental efficiency and birth weight and increase the placental expression of antioxidant enzymes in undernourished pregnancy. J Pineal Res. 2009;46(4):357–64.
12. Srinivasan V, Mohamed M, Kato H. Melatonin in bacterial and viral infections with focus on sepsis: a review. Recent Pat Endocr Metab Immune Drug Discov. 2012;6(1):30–9.
13. Huang SH, Cao XJ, Wei W. Melatonin decreases TLR3-mediated inflammatory factor expression via inhibition of NF-kappa B activation in respiratory syncytial virus-infected RAW264.7 macrophages. J Pineal Res. 2008;45(1):93–100.
14. Kendell RE, Juszczak E, Cole SK. Obstetric complications and schizophrenia: a case control study based on standardised obstetric records. Br J Psychiatry. 1996;168:55–61.
15. Lanoix D, Guerin P, Vaillancourt C. Placental melatonin production and melatonin receptor expression are altered in preeclampsia: new insights into the role of this hormone in pregnancy. J Pineal Res. 2012;53(4):417–25.
16. Bonnin A, Levitt P. Fetal, maternal, and placental sources of serotonin and new implications for developmental programming of the brain. Neuroscience. 2011;197:1–7.
17. Chung JH, Melsop KA, Gilbert WM, Caughey AB, Walker CK, Main EK. Increasing pre-pregnancy body mass index is predictive of a progressive escalation in adverse pregnancy outcomes. J Matern Fetal Neonatal Med. 2012;25(9):1635–9.
18. Lynch AM, Eckel RH, Murphy JR, Gibbs RS, West NA, Giclas PC, et al. Prepregnancy obesity and complement system activation in early pregnancy and the subsequent development of preeclampsia. Am J Obstet Gynecol. 2012;206(5):428.e1–8.
19. Chigusa Y, Tatsumi K, Kondoh E, Fujita K, Nishimura F, Mogami H, et al. Decreased lectin-like oxidized LDL receptor 1 (LOX-1) and low Nrf2 activation in placenta are involved in preeclampsia. J Clin Endocrinol Metab. 2012;97(10):E1862–70.
20. Gupta BB, Yanthan L, Singh KM. In vitro effects of 5-hydroxytryptophan, indoleamines and leptin on arylalkylamine N-acetyltransferase (AA-NAT) activity in pineal organ of the fish, Clarias gariepinus (Burchell, 1822) during different phases of the breeding cycle. Indian J Exp Biol. 2010;48(8):786–92.
21. Miller J, Gallo RL. Vitamin D and innate immunity. Dermatol Ther. 2010;23(1):13–22.
22. Bikle DD. Vitamin D, and immune function: understanding common pathways. Curr Osteoporos Rep. 2009;7(2):58–63.
23. McGrath J, Eyles D, Mowry B, Yolken R, Buka S. Low maternal vitamin D as a risk factor for schizophrenia: a pilot study using banked sera. Schizophr Res. 2003;63(1–2):73–8.
24. Hewison M. Vitamin D, and the immune system: new perspectives on an old theme. Endocrinol Metabol Clin North Am. 2010;39(2):365–79.
25. Proietti S, Cucina A, D'Anselmi F, Dinicola S, Pasqualato A, Lisi E, et al. Melatonin and vitamin D3 synergistically down-regulate Akt and MDM2 leading to TGFβ-1-dependent growth inhibition of breast cancer cells. J Pineal Res. 2011;50(2):150–8.
26. Park HJ, Park JK, Kim SK, Cho AR, Kim JW, Yim SV, et al. Association of polymorphism in the promoter of the melatonin receptor 1A gene with schizophrenia and with insomnia symptoms in schizophrenia patients. J Mol Neurosci. 2011;45(2):304–8.
27. Aufdenblatten M, Baumann M, Raio L, Dick B, Frey BM, Schneider H, et al. Prematurity is related to high placental cortisol in preeclampsia. Pediatr Res. 2009;65(2):198–202.
28. Causevic M, Mohaupt M. 11beta-hydroxysteroid dehydrogenase type 2 in pregnancy and preeclampsia. Mol Aspects Med. 2007;28(2):220–6.
29. Crupi R, Mazzon E, Marino A, La Spada G, Bramanti P, Cuzzocrea S, et al. Melatonin treatment mimics the antidepressant action in chronic corticosterone-treated mice. J Pineal Res. 2010;49(2):123–9.
30. Quiros I, Mayo JC, Garcia-Suarez O, Hevia D, Martin V, Rodríguez C, et al. Melatonin prevents the glucocorticoid receptor inhibition of cell proliferation and toxicity in hippocampal cells by reducing the glucocorticoid receptor nuclear translocation. J Steroid Biochem Mol Biol. 2008;110:116–24.
31. Chun RF, Adams JS, Hewison M. Review: back to the future: a new look at "old" vitamin D3. J Endocrinol. 2008;198:261–9.
32. Reynolds RM, Walker BR, Phillips DI, Dennison EM, Fraser R, Mackenzie SM, et al. Programming of hypertension: associations of plasma aldosterone in adult men and women with birthweight, cortisol, and blood pressure. Hypertension. 2009;53(6):932–6.
33. Rennie K, De Butte M, Pappas BA. Melatonin promotes neurogenesis in dentate gyrus in the pinealectomized rat. J Pineal Res. 2009;47(4):313–7.
34. Chen YC, Tain YL, Sheen JM, Huang LT. Melatonin utility in neonates and children. J Formos Med Assoc. 2012;111(2):57–66.
35. Gozdzik-Zelazny A, Borecki L, Pokorski M. Depressive symptoms in schizophrenic patients. Eur J Med Res. 2011;16(12):549–52.
36. Anderson G, Maes M, Berk M. Schizophrenia is primed for an increased expression of depression through activation of immuno-inflammatory, oxidative and nitrosative stress, and tryptophan catabolite pathways. Prog Neuropsychopharmacol Biol Psychiatry. 2013;42:101–14.

37. Laugeray A, Launay JM, Callebert J, Surget A, Belzung C, Barone PR. Peripheral and cerebral metabolic abnormalities of the tryptophan-kynurenine pathway in a murine model of major depression. Behav Brain Res. 2010;210(1):84–91.
38. Laugeray A, Launay JM, Callebert J, Surget A, Belzung C, Barone PR. Evidence for a key role of the peripheral kynurenine pathway in the modulation of anxiety- and depression-like behaviours in mice: focus on individual differences. Pharmacol Biochem Behav. 2011;98(1):161–8.
39. Shini S, Shini A, Kaiser P. Cytokine and chemokine gene expression profiles in heterophils from chickens treated with corticosterone. Stress. 2010;13(3):185–94.
40. Kristo C, Godang K, Ueland T, Lien E, Aukrust P, Froland SS, et al. Raised serum levels of interleukin-8 and interleukin-18 in relation to bone metabolism in endogenous Cushing's syndrome. Eur J Endocrinol. 2002;146(3):389–95.
41. Reale M, Patruno A, DeLutiis MA, Pesce M, Felaco M, Di Giannantonio M, et al. Dysregulation of chemo-cytokine production in schizophrenic patients versus healthy controls. BMC Neurosci. 2011;12:13.
42. Liu J, Liu J, Zhou Y, Li S, Li Y, Song X, et al. Association between promoter variants of interleukin-18 and schizophrenia in a Han Chinese population. DNA Cell Biol. 2011;30(11):913–7.
43. Anderson G. Neuronal-immune interactions in mediating stress effects in the etiology and course of schizophrenia: role of the amygdala in developmental co-ordination. Med Hypotheses. 2011;76(1):54–60.
44. Miller BJ, Buckley P, Seabolt W, Mellor A, Kirkpatrick B. Meta-analysis of cytokine alterations in schizophrenia: clinical status and antipsychotic effects. Biol Psychiatry. 2011;70:663–71.
45. Potvin S, Stip E, Sepehry AA, Gendron A, Bah R, Kouassi E. Inflammatory cytokine alterations in schizophrenia: a systematic quantitative review. Biol Psychiatry. 2008;63:801–8.
46. Drexhage RC, Hoogenboezem TA, Cohen D, Versnel MA, Nolen WA, van Beverens NJM, et al. An activated set point of T-cell and monocyte inflammatory networks in recent-onset schizophrenia patients involves both pro- and anti-inflammatory forces. Int J Neuropsychopharmacol. 2011;14:746–55.
47. Bošković M, Vovk T, Kores Plesničar B, Grabnar I. Oxidative stress in schizophrenia. Curr Neuropharmacol. 2011;9(2):301–12.
48. Wulff K, Dijk DJ, Middleton B, Foster RG, Joyce EM. Sleep and circadian rhythm disruption in schizophrenia. Br J Psychiatry. 2012;200(4):308–16.
49. Maldonado MD, Pérez-San-Gregorio MA, Reiter RJ. The role of melatonin in the immuno-neuro-psychology of mental disorders. Recent Pat CNS Drug Discov. 2009;4(1):61–9.
50. Maldonado MD, Reiter RJ, Pérez-San-Gregorio MA. Melatonin as a potential therapeutic agent in psychiatric illness. Hum Psychopharmacol. 2009;24(5):391–400.
51. Martín M, Macías M, León J, Escames G, Khaldy H, Acuña-Castroviejo D. Melatonin increases the activity of the oxidative phosphorylation enzymes and the production of ATP in rat brain and liver mitochondria. Int J Biochem Cell Biol. 2002;34(4):348–57.
52. Olcese JM, Cao C, Mori T, Mamcarz MB, Maxwell A, Runfeldt MJ, et al. Protection against cognitive deficits and markers of neurodegeneration by long-term oral administration of melatonin in a transgenic model of Alzheimer disease. J Pineal Res. 2009;47(1):82–96.
53. Tajes M, Gutierrez-Cuesta J, Ortuño-Sahagun D, Camins A, Pallàs M. Anti-aging properties of melatonin in an in vitro murine senescence model: involvement of the sirtuin 1 pathway. J Pineal Res. 2009;47(3):228–37.
54. Corbalán-Tutau D, Madrid JA, Nicolás F, Garaulet M. Daily profile in two circadian markers "melatonin and cortisol" and associations with metabolic syndrome components. Physiol Behav. 2012; (in press).
55. Monteleone P, Maj M, Fusco M, Kemali D, Reiter RJ. Depressed nocturnal plasma melatonin levels in drug-free paranoid schizophrenics. Schizophr Res. 1992;7(1):77–84.
56. Monteleone P, Natale M, La Rocca A, Maj M. Decreased nocturnal secretion of melatonin in drug-free schizophrenics: no change after subchronic treatment with antipsychotics. Neuropsychobiology. 1997;36(4):159–63.
57. Bersani G, Mameli M, Garavini A, Pancheri P, Nordio M. Reduction of night/day difference in melatonin blood levels as a possible disease-related index in schizophrenia. Neuro Endocrinol Lett. 2003;24(3–4):181–4.
58. Jiang HK, Wang JY. Diurnal melatonin and cortisol secretion profiles in medicated schizophrenic patients. J Formos Med Assoc. 1998;97(12):830–7.
59. Vigano D, Lissoni P, Rovelli F, Roselli MG, Malugani F, Gavazzeni C, et al. A study of light/dark rhythm of melatonin in relation to cortisol and prolactin secretion in schizophrenia. Neuro Endocrinol Lett. 2001;22(2):137–41.
60. Rao ML, Gross G, Strebel B, Halaris A, Huber G, Bräunig P, et al. Circadian rhythm of tryptophan, serotonin, melatonin, and pituitary hormones in schizophrenia. Biol Psychiatry. 1994;35(3):151–63.
61. Afonso P, Brissos S, Figueira ML, Paiva T. Discrepant nocturnal melatonin levels in monozygotic twins discordant for schizophrenia and its impact on sleep. Schizophr Res. 2010;120(1–3):227–8.
62. Sandyk R, Kay SR. The relationship of pineal calcification to cortical atrophy in schizophrenia. Int J Neurosci. 1991;57(3–4):179–91.
63. Menon RR, Barta PE, Aylward EH, Richards SS, Vaughn DD, Tien AY, et al. Posterior superior temporal gyrus in schizophrenia: grey matter changes and clinical correlates. Schizophr Res. 1995;16(2):127–35.
64. Xu MQ, St Clair D, He L. Meta-analysis of association between ApoE epsilon 4 allele and schizophrenia. Schizophr Res. 2006;84(2–3):228–35.

65. Esposito E, Cuzzocrea S. Antiinflammatory activity of melatonin in central nervous system. Curr Neuropharmacol. 2010;8(3):228–42.
66. Otalora BB, Popovic N, Gambini J, Popovic M, Viña J, Bonet-Costa V. Circadian system functionality, hippocampal oxidative stress, and spatial memory in the APPswe/PS1dE9 transgenic model of Alzheimer disease: effects of melatonin or ramelteon. Chronobiol Int. 2012;29(7):822–34.
67. Zmarowski A, Wu HQ, Brooks JM, Potter MC, Pellicciari R, Schwarcz R, et al. Astrocyte-derived kynurenic acid modulates basal and evoked cortical acetylcholine release. Eur J Neurosci. 2009;29(3):529–38.
68. Alexander KS, Wu HQ, Schwarcz R, Bruno JP. Acute elevations of brain kynurenic acid impair cognitive flexibility: normalization by the alpha7 positive modulator galantamine. Psychopharmacology (Berl). 2012;220(3):627–37.
69. Miller CL, Murakami P, Ruczinski I, Ross RG, Sinkus M, Sullivan B, et al. Two complex genotypes relevant to the kynurenine pathway and melanotropin function show association with schizophrenia and bipolar disorder. Schizophr Res. 2009;113(2–3):259–67.
70. Luchowska E, Kloc R, Olajossy B, Wnuk S, Wielosz M, Owe-Larsson B, et al. Beta-adrenergic enhancement of brain kynurenic acid production mediated via cAMP-related protein kinase A signalling. Prog Neuropsychopharmacol Biol Psychiatry. 2009;33(3):519–29.
71. Rimmele U, Spillmann M, Bärtschi C, Wolf OT, Weber CS, Ehlert U, et al. Melatonin improves memory acquisition under stress independent of stress hormone release. Psychopharmacology (Berl). 2009;202(4):663–72.
72. Mexal S, Horton WJ, Crouch EL, Maier SI, Wilkinson AL, Marsole M, et al. Diurnal variation in nicotine sensitivity in mice: role of genetic background and melatonin. Neuropharmacology. 2012;63(6):966–73.
73. Afonso P, Brissos S, Figueira ML, Paiva T. Schizophrenia patients with predominantly positive symptoms have more disturbed sleep- wake cycles measured by actigraphy. Psychiatry Res. 2011;189(1):62–6.
74. Suresh Kumar PN, Andrade C, Bhakta SG, Singh NM. Melatonin in schizophrenic outpatients with insomnia: a double-blind, placebo-controlled study. J Clin Psychiatry. 2007;68(2):237–41.
75. Bromundt V, Köster M, Georgiev-Kill A, Opwis K, Wirz-Justice A, Stoppe G, et al. Sleep-wake cycles and cognitive functioning in schizophrenia. Br J Psychiatry. 2011;198(4):269–76.
76. Afonso P, Figueira ML, Paiva T. Sleep-promoting action of the endogenous melatonin in schizophrenia compared to healthy controls. Int J Psychiatry Clin Pract. 2011;15(4):311–5.
77. Anderson G. Melatonin, agomelatine and alcoholism: relevance to alcohol related brain damage and comorbid psychosis. Addict Drugs Th Treat. 2011;10(2):84–90.
78. Graham SM, Howgate D, Anderson W, Howes C, Heliotis M, Mantalaris A, et al. Risk of osteoporosis and fracture incidence in patients on antipsychotic medication. Expert Opin Drug Saf. 2011;10(4):575–602.
79. Zhang L, Su P, Xu C, Chen C, Liang A, Du K, et al. Melatonin inhibits adipogenesis and enhances osteogenesis of human mesenchymal stem cells by suppressing PPARγ expression and enhancing Runx2 expression. J Pineal Res. 2010;49(4):364–72.
80. Maes M, Rief W. Diagnostic classifications in depression and somatization should include biomarkers, such as disorders in the tryptophan catabolite (TRYCAT) pathway. Psychiatry Res. 2012;196(2–3):243–9.
81. Nagane M, Suge R, Watanabe S. Relationship between psychosomatic complaints and circadian rhythm irregularity assessed by salivary levels of melatonin and growth hormone. J Circadian Rhythms. 2011;9:9.
82. Yousaf F, Seet E, Venkatraghavan L, Abrishami A, Chung F. Efficacy and safety of melatonin as an anxiolytic and analgesic in the perioperative period: a qualitative systematic review of randomized trials. Anesthesiology. 2010;113(4):968–76.
83. Miller BH, Zeier Z, Xi L, Lanz TA, Deng S, Strathmann J, et al. MicroRNA-132 dysregulation in schizophrenia has implications for both neurodevelopment and adult brain function. Proc Natl Acad Sci U S A. 2012;109(8):3125–30.
84. Lee SE, Kim SJ, Yoon HJ, Yu SY, Yang H, Jeong SI, et al. Genome-wide profiling in melatonin-exposed human breast cancer cell lines identifies differentially methylated genes involved in the anticancer effect of melatonin. J Pineal Res. 2012;54:80–8.
85. Chwastiak LA, Tek C. The unchanging mortality gap for people with schizophrenia. Lancet. 2009;374(9690):590–2.
86. Anderson G, Maes M. Melatonin: an overlooked factor in schizophrenia and in the inhibition of anti- psychotic side effects. Metab Brain Dis. 2012;27(2):113–9.
87. Chang HM, Wu UI, Lan CT. Melatonin preserves longevity protein (sirtuin 1) expression in the hippocampus of total sleep- deprived rats. J Pineal Res. 2009;47(3):211–20.
88. Cantó C, Auwerx J. Caloric restriction, SIRT1 and longevity. Trends Endocrinol Metab. 2009;20(7):325–31.
89. Kitagawa A, Ohta Y, Ohashi K. Melatonin improves metabolic syndrome induced by high fructose intake in rats. J Pineal Res. 2012;52(4):403–13.
90. Shieh JM. Melatonin ameliorates high fat diet-induced diabetes and stimulates glycogen synthesis via a PKCzeta-Akt-GSK-3b pathway in hepatic cells. J Pineal Res. 2009;47(4):339–44.
91. Sartori C, Dessen P, Mathieu C, Monney A, Bloch J, Nicod P, et al. Melatonin improves glucose homeostasis and endothelial vascular function in high-fat diet-fed insulin-resistant mice. Endocrinology. 2009;150(12):5311–7.
92. Relationship between insulin, leptin, and melatonin contents in patients with metabolic syndrome. Klin Med (Mosk). 2011;89(6):46–9.

93. Jonas M, Garfinkel D, Zisapel N, Laudon M, Grossman E. Impaired nocturnal melatonin secretion in non-dipper hypertensive patients. Blood Press. 2003;12:19–24.
94. Banks WA. Role of the blood–brain barrier in the evolution of feeding and cognition. Ann N Y Acad Sci. 2012;1264:13–19.
95. Ríos-Lugo MJ, Cano P, Jiménez-Ortega V, Fernández-Mateos MP, Scacchi PA, Cardinali DP, et al. Melatonin effect on plasma adiponectin, leptin, insulin, glucose, triglycerides and cholesterol in normal and high fat-fed rats. J Pineal Res. 2010;49(4):342–8.
96. Garza JC, Guo M, Zhang W, Lu XY. Leptin restores adult hippocampal neurogenesis in a chronic unpredictable stress model of depression and reverses glucocorticoid-induced inhibition of GSK- 3β/β-catenin signaling. Mol Psychiatry. 2012;17(8):790–808.
97. Venkatasubramanian G, Chittiprol S, Neelakantachar N, Shetty TK, Gangadhar BN. A longitudinal study on the impact of antipsychotic treatment on serum leptin in schizophrenia. Clin Neuropharmacol. 2010;33(6):288–92.
98. Avraham Y, Davidi N, Lassri V, Vorobiev L, Kabesa M, Dayan M, et al. Leptin induces neuroprotection neurogenesis and angiogenesis after stroke. Curr Neurovasc Res. 2011;8(4):313–22.
99. Zeki Al Hazzouri A, Stone KL, Haan MN, Yaffe K. Leptin, mild cognitive impairment, and dementia among elderly women. J Gerontol A Biol Sci Med Sci. 2013;68(2):175–80.
100. Johnston JM, Greco SJ, Hamzelou A, Ashford JW, Tezapsidis N. Repositioning leptin as a therapy for Alzheimer's disease. Therapy. 2011;8(5):481–90.
101. Guo M, Lu Y, Garza JC, Li Y, Chua SC, Zhang W, et al. Forebrain glutamatergic neurons mediate leptin action on depression-like behaviors and synaptic depression. Transl Psychiatry. 2012;2:e83.
102. Hosoi T, Miyahara T, Kayano T, Yokoyama S, Ozawa K. Fluvoxamine attenuated endoplasmic reticulum stress-induced leptin resistance. Front Endocrinol (Lausanne). 2012;3:12.
103. Raskind MA, Burke BL, Crites NJ, Tapp AM, Rasmussen DD. Olanzapine-induced weight gain and increased visceral adiposity is blocked by melatonin replacement therapy in rats. Neuropsychopharmacology. 2007;32(2):284–8.
104. Kilzieh N. Principal Investigator. ClinicalTrials.gov Identifier: NCT00512070; conference presentation.
105. Mann K, Rossbach W, Müller MJ, Müller-Siecheneder F, Pott T, Linde I, et al. Nocturnal hormone profiles in patients with schizophrenia treated with olanzapine. Psychoneuroendocrinology. 2006;31(2):256–64.
106. Borba CP, Fan X, Copeland PM, Paiva A, Freudenreich O, Henderson DC. Placebo-controlled pilot study of ramelteon for adiposity and lipids in patients with schizophrenia. J Clin Psychopharmacol. 2011;31(5):653–8.
107. McKenna JT, Christie MA, Jeffrey BA, McCoy JG, Lee E, Connolly NP, et al. Chronic ramelteon treatment in a mouse model of Alzheimer's disease. Arch Ital Biol. 2012;150(1):5–14.
108. Chenu F, El Mansari M, Blier P. Electrophysiological effects of repeated administration of agomelatine on the dopamine, norepinephrine, and serotonin systems in the rat brain. Neuropsychopharmacology. 2013;38(2):275–84.
109. Reagan LP, Reznikov LR, Evans AN, Gabriel C, Mocaër E, Fadel JR. The antidepressant agomelatine inhibits stress-mediated changes in amino acid efflux in the rat hippocampus and amygdala. Brain Res. 2012;1466:91–8.
110. Morley-Fletcher S, Mairesse J, Soumier A, Banasr M, Fagioli F, Gabriel C, et al. Chronic agomelatine treatment corrects behavioral, cellular, and biochemical abnormalities induced by prenatal stress in rats. Psychopharmacology (Berl). 2011;217(3):301–13.
111. Tardito D, Molteni R, Popoli M, Racagni G. Synergistic mechanisms involved in the antidepressant effects of agomelatine. Eur Neuropsychopharmacol. 2012;22 Suppl 3:S482–6.
112. Dodd S, Ratheesh A, Maes M, Anderson G, Dean O, Sarris J, et al. Putative neuroprotective agents in major psychoses. Prog Neuropsychopharmacol Biol Psychiatry. 2013;42:135–45.
113. Condray R, Dougherty GG, Keshavan MS, Reddy RD, Haas GL, Montrose DM, et al. 3-hydroxykynurenine and clinical symptoms in first-episode neuroleptic-naive patients with schizophrenia. Int J Neuropsychopharmacol. 2011;14:756–67.
114. Myint AM, Schwarz MJ, Verkerk R, Mueller HH, Zach J, Scharpé S. Reversal of imbalance between kynurenic acid and 3-hydroxykynurenine by antipsychotics in medication-naïve and medication-free schizophrenic patients. Brain Behav Immun. 2011;25(8):1576–81.
115. Kuo CJ, Yang SY, Liao YT, Chen WJ, Lee WC, Shau WY. Second-generation antipsychotic medications and risk of pneumonia in schizophrenia. Schizophr Bull. 2013;39(3):648–57.
116. Leow L, Simpson T, Cursons R, Karalus N, Hancox RJ. Vitamin D, innate immunity and outcomes in community acquired pneumonia. Respirology. 2011;16(4):611.
117. Lee YD, Kim JY, Lee KH, Kwak YJ, Lee SK, Kim OS, et al. Melatonin attenuates lipopolysaccharide-induced acute lung inflammation in sleep-deprived mice. J Pineal Res. 2009;46(1):53–7.
118. Shilo L, Dagan Y, Smorjik Y, Weinberg U, Dolev S, Komptel B, et al. Effect of melatonin on sleep quality of COPD intensive care patients: a pilot study. Chronobiol Int. 2000;17(1):71–6.
119. Maes M, Meltzer HY, Bosmans E. Immune-inflammatory markers in schizophrenia: comparison to normal controls and effects of clozapine. Acta Psychiatr Scand. 1994;89:346–51.
120. Utsunomiya K, Shinkai T, Sakata S, Yamada K, Chen HI, De Luca V, et al. Genetic association between the dopamine D3 receptor gene polymorphism (Ser9Gly) and tardive dyskinesia in patients

with schizophrenia: a reevaluation in East Asian populations. Neurosci Lett. 2012;507(1):52–6.

121. Wang F, Fan H, Sun H, Yang F, Luo Y, Liu H, et al. Association between TNF-α promoter-308A/G polymorphism and tardive dyskinesian Chinese Han patients with schizophrenia. Prog Neuropsychopharmacol Biol Psychiatry. 2012;37(1):106–10.
122. Shamir E, Barak Y, Plopsky I, Zisapel N, Elizur A, Weizman A. Is melatonin treatment effective for tardive dyskinesia? J Clin Psychiatry. 2000; 61(8):556–8.
123. Shamir E, Barak Y, Shalman I, Laudon M, Zisapel N, Tarrasch R, et al. Melatonin treatment for tardive dyskinesia: a double-blind, placebo-controlled, crossover study. Arch Gen Psychiatry. 2001;58(11): 1049–52.
124. Lai IC, Chen ML, Wang YC, Chen JY, Liao DL, Bai YM. Analysis of genetic variations in the human melatonin receptor (MTNR1A, MTNR1B) genes and antipsychotics-induced tardive dyskinesia in schizophrenia. World J Biol Psychiatry. 2011;12(2):143–8.
125. Lerner V, Miodownik C. Motor symptoms of schizophrenia: is tardive dyskinesia a symptom or side effect? A modern treatment. Curr Psychiatry Rep. 2011;13(4):295–304.

Neurobiology of Monoaminergic Neurotransmission and Antidepressants

23

Francisco López-Muñoz and Cecilio Álamo

Abstract

Pathophysiological mechanisms underlying depression are complex and are at multiple levels of analysis. But, during the 1960s, monoamine theories of depression flourished, postulating that a fundamental cause of depression was a functional deficit in noradrenergic and serotonergic neurotransmission in certain areas of the brain. These hypotheses were developed based on the fact that certain drugs that lessened depressive symptoms had monoaminergic properties, like blocking the serotonin transporter (5-HTT) or inhibiting MAO enzymes. Thus, any sort of alteration in monoamine functioning, whether in its synthesis, storage, release, or biotransformation, not to mention changes in its reuptake or monoamine receptor sensitivity, was related to the manifestation of characteristic depressive and behavioral symptoms (e.g., mood, alertness, motivation, fatigue, agitation, and psychomotor retardation).

It is generally accepted that a variety of genetic, environmental, and neurobiological factors are implicated in depression. The 5-HTT gene (SLC6A4) and other genes involved in the serotonergic system (polymorphisms on TPH2, 5-HT_{1A} or COMT genes), norepinephrine transporter (NET, SLC6A2), and dopamine transporter (DAT, SLC6A) are candidates for susceptibility to depression. Many antidepressant medications act on that system. This chapter analyzes the validity of the monoamine hypothesis of depression, its intersections with other neurobiological mechanisms, and antidepressants' influence on such mechanisms. The monoamine

F. López-Muñoz, MD, PhD (✉)
Faculty of Health Sciences,
Camilo José Cela University and Hospital 12 de Octubre Research Institute, C/Castillo de Alarcón, 49, Urb. Villafranca del Castillo,
Villanueva de la Cañada, Madrid 28692, Spain
e-mail: francisco.lopez.munoz@gmail.com

C. Álamo, MD, PhD
Department of Pharmacology, Faculty of Medicine,
University of Alcalá, Serrano Galvache 42, 9ºC.,
Madrid 28033, Spain
e-mail: cecilioalamo@hotmail.com

V. Srinivasan et al. (eds.), *Melatonin and Melatonergic Drugs in Clinical Practice*,
DOI 10.1007/978-81-322-0825-9_23, © Springer India 2014

hypothesis of depression is critically discussed. Specifically, we wish to add to the body of knowledge about monoamines in the pathophysiology of depression and to suggest other neurobiological aspects that could help improve the treatment of such disorders.

Keywords
Antidepressants • Depression • Dopamine • Genetic • Neurotransmission • Noradrenaline • Serotonin

Introduction

Our understanding of the pathophysiology of depression has evolved substantially in the last century. Until the mid-nineteenth century, etiological hypotheses on melancholy and depression postulated that such mental disorders were the result of the humors' dysregulation, were the result of mechanical alterations in the correct circulation of biological fluids, or were considered diseases of the soul [1, 2]. However, great advances took place during the second half of the nineteenth century in the field of neurobiology and in our knowledge of the structure of the nervous system, and positivism took hold in psychiatry, which definitively debunked these postulates. These developments led to a process that has been called "mental illness somatization," in which mental disorders came to be regarded as the products of an organic lesion [3]. Accordingly, the affective disorders' origins were associated, for example, with a local effect on the brain from a spasm of the dura mater (*status striatus*), a state of exhaustion or decreased brain energy, or a hormonal or metabolic alteration. In the first half of the twentieth century, the discovery of the chemical messengers responsible for interneuronal communication [4], and the clinical introduction of the main groups of psychotropic drugs in the 1950s, considered the "golden decade" of psychopharmacology, brought about a veritable revolution in the field of psychiatry [5].

Despite criticism of antidepressants from dominant voices in the field of psychoanalysis, these drugs were shown to markedly reduce symptoms, especially after a period of 2 or 3 weeks. Thus, support began to grow within the scientific community for the notion that these drugs might correct a kind of specific "chemical imbalance," the underlying cause of the illness. Furthermore, this concept of "chemical imbalance" revolutionized the view held by the most traditional sectors of society about mental illness, entrenched in pseudo-medieval conceptions like states of possession, and even by psychiatrists themselves, some of whom continued to see psychiatric patients as deranged individuals with moral defects, needful of moral therapy. In addition, the discovery of the mechanisms of neurotransmission, and the antidepressants' impact on them, laid the groundwork for what came to be known as "biological psychiatry" [6]. As a consequence, what is referred to as the "monoamine hypothesis of depression" began to take shape, according to which "some, if not all, depressions are associated with an absolute or relative deficiency of monoamines at functionally important receptor sites in the brain." The corollary that antidepressants work by correcting these deficiencies, building on this theory, has provided the major neurobiological account of depression [7].

Until some decades ago, that was the lone etiopathogenic hypothesis of depression. However, in recent years, its predominance has been eclipsed by new conceptions that incorporate several areas of neuroscience [8]. It is generally accepted that a variety of genetic, environmental, and neurobiological factors are implicated in depression. Genetic variations may be responsible for a person's vulnerability to environmental factors like stress and mediating factors like levels of corticosteroids, neurotrophins, and cytokines. As researchers seek new therapeutic alternatives, additional mechanisms have been implicated, for example, altered glutamatergic neurotransmission, cannabinoid systems, endogenous opioid systems, and neurokinin-1 receptor antagonism, among other mechanisms [2]. Nevertheless, the pharmaceutical industry's many costly efforts to discover new antidepressants to act via the aforementioned extra-aminergic mechanisms have been fruitless [7]. To date, agomelatine has yielded the best, really the only, such results of note. This agent is the first antidepressant with proven clinical efficacy that approaches the treatment of depression from a different pharmacological perspective than other drugs employed until now. This agent's primary mechanism is its agonistic action at MT_1 and MT_2 melatonin receptors, but it may also indirectly increase monoamine presence [9, 10].

In recent years, some authors have pointed out weaknesses in the amine hypothesis of depression based on the fact that the antidepressant tianeptine does not increase monoamine presence [11]. However, given the role of other chemical mediators and neurotransmitters in the pathophysiology of depression, there continues to be consensus that monoamine neurotransmitters, especially serotonin (5-HT), noradrenaline (NA), and to a lesser extent dopamine (DA), participate directly or indirectly in the pathophysiological and therapeutic mechanisms of depression [12]. Moreover, antidepressant effect seems to be the result of changes to the mechanisms of monoamine neurotransmission. Bear in mind that the current monoamine hypothesis of depression does not rule out other hypotheses; instead, it should be viewed as complementary to other more recently proposed hypotheses.

This chapter will analyze the validity of the monoamine hypothesis of depression, its intersections with other neurobiological mechanisms, and antidepressants' influence on such mechanisms. Specifically, we wish to add to the body of knowledge about monoamines in the pathophysiology of depression and to suggest neurobiological aspects that could help improve the treatment of such disorders.

Challenges to the Study of Depressive Disorders' Pathophysiology

For certain reasons, it is inherently difficult to determine the pathophysiology of psychiatric disorders, particularly depression. The pathophysiological mechanisms that give rise to major depression are complex and must be understood at multiple levels of analysis. It is perhaps major depression that best illustrates the complex interplay of the environment, genetics, neurobiology, and psychological mechanisms that synergistically interact to produce this debilitating disorder. Additionally, functions altered by depression like cognitive processes and emotions and executive functions, to which cognitive and behavioral processes are definitively, directly attributable, together exhibit a neurobiology that is hard to circumscribe. On another note, the human brain seems to be especially discreet in the curious eyes and instruments of researchers, not only because of its bony cortex. In addition, for practical and ethical reasons, experimental neurobiology is limited to noninvasive tests like neuroimaging, indirect research methods, and postmortem studies, which have obvious limitations. Also, it is hard to extrapolate knowledge of depression's pathophysiology from animal models even though they are to some extent valid in the development of new antidepressants. On another note, genetic risk factors have proven monumentally complex; the genes involved have not managed to reproduce depressive profiles in laboratory animals. Nor are thoroughly validated, objective, biological markers available with which to precisely define phenotypes that can be used in genetics studies or other types of research [2, 12].

Genetic Aspects of Depression Related to the Monoamine Hypothesis

Classifying the genes responsible for inheritable components of depression is crucial to advancing our understanding of the underlying neurobiology and pathology of this complex psychiatric disorder. In contrast to the very solid evidence from epidemiological studies on broad risk factor domains, there is no solid evidence for specific genes and specific gene-by-environment interactions in the pathogenesis of major depressive disorders (MDD) [13]. Unipolar depression is not as robustly inheritable as mental pathologies such as schizophrenia, bipolar disorder, and attention deficit hyperactivity disorder (ADHD). However, epidemiological data on unipolar depression collected from monozygotic and dizygotic twins indicate that depression is inherited approximately 37.5 % of the time and that its lifetime prevalence is around 10–15 % [14]. Furthermore, studies indicate that genetic factors contribute30–40 % of the time to the development of depression [15].

The serotonin transporter (5-HTT) gene and other genes involved in the serotonergic system are candidates for susceptibility to depression in light of the fact that many antidepressant medications act on that system. Numerous studies have focused on the functional insertion/deletion promoter variant (serotonin transporter-linked polymorphic region [5-HTTLPR]) on the serotonin transporter gene (SLC6A4). Meta-analyses suggest small, positive associations between the polymorphism in the 5-HTTLPR and bipolar disorder, suicidal behavior, depression-related personality traits, and stress vulnerability, but not yet to MDD itself.

Caspi et al. [16] reported a positive association between one's number of stressful life events and their probability of depression that was statistically stronger in S carriers than L homozygotes. This association demonstrated that among participants who had experienced more than four stressful life events, S carriers were twice as likely as L homozygotes to develop depression. While the researchers noted that their results did not prove a direct association between the 5-HTT genotype and depression, they concluded that S carriers were more likely to develop depression in response to stressful life events. Furthermore, stress vulnerability has been found to be associated with the serotonin transporter gene and compromised serotonin transporter function, not only in human studies but also in multiple nonhuman experiments [17, 18].

Although this interaction is highly plausible, clinically and neurobiologically speaking, recent meta-analysis yielded no evidence that the serotonin transporter gene alone, or in interaction with psychological stress, was associated with risk of depression [19, 20]. However, early stress exposure's ability to alter the brain's susceptibility to depression may depend, in part, on the presence of certain genetic vulnerability genotypes [21], for example, poor transcriptional activity of the S allele ("risk allele"). This polymorphism's frequency in the general population is relatively high, and it may increase susceptibility to not only negative but also positive environmental events, either hindering or promoting adaptation [22]. This hypothesis is also supported by the fact that among primates, humans and rhesus macaques were best at adapting to diverse ecological challenges, and those are the two primate species that carry this polymorphism [23]. In conclusion, studies assessing the association between 5-HTTLPR and depression have generated inconsistent results [24].

Tryptophan hydroxylase (TPH) is the rate-limiting enzyme in the biosynthesis of serotonin. Changes in the metabolism of the essential amino acid tryptophan play an important role in the brain-endocrine-immune system interaction, which is hypothesized to be involved in the pathophysiology of MDD. A polymorphism in intron 7 of TPH1, 218A/C, is associated with somatic anxiety symptoms in depression, but not with major depression [18, 25]. Another potential functional serotonergic system candidate gene is TPH2 polymorphism. This would result in the production of less serotonin, and initial findings show TPH2 single nucleotide polymorphisms (SNPs) related to this truncated transcript are associated with MDD but not directly with suicide [26].

5-HT_{1A} autoreceptors act on serotonergic neurons in the raphe nuclei and prevent serotonin release through negative feedback. Depressed individuals have a higher number of 5-HT_{1A}autoreceptors [27]. A functional promoter polymorphism (−1019C/G, rs6295) on the 5-HT_{1A} gene has been associated with depression, anxiety, coping with stress, impulsivity, and antidepressant therapy response [22, 28].

There are several SNPs at this gene's 5-HT_{2A} receptor, including polymorphisms in the promoter region. With respect to a possible direct impact of 5-HT_{2A} variation on depression, previous studies have yielded inconsistent results [28]. However, several studies have found evidence for associations between at least one of these 5-HT_{2A} SNPs and depression [18] or antidepressant drug response [29].

Catechol-*O*-methyltransferase (COMT) polymorphism (Val/Val genotype) was associated with early-onset MDD in one European study, but other studies with fewer participants reported conflicting results [18]. Genetic variation in the COMT gene, which modulates COMT activity, is associated with response to treatment with several antidepressants [30].

Although several lines of evidence suggest an association between dopamine and MDD, few studies have directly explored polymorphisms in main dopaminergic genes such as DAT1. The SNP rs40184, which plays a genetic role in ADHD and bipolar disorder, has a demonstrated gene-by-environment interaction in the etiology of MDD [31].

To date, studies have focused primarily on genetic links to non-aminergic mechanisms. For example, MDD has been associated with polymorphisms in the glucocorticoid receptor gene, the monoamine oxidase A gene, the gene for glycogen synthase kinase-3β, and a group-2 metabotropic glutamate receptor gene (GRM3) [30].

That being said, despite all the data discussed above, Wray et al. [20] showed that no SNPs achieved genome-wide significance, neither in the MDD2000+ Study nor in a meta-analysis of two other studies totaling 5,763 clinical cases and 6,901 controls. These analyses and meta-analyses represent the largest and most powerful investigation into the genetic architecture of MDD to date. Their results imply that common variables with intermediate and large effects do not have main effects on the genetic architecture of major depression.

Genetic Aspects Linked to Antidepressant Response

Genetic factors account for about 50 % of antidepressant response [32]. However, thus far, pharmacodynamic evidence remains partial and sparse. Replication rate does not yet allow useful genetic chips to be designed that can help clinicians find the correct drug for a specific patient [33].

The serotonin transporter (5-HTT, SLC6A4), norepinephrine transporter (NET, SLC6A2), and dopamine transporter (DAT, SLC6A) are involved in the active reuptake of serotonin, noradrenaline, and dopamine from the synaptic cleft. NET and 5-HTT are the main targets of many antidepressant agents. Thus, the NET and 5-HTTgenes constitute promising a priori candidate genes to mediate antidepressant treatment response.

While the exact nature of the 5-HTT genotype's link to depression continues to be a complex area of research, it has been established that it can significantly influence individual response to antidepressant medications. A recent meta-analysis of 15 studies confirmed the role of 5-HTTLPR in antidepressant response. People with the 5-HTTLPR S allele, who are at an increased risk of depression, showed slower improvement of depressive "core" and somatic anxiety symptoms [34]. Additionally, they showed worse therapeutic response to SSRIs, the most frequently used antidepressant agents; they delayed more in taking effect and yielded lower rates of response and remission, worse tolerability, and more frequent side effects [35, 36]. Furthermore, antidepressants with a different mechanism of action (e.g., selective noradrenaline agents) and psychotherapy were both found to be more effective in such individuals [37]. These findings have generally been replicated in studies of white populations, but opposing or inconsistent findings have also been reported. On the other hand, studies of Asian populations have usually reported conflicting results. It is still possible that a number of other unknown alleles within this genetic region may affect the expression of 5-HTT [33]. An SNP of the SLC6A4 gene promoter (rs25531) may also influence treatment response [38]. In conclusion, more research is needed in varied cultural populations before we can conclude that the S allele is associated with poorer response to SSRIs only in certain populations; that finding would certainly have significant implications for the future development of antidepressant medications [24, 39].

On the other hand, it has recently been found that response to noradrenaline reuptake inhibitors (NRIs) is associated with G1287A polymorphism (rs5569), the GG genotype being associated with better response [40]. However, Uher et al. [41] did not confirm the role of rs5569 in response to nortryptyline treatment. Meanwhile, Baffa et al. [42] analyzed seven polymorphisms in the NET gene promoter in terms of antidepressant treatment response. None of the seven investigated NET polymorphisms had an impact on overall treatment response. However, they did find that an additional –/CT insertion/deletion (ins/del) polymorphism (rs58532686) was significantly associated with melancholic depression, such that 12 patients carrying the deletion responded better to treatment [42].

The dopamine/noradrenaline reuptake inhibitor bupropion, and the SSRI sertraline, modulate the activity of the dopamine transporter. A 40-base pair VNTR polymorphism in the SLC6A3 gene has been associated with expression levels of the DAT. There is an association between the number of repeats and individual response to AD drugs indicating that the 9/10 and 9/9 genotypes have a higher risk of poorer, slower response to various AD drugs compared to the 10/10 genotype. Moreover, that genotype seems to be associated with late-life depression that responds preferentially to methylphenidate in conjunction with SSRI treatment [43].

The TPH gene encoding the rate-limiting enzyme in serotonin synthesis has been studied intensively in people with psychiatric disorders, yielding mixed results. The TPH2 form is expressed solely in neuronal cell types and is the predominant isoform in the CNS. Several studies have found that different genetic variations of the TPH2 gene (e.g., the functional SNP Arg441His, rs1843809, rs10897346, rs1386494) are associated with response to treatment with antidepressants or electroconvulsive therapy (ECT). However, SNPs of the TPH2 gene have also produced many negative results [38, 43]. Independent studies have reported no effects of the TPH1218A>C SNP on the efficacy of SSRI therapy or related side effects [44].

The COMT enzyme is involved in the catabolic pathways of NE and DA and can indirectly affect brain 5-HT tone because of the interactions between DA and 5-HT. The COMT gene has several allelic variants, the most widely studied of which is rs4680. The Met allele results in a three- to fourfold lower enzymatic activity than the Val allele. The Met allele was associated with better response to paroxetine, fluoxetine, fluvoxamine, and milnacipran treatments. The Val variant has been associated with higher risk of suicidal behavior and personality disorder traits and with worse response to mirtazapine and citalopram [33]. The effects of other SNPs in the COMT gene have shown inconclusive results in terms of antidepressant response [43, 45].

Monoamine oxidase A (MAO-A) is a major degrading enzyme in the metabolic pathways of monoamine neurotransmitters (NE, DA, 5-HT). One polymorphism in the promoter region of the MAO-A gene, consisting of a repetitive sequence (VNTR), has been linked to variations in biological activity and consequently serotonin concentrations [46]. Since the activity of MAO-A influences neurotransmitter concentrations, VNTR may affect antidepressant response. However, the current literature reports no such connection to antidepressant response or adverse effects [33, 38]. Another polymorphism (rs6323), associated with diminished MAO-A activity, has been associated with mirtazapine response in girls and women [38].

Monoamine receptors are among the most plausible candidates for modulation of antidepressant response, since most antidepressant drugs act to increase monoamine concentration in the synaptic cleft. Both pre- and post-synaptic 5-HT_{1A} receptors are present in different brain regions. The 5-HT_{1A}autoreceptor diminishes the release of 5-HT in the prefrontal cortex. Several antidepressant compounds desensitize raphe 5-HT_{1A}autoreceptors, resulting in enhanced

5-HT neurotransmission, which is thought to be connected to those drugs' antidepressant effects. One of the most extensively investigated functional polymorphisms, in 1019C>G (rs6295), lies in the promoter region of the gene for the 5-HT_{1A} receptor. The 1019G allele induces upregulation of the receptor's expression and may counteract antidepressant drugs' therapeutic effects by increasing the number of inhibitory 5-HT_{1A} autoreceptors on cell surfaces. This hypothesis has been partially confirmed by a series of SSRI studies [33, 38], but negative results were also reported. It is noteworthy that some studies suggest the effect of rs6295 on antidepressant response is confined to females and patients with melancholic depression [33, 47, 48]. Other variants of this gene (rs10042486 and rs1364043) were found to be linked to better antidepressant response [49], while others' roles (rs1800042) were dubious [33, 38].

The 5-HT_{2A} receptor is a post-synaptic receptor expressed widely throughout the CNS that plays a role in mediating anxiety, sleep, and sexual function. Several research findings suggest 5-HT_{2A} is involved in the pathophysiology and treatment of depression. These receptors are downregulated during antidepressant treatment, and in animal models, 5-HT_{2A} antagonists have been shown to have antidepressant effects and to diminish stress-induced reduction in brain-derived neurotrophic factor (BDNF) expression [43]. Three important, common SNPs of the 5-HT_{2A} gene (rs6313, rs6311, and rs6314) are linked to responses to antidepressant treatment, but negative results also exist. Also, another genetic variant of the 5-HT_{2A} gene (rs7997012) is associated with successful antidepressant treatment; however, the results have been somewhat ambiguous [33, 38, 50]. Several studies found significant associations between rs6311 or rs6313 and the occurrence of adverse drugs reactions [38]. Inconsistent results were reported between Asian and Caucasian samples. These findings suggest these SNPs could be useful in predicting SSRI intolerance and may be indicators of SSRI treatment response in individuals of Asian heritage [51].

5-HT_3 receptors are expressed throughout the CNS and peripheral nervous system and mediate a variety of physiological functions. The 5-HT_{3A} and 5-HT_{3B} genes have been most widely characterized and identified as having genetic polymorphisms [33]. Some studies link certain polymorphisms to SSRI responses and adverse effects, particularly vomiting [38, 52]. However, all these studies focused solely on SSRIs and were conducted in Japanese samples only. Given the small number of studies performed, and this lack of diversity in the studied group, further research is needed [43].

The 5-HT_6 receptor gene stands as an interesting candidate gene considering that some of this receptor's specific ligands have yielded antidepressant effects in animal models. Furthermore, the 5-HT_6 receptor influences the release of several neurotransmitters (ACh, NE, GABA, DA), as well as BDNF. According to some studies but not others, within the 5-HT_6 receptor gene is a silent SNP (rs1805054) associated with treatment response to antidepressant drugs [38].

Pharmacological treatment of depression leads to downregulation of β receptors [1]. The SNP (rs1801253) in the ADRβ1 gene has been linked to increased adenylate cyclase activation and might be responsible for faster antidepressant treatment response [53]. Nevertheless, data from the STAR*D Study was unable to confirm the relevance of this gene in modulating responses to citalopram treatment [33].

With respect to DA receptors, functional polymorphism in the DRD2 gene (rs1801028) showed no significant influence on antidepressant response in some studies [33]. Likewise, other studies reported no association between DRD4 polymorphism and antidepressant action [33]. However, in one study, DRD4 exon 3 variants exerted a significant modulation effect on various antidepressant drugs [54].

Nevertheless, in a large pharmacogenetic analysis that included 1,790 antidepressant-treated individuals with MDD, none of the more than 500,000 genetic markers studied predicted treatment outcomes after applying a genome-wide correction. The study's results suggest that single-marker prediction will not enable personalized prescriptions for the antidepressants currently available. Future studies may need to combine clinical, genetic, epigenetic, transcriptomic, and proteomic information to form clinically meaningful predictions of how an individual with major depression will respond to antidepressant treatment [55].

Whichever way we look at it, whether the risk variants are common or rare, it seems MDD will pose a much greater challenge in this case than less prevalent but more inheritable psychiatric disorders. While there is no question that genetic vulnerability plays a role in unipolar depression, it definitely seems to be more highly correlated with particular features and symptoms of depression, like early onset, severity, concomitant anxiety, and stress response, than with the fact of having a depressive profile. It is quite apparent that depression is an illness with a complex genetic component; rather than owing to alterations in just one gene, several genes participate and various life events intervene, modifying gene expression.

Monoamine Theories of Depression

During the 1960s, monoamine theories of depression flourished, postulating that depression's fundamental cause was a functional deficit in noradrenergic and serotonergic neurotransmission in certain areas of the brain. In general terms, the monoamine disorder hypothesis proposes that forebrain levels of monoamine neurotransmitters are depleted in depressive disorder – particularly 5-HT, NE, and to a lesser extent DA. These hypotheses were developed based on the fact that certain drugs that lessened symptoms had monoaminergic properties, like blocking the serotonin transporter or inhibiting MAO enzymes [56]. However, these drugs' efficacy was also limited during acute treatment [57, 58], which is one reason researchers are investigating other neurochemicals' respective roles in depression [12].

That being said, considering monoamine neurons' origin and distribution throughout multiple areas of the brain, there seems to be consensus that the monoamine neurotransmitters – particularly 5-HT, NE, and to a lesser extent DA – are directly or indirectly involved in the biochemical pathways toward depression [12]. Thus, any sort of alteration in monoamine functioning, whether in its synthesis, storage, release, or biotransformation, not to mention changes in its reuptake or monoamine receptor sensitivity, will have an impact on the manifestation of characteristic depressive and behavioral symptoms, such as mood state, alertness, motivation, fatigue, agitation, and psychomotor retardation [59]. Figure 23.1 displays the main connections between monoamines and behavioral symptoms that can be involved in depression.

Despite the available evidence that depression involves monoamine alteration, no such biological alteration has been employed, so far, as a basis for diagnosis. Therefore, the current monoamine hypothesis seems to implicate monoamines more in the mechanisms of initial antidepressant activity than in the origin of depression.

Noradrenaline Hypothesis of Depression

In 1965, Schildkraut proposed the "catecholamine hypothesis" of depression transcribed here: "some depressions, if not all, are associated with an absolute or relative deficit of catecholamines, particularly noradrenaline, in important adrenergic receptors in the brain. Contrariwise, elation may be associated with an excess of such amines" [60]. Schildkraut built this theory on the observation that tricyclic antidepressants (TCAs) and monoamine oxidase inhibitors (MAOIs) boost the presence of noradrenaline at the synaptic cleft, either by blocking synaptic reuptake of noradrenaline or by inhibiting the system through which MAO is metabolized. This so-called noradrenaline hypothesis of depression set off an avalanche of studies on the role of the noradrenaline system in the genesis of affective and other psychiatric disorders.

It is now generally agreed that this original hypothesis is insufficient as a neurobiological basis for depressive disorders, with the true picture likely much more complex and heterogeneous, involving both monoaminergic and

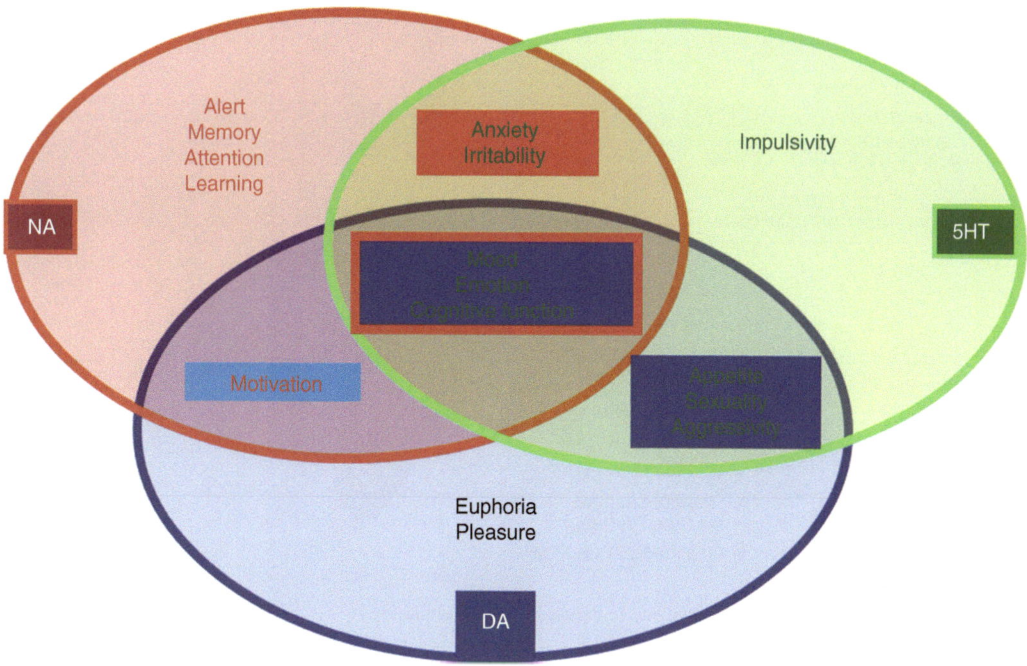

Fig. 23.1 Aspects of overall CNS functioning and its relation with different monoamines

non-monoaminergic players. Nevertheless, the concept of monoamine dysfunction remains a useful and well-regarded component of the neurobiological picture and has stimulated an extensive, productive line of research inquiry into the central noradrenergic system's function in depressive disorders [61].

The noradrenaline system is anatomically based in the brainstem nucleus known as the locus coeruleus (LC), which is the primary source of central NE synthesis; its noradrenergic projections reach virtually all areas of the brain [62]. Some of the symptoms that typically serve to diagnose depression seem to have implications for noradrenergic functioning. Hence, cognitive dysfunction could be tied to noradrenaline projections from the LC to the prefrontal cortex, a key structure in attention, working memory, decision-making, and skill acquisition. Meanwhile, the hypothalamus is key in regulating homeostatic functions, such that a noradrenergic innervation deficit could be responsible for the vegetative symptoms of depression, as well as changes in weight, appetite, and sleep schedule. Physical fatigue is one possible side effect of noradrenaline dysfunction in the cerebellum, which is essential to human motor control [59, 63] (Fig. 23.2).

Numerous subsequent studies carried out with patients suffering from affective disorders attempted to validate the catecholamine deficiency hypothesis by measuring the concentration of catecholamine and its major metabolites, 3-methoxy-4-hydroxyphenylglycol (MHPG) and homovanillic acid (HVA), in patients' cerebrospinal fluid (CSF), urine, and blood plasma. These studies' results remain controversial to this day. Additionally, the concentration of noradrenergic metabolites in the urine has been measured to predict responses to noradrenergic antidepressants and to classify subtypes of depression. However, this approach has so far not entered into clinical practice [64].

However, there are findings to suggest, at least in some types of depression, hyperfunctioning of α_2-adrenergic receptors, which could slow the neurotransmitter's synthesis and release and bring about a functional noradrenergic deficit. There is some evidence that upregulation of α_2-adrenergic receptors, in terms of either absolute

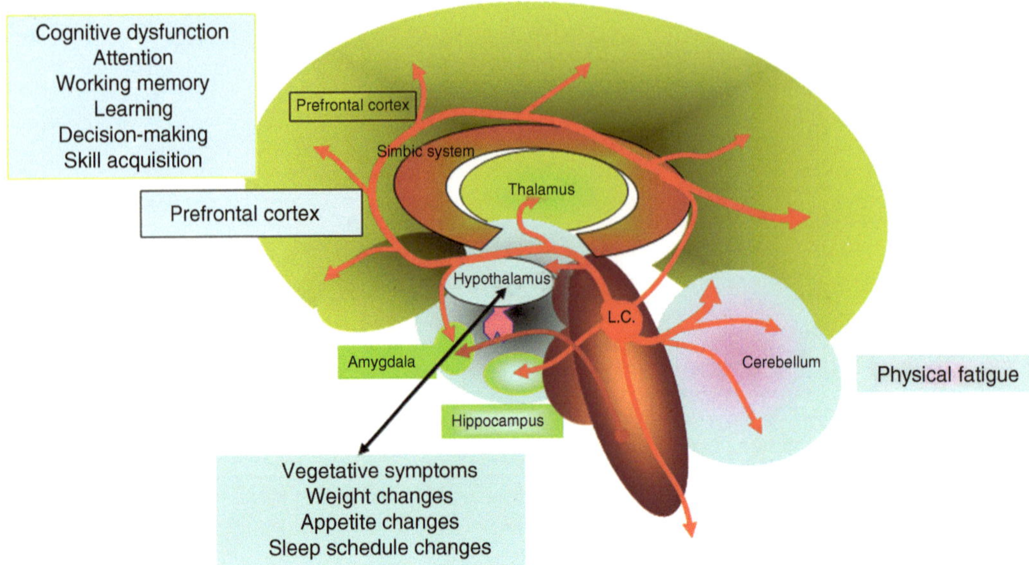

Fig. 23.2 Noradrenaline pathways involved in depressive symptomatology

level of expression or overall receptor activity, represents a valid component of the physiological view on depressive disorders. This α_2-adrenergic receptor dysregulation would have clear consequences to noradrenergic neurotransmission in the brain, given those receptors' important role in regulating the noradrenergic system [61]. Other components of the receptor system, including G proteins, G protein-coupled receptor kinases (GRKs), arrestin, and spinophilin, may contribute to α_2-adrenergic receptor dysfunction [65]. In fact, some data suggest coordinated changes in both the receptor and its partner proteins in the neurobiology of depression and in response to antidepressant therapy.

Furthermore, indirect assessment of central adrenaline receptor functioning using neuroendocrine tests (TSH, TRH, and GH release) has confirmed apparent hyperfunctioning at α_2-adrenergic receptors. Consistent with this hypothesis is the fact that in treating chronic depression, antidepressants reduce α_2-adrenaline hyperfunctioning and that those receptors' antagonists, like mianserin and mirtazapine, behave like comparable antidepressant agents (Fig. 23.3). As β-adrenoceptors are negatively regulated by the presence of NE, decreased NE may promote the upregulation of cortical β-adrenoceptors. In fact, this upregulation is observed in at least 25 % of the patients with MDD [2].

A key element of noradrenergic functioning is the NE transporter, which is responsible for presynaptic reuptake of NE. For many antidepressant drugs (TCAs, NRIs), their pharmacological action lies in inhibiting NE transport by interacting with the transporter. This happens quickly and can be observed if even a single dose is administered, even though it takes several weeks of continuous treatment to yield therapeutic effects. Some have postulated that the underlying mechanism that brings about an antidepressant effect is more the result of downregulation than inhibition of the NE transporter. NET downregulation is associated with an antidepressant effect on behavior, even when no detectable drug is present to inhibit NE reuptake. Desipramine-induced downregulation of the NET, and persistent antidepressant-like effects on behavior, develops gradually with repeated treatment, which is consistent with the idea that one is responding clinically to antidepressants. This suggests that neural adaptation resulting in enhanced monoamine neurotransmission may be a key mechanism mediating antidepressant action [66]. Human genetics studies have shown that variations in the gene coding

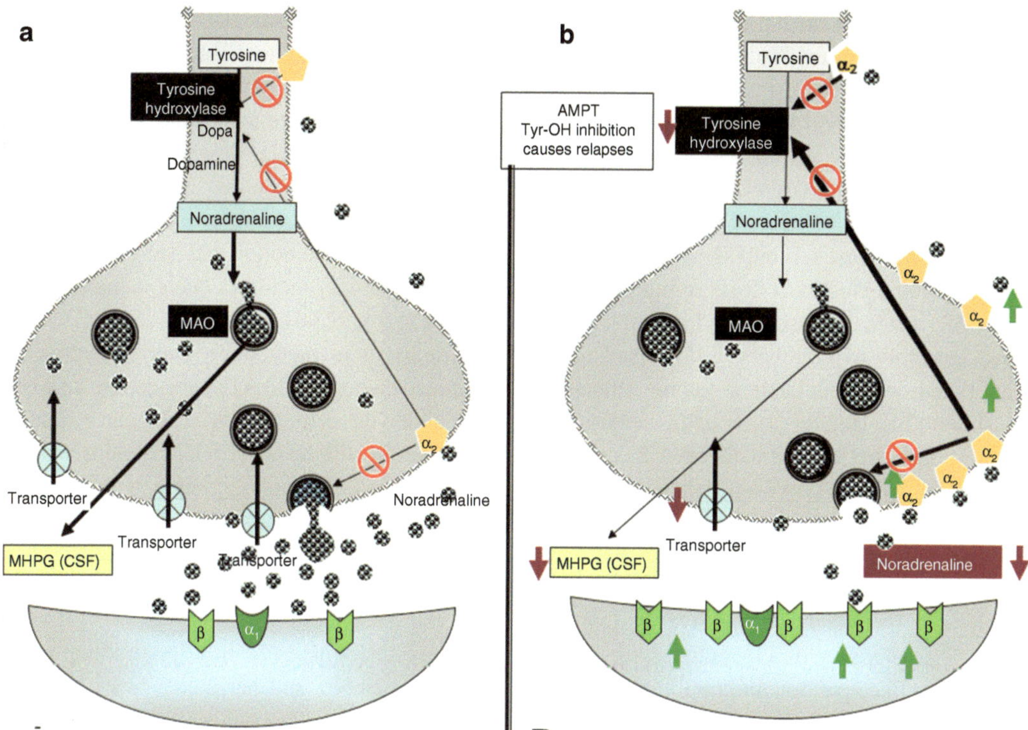

Fig. 23.3 Normal noradrenaline neurotransmission (**a**) and the major changes detected in depression (**b**). *MAO* monoamine oxidase, *MHPG* 3-methoxy-4-hydroxyphenylglycol in the CSF

for NET that alter neurotransmitter release are linked to individual differences in behavior and susceptibility to depression. The polymorphism NET-T182C, for example, is associated with increased susceptibility to depression [67]. In addition, decreased NE transporter binding has been reported in the LC of postmortem samples of subjects diagnosed with MDD [68, 69].

Furthermore, studies of depressed patients in remission and no longer taking medication have shown that a drastic reduction of NE levels (by inhibiting the key synthetic enzyme TH with α-methyl-p-tyrosine) results in the rapid reappearance of depressive symptoms. Interestingly, however, catecholamine depletion in healthy control volunteers did not result in depressed mood [70, 71]. These data reiterate that NE plays a role in the mechanism of antidepressant action, but its role in depression appears to be more complex.

In conclusion, some lines of evidence (genetics, anatomy, biochemical differences in postmortem brains, depletion of NE, and agents that specifically increase NE activity in depressed patients) suggest that NE is of major importance in the pathophysiology and treatment of depressive disorder [69].

Serotonin Hypothesis of Depression

In its original formulation, the 5-HT hypothesis postulated that a 5-HT deficit was the primary cause and could be reversed by antidepressants to restore normal functioning in depressed patients. Indeed, a variety of functional deficits of 5-HT neurotransmission in brain circuits known to regulate emotions, whether primary or secondary, have consistently been associated with aspects of the pathophysiology of depression [8].

The "serotonin hypothesis" of depression was initially developed by Brodie et al. [72], who reported a correlation between the depletion of serotonin induced by reserpine, with the onset of depressive symptoms. Also, the inhibition of serotonin synthesis with p-chloro-phenyl-alanine (PCPA) favored the onset of depression. Similarly, iproniazid, a tuberculostatic that inhibits MAO and increases cerebral 5-HT levels, displayed antidepressant activity in tuberculosis patients also suffering from depression [56]. Furthermore, the 5-HT precursor 5-hydroxytryptophan (5-HTP) was found to boost cerebral serotonin levels [73] and had antidepressant effects in humans. Thus, in 1968, Arvid Carlsson and his colleagues at the University of Gothenburg described for the first time how TCAs block serotonin reuptake in the brain [74], leading Lapin and Oxenkrug [75] to postulate the serotonin theory of depression that stems from a serotonin deficit at the intersynaptic level in certain regions of the brain.

With that in mind, the trajectory of different serotonin projections originating in the raphe nuclei may be linked to depressive symptomatology. Characteristic psychomotor symptoms of depression like agitation and inhibited movement and thought may be tied to dysfunctional serotonin innervation in the striate nucleus, which is known for its motor regulatory function. Anhedonia and loss of interest could be tied to serotonin innervation in the nucleus accumbens, whose function is closely related to pleasant sensations. Dysfunction in the ventral prefrontal cortex may be linked to depressed mood and suicidal ideation, the latter of which is also linked to serotonergic dysfunction in the amygdala. Serotonin innervation in the hippocampus may be tied to vegetative symptoms as well as altered appetite, weight, and sleep, which are features of depression. Moreover, methodological variables aside, most results to date have supported the notion that decreased cerebral serotonin activity increases one's vulnerability to MDD [2] (Fig. 23.4).

Serotonin is metabolized into 5-hydroxyindoleacetic acid (5-HIAA) by the actions of MAO and aldehyde dehydrogenase. In early studies, decreases in CSF levels of 5-HIAA were reported in depressive patients, compared to patients with neurological disorders without depression [76]. However, several subsequent studies were inconclusive. Further research has suggested a bimodal distribution of CSF levels of 5-HIAA in depressed patients [77]. In a longitudinal study, Träskman-Bendz and her colleagues [78] replicated this finding, observing a significant increase in 5-HIAA levels after recovery in a subset of depressed patients who exhibited lower CSF concentrations of it before improving. Many studies of depressed individuals have reported low CSF 5-HIAA levels in patients who have attempted suicide [79] or have suicidal ideation [80],

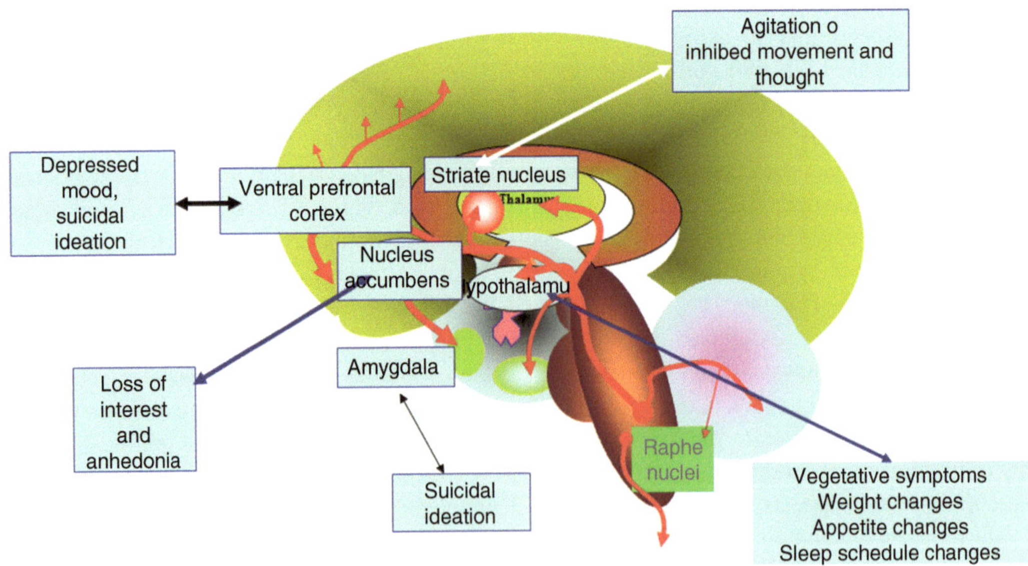

Fig. 23.4 Serotonergic pathways involved in depressive symptomatology

compared to depressed, non-suicidal patients and healthy controls. However, other studies of patients suffering from affective disorders have found no association between suicide attempt and low CSF 5-HIAA levels [81]. Altogether, low CSF 5-HIAA is linked to a higher probability of suicidal ideation or suicide attempt, which are sometimes comorbid with depression, but not always. High variability in CSF levels in healthy subjects may contribute to the variability of research results in this area. Furthermore, CSF levels can be affected by environmental factors such as daily diet or the time of day tested [82].

In postmortem studies of depressed patients, significant reductions in serotonin were reported in the brain stem, nucleus accumbens, caudate, putamen, substantia nigra, and amygdala. Moreover, this deficit in tissue serotonin content was not observed in brain tissue from depressed cases in remission, suggesting treatment had restored serotonin levels. Similarly, decreased tissue levels of 5-HIAA were also observed in depressed patients. These results, from studies of postmortem human brain tissue, support the hypothesis that depression involves impairment of the serotonin system. However, other postmortem findings about neurochemical levels in the brain failed to detect changes in serotonin and 5-HIAA levels in depressed patients [83]. While a correlation between low CSF 5-HIAA and major depression is reported only inconsistently, the correlation between low CSF 5-HIAA and suicidality, aggression, and impulsivity is more robust [84].

Serotonin can be depleted experimentally in humans given oral treatments. A drink containing all the amino acids except tryptophan stimulates the liver to synthesize proteins to rapidly deplete plasma levels of tryptophan. Tryptophan is rate-limiting for serotonin synthesis in the brain. This oral tryptophan depletion does not induce depression in healthy subjects, nor does it increase the severity of depressed mood in patients who have been clinically diagnosed with depression, but who are not currently receiving antidepressant treatment. However, it does cause relapse in depressed patients who have been successfully treated with an SSRI [70, 85], presumably by lowering cerebral 5-HT. Moreover, in response to tryptophan depletion, S allele carriers of the 5-HTTLPR SERT-gene polymorphism tend to be more vulnerable to relapse into a depressive state, tend to perform worse on motivational tasks, and tend to respond more slowly to antidepressants [86]. However, tryptophan depletion seems a somewhat nonselective tool to probe the 5-HT deficiency hypothesis. It can affect general protein synthesis. Also, less than 1 % of dietary tryptophan is converted into 5-HT, whereas 95 % is metabolized into the neuroactive substances quinolinic acid and kynurenic acid, which affect cholinergic and glutamatergic receptors, respectively, that can affect the brain and mood [84].

The serotonin transporter (5-HTT), the molecular target of a variety of antidepressants, has been investigated in postmortem human brains. Most studies have observed a significant decrease in 5-HTT in depressed patients in many serotonin-rich brain regions, including the hippocampus, putamen, occipital cortex, frontal cortex, prefrontal cortex, and dorsal raphe nuclei. However, other studies have reported no significant alteration in 5-HTT in the hippocampus, frontal cortex, midbrain, or prefrontal cortex [2, 83] (Fig. 23.5). In vivo visualization and measurement of 5-HTT using positron emission tomography (PET) and single-photon emission computerized tomography (SPECT) have revealed a significant decrease in 5 HTT binding potential in the midbrain region, amygdala, hippocampus, thalamus, putamen, and anterior cingulate cortex [83, 87] among depressed patients, as compared to healthy subjects. In contrast, other studies have reported increases in 5-HTT binding in the thalamus, dorsal cingulate cortex [88], and medial-frontal cortex in depressed patients [89]. Furthermore, subjects with a history of suicide attempt showed a markedly lower 5-HTT binding potential in the midbrain and increased 5-HTT binding in the anterior cingulate cortex, compared to depressed patients without suicidal histories as well as healthy controls [89]. These results are in line with the hypothesis that individuals with suicidal tendencies might represent a specific subset of depressed patients exhibiting serotonergic dysfunction. In addition,

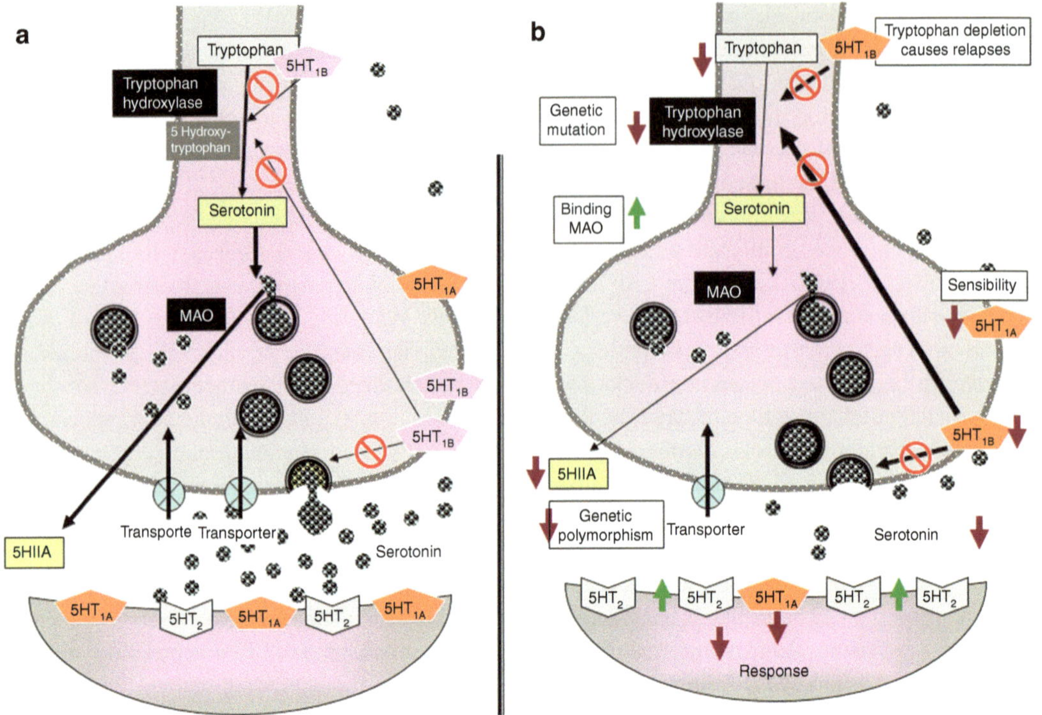

Fig. 23.5 Normal serotonin neurotransmission (**a**) and the major changes detected in depression (**b**). *MAO* monoamine oxidase, *5-HIIA* 5-hydroxyindoleacetic acid

environmental factors like abuse-induced stress and maternal separation were associated with significant decreases in 5-HTT binding in all brain regions. Such factors can modulate the serotonin system and may therefore be risk factors for developing depression [83].

In general, results from studies of 5-HT$_{1A}$ binding are variable. The 5-HT$_{1A}$ receptor is located both presynaptically and post-synaptically to regulate serotonin function. This receptor can be evaluated in depressive patients by injecting certain agonists and measuring specific neuroendocrine responses, such as elevated prolactin level. Results suggest the sensitivity of the hippocampal 5-HT$_{1A}$ receptor is lower in patients with depression, indicating that general upregulation of 5-HT receptors (hypothetically as compensation for lower levels of extracellular 5-HT) fails to occur in depression [90]. In fact, some groups have reported an overall decrease in 5-HT$_{1A}$ binding in antidepressant-näive depressed patients [91]. On the other hand, others have observed a global increase in 5-HT$_{1A}$ binding [92].

The relationship between 5-HT$_{1A}$ binding potential and the severity of depression has also been taken into consideration; findings have indicated a high correlation [93], but not consistently so [91]. Antidepressant-naïve depressed patients showed increased 5-HT$_{1A}$ binding potential compared to healthy controls, but no change registered in depressed patients with a history of antidepressant exposure compared to healthy individuals [27, 92].

The 5-HT$_{1B}$ regulatory autoreceptor, which interacts with the p11 protein, regulates serotonin release. The p-11 protein, which increases the receptor's efficiency, is less present in the brains of depressive patients postmortem [94] (Fig. 23.5).

Increased cortical 5-HT$_{2A}$ receptors have also been repeatedly associated with depression. This link between increased frontal 5-HT$_{2A}$ receptors and suicidality has been widely cited [95]. Recent data indicate that increased 5-HT$_{2A}$ receptors could in fact reflect 5-HT deficiency. However, several groups argue there is no association between frontal cortex 5-HT$_{2A}$ receptor levels and suicide. Investigations into other brain regions, including the hippocampus and amygdala, have also produced inconsistent findings. These discrepancies could be attributed to the hypothesis that elevated 5-HT_{2A} receptor levels more strongly correlate with aggression and that both age [96] and antidepressant treatment may alter 5-HT_{2A} receptor levels. However, other authors indicate 5-HT_{2A} receptor levels are not closely associated with depression or suicidality [84].

The rate-limiting step in 5-HT synthesis is converting tryptophan into 5-HTP, catalyzed by TH. TH exists in two isoforms [1, 2]. TH1 is largely responsible for 5-HT synthesis in the periphery and in the pineal gland. TH2 is expressed in the brain exclusively in serotonin neurons of the midbrain [97]. At this moment, the evidence for associations between functional polymorphisms in TH2 and depression and other psychiatric disorders is growing. It seems quite reasonable that TH2 gene variants leading to impaired TH2 function could result in reduced 5-HT synthesis and consequently cerebral 5-HT deficit. Polymorphisms in TH2 alone, or in conjunction with other genetic vulnerability factors, could predispose someone to depression that could then be precipitated by life stressors [84].

In conclusion, as in the case of the noradrenaline hypothesis, there is a multitude of evidence about serotonin dysfunction in depression. Nevertheless, the data are not specific enough for this mechanism alone to explain the origin of this pathology. That being said, clinical evidence points to the presence of 5-HT deficiency in at least some depressed individuals, perhaps most convincingly when suicidality or aggression is present.

Dopamine Hypothesis of Depression

Multiple data sources support the role of low dopamine neurotransmission in MDD. Dopamine is considered a neurotransmitter that is involved in motivation and pleasant experiences, and the inability to perceive pleasure, or anhedonia, is one of the most important signs of a depressive state. In fact, patients with Parkinson's disease, which destroys dopamine neurons, frequently suffer from depression.

However, research on DA's role in depression has been largely overshadowed by research on NE- and circuits containing 5HT (Fig. 23.6). The physiological alterations underlying reduced DA signaling could result from

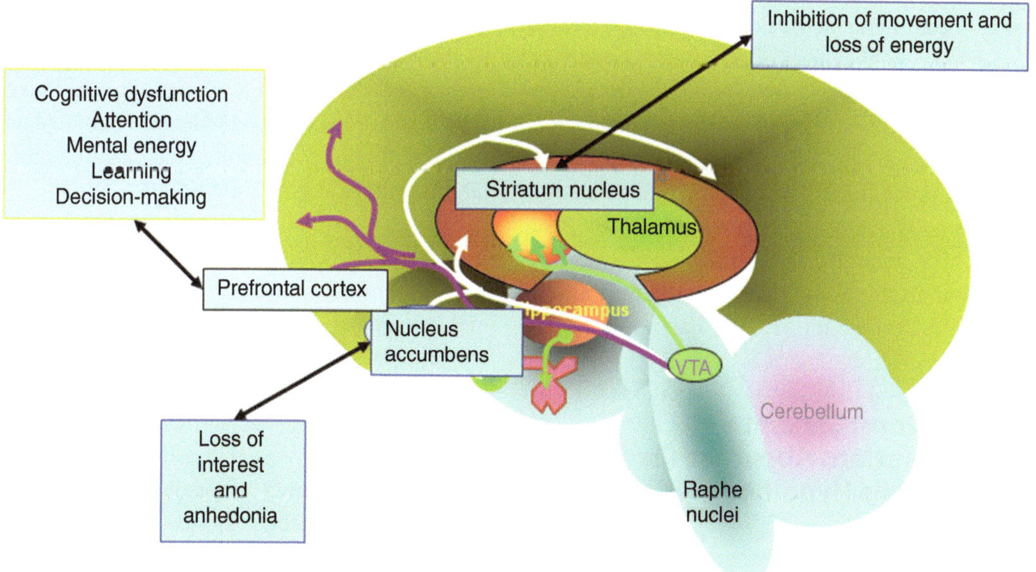

Fig. 23.6 Dopamine pathways involved in depressive symptomatology

either diminished DA release from presynaptic neurons or from impaired signal transduction. The latter could be due to changes in receptor number or function and/or altered intracellular signal processing [2, 98].

The majority of studies examining the concentration of DA metabolites in CSF, primarily HVA, found lower concentrations in depressed patients than in controls. However, discrepant results have also appeared. Apomorphine, a DA agonist, has been used as a probe to assess DA receptor responsiveness in depression. Apomorphine stimulates the release of growth hormone – releasing hormone and prolactin. Most such studies have found no difference between depressed and healthy control subjects in terms of growth hormone or prolactin response to apomorphine [98].

Relatively few postmortem studies of the DA system have been conducted in depressed patients and they have, not surprisingly, generated conflicting results. That is due at least in part to methodological variability and to some studies' inclusion of suicide victims. Studies of DAT expression have also found conflicting results, but the most comprehensive PET study observed reduced DAT binding in depression [99].

Anhedonia appears to be a particularly central feature of MDD. Reward is mediated by dopamine projections to the nucleus accumbens, suggesting that mesolimbic neurocircuitry plays a crucial role in the pathogenesis of depression. Functional brain imaging during a dopamine challenge has emphasized that when experiencing anhedonia, dopaminergic circuitry is involved in altered reward processing. The efficacy of medications that directly act on DA neurons or receptors, such as MAOIs, bupropion, and pramipexole, suggests that some subtypes of depression stem primarily from DA dysfunction [2, 100, 101].

Conclusions: General Considerations About the Classical Monoamine Hypothesis of Depression

The main systems of neurotransmission involved in depression are, as discussed above, noradrenaline, serotonin, and dopamine. According to some authors, alteration in some of these systems may be an underlying cause of affective disorders. However, there are data to indicate that these alterations in monoamine functioning are not enough to explain the origin of a pathology as complex as depression – or better put, depressions – especially when each monoamine is considered individually [2, 85].

With the exceptions discussed above, neurobiochemical findings in depressed patients have led us to hypothesize a distinction between the subgroups "noradrenaline depressions" and "serotonin depressions." In the first case, there is a drop in noradrenaline metabolism; that is, MHPG levels are low in the CSF. In the second case, there is a drop in serotonin metabolism, with distinctly low CSF levels of 5-HIAA, serotonin's primary metabolite [2, 85]. That hypothesis, while it has yet to be confirmed, has a series of therapeutic implications. For example, noradrenaline depressions are marked by a loss of emotionality, which manifests itself as altered mood or sadness, loss of interest and energy, psychomotor slowing, tiredness, anhedonia, and a motivation. Conversely, in serotonin depressions, added to the sadness and low mood are associated anxiety, irritability, impulsiveness, and feelings of guilt and fear. It stands to reason that antidepressants with noradrenaline and dopamine profiles more effectively treat the first type of depression, while serotonin-based antidepressants should more effectively treat the second type. However, such distinctions have yet to be substantiated and what therapy to apply in a given case remains a largely empirical question [59].

These explanations seem in many lights incomplete. If heightened monoamine tone were the only mechanism involved, administering antidepressants, which inhibit monoamine reuptake almost immediately, should yield an instantaneous response. On the contrary, experience tells us that clinical improvement occurs gradually and, generally speaking, is never observed in less than 2 weeks of beginning antidepressant treatment. Along those lines, one might reason that secondary or tertiary biochemical changes resulting from increased synaptic concentrations of 5-HT and/or NE in the CNS would combat the biochemical anomalies responsible for depressive disorders. Logically, increased synaptic concentrations of 5-HT and/or NE may essentially flip the switch, turning on the CNS "hard drive" and yielding secondary or tertiary biochemical changes in the CNS that counteract the biochemical anomaly or anomalies responsible for depressive disorders [1, 102].

The receptor adaptation theory about the physiopathogenesis of depression emerged in the 1980s. The theory hinges mainly on the delayed onset of antidepressant action and several receptors' adaptation in terms of number and functioning. On a related note, most antidepressants downregulate the excess activity at the β-adrenergic and/or 5-HT_2 receptors exhibited by depressive patients. Likewise, some experimental studies have demonstrated that antidepressants desensitize dopamine receptors, decrease the density of α_2-presynaptic adrenaline receptors, and desensitize the adenylate cyclase system coupled to β-adrenergic receptors, which may also contribute to its antidepressant activity. These adaptive changes do not occur immediately, which could explain the delay in clinical improvement displayed by all antidepressants [103]. On the other hand, the fact that this regulatory phenomenon is not universal for all antidepressants and that antagonists of these receptors lack antidepressant effects and even induce depression in some individuals [104] calls into question the notion that this adaptive receptor mechanism could be solely responsible for the antidepressants' therapeutic effects.

On a similar note, some authors believe depressive patients exhibit hyperfunctioning mediated by β-adrenergic and/or 5-HT_2 receptors that is downregulated by antidepressant treatment [105, 106]. Along those lines, it is known that one effect of TCAs, like amitriptyline and clomipramine, and MAOIs is that they downregulate β-adrenergic receptors. SSRIs, however, generally do not produce this effect, and differences have been established between different SSRIs. Hence, while fluvoxamine, fluoxetine, and paroxetine downregulate β-adrenergic receptors, sertraline and citalopram are not part of this phenomenon.

Some experimental studies have demonstrated that antidepressants desensitize dopamine autoreceptors, decrease the density of presynaptic α_2-adrenergicreceptors, and desensitize the adenylate cyclase system coupled to β-adrenergic receptors, a phenomenon that may also contribute to antidepressant activity. Consistent with that hypothesis is the fact that antagonists of α_2-adrenergic receptors like mianserin and mirtazapine behave like comparable antidepressants [107].

Other receptors, too, are susceptible to regulation in response to chronically administering antidepressants. In the 1990s, Blier and De Montigny [108] involved the 5-HT_{1A} receptor in the common mechanism behind antidepressant activity based on a series of experimental and clinical results. Likewise, SSRIs' delayed effectiveness is known to be an outcome of the time they need to desensitize the 5-HT_{1A} autoreceptors in the cell body of serotonin neurons. Desensitizing these autoreceptors enables postsynaptic serotonin neurotransmission to be potentiated. In that way, it has been demonstrated that the various groups of antidepressant treatments, including ECT, increase serotonin transmission at the 5-HT_{1A} receptors through several mechanisms, mainly in the hippocampus and other areas of the CNS. TCAs and ECT thus increase the sensitivity of 5-HT_{1A} receptors [109, 110], while MAOIs and SSRIs desensitize presynaptic 5-HT_{1A} and 5-HT_{1D} receptors, facilitating the release of 5-HT and therefore its interaction with postsynaptic 5-HT_{1A} receptors [107, 111, 112].

Despite these considerations, it is important to emphasize that currently there is no convincing evidence that regulation of adrenaline and serotonin receptors is solely responsible, per se, for the antidepressants' therapeutic effects. Therefore, rather than arrive at the conclusion that receptor regulation is the mechanism responsible for the action of antidepressant agents, it seems more plausible to interpret such regulation as a sign of a more complicated adaptive mechanism. It is believed that this serotonergic mechanism may be necessary, but that the intervention of other factors should be taken into consideration in accounting for antidepressant effect [107].

In light of the results we possess about different markers of monoamine functioning, and considering the therapeutic results of antidepressant treatments, which are more or less selective of that system, we emphasize that only 2 out of 3 patients respond to antidepressant treatment and a third respond to a placebo. It is possible that the pathophysiology of depression is not linked to monoaminergic mechanisms in 2 out of 3 cases. Moreover, it has been proposed that alteration in these systems of neurotransmission may be, rather than the cause, reasons for vulnerability to depression. In fact, numerous studies have demonstrated that monoamine depletion does not spark depressive symptoms in healthy control subjects, yet it causes depressive relapse in subjects with a prior history of depression or who are under antidepressant treatment. Perhaps depressive subjects exhibit an altered ability to recognize the neurotransmitter and put it to use, an alteration not experienced by healthy subjects. In depressive individuals, certain neurons in the circuits that regulate emotion are unable to maintain normal functioning when monoamine levels drop; this does not occur in healthy individuals [2, 107].

By way of conclusion, we argue that since the monoamine hypothesis of depression does not fully explain the etiopathology of depression, intraneuronal transduction mechanisms of receptor signaling must be involved.

References

1. Álamo C, López-Muñoz F. New antidepressant drugs: beyond monoaminergic mechanisms. Curr Pharm Des. 2009;15:1559–62.
2. Álamo C, López-Muñoz F, García-García P. Trastornos del estado de ánimo. In: Consejo General de Colegios Oficiales de Farmacéuticos, editor. Principios de fisiopatología para la atención farmacéutica, Módulo IV. Madrid: CGCOF; 2009. p. 97–138.
3. Alexander F, Selesnick S. Historia de la Psiquiatría. Barcelona: Ed. Expaxs; 1970.
4. López-Muñoz F, Alamo C. Historical evolution of the neurotransmission concept. J Neural Transm. 2009;116:515–33.
5. López-Muñoz F, Alamo C, Cuenca E. La "Década de Oro" de la Psicofarmacología (1950–1960): Trascendencia histórica de la introducción clínica de los psicofármacos clásicos. Psiquiatria.com (Electronic Journal). 2000;4(3). http://www.psiquiatria.com/psiquiatria/revista/47/1800/?++interactivo.
6. López-Muñoz F, Alamo C, Cuenca E. Historia de la Psicofarmacología. In: Vallejo J, Leal C, editors. Tratado de Psiquiatría. Barcelona: Ars Medica; 2005. p. 1709–36.
7. Willner P, Scheel-Krüger J, Belzung C. The neurobiology of depression and antidepressant action. Neurosci Biobehav Rev. 2012; doi:10.1016/j.neubiorev.2012.12.007. pii:S0149-7634(12)00216-3.
8. Albert PR, Benkelfat C, Descarries L. The neurobiology of depression—revisiting the serotonin hypothesis. I. Cellular and molecular mechanisms. Philos Trans R Soc Lond B Biol Sci. 2012;367:2378–81.
9. Álamo C, López-Muñoz F, Armada MJ. Agomelatina: un nuevo enfoque farmacológico en el tratamiento de la depresión con traducción clínica. Psiquiatr Biol. 2008;15:125–39.
10. Chenu F, El Mansari M, Blier P. Electrophysiological effects of repeated administration of agomelatine on the dopamine, norepinephrine, and serotonin systems in the rat brain. Neuropsychopharmacology. 2013;38:275–84.
11. Brink CB, Harvey BH, Brand L. Tianeptine: a novel atypical antidepressant that may provide new insights into the biomolecular basis of depression. Recent Pat CNS Drug Discov. 2006;1:29–41.
12. Krishnan V, Nestler EJ. The molecular neurobiology of depression. Nature. 2008;455:894–902.
13. Hasler G. Pathophysiology of depression: do we have any solid evidence of interest to clinicians? World Psychiatry. 2010;9:155–61.
14. Kendler KS, Gatz M, Gardner CO, Pedersen NL. A Swedish national twin study of lifetime major depression. Am J Psychiatry. 2006;163:109–14.
15. Dick DM, Riley B, Kendler KS. Nature and nurture in neuropsychiatric genetics: where do we stand? Dialogues Clin Neurosci. 2010;12:7–23.
16. Caspi A, Sugden K, Moffitt TE, et al. Influence of life stress on depression: moderation by a polymorphism in the 5-HTT gene. Science. 2003;301:386–9.
17. Caspi A, Hariri AR, Holmes A, Uher R, Moffitt TE. Genetic sensitivity to the environment: the case of the serotonin transporter gene and its implications for studying complex diseases and traits. Am J Psychiatry. 2010;167:509–27.
18. Tamatam A, Khanum F, Bawa AS. Genetic biomarkers of depression. Indian J Hum Genet. 2012;18:20–33.
19. Risch N, Herrell R, Lehner T, et al. Interaction between the serotonin transporter gene (5-HTTLPR), stressful life events, and risk of depression: a meta-analysis. JAMA. 2009;301:2462–71.
20. Wray NR, Pergadia ML, Blackwood DHR, et al. Genome-wide association study of major depressive disorder: new results, meta-analysis, and lessons learned. Mol Psychiatry. 2012;17:36–48.
21. Palazidou E. The neurobiology of depression. Br Med Bull. 2012;101:127–45.
22. Bagdy G, Juhasz G, Gonda X. A new clinical evidence-based gene-environment interaction model of depression. Neuropsychopharmacol Hung. 2012;14:213–20.
23. Belsky J, Jonassaint C, Pluess M, Stanton M, Brummett B, Williams R. Vulnerability genes or plasticity genes? Mol Psychiatry. 2009;14:746–54.

24. Kenna GA, Roder-Hanna N, Leggio L, et al. Association of the 5-HTT gene-linked promoter region (5-HTTLPR) polymorphism with psychiatric disorders: review of psychopathology and pharmacotherapy. Pharmacogenics Pers Med. 2012;5: 19–35.
25. Du L, Bakish D, Hrdina PD. Tryptophan hydroxylase gene 218A/C polymorphism is associated with somatic anxiety in major depressive disorder. J Affect Disord. 2001;65:37–44.
26. Mann JJ, Currie DM. Stress, genetics and epigenetic effects on the neurobiology of suicidal behavior and depression. Eur Psychiatry. 2010;25:268–71.
27. Parsey RV, Oquendo MA, Ogden RT, et al. Altered serotonin 1A binding in major depression: a (carbonyl-C-11) WAY100635 positron emission tomography study. Biol Psychiatry. 2006;59:106–13.
28. Lebe M, Hasenbring MI, Schmieder K, et al. Association of serotonin-1A and -2A receptor promoter polymorphisms with depressive symptoms, functional recovery, and pain in patients 6 months after lumbar disc surgery. Pain. 2013;154:377–84.
29. Lucae S, Ising M, Horstmann S, et al. HTR2A gene variation is involved in antidepressant treatment response. Eur Neuropsychopharmacol. 2010;20:65–8.
30. Kupfer DJ, Frank E, Phillips ML. Major depressive disorder: new clinical, neurobiological, and treatment perspectives. Lancet. 2012;379:1045–55.
31. Haeffel GJ, Getchell M, Koposov RA, Yrigollen CM. Association between polymorphisms in the dopamine transporter gene and depression: evidence for a gene-environment interaction in a sample of juvenile detainees. Psychol Sci. 2008;19:62–9.
32. Porcelli S, Fabbri C, Serretti A. Meta-analysis of serotonin transporter gene promoter polymorphism (5-HTTLPR) association with antidepressant efficacy. Eur Neuropsychopharmacol. 2012;22:239–58.
33. Porcelli S, Drago A, Fabbri C, et al. Pharmacogenetics of antidepressant response. J Psychiatry Neurosci. 2011;36:87–113.
34. Serretti A, Kato M, de Ronchi D. Kinoshita T- meta-analysis of serotonin transporter gene promoter polymorphism (5 HTTLPR) association with selective serotonin reuptake inhibitor efficacy in depressed patients. Mol Psychiatry. 2007;12:247–57.
35. Hu XZ, Rush AJ, Charney D, et al. Association between a functional serotonin transporter promoter polymorphism and citalopram treatment in adult outpatients with major depression. Arch Gen Psychiatry. 2007;64:783–92.
36. Laje G, Perlis RH, Rush AJ, McMahon FJ. Pharmacogenetics studies in STAR*D: strengths, limitations, and results. Psychiatr Serv. 2009;60:1446–57.
37. Rundell JR, Staab JP, Shinozaki G, McAlpine D. Serotonin transporter gene promotor polymorphism (5-HTTLPR) associations with number of psychotropic medication trials in a tertiary care outpatient psychiatric consultation practice. Psychosomatics. 2011;52:147–53.
38. Narasimhan S, Lohoff FW. Pharmacogenetics of antidepressant drugs: current clinical practice and future directions. Pharmacogenomics. 2012;13:441–64.
39. White KJ, Walline CC, Barker EL. Serotonin transporters: implications for antidepressant drug development. AAPS J. 2005;7:421–33.
40. Kim H, Lim SW, Kim S, et al. Monoamine transporter gene polymorphisms and antidepressant response in Koreans with late-life depression. JAMA. 2006;296:1609–18.
41. Uher R, Huezo-Diaz P, Perroud N, et al. Genetic predictors of response to antidepressants in the GENDEP project. Pharmacogenomics J. 2009;9:225–33.
42. Baffa A, Hohoff C, Baune BT, et al. Norepinephrine and serotonin transporter genes: impact on treatment response in depression. Neuropsychobiology. 2010;62:121–31.
43. Weizman S, Gonda X, Dome P, Faludi G. Pharmacogenetics of antidepressive drugs: a way towards personalized treatment of major depressive disorder. Neuropsychopharmacol Hung. 2012;14:87–101.
44. Serretti A, Kato M, Kennedy JL. Pharmacogenetic studies in depression: a proposal for methodologic guidelines. Pharmacogenomics J. 2008;8:90–100.
45. Perlis RH, Fijal B, Adams DH, et al. Variation in catechol-O-methyltransferase is associated with duloxetine response in a clinical trial for major depressive disorder. Biol Psychiatry. 2009;65:785–91.
46. Sabol SZ, Hu S, Hamer D. A functional polymorphism in the monoamine oxidase A gene promoter. Hum Genet. 1998;103:273–9.
47. Yu YW, Tsai SJ, Liou YJ, et al. Association study of two serotonin 1A receptor gene polymorphisms and fluoxetine treatment response in Chinese major depressive disorders. Eur Neuropsychopharmacol. 2006;16:498–503.
48. Baune BT, Hohoff C, Mortensen L. Serotonin transporter polymorphism (5-HTTLPR) association with melancholic depression: a female specific effect? Depress Anxiety. 2008;25:920–5.
49. Kato M, Fukuda T, Wakeno M, et al. Effect of 5-HT1A gene polymorphisms on antidepressant response in major depressive disorder. Am J Med Genet B Neuropsychiatr Genet. 2009;150B:115–23.
50. Horstmann S, Binder EB. Pharmacogenomics of antidepressant drugs. Pharmacol Ther. 2009;124:57–73.
51. Kato M, Serretti A. Review and meta-analysis of antidepressant pharmacogenetic findings in major depressive disorder. Mol Psychiatry. 2010;15:473–500.
52. Kato M, Fukuda T, Wakeno M, et al. Effects of the serotonin type 2A, 3A and 3B receptor and the serotonin transporter genes on paroxetine and fluvoxamine efficacy and adverse drug reactions in depressed Japanese patients. Neuropsychobiology. 2006;53:186–95.
53. Zill P, Baghai TC, Engel R, et al. Beta-1-adrenergic receptor gene in major depression: influence on antidepressant treatment response. Am J Med Genet B Neuropsychiatr Genet. 2003;120B:85–9.

54. Garriock HA, Delgado P, Kling MA, et al. Number of risk genotypes is a risk factor for major depressive disorder: a case–control study. Behav Brain Funct. 2006;2:24.
55. Tansey KE, Guipponi M, Perroud N, et al. Genetic predictors of response to serotonergic and noradrenergic antidepressants in major depressive disorder: a genome-wide analysis of individual-level data and a meta-analysis. PLOS Med. 2012;9(10):e1001326.
56. López-Muñoz F, Alamo C. Monoaminergic neurotransmission: the history of the discovery of antidepressants from 1950s until today. Curr Pharm Des. 2009;15:1563–86.
57. Kirsch I, Deacon BJ, Huedo-Medina TB, et al. Initial severity and antidepressant benefits: a meta-analysis of data submitted to the Food and Drug Administration. PLoS Med. 2008;5:260–8.
58. Fournier JC, De Rubeis RJ, Hollon SD, et al. Antidepressant drug effects and depression severity: a patient-level meta-analysis. JAMA. 2010;303:47–53.
59. Nutt DJ. Relationship of neurotransmitters to the symptoms of major depressive disorder. J Clin Psychiatry. 2008;69(Suppl E1):4–7.
60. Schildkraut JJ. The catecholamine hypothesis of affective disorders: a review of supporting evidence. Am J Psychiatry. 1965;122:509–22.
61. Cottingham C, Wang Q. Alpha-2 adrenergic receptor dysregulation in depressive disorders: implications for the neurobiology of depression and antidepressant therapy. Neurosci Biobehav Rev. 2012;36:2214–25.
62. Sara SJ. The locus coeruleus and noradrenergic modulation of cognition. Nat Rev Neurosci. 2009;10:211–23.
63. Drevets WC, Bogers W, Raichle ME. Functional anatomical correlates of antidepressant drug treatment assessed using PET measures of regional glucose metabolism. Eur Neuropsychopharmacol. 2002;12:527–44.
64. Kern N, Sheldrick AJ, Schmidt FM, Minkwitz J. Neurobiology of depression and novel antidepressant drug targets. Curr Pharm Des. 2012;18:5791–801.
65. González-Maeso J, Meana JJ. Heterotrimeric G proteins: insights into the neurobiology of mood disorders. Curr Neuropharmacol. 2006;4:127–38.
66. Zhao Z, Zhang HT, Bootzin E, et al. Association of changes in norepinephrine and serotonin transporter expression with the long-term behavioral effects of antidepressant drugs. Neuropsychopharmacology. 2009;34:1467–81.
67. Lin Z, Madras BK. Human genetics and pharmacology of neurotransmitter transporters. Handb Exp Pharmacol. 2006;175:327–71.
68. Klimek V, Stockmeier C, Overholser J, et al. Reduced levels of norepinephrine transporters in the locus coeruleus in major depression. J Neurosci. 1997;17:8451–8.
69. Moret C, Briley M. The importance of norepinephrine in depression. Neuropsychiatr Dis Treat. 2011;7 Suppl 1:9–13.
70. Delgado PL, Moreno FA. Role of norepinephrine in depression. J Clin Psychiatry. 2000;61 Suppl 1:5–12.
71. Ruhe HG, Mason NS, Schene AH. Mood is indirectly related to serotonin, norepinephrine and dopamine levels in humans: a meta-analysis of monoamine depletion studies. Mol Psychiatry. 2007;12:331–59.
72. Brodie BB, Pletscher AP, Shore PA. Evidence that serotonin has a role in brain function. Science. 1955;122:968.
73. Udenfriend S, Weissbach H, Bogdanski DF. Increase in tissue serotonin following administration of its precursor 5-hydroxytryptophan. J Biol Chem. 1957;224:803–10.
74. Carlsson A, Fuxe K, Ungerstedt U. The effect of imipramine on central 5hydroxytryptamine neurons. J Pharm Pharmacol. 1968;20:150–1.
75. Lapin JP, Oxenkrug GF. Intensification of the central serotonergic processes as a possible determinal of the thymoleptic effect. Lancet. 1969;i:132–6.
76. Ashcroft GW, Sharman DF. 5-hydroxyindoles in human cerebrospinal fluids. Nature. 1960;186:1050–1.
77. Asberg M, Thorén P, Träskman L, Bertilsson L, Ringberger V. "Serotonin depression" – a biochemical subgroup within the affective disorders? Science. 1976;1976(191):478–80.
78. Träskman-Bendz L, Asberg M, Bertilsson L, Thorén P. CSF monoamine metabolites of depressed patients during illness and after recovery. Acta Psychiatr Scand. 1984;69:333–42.
79. Samuelsson M, Jokinen J, Nordström A-L, Nordström P. CSF 5-HIAA, suicide intent and hopelessness in the prediction of early suicide in male high-risk suicide attempters. Acta Psychiatr Scand. 2006;113:44–7.
80. López-Ibor JJ, Saiz-Ruiz J, Pérez de los Cobos JC. Biological correlations of suicide and aggressivity in major depressions (with melancholia): 5-hydroxyindoleacetic acid and cortisol in cerebral spinal fluid, dexamethasone suppression test and therapeutic response to 5-hydroxytryptophan. Neuropsychobiology. 1985;14:67–74.
81. Sullivan GM, Oquendo MA, Huang Y-Y, Mann JJ. Elevated cerebrospinal fluid 5-hydroxyindoleacetic acid levels in women with comorbid depression and panic disorder. Int J Neuropsychopharmacol. 2006;9:547–56.
82. Kennedy JS, Gwirtsman HE, Schmidt DE, et al. Serial cerebrospinal fluid tryptophan and 5-hydroxy indoleacetic acid concentrations in healthy human subjects. Life Sci. 2002;71:1703–15.
83. Altieri YS, Singh E, Sibille Y, Andrews AM. Serotonergic pathways in depression. In: López-Muñoz F, Álamo C, editors. Neurobiology of depression. Boca Raton: Taylor & Francis/CRC Press; 2012. p. 143–70.
84. Jacobsen JPR, Medvedev IO, Caron MG. The 5-HT deficiency theory of depression: perspectives from a naturalistic 5-HT deficiency model, the tryptophan hydroxylase 2Arg439His knockin mouse. Philos Trans R Soc Lond B Biol Sci. 2012;367:2444–59.
85. Belmaker RH, Agam G. Major depressive disorders. N Engl J Med. 2008;358:55–68.
86. Walderhaug E, Magnusson A, Neumeister A, et al. Interactive effects of sex and 5-HTTLPR on mood and impulsivity during tryptophan depletion in healthy people. Biol Psychiatry. 2007;62:593–9.

87. Oquendo MA, Hastings RS, Huang Y-Y, et al. Brain serotonin transporter binding in depressed patients with bipolar disorder using positron emission tomography. Arch Gen Psychiatry. 2007;64:201–8.
88. Miller JM, Kinnally EL, Ogden RT, et al. Reported childhood abuse is associated with low serotonin transporter binding in vivo in major depressive disorder. Synapse. 2009;63:565–73.
89. Cannon DM, Ichise M, Fromm SJ, et al. Serotonin transporter binding in bipolar disorder assessed using [11C]DASB and positron emission tomography. Biol Psychiatry. 2006;60:207–17.
90. Pitchot W, Hansenne M, Pinto E, et al. 5-hydroxytryptamine 1A receptors, major depression, and suicidal behavior. Biol Psychiatry. 2005;58:854–8.
91. Hirvonen J, Karlsson H, Kajander J, et al. Decreased brain serotonin 5-HT1A receptor availability in medication-naive patients with major depressive disorder: an in-vivo imaging study using PET and [carbonyl-11C]WAY-100635. Int J Neuropsychopharmacol. 2008;11:465–76.
92. Miller JM, Brennan KG, Ogden TR, et al. Elevated serotonin 1A binding in remitted major depressive disorder: evidence for a trait biological abnormality. Neuropsychopharmacology. 2009;34:2275–84.
93. Meltzer CC, Price JC, Mathis CA, et al. Serotonin 1A receptor binding and treatment response in late-life depression. Neuropsychopharmacology. 2004;29:2258–65.
94. Svenningsson P, Chergui K, Rachleff I, et al. Alterations in 5-HT1B receptor function by p11 in depression-like states. Science. 2006;311:77–80.
95. Stanley M, Mann JJ. Increased serotonin-2 binding sites in frontal cortex of suicide victims. Lancet. 1983;i:214–6.
96. Oquendo MA, Russo SA, Underwood MD, et al. Higher postmortem prefrontal 5-HT2A receptor binding correlates with lifetime aggression in suicide. Biol Psychiatry. 2006;59:235–43.
97. Gutknecht L, Kriegebaum C, Waider J, et al. Spatio-temporal expression of tryptophan hydroxylase isoforms in murine and human brain: convergent data from Tph2 knockout mice. Eur Neuropsychopharmacol. 2009;19:266–82.
98. Dunlop BW, Nemeroff CB. The role of dopamine in the pathophysiology of depression. Arch Gen Psychiatry. 2007;64:327–37.
99. Klimek V, Schenck JE, Han H, Stockmeier CA, Ordway GA. Dopaminergic abnormalities in amygdaloid nucleus in major depression: a postmortem study. Biol Psychiatry. 2002;52:740–8.
100. Stein D. Depression, anhedonia, and psychomotor symptoms: the role of dopaminergic neurocircuitry. CNS Spectr. 2008;13:561–5.
101. Tremblay LK, Naranjo CA, Graham SJ, et al. Functional neuroanatomical substrates of altered reward processing in major depressive disorder revealed by a dopaminergic probe. Arch Gen Psychiatry. 2005;62:1228–36.
102. Machado-Vieira R, Salvadore G, Luckenbaugh DA, Manji HK, Zarate CA. Rapid onset of antidepressant action: a new paradigm in the research and treatment of major depressive disorder. J Clin Psychiatry. 2008;69:946–58.
103. Sulser F, Vetulani J, Mobley P. Mode of action of antidepressant drugs. Biochem Pharmacol. 1978;27:257–61.
104. Paykel ES, Fleminger R, Watson JP. Psychiatric side effects of antihypertensive drugs other than reserpine. J Clin Psychopharmacol. 1982;2:14–39.
105. Stahl S. 5HT1A receptors and pharmacotherapy. Is serotonin receptor down-regulation linked to the mechanism of action of antidepressant drugs? Psychopharmacol Bull. 1994;30:39–43.
106. Wang Z, Crowe RR, Tanna VL, Winokur G. Alpha 2 adrenergic receptor subtypes in depression: a candidate gene study. J Affect Disord. 1992;25:191–6.
107. Álamo C, Guerra JA, López-Muñoz F. Psicofármacos antidepresivos. In: Chinchilla A, editor. Tratado de terapéutica psiquiátrica. Madrid: Nature Publishing Group; 2010. p. 41–87.
108. Blier P, De Montigny C. Current advances and trends in the treatment of depression. Trends Pharm Sci. 1994;15:220–6.
109. Celada P, Puig M, Amargos-Bosch M, Adell A, Artigas F. The therapeutic role of 5-HT1A and 5-HT2A receptors in depression. J Psychiatry Neurosci. 2004;29:252–65.
110. Savitz J, Lucki I, Drevets WC. 5-HT(1A) receptor function in major depressive disorder. Prog Neurobiol. 2009;88:17–31.
111. Berendsen HH. Interactions between 5-hydroxytryptamine receptor subtypes: is a disturbed receptor balance contributing to the symptomatology of depression in humans? Pharmacol Ther. 1995;66:17–37.
112. Bourin M, David DJ, Jolliet P, Gardier A. Mechanism of action of antidepressants and therapeutic perspectives. Therapie. 2002;57:385–96.

Melatonergic Drug: Ramelteon and Its Therapeutic Applications in Insomnia

24

V. Srinivasan, Rahimah Zakaria, Timo Partonen, Edward C. Lauterbach, Preetha Sharone Kuppuswamy, Amnon Brzezinski, Zahiruddin Othman, and Atul Prasad

Abstract

The efficacy of melatonin in promoting and maintaining sleep has been demonstrated in most of the clinical studies. However, because of its short half-life, its sustained effect in improving sleep quality could not be demonstrated uniformly in all the studies that have been undertaken so far. The development of slow-release melatonin preparation Circadin has been found effective in reducing sleep onset time and also for improving sleep quality. This was followed by the introduction of another melatonergic drug ramelteon a melatonin receptor agonist that has high selectivity for

V. Srinivasan, MSc, PhD, MAMS (✉)
Sri Sathya Sai Medical Educational and Research Foundation, An International Medical Sciences Research Study Center, Prasanthi Nilayam, 40-Kovai Thirunagar Extn, Goldwins, Coimbatore, TN 641014, India

National Health Service, Department of Mental Health, Psychiatric Service of Diagnosis and Treatment, Hospital "G. Mazzini", ASL 4, Teramo, Italy

Department of Neuroscience and Imaging, University "G.D' Annunzio", Chieti 66013, Italy
e-mail: sainivasan@yahoo.com, venkataramanujamsrinivasan6@gmail.com

R. Zakaria, MBBS, MSc, PhD (Physiology)
Department of Physiology, School of Medical Sciences, Universiti Sains Malaysia, Kubang Kerian, Kelantan 16150, Malaysia
e-mail: rahimah@kck.usm.my

T. Partonen, MD, PhD
Department of Mental Health and Substance Abuse Services, National Institute for Health and Welfare, Mannerheimintie 166, FI-00300 Helsinki, Finland
e-mail: timo.partonen@thl.fi

E.C. Lauterbach, MD
Department of Psychiatry and Behavioral Sciences, and the Department of Internal Medicine, Neurology Section, Mercer University School of Medicine, 655 First Street, Macon, GA 31201, USA
e-mail: eclbgnp@earthlink.net

P.S. Kuppuswamy, MD
Department of Psychiatry and Psychology, Mayo Clinic College of Medicine, 200 First Street SW, Rochester, MN 55905, USA
e-mail: preethasharone@gmail.com

A. Brzezinski, MD
Department of Obstetrics and Gynecology, Hadassah Hebrew-University Medical Center, Ein-Kerem, Jerusalem 91120, Israel
e-mail: amnonbrz@gmail.com

Z. Othman, MD, MMed (Psychiatry)
Department of Psychiatry, School of Medical Sciences, Hospital Universiti Sains Malaysia, Kubang Kerian, Kelantan, 16150, Malaysia
e-mail: zahir@kb.usm.my

A. Prasad, MBBS, DM (Neurology)
Department of Neurology, Dr BL Kapur Superspeciality Hospital, Pusa Road, New Delhi, DL 110005, India
e-mail: prasad.atul@gmail.com

V. Srinivasan et al. (eds.), *Melatonin and Melatonergic Drugs in Clinical Practice*, DOI 10.1007/978-81-322-0825-9_24, © Springer India 2014

MT_1 receptors than MT_2 receptors and therefore targets *sleep onset* more specifically than melatonin. Clinical trials undertaken in different countries of European region and Japan have conclusively demonstrated that ramelteon in various doses (from 4 to 32 mg/day) reduced sleep onset latency, increased total sleep time, and sleep efficiency and quality in patients suffering from chronic insomnia. Besides acting as a sedative-hypnotic drug, ramelteon also demonstrated its ability as a drug with chronobiotic properties and has been found useful in resetting the disturbed circadian rhythms. The action of ramelteon in improving sleep efficiency is dose independent and hence acts differently from melatonin. It has a promising value in treating patients with chronic insomnia as it does not have any of the adverse effects like next-day hangover and dependence associated with the usage of other conventional hypnotic drugs.

Keywords
Ramelteon • Sleep onset latency • Total sleep time • Sleep efficiency • Sleep quality

Introduction

Melatonin (*N*-acetyl-5-methoxytryptamine), first identified by Lerner et al., is the major neurohormone secreted from the pineal gland mainly during the dark hours of the night and is released in higher concentrations into the cerebrospinal fluid [1, 2]. The circadian pattern of pineal melatonin secretion is regulated by suprachiasmatic nucleus (SCN) of the hypothalamus. The SCN has extensive efferent projections to the subparaventricular zone of the hypothalamus from where these fibers proceed further to terminate in the areas involved in sleep-wake regulation [3]. Sleep regulation involves interaction of two separate mechanisms, namely, an endogenous biological clock that drives the circadian rhythm of the sleep-wake cycle (process-C) and a homeostatic process (process-S) that influences sleep propensity that is determined by the duration of previous sleep episodes [4]. These processes interact continuously and are involved in the determination of consolidated bouts of sleep at night and consolidated bouts of wakefulness during daytime. Melatonin has a role in sleep regulation, since its nocturnal rise/increase leads to "opening of the sleep gate" and augmentation of sleep propensity [5].

The importance of melatonin in both the initiation and maintenance of sleep has been demonstrated [6]. In diurnal animals and in human beings, the onset of melatonin secretion has been shown to coincide with the timing of an increase in nocturnal sleep propensity [7]. Since melatonin has both hypnotic and chronobiotic properties, it has been used in the treatment of age-related insomnia and other primary and secondary insomnias [8]. Also, prolonged-release melatonin formulations are available that are effective in treating insomnias [9].

Melatonin has also been used successfully for the treatment of circadian rhythm sleep disorders like jet-lag, shift-work disorder, and delayed sleep phase syndrome [10, 11]. The high density of MT_1 and MT_2 melatonin receptors in the hypothalamic SCN confirms that melatonin regulates sleep and the sleep-wakefulness cycle by acting on both these receptors [12, 13].

As melatonin has a short half-life (less than 30 min), its efficacy in promoting and maintaining sleep has been inconsistent in the studies that have been undertaken so far. Hence, the need for the development of melatonin agonists with a longer duration of action on sleep regulatory structures in the brain is evident [14]. Recently, the melatonergic chrono-hypnotic drug ramelteon has been introduced for the treatment of primary insomnia and has been effective in improving sleep quality and efficiency when compared to melatonin or slow-release preparations [15].

Insomnia

Insomnia is a sleep disorder characterized by poor quality of sleep with symptoms like difficulty in falling asleep, frequent nocturnal awakenings, and early morning awakenings, resulting in fatigue, reduced alertness, irritability, and impaired concentration, memory, and performance with a major negative impact on quality of life [16, 17]. It is more common among elderly people and is a major cause of impaired physical and mental health in this aged population [18]. Nearly 30–40 % of the adult population suffers from mild to severe insomnia. Due to its numerous effects on psychological and physiological well-being, insomnia also has serious social consequences, especially motor vehicle accidents and reduced work performance and productivity. Insomnia can be treated with lifestyle modifications, behavioral techniques including sleep hygiene, relaxation and distraction techniques, cognitive-behavioral therapy, and pharmacological interventions that include both benzodiazepines and nonbenzodiazepine drugs [9, 19].

Sleep and Melatonin

The role of melatonin in the control of sleep has been investigated in both diurnal and nocturnal species. Local injection of pharmacological amounts of melatonin (1–50 μg) in the medial preoptic area of the rat hypothalamus during daytime increased total sleep time in a dose-dependent manner mainly by increasing non-rapid eye movement (NREM) sleep [20]. Melatonin has been shown to induce sleep by altering the functions of the $GABA_A$-benzodiazepine receptor complex [21]. In diurnal species, suppression of electrical activity in the SCN is suggested as a possible mechanism by which melatonin regulates sleep. This effect is absent in MT_1 knockout mice, thereby demonstrating the importance of MT_1 receptors in melatonin's acute inhibitory effects on SCN electrical activity [22]. The MT_1 and MT_2 melatonin receptor subtypes are complementary in their actions and, to some extent, mutually substitute for each other. The suppression of neuronal (GABAergic) activity by melatonin is one of the possible mechanisms by which this hormone contributes to the regulation of sleep.

As melatonin deficiency is suggested as a *cause rather than a marker* for insomnia in the elderly, melatonin replacement therapy has been advocated for treating insomnia in the geriatric population. Because melatonin is a natural hypnotic, it is suitable for long-term use in elderly people due to its low toxicity and limited side effect profile. It has also been proven to be beneficial since it significantly improved total sleep time (TST) and sleep quality and reduced sleep onset latency (SOL) [23–28].

Reduced production of endogenous melatonin seems to be a prerequisite for effective exogenous melatonin treatment of sleep disorders in the geriatric population. A meta-analysis on the effects of melatonin in sleep disturbances in all age groups (including young adults with presumably normal melatonin levels) by one of the authors of this review revealed significant and clinically meaningful effects of exogenous melatonin on sleep quality, efficiency, and latency [28]. However, another meta-analytical study did not find melatonin to be effective in increasing sleep efficacy (SE) or in reducing SOL in geriatric patients [29].

The relationship between sleep disturbances and low nocturnal melatonin production was investigated in a large population of insomniacs aged 55 years or more. Elderly patients with insomnia with sleep problems excreted 9.0 ± 8.3 μg of the urinary melatonin metabolite 6-sulfatoxymelatonin per night, whereas age-matched healthy controls excreted 18.1 ± 12.7 μg of 6-sulfatoxymelatonin per night, and younger subjects excreted 24.2 ± 11.9 μg of 6-sulfatoxymelatonin per night. It was also observed that half of the elderly insomniacs excreted less than 8.0 μg of 6-sulfatoxymelatonin per night. Within this subpopulation of 372 subjects, 112 had urinary 6-sulphatoxy melatonin values lower than 3.5 μg per night [5].

Studies carried out using 0.3–1 mg doses of melatonin that attained "physiological melatonin levels" or "physiological" melatonin blood levels have shown that melatonin reduced sleep latency (SL) and increased SE when administered to healthy human subjects during the evening [23]. However, in most studies, higher amounts of melatonin (2–6 mg) are needed to be given in order to obtain similar effects. Brain imaging studies in awake subjects show that melatonin modulates the brain activity pattern to one resembling actual sleep [30]. Despite clinical studies, the general efficacy of melatonin as a sleep-promoting substance has been a subject of debate [31]. A possible explanation for this is that administered melatonin doses are too low. The reported lack of efficacy of melatonin could be related to the extremely short half-life of the fast-release melatonin preparations, and this prompted the development of active slow-release formulations [32]. Circadin®, a 2 mg controlled-release preparation of melatonin developed by Neurim (Tel Aviv, Israel), was approved by the European Medicines Agency (EMEA) as a monotherapy for short-term treatment of primary insomnia in elderly subjects in 2007. Circadin®, a slow-release melatonin preparation, has been shown to improve the quality of sleep and morning alertness, to reduce SOL, and to ameliorate quality of life in the middle-aged and elderly patients with insomnia [33, 34]. Generally, patients who have low melatonin levels responded better to melatonin replacement therapy compared to other patients with insomnia. An unknown aspect of melatonin activity in brain with regard to its hypnotic and chronobiotic activities is the extent to which it desensitizes its membrane MT_1 and MT_2 receptors. Since MT_1 and MT_2 melatonin receptors are G protein-coupled receptors, desensitization is an expected normal phenomenon in these receptors. Gerdin et al. demonstrated the desensitization of endogenous MT_2 melatonin receptors by physiological melatonin concentrations simulating the nocturnal surge in the rat SCN [35]. This finding questioned the efficacy of using supraphysiological doses of melatonin to treat insomnia. However, in a study conducted on SCN neurons, neither in vivo studies (intraperitoneal or iontophoretic application of melatonin) nor in vitro studies on SCN neuronal cells revealed any desensitization phenomenon [36]. Also, the melatonin receptor concentration has been shown to increase in parallel with the increase of melatonin concentration, which raises doubt over the theory of receptor desensitization phenomenon after long-term use of either melatonin or its agonists [37].

Ramelteon: The Melatonergic Drug for Insomnia

Ramelteon (Rozerem®, Takeda Pharmaceuticals, Japan) is a melatonergic hypnotic medication that has been demonstrated to be effective and safe in clinical trials. It is a tricyclic synthetic analog of melatonin, chemically designated as (*S*)-*N*-[2-(1, 6,7,8-tetrahydro-2*H*-indeno[5,4-*b*] furan-8-yl)-ethyl]propionamide. In 2005, the Food and Drug Administration (FDA) approved its use for the treatment of insomnia. Ramelteon is a selective MT_1/MT_2 receptor agonist without significant affinity for other receptor sites [38, 39]. In vitro binding studies have shown that ramelteon's affinity for MT_1 and MT_2 receptors is 3–16 times higher than that of melatonin. The selectivity of ramelteon for MT_1 has been found to be greater than that of MT_2 receptors. The selectivity of MT_1 receptors by ramelteon suggests that it targets sleep onset more specifically than melatonin itself [40].

Pharmacokinetics of Ramelteon

Ramelteon is usually administered by the oral route and is absorbed rapidly by the gastrointestinal tract (84 %). The half-life of circulating ramelteon is in the range of 1–2 h, which is much longer than that of melatonin. The influence of age and gender on the pharmacokinetics and the pharmacodynamics of ramelteon was evaluated in healthy volunteers (young: 18–34 years; elderly: 63–79 years) after administration of a single dose of ramelteon. Compared to young individuals, the clearance of ramelteon was significantly reduced in elderly individuals. No significant effect of gender was observed [41].

Ramelteon is extensively metabolized into active metabolites primarily via oxidation to hydroxyl and carbonyl species, with secondary metabolism to form glucuronide conjugates. Cytochrome P450 1A2 is the major hepatic enzyme involved in ramelteon metabolism. Four principal metabolites of ramelteon (M-I, M-II, M-III, M-IV) have been identified. Among these, M-II has been found to occur in much higher concentrations with systemic levels 20–100-fold greater than ramelteon itself. Although the activity of M-II is 30-fold lower than that of ramelteon, its exposure exceeds that of ramelteon by a factor of 30. Hence, it is suggested that M-II may contribute significantly to the net clinical effect of ramelteon intake [39].

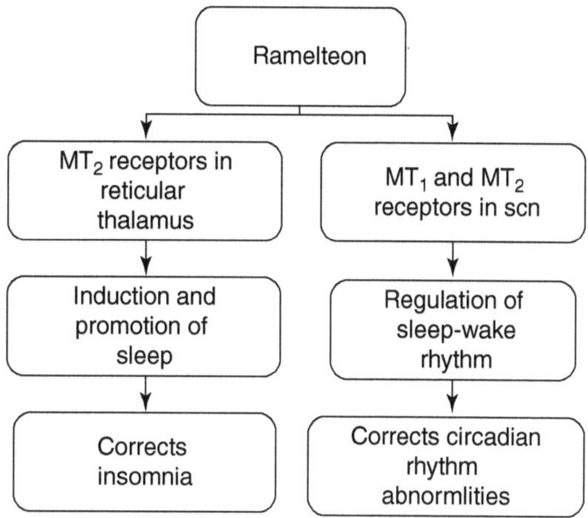

Fig. 24.1 Ramelteon acts specificity on MT_1 and MT_2 melatonin receptors indicates that its sleep-related site of action is probably in the SCN

Mechanism of Ramelteon Sedative-Hypnotic Action

Although MT_1 and MT_2 receptors are widely distributed in the brain outside of the SCN, the high density of melatonin receptors in the SCN and their relationship to the circadian pacemaker function and especially to the sleep-wake cycle are highly suggestive of the SCN melatonin receptor role in sleep regulation [42, 43]. Ramelteon's specificity for MT_1 and MT_2 melatonin receptors indicates that its sleep-related site of action is probably in the SCN (Fig. 24.1) [22].

A "sleep-switch" model to describe the regulation of sleep-wakefulness was originally proposed by Saper and his colleagues [3]. It consists of "flip-flop" reciprocal inhibitions among sleep-associated activities in the ventrolateral preoptic nucleus and wakefulness-associated activities in the locus coeruleus, dorsal raphe, and tuberomammillary nuclei. The SCN has an active role both in promoting wakefulness and in promoting sleep, and this depends upon a complex neuronal network and also involves a number of neurotransmitters [and neuropeptides] like GABA, glutamate, arginine vasopressin, and somatostatin [44, 45].

Ramelteon may accelerate sleep onset by influencing the hypothalamic sleep-switch downstream from the SCN in the same way as melatonin [46, 47]. Ramelteon promotes sleep onset through inhibition of SCN electrical activity and the consequent inhibition of the circadian wake signal, thereby activating the specific sleep-circuit pathway [46].

Clinical Studies on Ramelteon in Insomnia

The first study of the effects of ramelteon on sleep was conducted by Roth and his colleagues in 2005 [48]. In this study involving 117 patients (aged 16–64 years) drawn from 13 centers in Europe, the efficacy, safety, and dose response of ramelteon were examined. Each patient was randomized to a dosing sequence of 4, 8, 16, or 32 mg of ramelteon. All doses of ramelteon produced a statistically significant reduction in latency to persistent sleep (LPS) and increased TST as shown by polysomnography (PSG) [48].

In a follow-up study, the same group of investigators administered ramelteon for a period of 5 weeks to 829 patients (>65 years). In this double-blind study, ramelteon at doses of either 4 or 8 mg/day brought about a significant reduction in SOL (16–35 %). TST was increased by both doses of ramelteon [49]. In another randomized, multicenter double-blind, placebo-controlled crossover study including 107 patients, ramelteon was administered in doses of 4–32 mg/day. The treatment decreased LPS and increased TST significantly as measured objectively with PSG [50].

A short-term evaluation of the efficacy of ramelteon was performed in 100 elderly patients by administering 4 and 8 mg doses in a 2-night/3-day period crossover design. LPS decreased, and TST and SE improved as compared to placebo [51]. Likewise, the efficacy of ramelteon in reducing SOL and in increasing TST and SE was evaluated in 371 patients administered with 8 or 16 mg of ramelteon for 5 weeks in a double-blind placebo-controlled study. The results were consistent in confirming the efficacy of ramelteon to reduce SOL and to increase SE and TST [52].

A long-term evaluation of the efficacy of ramelteon was conducted in 1,213 adult and elderly patients with chronic insomnia [53]. The adult patients aged 18–64 years were given ramelteon 16 mg, and the elderly patients aged 65 and older were given 8 mg. Five hundred ninety-seven patients remained in the study at 6 months, and 473 patients completed the full 12 months [54]. Both elderly and adult patients experienced improvement at month 1 (34.0 and 35.1 %, respectively), month 6 (44.7 and 49.1 %), and month 12 (50.3 and 52.1 %) [53]. TST estimates also showed steady improvement for elderly and adult patients at month 1 (15.2 and 16.9 %), month 6 (21.6 and 22.7 %), and month 12 (25.5 and 23.9 %).

In a post hoc analysis of a previously published 5-week, randomized, double-blind, placebo-controlled study involving 405 patients with chronic insomnia aged 18–64 years, rapid onset of action of 8 mg of ramelteon caused significant reductions in SOL within a week (63 % for ramelteon vs. 39.7 % for placebo, $p<0.001$). This reduction in LPS was sustained throughout the 5 weeks of study (63 and 65.9 % ramelteon vs. 41.2 and 48.9 % placebo at the end of the third and fifth week, respectively) [55]. Reduction in LPS after ramelteon was also noted in healthy human subjects in a 6-week-long study using an 8 mg dose; in this study of healthy human subjects, ramelteon also increased TST [56]. In another 6-month study performed in 451 adults suffering from chronic insomnia drawn from different centers across the globe (mainly the USA, Europe, Russia, and Australia), ramelteon consistently reduced LPS when compared to placebo [57]. The baseline LPS decreased from 70.7 to 32.0 min at week 1 (with ramelteon), and this reduction in LPS was maintained at months 1, 3, 5, and 6. No adverse effects like next-morning residual effects, rebound insomnia, or withdrawal effects were noted [57].

In a double-blind placebo-controlled study involving a large number of Japanese patients with chronic insomnia ($n=1,130$), the efficacy and safety of 4 and 8 mg ramelteon doses were evaluated. At a 4 mg dose of ramelteon, no statistically significant differences were found in subjective SOL when compared with the placebo group, while with 8 mg of ramelteon, a significant increase in TST and a decrease in SOL were observed [58].

The same investigators evaluated the efficacy and safety of ramelteon in 190 Japanese adults with chronic insomnia treated for a period of 24 weeks. TST significantly increased with ramelteon 8 mg/day dose, and this was maintained for 20 weeks. In this study, ramelteon was well tolerated, and it did not cause residual effects, rebound insomnia, withdrawal symptoms, or dependence even after 24 weeks of continuous treatment [59]. In all clinical studies undertaken so far to evaluate the efficacy and safety of ramelteon in various doses ranging from 4 to 32 mg/day in patients with chronic insomnia, the drug reduced SOL and increased sleep duration (Table 24.1).

Besides acting as a sedative-hypnotic drug, ramelteon also exhibited chronobiotic properties. In a study conducted in 75 healthy human subjects, the administration of ramelteon at doses of 1, 2, 4, and 8 mg for 6 days caused significant advancement of dim-light melatonin offset [62]. As a melatonergic hypnotic and chronobiotic drug, ramelteon has a unique place in the development of novel drugs for the treatment of insomnia [63].

Interestingly, a recent randomized, placebo-controlled study suggested that ramelteon can be also beneficial for the treatment of ambulatory

Table 24.1 Clinical studies with ramelteon for chronic insomnia

Dosage (mg/day)	Duration of administration	Number of insomnia patients	Sleep onset latency	Sleep efficacy and quality	Total sleep time	Reference
4 and 8	5 weeks	829 (mean age: 72.4 years)	Reduced	Enhanced	Increased at the end of first week, third week, and fifth week	[49]
4, 8, 16, and 32	2 days	107 (mean age: 37.7 years)	Reduction in latency to persistent sleep	Increased	Increased	[50]
4	5 weeks	100 elderly patients	Reduced	Increased	Increased	[51]
8 and 16	5 weeks	371 patients with chronic insomnia	Reduced	Increased	Increased at all doses	[52]
8	5 weeks	270 patients with chronic insomnia	63 % reduction in week 1 and 3, 65.9 % reduction at week 5	–	–	[55]
8	6 weeks	20 healthy peri- and postmenopausal women	Reduced	Increased	Increased	[56]
8	6 months	451 adults with chronic insomnia	Reduced latency to persistent sleep consistently	–	–	[57]
8 and 16	5 weeks	289 patients with chronic insomnia (mean age: 65 years)	Reduced	Increased	Increased	[60]
4 and 8	2 weeks	1,130 adults	Reduced with 8 mg only	Increased in the first week	Increased	[58]
4, 8, and16	24 weeks	190 adults with chronic insomnia	Reduces sleep latency	Increased	Increased up to 20 weeks and maintained	[59]
8	2 nights	65 patients with insomnia	Reduced	Increased	Increased	[61]

bipolar I disorder patients suffering from manic symptoms and sleep disturbances. Twenty-one outpatients with bipolar I disorder with mild-to-moderate manic symptoms and sleep disturbances were randomized to receive either ramelteon ($N=10$) or placebo ($N=11$) in an 8-week, double-blind, fixed-dose (8 mg/day) study. Ramelteon and placebo had similar rates of reduction in ratings of symptoms of insomnia, mania, and global severity of illness. However, ramelteon was associated with improvement in a global rating of depressive symptoms. It was also well tolerated and associated with no serious adverse events [64].

Conclusion

Melatonin exhibits both hypnotic and chronobiotic properties and thus has been used for inducing sleep and for treating sleep disorders in children, adults, and elderly people. The results of endogenous melatonin's action in insomnia have not been consistent due to its short half-life and rapid metabolism.

Ramelteon (Rozerem®), a melatonergic drug with rapid onset and sustained duration of action, has been effective in treating sleep disorders and sleep disturbances associated with depressive disorders. The melatonergic agonist ramelteon has shown promising results in the treatment and management of insomnia as revealed in the numerous clinical trials that were undertaken in Europe, the USA, and Japan. This melatonergic drug, by acting through MT_1 and MT_2 melatonergic receptors in brain, particularly in the SCN, has demonstrated its superior efficacy in promoting sleep with its rapid onset of action. Moreover, it did not exhibit any adverse side effects that have been associated with the use of benzodiazepine and nonbenzodiazepine sedative drugs that are commonly used today.

Ramelteon exerts a promising effect on sleep by enhancing daytime alertness and sleep quality and by displaying an effective sleep-inducing effect. Because melatonin and ramelteon act in a natural way in promoting sleep, their long-term use is not associated with any side effects like dependency, next-day hangover, memory impairment, cognitive dysfunction, or psychomotor retardation. Agomelatine, the melatonergic antidepressant, is effective in treating patients with major depressive disorders and other mood disorders, partly attributable to its property of improving the sleep quality and efficiency. Melatonergic drugs have a place in the treatment of sleep disorders, and large clinical trials are needed to prove their efficacy and long-term safety.

References

1. Lerner AB, Case JD, Takahashi Y, Lee TH, Mori N. Isolation of melatonin a pineal factor that lightens melanocytes. J Am Chem Soc. 1958;80:2587.
2. Tricoire H, Moller H, Chemineau P, Malpaux B. Origin of cerebrospinal fluid melatonin and possible function in the integration of photoperiod. Reprod Suppl. 2003;61:311–21.
3. Saper CB, Scammell TE, Lu J. Hypothalamic regulation of sleep and circadian rhythms. Nature. 2005;437: 1257–63.
4. Borbely AA. A two process model of sleep regulation. Hum Neurobiol. 1982;1:195–204.
5. Dijk DJ, Cajochen C. Melatonin and the circadian regulation of sleep initiation, consolidation, structure and sleep EEG. J Biol Rhythms. 1997;12:627–35.
6. Cajochen C, Jewett ME, Dijk DJ. Human circadian melatonin rhythm phase delay during a fixed sleep-wake schedule interspersed with nights of sleep deprivation. J Pineal Res. 2003;35:149–57.
7. Lavie P. Melatonin: role in gating nocturnal rise in sleep propensity. J Biol Rhythms. 1997;12:657–65.
8. Zhdanova IV, Wurtman RJ, Regan MM, Taylor JA, Shi JP, Leclair OU. Melatonin treatment for age-related insomnia. J Clin Endocrinol Metab. 2001;86: 4727–30.
9. Wilson SJ, Nutt DJ, Alford C, Argyropoulos SV, Baldwin DS, Bateson AN, Britton TC, Crowe C, Dijk DJ, Espie CA, Gringras P, Hajak G, Idzikowski C, Krystal AD, Nash JR, Selsick H, Sharpley AL, Wade AG. British Association for Psychopharmacology consensus statement on evidence-based treatment of insomnia, parasomnias and circadian rhythm disorders. J Psychopharmacol. 2010;24:1577–601.
10. Arendt J, Skene DJ, Middleton B, Lockley SW, Deacon S. Efficacy of melatonin treatment in jet lag, shift work, and blindness. J Biol Rhythms. 1997;12: 604–17.
11. Srinivasan V, Singh J, Pandi-Perumal SR, Brown GM, Spence DW, Cardinali DP. Jet lag, circadian rhythm sleep disturbances, and depression: the role of melatonin and its analogs. Adv Ther. 2010;27:796–813.
12. Reppert SM, Weaver DR, Ebisawa T. Cloning and characterization of a mammalian melatonin receptor that mediates reproductive and circadian responses. Neuron. 1994;13:1177–85.
13. Dubocovich ML, Delagrange P, Krause DN, Sugden D, Cardinali DP, Olcese J. International Union of Basic and Clinical Pharmacology. LXXV. Nomenclature, classification, and pharmacology of G protein-coupled melatonin receptors. Pharmacol Rev. 2010;62:343–80.
14. Turek FW, Gillette MU. Melatonin, sleep, and circadian rhythms: rationale for development of specific melatonin agonists. Sleep Med. 2004;5:523–32.
15. Srinivasan V, Zakaria R, Othman Z, Brzezinski A, Prasad A, Brown GM. Melatonergic drugs for insomnia and sleep disturbances of mood disorders. CNS Neurol Disord Drug Targets. 2012;11:180–9.
16. Cricco M, Simonsick EM, Foley DJ. The impact of insomnia on cognitive functioning in older adults. J Am Geriatr Soc. 2001;49:1185–9.
17. Bastien CH. Insomnia: neurophysiological and neuropsychological approaches. Neuropsychol Rev. 2011;21:22–40.
18. Van Someren J. Circadian and sleep disturbances in the elderly. Exp Gerontol. 2000;35:1229–37.
19. Montgomery P, Dennis J. A systematic review of non-pharmacological therapies for sleep problems in later life. Sleep Med Rev. 2004;8:47–62.
20. Mendelson WB. Melatonin microinjection into the medial preoptic area increases sleep in the rat. Life Sci. 2002;71:2067–70.
21. Golombek DA, Pevet P, Cardinali DP. Melatonin effect on behavior: possible mediation by the central GABAergic system. Neurosci Biobehav Rev. 1996;20:403–12.
22. Liu C, Weaver DR, Jin X, Shearman LP, Pieschl RL, Gribkoff VK, Reppert SM. Molecular dissection of two distinct actions of melatonin on the suprachiasmatic circadian clock. Neuron. 1997;19:91–102.
23. Dollins AB, Zhdanova IV, Wurtman RJ, Lynch HJ, Deng MH. Effect of inducing nocturnal serum melatonin concentrations in daytime on sleep, mood, body temperature, and performance. Proc Natl Acad Sci U S A. 1994;91:1824–8.

24. Garfinkel D, Laudon M, Nof D, Zisapel N. Improvement of sleep quality in elderly people by controlled-release melatonin. Lancet. 1995;346:541–4.
25. Zhdanova IV, Wurtman RJ, Lynch HJ, Ives JR, Dollins AB, Morabito C, Matheson JK, Schomer DL. Sleep-inducing effects of low doses of melatonin ingested in the evening. Clin Pharmacol Ther. 1995;57:552–8.
26. Zhdanova IV, Wurtman RJ, Morabito C, Piotrovska VR, Lynch HJ. Effects of low oral doses of melatonin, given 2–4 hours before habitual bedtime, on sleep in normal young humans. Sleep. 1996;19:423–31.
27. Monti JM, Alvarino F, Cardinali D, Savio I, Pintos A. Polysomnographic study of the effect of melatonin on sleep in elderly patients with chronic primary insomnia. Arch Gerontol Geriatr. 1999;28:85–98.
28. Brzezinski A, Vangel MG, Wurtman RJ, Norrie G, Zhdanova I, Ben-Shushan A, Ford I. Effects of exogenous melatonin on sleep: a meta-analysis. Sleep Med Rev. 2005;9:41–50.
29. Buscemi N, Vandermeer B, Hooton N, Pandya R, Tjosvold L, Hartling L, Vohra S, Klassen TP, Baker G. Efficacy and safety of exogenous melatonin for secondary sleep disorders and sleep disorders accompanying sleep restriction: meta-analysis. BMJ. 2006;332:385–93.
30. Gorfine T, Assaf Y, Goshen-Gottstein Y, Yeshurun Y, Zisapel N. Sleep-anticipating effects of melatonin in the human brain. Neuroimage. 2006;31:410–8.
31. Mendelson WB. A critical evaluation of the hypnotic efficacy of melatonin. Sleep. 1997;20:916–9.
32. Dalton EJ, Rotondi D, Levitan RD, Kennedy SH, Brown GM. Use of slow-release melatonin in treatment-resistant depression. J Psychiatry Neurosci. 2000;25:48–52.
33. Lemoine P, Guilleminault C, Alvarez E. Improvement in subjective sleep in major depressive disorder with a novel antidepressant, agomelatine: randomized, double-blind comparison with venlafaxine. J Clin Psychiatry. 2007;68:1723–32.
34. Wade AG, Crawford G, Ford I, McConnachie A, Nir T, Laudon M, Zisapel N. Prolonged release melatonin in the treatment of primary insomnia: evaluation of the age cut-off for short- and long-term response. Curr Med Res Opin. 2011;27:87–98.
35. Gerdin MJ, Masana MI, Rivera-Bermudez MA, Hudson RL, Earnest DJ, Gillette MU, Dubocovich ML. Melatonin desensitizes endogenous MT_2 melatonin receptors in the rat suprachiasmatic nucleus: relevance for defining the periods of sensitivity of the mammalian circadian clock to melatonin. FASEB J. 2004;18:1646–56.
36. Ying SW, Rusak B, Mocaer B. Chronic exposure to melatonin receptor agonists does not alter their effects on suprachiasmatic nucleus neurons. Eur J Pharmacol. 1998;342:29–37.
37. Masana MI, Benloucif S, Dubocovich L. Circadian rhythm of MT1 melatonin receptor in the suprachiasmatic nucleus of the C3H/HeN mouse. J Pineal Res. 2000;28:185–92.
38. Kato K, Hirai K, Nishiyama K, Uchikawa O, Fukatsu K, Ohkawa S, Kawamata Y, Hinuma S, Miyamoto M. Neurochemical properties of ramelteon (TAK-375), a selective MT1/MT2 receptor agonist. Neuropharmacology. 2005;48:301–10.
39. Miyamoto M. Pharmacology of ramelteon, a selective MT1/MT2 receptor agonist: a novel therapeutic drug for sleep disorders. CNS Neurosci Ther. 2009;15:32–51.
40. Cajochen C. TAK-375 Takeda. Curr Opin Investig Drugs. 2005;6:114–21.
41. Greenblatt DJ, Harmatz JS, Karim A. Age and gender effects on the pharmacokinetics and pharmacodynamics of ramelteon, a hypnotic agent acting via melatonin receptors MT1 and MT2. J Clin Pharmacol. 2007;47:485–96.
42. Wu YH, Zhou JN, Balesar R, Unmehopa U, Bao A, Jockers R, Van Heerikhuize J, Swaab DF. Distribution of MT1 melatonin receptor immunoreactivity in the human hypothalamus and pituitary gland: colocalization of MT1 with vasopressin, oxytocin, and corticotropin-releasing hormone. J Comp Neurol. 2006;499:897–910.
43. Reppert SM, Weaver DR, Rivkees SA, Stopa EG. Putative melatonin receptors in a human biological clock. Science. 1988;242(4875):78–81.
44. Kalsbeek A, Perreau-Lenz S, Buijs RM. A network of (autonomic) clock outputs. Chronobiol Int. 2006;23:521–35.
45. Reghunandanan V, Reghunandanan R. Neurotransmitters of the suprachiasmatic nuclei. J Circadian Rhythms. 2006;4:2.
46. Saper CB, Lu J, Chou TC, Gooley J. The hypothalamic integrator for circadian rhythms. Trends Neurosci. 2005;28:152–7.
47. Fuller PM, Gooley JJ, Saper CB. Neurobiology of the sleep-wake cycle: sleep architecture, circadian regulation, and regulatory feedback. J Biol Rhythms. 2006;21:482–93.
48. Roth T, Stubbs C, Walsh JK. Ramelteon (TAK-375), a selective MT1/MT2-receptor agonist, reduces latency to persistent sleep in a model of transient insomnia related to a novel sleep environment. Sleep. 2005;28:303–7.
49. Roth T, Seiden D, Sainati S, Wang-Weigand S, Zhang J, Zee P. Effects of ramelteon on patient-reported sleep latency in older adults with chronic insomnia. Sleep Med. 2006;7:312–8.
50. Erman M, Seiden D, Zammit G, Sainati S, Zhang J. An efficacy, safety, and dose–response study of ramelteon in patients with chronic primary insomnia. Sleep Med. 2006;7:17–24.
51. Roth T, Seiden D, Wang-Weigand S, Zhang J. A 2-night, 3-period, crossover study of ramelteon's efficacy and safety in older adults with chronic insomnia. Curr Med Res Opin. 2007;23:1005–14.
52. Zammit G, Erman M, Wang-Weigand S, Sainati S, Zhang J, Roth T. Evaluation of the efficacy and safety of ramelteon in subjects with chronic insomnia. J Clin Sleep Med. 2007;3:495–504.

53. DeMicco M, Wang-Weigand S, Zhang J. Long-term therapeutic effects of ramelteon treatment in adults with chronic insomnia: a 1 year study. Sleep. 2006;29(Abstract Suppl):A234.
54. Richardson GS, Wang-Weigand S, Zhang J, DeMicco M. Long-term safety of ramelteon treatment in adults with chronic insomnia: a 1-year study. Sleep. 2006;29(Abstract Suppl):A233.
55. Mini L, Wang-Weigand S, Zhang J. Ramelteon 8 mg/d versus placebo in patients with chronic insomnia: post hoc analysis of a 5-week trial using 50% or greater reduction in latency to persistent sleep as a measure of treatment effect. Clin Ther. 2008;30:1316–23.
56. Dobkin RD, Menza M, Bienfait KL, Allen LA, Marin H, Gara MA. Ramelteon for the treatment of insomnia in menopausal women. Menopause Int. 2009;15:13–8.
57. Mayer G, Wang-Weigand S, Roth-Schechter B, Lehmann R, Staner C, Partinen M. Efficacy and safety of 6-month nightly ramelteon administration in adults with chronic primary insomnia. Sleep. 2009;32:351–60.
58. Uchimura N, Ogawa A, Hamamura M, Hashimoto T, Nagata H, Uchiyama M. Efficacy and safety of ramelteon in Japanese adults with chronic insomnia: a randomized, double-blind, placebo-controlled study. Expert Rev Neurother. 2011;11:215–24.
59. Uchiyama M, Hamamura M, Kuwano T, Nagata H, Hashimoto T, Ogawa A, Uchimura N. Long-term safety and efficacy of ramelteon in Japanese patients with chronic insomnia. Sleep Med. 2011;12:127–33.
60. Zammit G, Schwartz H, Roth T, Wang-Weigand S. The effects of ramelteon in a first-night model of transient insomnia. Sleep Med. 2009;10(1):55–9.
61. Kohsaka M, Kanemura T, Taniguchi M, Kuwahara H, Mikami A, Kamikawa K, Uno H, Ogawa A, Murasaki M, Sugita Y. Efficacy and tolerability of ramelteon in a double-blind, placebo-controlled, crossover study in Japanese patients with chronic primary insomnia. Expert Rev Neurother. 2011;11(10):1389–97.
62. Richardson GS, Zee PC, Wang-Weigand S, Rodriguez L, Peng X. Circadian phase-shifting effects of repeated ramelteon administration in healthy adults. J Clin Sleep Med. 2008;4:456–61.
63. Srinivasan V, Pandi-Perumal SR, Trahkt I, Spence DW, Poeggeler B, Hardeland R, Cardinali DP. Melatonin and melatonergic drugs on sleep: possible mechanisms of action. Int J Neurosci. 2009;119:821–46.
64. McElroy SL, Winstanley EL, Martens B, Patel NC, Mori N, Moeller D, McCoy J, Keck Jr PE. A randomized, placebo-controlled study of adjunctive ramelteon in ambulatory bipolar I disorder with manic symptoms and sleep disturbance. Int Clin Psychopharmacol. 2011;26(1):48–53.

Melatonin's Neuroprotective Actions on Hippocampal Neurons

25

Pooja Suhalka, Chhavi Sharma, Neha Jaiswal, Piyu Sukhwal, Reena Chittora, Ayushi Jain, and Maheep Bhatnagar

Abstract

Melatonin is the pineal hormone, is an indoleamine, and has a persuasive role in the biological regulation of circadian rhythm, sleep–mood disorders, immunoregulation, cancer, neurodegenerative disorders, and aging. It passively diffuses into the bloodstream, exerting maximum effectiveness and protective action. This protective action is due to direct free radical scavenging and indirect antioxidative effects, especially in cases of neurodegenerative disorders like Alzheimer's and Parkinson's disease whose pathogenesis is associated with the cytotoxic effects of free radicals. Melatonin also promotes neurogenesis in adults, thus affecting hippocampal functions and enhancing cognitive and behavioral activities. Therapeutic trials with melatonin have been effective also in slowing down the progression of some neurodegenerative disorders. Studies suggest that melatonin have clinical potential for the treatment of neurodegenerative diseases.

Keywords

Hippocampus • Melatonin • Neuroprotection • Oxygen free radicals • Neurodegenerative diseases • Adult neurogenesis

Abbreviations

4-HNE	4-Hydroxy-2-nonenal
Akt	Protein kinase B (PKB)
CA1	Cornu ammonis 1
Ca^{2+}	Calcium^{2+} ion
CA3	Cornu ammonis 3
CAT	Catalase
GABA	Gamma-aminobutyric acid
GPx	Glutathione peroxidase
GSH	Reduced glutathione

P. Suhalka, PhD • C. Sharma, MSc
N. Jaiswal, MSc • P. Sukhwal, PhD
R. Chittora, MSc • A. Jain, PhD
M. Bhatnagar, PhD (✉)
Department of Zoology,
University College of Science, MLSU,
Durga Nursery Road, Udaipur, Rajasthan 313001, India
e-mail: poojasuhalka@gmail.com;
csharma134@gmail.com; jaisneha411@gmail.com;
sukhwalpiyu@gmail.com; reenachittora89@gmail.com;
ayushibiotec@yahoo.com; mbhatnagar@yahoo.com

V. Srinivasan et al. (eds.), *Melatonin and Melatonergic Drugs in Clinical Practice*,
DOI 10.1007/978-81-322-0825-9_25, © Springer India 2014

KA	Kainic acid kainate
MDA	Malondialdehyde
MT1	Melatonin receptor 1
MT2	Melatonin receptor 2
NADPH-d	Nicotinamide adenine dinucleotide phosphate-diaphorase
NMDA	*N*-methyl-D-aspartate
nNOS	Neuronal nitric oxide synthase
NO	Nitric oxide
PI3K	Phosphatidylinositide 3-kinases
ROS	Reactive oxygen species
SOD	Superoxide dismutase

Introduction

Melatonin, a derivative of the essential amino acid tryptophan, was first identified in bovine pineal, and for that reason, it has been portrayed exclusively as a hormone. It is released during the night as part of our time-reliant biorhythms to help sleep and recuperation from fatigue. This hormone is assumed to intervene with photoperiodicity, is light sensitive, and is subject to oxidation. It is a powerful hormone produced in the pineal gland and secreted into cerebrospinal fluid. It is also found in many plants from bananas to morello cherries and in most of cereals. This neurologically and endocrinologically dynamic substance is able to retune the biological clock and improve symptoms of depressive mood, jet lag, panic disorders, common colds, and cancers and even portrayed as a pacemaker of aging in humans. Melatonin is a potent antioxidant as well. It reinforces the immune system and stabilizes the nervous system. Melatonin plays a significant role in the proliferation of neuronal cells. Recently it has been called a "wonder drug" helpful for treating all illnesses ranging from AIDS to Alzheimer's.

The pineal gland produces melatonin from serotonin, which is a neurotransmitter derived from the amino acid tryptophan. Inside the pineal gland, serotonin is acetylated and subsequently methylated to yield melatonin [1]. Melatonin is well known for its functional exchanges with the neuroendocrine axis and with circadian biorhythms [2]. Recently, it has been revealed that it has neuroprotective and neuroregenerative effects as observed in models of neuronal cell deaths in which excitotoxins are involved [3]. Melatonin plays a vital role in different physiological processes including regulation of sleep promotion, circadian rhythms [4], and reproduction [5]. It also has an anti-inflammatory action, reducing damage as a result of ischemia or reperfusion injury in stroke models [6]. Melatonin is also efficient in defending the nuclear DNA and its allied histone proteins [7].

Powerful Antioxidant Effects

It was "Lanas" who first recommended that melatonin may perhaps have a role in scavenging free radicals [8]. Melatonin has been shown to be highly effective in reducing oxidative damage in the central nervous system [9]. This efficiency is derived from its capability to directly scavenge numerous free radicals [2] and to act as an indirect antioxidant [10]. In particular, melatonin detoxifies free radicals via electron donation [11]. Its function as a free radical scavenger is likely facilitated by the ease with which it traverses the morphological barriers, such as blood–brain barriers to enter nerve cells and subcellular compartments [12]. It can scavenges hydroxyl, carbonate, and a variety of organic radicals, peroxynitrite, and additional reactive nitrogen species [13]. Melatonin also augments the antioxidant potential of cells by stimulating the synthesis of antioxidant enzymes, specifically superoxide dismutase, glutathione reductase, and glutathione peroxidase, and by augmenting glutathione levels [14]. Tan et al. in 1993 provided classic evidence that melatonin functions as a direct scavenger of the hydroxyl radical (OH^-) [15]. OH^- is widely accepted as the most destructive molecule endogenously formed in aerobic organisms. The OH^- radical mutilates any molecule in the vicinity of where it is produced [15]. Melatonin not only initiates the "antioxidant cascade" but also effectively scavenges the resultant metabolite. Melatonin as an antioxidant protects membrane lipids, cytosolic proteins, and nuclear DNA from oxidative damage, but also it is reported to modify the actions of enzymes that improve the total anti-oxidative protection capacity of an organism [16].

The Life Extender Role

Increased melatonin has significantly extended the life span of test animals. Systemic administration of melatonin improved neuronal survival rate, stimulated the neurogenesis, and facilitated behavioral revival after transient focal cerebral ischemia in mice [17]. It was also shown that melatonin enhanced cell proliferation in the dentate gyrus sub region of maternally separated rats [18]. Melatonin has antidepressant properties and thus can be recommended to improve the quality of life of cancer patients on chemotherapy [19]. It has been also proven that melatonin enhances the quality of sleep and is supportive in maintaining biorhythms [4].

How Melatonin Works

Melatonin possibly works via electron contribution to directly detoxify free radicals. In vitro and in vivo experiments have proven that melatonin protects cells, tissues, and organs against oxidative damage induced by a variety of free radical-generating processes and agents, including cyanide poisoning, ischemia–reperfusion, glutathione depletion, MPTP (1 methyl-4-phenyl 1,2,3,6-tetrahydropyridine), and kainic acid (KA)-induced excitotoxicity [20]. The discovery of diverse targets in cells proposes a variety of methods of action for this complex process which appears to fall into three categories:

1. Receptor mediated
2. Protein mediated
3. Nonprotein mediated

Neurodegenerative Diseases and Melatonin

Melatonin's adaptability and the complexity of its actions make it an extremely efficient pharmacological agent for neuroregeneration, neuroprotection, and the treatment and cure of neurodegenerative disorders, brain tumors, and cancers [21], because it is one of the safest products, with no pragmatic side effects or consequences. Recent research has shown that melatonin averted delayed death of hippocampal neurons stimulated by enhanced excitatory nitridergic and other neurotransmission pathways [22]. Researchers are studying mechanisms of plasticity of neurons and stressor toxicity through aging and the function of melatonin during these courses. Kilic et al. 2004 reported that pretreatment of melatonin exerts anti-inflammatory activity reducing ischemia/reperfusion injury in rat middle brain cerebral artery occlusion model.

Fluctuations in the concentration of melatonin are particularly prominent in brain ventricles [2], where levels of melatonin can be approximately 75-fold more than in peripheral plasma [23]. One of the brain structures that might be chiefly susceptible to melatonin's action is the hippocampus. Because of its proximity to ventricles, the hippocampus is bathed in variable levels of melatonin, which appear to manipulate the physiology of the hippocampus [24, 25]. The hippocampus has a role in cognitive and learning behavior, and damage to the hippocampus during the developmental phase of brain maturation results in neurodegenerative alterations in later life.

Melatonin has pleiotropic neurobiological procedures reconciled through cell membrane receptors [26, 27] and by means of intracellular signaling cascades [28–30]. Additionally, it is involved in the control of a variety of physiological functions like synchronization of other circadian rhythms, as well as that of the central pacemaker, the suprachiasmatic nucleus (SCN) [31–34], immune function [35, 36], sleep regulation [4, 37], blood pressure regulation [38, 39], growth inhibition of malignant cells [40], modulation of mood and behavior [41–43], and retinal functions [44–46].

Animal studies established effects of melatonin in the hippocampus, chiefly suggesting its participation in synaptic plasticity. Even though melatonin influences all parts of the brain, still the hippocampus is the most studied region.

The efficiency of melatonin's inhibition of oxidative stress was projected in various neurodegenerative disorders, the pathogenesis of which is linked with the cytotoxic action of free oxygen radicals, such as in Parkinson's or Alzheimer's disease [47]. Alzheimer's disease (AD), which is the most common reason of cognitive decline in the elderly population, is neuropathologically distinguished by progressive development of insoluble amyloid plaques, consisting of amyloid β-peptide (Aβ), and neurofibrillary tangles, predominantly in neurons of the hippocampus and cerebral cortex [48, 49]. Melatonin is a highly effective antioxidant which scavenges hydroxyl, and possibly peroxyl radicals [14, 50]. A related detoxifying consequence of melatonin is also identified for nitric oxide, hydrogen peroxide, and peroxynitrite [11, 51].

Additionally, melatonin enhances the actions of antioxidizing enzymes like glutathione peroxidase, superoxide dismutase, and glutathione reductase and defends against glutamate excitotoxicity. Cell culture experimentation have shown that melatonin prevents Aβ-induced neurotoxicity [52]. There is a large reduction in melatonin secretion occurring with age; in addition, the reduction in melatonin levels in AD patients may perhaps correlate with dementia severity [50, 53]. The experimental evidence related to the neuroprotective role of melatonin focused on research aimed at models of Alzheimer's disease, Huntington's disease [54], and parkinsonism [55]. The decline in the production of melatonin in aged persons has been recommended as one of the primary causative factors for the development of age-associated neurodegenerative diseases [56], such as Alzheimer's disease [57].

Melatonin conserves mitochondrial homeostasis, decreases free radical generation by enhancing mitochondrial glutathione levels, and safeguards proton potential [58] and ATP synthesis by stimulating complex I and IV activities [9]. Therapeutic trials using melatonin have been effective in slowing down the progression of Alzheimer's disease but not Parkinson's disease. Melatonin's effectiveness in fighting free radical damage in the brain recommends that it may be a valuable curative agent in treatment of cerebral edema following traumatic brain injury. Different levels of melatonin concentrations observed at various stages of neurodegenerative diseases though associated with secretion patterns and age are being studied for the commencement of neurodegenerative diseases [59–61]. Melatonin's pharmacological function as a mediator against neuronal loss in investigational models of Alzheimer's disease, Huntington's disease, and Parkinson's disease needs to be substantiated before the drug can establish its place in neurology clinics [62].

Melatonin's action as a free radical scavenger and antioxidant [63, 64] protects hippocampal neurons in vivo against KA-induced injury in mice [65–67]. As well, melatonin is also efficient in reducing the detrimental action of singlet oxygen-induced apoptosis [68] and brain ischemia-stimulated nitric oxide and cyclic-GMP production [69]. Pinealectomized rats deficient in melatonin were more vulnerable to excitotoxicity and focal ischemia [70]. Adverse results of pinealectomy were reversed by melatonin treatment [71]. Melatonin upregulated levels of glial cell line-derived neurotrophic factor (GDNF) [72]. Furthermore, melatonin caused activation of serine or threonine kinase and Akt (also known as protein kinase B (PKB), a serine/threonine-specific protein kinase) by acting on melatonin receptors [73]. Akt, which is a downstream effecter of PI3K, is a critical intermediary of neuronal endurance in pathological neuronal cell death, such as excitotoxic damage [74, 75]. Melatonin defends against cell death by varying activities of enzymes which recover the total antioxidative protection capability of the organism, such as glutathione peroxidase, superoxide dismutase, and glutathione reductase [76].

These characteristics possibly underline protection by melatonin of cultured neurons in the presence of KA [77] or oxidative stress [63, 68] and of neurons in vivo following ischemic injury [78] or systemic administration of KA [79]. Melatonin altered the behavioral reaction of rats against neurotoxicity of KA and also barred neuromorphological damages in rats [20, 65, 79]. Concurrent administration of melatonin possibly may effectively neutralize the lethal effects of cadmium by reducing hydroxyl radicals and avert loss of cholinergic neurons of the hippocampus [80]. Melatonin is also able to ameliorate other trace elements in the hippocampus region which serve as cofactors of antioxidant enzymes.

In additional to melatonin-induced inhibition of apoptosis and necrosis [66, 81–84], some studies have focused on the function of autophagy in neuroprotection induced by melatonin. Melatonin has been found to put forth its neuroprotection by enhancing autophagy in ischemia–reperfusion injury [85]. On the contrary, melatonin apparently attenuated methamphetamine-induced neurotoxicity by inhibition of autophagy [86].

Recent studies explored whether or not systemic administration of melatonin-induced endogenous neurogenesis improved neuronal survival and assisted behavioral recovery following focal cerebral ischemia in mice. Neurogenesis in the adult hippocampus contributes to functioning of the hippocampus by allowing lifetime adaptations of the mossy fiber system [87]. Numerous theories are now suggesting that linkage failure of hippocampal neurogenesis in adults contributes to neuropsychiatric disorders, particularly schizophrenia and depression, but also dementia [88, 89]. Circadian rhythm regulation of adult hippocampal neurogenesis is affected by manipulation of sleep cycles and is reduced in animal models of these disorders. The results of these studies link the disturbed regulation of circadian production of melatonin and neuropsychiatric disorders [90, 91]. These results establish that, in all the assessed regions of the brain, including the cortex, hippocampus, striatum, and subventricular zone, the number of proliferating cells of neural ancestry is considerably higher for animals treated with melatonin than for control groups. The number of neurons surviving was also appreciably higher in animals treated with melatonin [17]. Numerous studies are being carried out to investigate the role of melatonin in the early developmental proceedings of apoptosis, adult neurogenesis, and neurophilic movement in the adult hippocampus. Functions of the hippocampus in adults are positively influenced by adult hippocampal neurogenesis, and inherent regulators of neurogenesis play a fundamental role in it. Early postnatal study in rats revealed that melatonin altered proliferative activity in dentate gyrus subregion [18]. Melatonin promoted proliferation and differentiation of brain neural stem cells in rat embryos [92, 93].

So far, it has been established that melatonin can control synaptic plasticity measured in hippocampal neurons [94, 95], it is best recognized for its function in regulation of seasonal reproduction. Nevertheless, this hormone may well serve additional functions. Melatonin receptors were certainly found in the hippocampus of a variety of animals [96 101]. Two subtypes of mammalian melatonin receptors have been replicated and distinguished, the MT1 and MT2 receptor subtypes [102]. Among supplementary actions, these receptors are negatively coupled to the adenylyl cyclase (AC)–protein kinase A (PKA) cascade [102]. The transcripts for melatonin receptors are present in the hippocampus [100, 103, 104]. Since the hippocampus serves a major role in memory development [105, 106], the impact of melatonin on neurons in the hippocampus may have comprehensive consequences. These findings stimulate questions about the physiological function of melatonin in the hippocampus. The conditions in the hippocampus appear to be particularly complex because there is proof for melatonin exerting both inhibitory and excitatory actions. Zeise and Semm discovered that the application of melatonin lessened the excitability of granular neurons of CA3 and dentate gyrus [107]. A recent finding on CA1 neurons showed that the application of melatonin produced a sluggish increase in the firing rate during the night but not during the day [104]. This increase in firing rate could be due to regulation of CA1 neurons; the relevance of melatonin has been shown to reduce the amplitude of GABA currents in these neurons [100]. Some reports also stated that the administration of melatonin produced biphasic regulation of evoked potentials evident from the CA1 region of a mouse hippocampus [24, 25].

Mechanism of Neuroprotective Action of Melatonin

Free radicals are chemical species generated in normal cells. Each cell is well equipped with endogenous scavenging and antioxidant systems. However, large amounts of free radicals and ROS generated in neurotoxicity can overcome cellular defenses and induce tissue damage. The high reactivity of ROS can trigger disorders in biological systems. ROS can disrupt cellular functions by exerting multiple damaging reactions to proteins, lipids, carbohydrates, and nucleic acids. The augmented production of ROS is therefore a potential risk to cellular homeostasis and neuronal survival, if the balance of oxygen species is not maintained by endogenous antioxidant mechanisms [108]. Sustained neuronal excitation damages neurons progressively due to the disturbed antioxidant pool and increased vulnerability to ROS, Ca^{2+} overload, and nitric oxide. The measurement of free radical damage in neurodegeneration induced by KA is important to facilitate understanding of the cellular and molecular mechanisms that play critical roles in neuronal damage. Since neurons are susceptible to ROS damage due to their relatively low levels of antioxidant defense, melatonin has an important role in regulating neuronal loss.

Melatonin, at physiological concentrations, is effective in both lipid and aqueous phases as a potent free radical scavenger [12]. In a number of studies, it was shown that pretreatment with melatonin was found to be highly effective in protecting cells against the damage induced in various pathological conditions [54, 109]. In vivo studies in our laboratory [110] demonstrated the free radical scavenging efficacy of melatonin. These observations were further confirmed by an in vitro model for neurotoxicity. Our data [110] showed the neuroprotective effects of melatonin treatment on KA-induced neuronal injury through scavenging ROS, limiting effect on lipid peroxidation, restoring antioxidant enzymes activity, and preventing mitochondrial dysfunction. The antioxidant enzymes, such as CAT, SOD, GPx, and reduced glutathione (GSH), create a mutually supportive team for defense against reactive oxygen species (ROS). The overload of free radicals observed in KA-treated groups contributed to a significant decrease in GPx, CAT, and SOD activity. Decreased concentration of these enzymes signifies an index of cellular damage prior to neuronal loss. Consistent with our results, the reduction in GSH level under neurotoxicity reported earlier in mouse brain can be attributed to ROS-induced changes in protein structures and activity [110]. KA decreases the available reserve of GSH and significantly induces more free radical generation where melatonin plays role in upholding the GSH levels. We proved that excitotoxicity increases most of the oxidative stress markers studied and induced significant morphological brain damage [110]. We also showed that daily administration of melatonin (20 mg/kg BW i.p.) in vivo prevented the oxidative biomolecules damage in the rat brain and concurrently the upregulation of different antioxidant enzymes [110]. Vitamin C, a potent antioxidant, can become a toxic prooxidant when exposed to free ion, and most antioxidants become weak free radicals after neutralizing a free radical. But melatonin donates two electrons, instead of donating one electron, thereby ensuring that melatonin does not become a free radical [111]. Oxygen free radical starts the destruction of cellular membranes by disrupting phospholipids and generating reactive aldehydes like MDA and 4-HNE, due to which neurons becomes more vulnerable to excitotoxicity.

An important consequence of free radical damage to cells is carbonyl modifications of proteins which may affect a variety of cellular functions involving proteins, namely, receptors, signal transduction mechanisms, transport systems and enzymes, and peroxidation of polyunsaturated fatty acids (PUFA), which results in the formation of lipid peroxides and aldehydes [112]. In the model of KA-induced in vivo neuronal death, a pronounced increase in hippocampal neuronal degeneration marked by a sharp increase in lipid peroxidation and protein carbonyl after KA injection was observed. The death of hippocampal neurons occurring as a result of excitotoxicity suggests the role of increased free radical production. Progressive impairment of the antioxidant reserves of the brain is contributed by an increase in oxidative stress. GSH is an important antioxidant which acts both as a nucleophilic scavenger of toxic compounds and as a substrate in the GPx-mediated destruction of hydroperoxides [113] and limits oxidative damage caused by ROS, many of which are generated as a consequence of normal metabolic activity. The reduction of GSH would be expected to negotiate this pathway and may thereby allow H_2O_2 to accumulate to toxic levels. Since antioxidant enzymes are relatively deficient in the brain [114], brain tissues are mainly vulnerable to this effect. The brain has a relatively low H_2O_2-metabolizing enzyme catalase [115]. Increasing oxidative stress may slowly damage neurons over a period of years, eventually leading to decreased membrane rigidity and neuronal cell death [116]. Studies from our laboratory also have suggested that plant extracts which are high in total antioxidant activity prevented the onset of the deleterious effects of certain compounds in the hippocampus [117].

However, previous studies showed that melatonin can inhibit KA-induced neuronal depolarization and injury [65, 66], selectively decrease the response of NMDA receptors, and attenuate the spread of neuronal activation [118]. The attenuation of neuronal activation by melatonin-mediated regulation of Ca^{2+} ions can be suggested as a mechanism for its neuroprotective action because the spread of neuronal activation is known to play a crucial role in the induction of remote brain damage after focal intracerebral KA injections [119]. The in vivo and in vitro studies [110] mainly demonstrate the decrease of antioxidant enzymes activity in KA-induced oxidative stress model and the reversal of these changes following melatonin treatment. The in vivo results were supported by the same result of in vitro assays for enzymatic and nonenzymatic antioxidant, ROS generation, and lipid peroxidation, concerning them the markers of oxidative stress and toxicity.

Our finding [110] suggests that melatonin efficiently interacts with various organic radicals, reactive oxygen, and nitrogen species as well as maintains and regulates antioxidant enzymes (glutathione peroxidase, glutathione reductase, superoxide dismutase, and catalase).

Neuroprotective Effect of Melatonin on Cellular and Morphological Changes

Excitotoxicity in the brain is characterized by disruption of axons and cell bodies, followed by little or no axonal regeneration and virtually no recovery of function by the lesioned tissue. Results demonstrate structural damage that KA causes in the CA1 and CA3 regions of the hippocampus, the part of the brain responsible for memory processing and learning and memory [120]. From the histology studies, it seems that melatonin not only protects neurons from structural damage induced by KA, but cells treated with melatonin seem healthier than cells from controls. Since the mammalian hippocampus plays an essential role in a diverse set of cognitive functions, such as memory and novelty detection [121–123], the antioxidant properties of melatonin studied in this work may play an important role in improving cognitive function, memory, and learning against excitotoxicity.

Effects of Melatonin on Brain-Derived Neurotrophic Factor (BDNF) and Glial Fibrillary Acidic Protein (GFAP) in In Vivo Model System of Excitotoxicity

Neurotrophins have broader biological effects on neurons than just regulation of cell death. They also regulate subcellular processes underlying neuronal plasticity and maintenance of structural neuronal integrity. Since neurotoxicity is accompanied by extensive structural damage and reactive plasticity, neurotrophic therapy might be advantageous in this regard. Our immunohistochemical studies on the distribution of brain-derived neurotrophic factor (BDNF) and glial fibrillary acidic protein (GFAP) immunoreactivity in the brain of mice exposed with KA neurotoxin and melatonin provide strong verification that this bioactive molecule alters their expression [110]. Activated microglia as well as activated macrophages which permeate the CNS in the repercussion of excitotoxicity or lesions are known to generate enhanced production of ROS which could account for the neuronal damage. The effects of KA on the expression of neurotrophin like BDNF and glial protein like GFAP depend on the excitotoxicity paradigms created and the brain regions observed. Melatonin treatment increased BDNF expression in the hippocampus after KA administration. KA administration reduces BDNF immunoreactivity possibly due to persistent polarization and neuronal death. Modifications of neurotrophins were also established in a number of studies following various kinds of brain insults such as epilepsy, hypoglycemia, ischemia, and trauma [110]. Activation of non-NMDA and NMDA receptors plays an important role in upregulating the expression of BDNF and NGF in the hippocampus of adult rats and cultured neurons [124]. Thus, it was concluded that melatonin administration regulated BDNF and GFAP expression in the hippocampus after kainate treatment.

The Effect of Melatonin Treatment on Changes in the Distribution of Nitrergic Neurons and Free Cytosolic Calcium Level

In this investigation, we verified that treatment with KA acid increased the number of NADPH-d positive neurons, in all examined areas of the hippocampus [110]. It is evident that nNOS activity in kainate-treated group is not regionally homogenous, and hippocampal CA1 and CA3 regions show enhanced production of NO when compared to the control group. Our data were consistent with earlier reports showing that the CA1 and CA3 zones, which are most vulnerable to neuronal injury following KA treatment, never recovered protein synthesis, signifying that a prolonged deficit in protein synthesis correlates with selective vulnerability of different nuclei [125–127]. This also supports the view that KA causes a rise in the level of ROS, a rapid increase in Ca^{2+} overload, enhanced NO production, generalized depolarization, progressive proteolysis, and loss of membrane integrity, which ultimately results in neurodegeneration [128, 129]. While KA has been widely used as a model of temporal lobe epilepsy and selective hippocampal neurodegeneration, few attempts have been made to characterize the role of calcium imbalance and nNOS activity associated with this limbic seizure model. Although the mechanism of neurotoxic effects of NO in KA-induced injury is not clearly known, it is attributed to the oxidative effects and calcium imbalance. Our results show that melatonin co-treatment against KA toxicity, decreased the density of nitrergic elements in all the examined hippocampal subregions [110]. Melatonin administration decreased nNOS activity, calcium overload, and KA-induced neurodegeneration. The underlying mechanism of neuroprotection by melatonin is attributed to its potent free radical scavenging ability and maintenance of calcium homeostasis [130, 131]. Furthermore melatonin inhibits the production of NO and may contribute to its neuroprotective properties in various pathophysiological conditions [132]. Many studies have shown that nicotinamide adenine dinucleotide phosphate-diaphorase (NADPH-d) may correspond to the neuronal NOS, and it is therefore suggested that neurons containing NADPH-d are likely to be capable of producing NO [128]. The method used to demonstrate nitrergic elements in the brain is based on histochemical reaction for NADPH-d. The relatively simple NADPH-d histochemical technique was widely used to identify NO-producing elements in the brain of representatives of all vertebrate classes [126]. It has been repeatedly proven that NADPH-d activity and NOS immunoreactivity in the nervous system is widely co-localized in the same sets of neurons [133]. KA administration brought about enhanced release of NO in all examined regions of the hippocampus which was significantly observed in CA1 and CA3 areas of the hippocampus, causing maximum injury to the neurons. The principal cell type of CA1 and CA3 regions is the pyramidal cell

(Lorente de No- 1934). CA3 pyramidal neurons are among the most responsive neurons to KA in the brain [134]. It is well established that protracted seizure activity can lead to irreversible brain damage, by both necrotic and apoptotic types of cell death, which has been recently reported as a consequence of seizures [135]. Intraperitoneal administration of KA results in the death of neurons in the CA1 and CA3 areas due to excitotoxicity as evident from our results. The altered cellular processes caused by KA administration include the following: enhanced ROS production, excessive Ca^{2+} overload, NOS activation, neuronal cell loss, and glial reactivation [136]. The number of NADPH-d positive neurons in dorsal and ventral blades of the dentate gyrus increased after KA administration, but these changes were not as evident as in CA1 and CA3 regions of the hippocampus. Our results show a regulatory effect of melatonin on nNOS activity and intracellular Ca^{2+} that could be explained by melatonin's neuroprotective role [110]. It is a potent free radical scavenger, an antioxidant that protects cells against the damage induced in different pathological conditions [130]. NADPH-d positive neurons are probably interneurons. The reason for the alteration in the number of NADPH-d neurons can also be a result of changes in gene expression by melatonin [137]. Our findings also suggest that Ca^{2+} overload-induced higher expression of nNOS contributes to the sustained neuronal excitation and ultimately in enhanced activity of nNOS [110]. In fact, NOS gene expression activated by hypoxia in central and peripheral neurons has recently been observed [138]. In conclusion, melatonin possesses neuroprotective properties against KA-induced toxicity and indicates its efficiency to regulate Ca^{2+} and NO levels in different regions of the hippocampus. The changes in the density of nitrergic neurons in KA- and melatonin-exposed animals are region specific in rat brain. Based on our findings, it seems that melatonin has a noteworthy role to play and regulate neuronal loss in excitotoxicity.

Contemporary knowledge of the mechanism(s) by which melatonin influences physiology in the course of activation of definite membrane receptors is exhilarating but still in its infancy. Better understanding of these processes will aid discovery and development of melatonergic agents for treatment of circadian, sleep, and neurodegenerative disorders. Taking into consideration melatonin's high efficiency in reducing oxidative damage in animals and its noticeable prospective for improving human health, it should be solemnly considered for use in clinical trials and may be dosed as a single molecule or in combination with additional antioxidants [139].

Nonetheless, exact molecular and cellular mechanisms for protective properties of melatonin are not entirely understood. Cell protection machinery sustained by melatonin seems to comprise the main apparatus in self-defense machinery of the cell. Moreover, melatonin may also play an essential role in modulating neuronal excitability in the hippocampus. Robust verifications in literature support the role of melatonin as a protection factor in various types of cells and tissues examined under various experimental situations simulating physiological and stressful conditions. This may correspond to a key homeostatic role for this molecule that too suggests appealing therapeutic perspectives.

References

1. Claustrat B, Brun J, Chazot G. The basic physiology and pathophysiology of melatonin. Sleep Med Rev. 2005;9:11–24.
2. Reiter RJ, Tan DX. Role of CSF in the transport of melatonin. J Pineal Res. 2002;33:61.
3. Zizapel N. Melatonin-dopamine interactions: from basic neurochemistry to a clinical setting. Cell Mol Neurobiol. 2001;21:605–16.
4. Wurtman RJ, Zhdanova I. Improvement of sleep quality by melatonin. Lancet. 1995;346:1491.
5. Reiter RJ. The pineal and its hormone in the control of reproduction in mammals. Endocr Rev. 1980;1: 109–31.
6. Reiter RJ, Tan DX. Melatonin: a novel protective agent against oxidative injury of the ischemic/reperfused heart. Cardiovasc Res. 2003;58:10–9.
7. Anton Tay F, Dfaz JL, Fernandez-guardiola A. On the effect of melatonin upon human brain: it's possible therapeutic implications. Life Sci. 1971;10:841–50.
8. Lanas O, Olinescu R, Badescu I. Melatonin involvement in oxidation processes. Endocrinologie. 1991;29:147–53.

9. Reiter RJ. Cytoprotective properties of melatonin: presumed association with oxidative damage and aging. Nutrition. 1998;14:691–6.
10. Srinivasan V. Melatonin, oxidative stress and ageing. Curr Sci. 1999;76:46–54.
11. Tan DX, Manchester LC, Reiter RJ, et al. Significance of melatonin in antioxidative defense system: reactions and products. Biol Signals Recept. 2000;9:137–59.
12. Reiter RJ, Tan D-X, Leon J, Kilic U, Kilic E. When melatonin gets on your nerves: its beneficial actions in experimental models of stroke. Exp Biol Med (Maywood). 2005;230:104–17.
13. Tan DX, Reiter RJ, Manchester LC, et al. Chemical and physical properties and potential mechanisms: melatonin as a broad spectrum antioxidant and free radical scavenger. Curr Top Med Chem. 2002; 2:181–97.
14. Reiter RJ. Oxidative damage in the central nervous system: protection by melatonin. Prog Neurobiol. 1998;56:359–84.
15. Tan DX, Chen LD, Poeggeler B, et al. Melatonin: a potent endogenous hydroxyl radical scavenger. Endocr J. 1993;1:57–60.
16. Reiter RJ, Acuna-Castroviejo D, Tan DX, Burkhardt S. Free radical–mediated molecular damage. Mechanisms for the protective actions of melatonin in the central nervous system. Ann N Y Acad Sci. 2001;939:200–15.
17. Kilic E, Kilic V, Yulug B, et al. Melatonin reduces disseminates neuronal death after mild focal ischemia in mice via inhibition of caspase-3 and is suitable as an add-on treatment to tissue-plasminogen activator. J Pineal Res. 2004;36:171–6.
18. Kim M, Kim HK, Kim BS, Yim S. Melatonin increases cell proliferation in the dentate gyrus of maternally separated rats. J Pineal Res. 2004;37:193–7.
19. Lissoni P, Barni S, Meregalli S, et al. Modulation of cancer endocrine therapy by melatonin: a phase II study of tamoxifen plus melatonin in metastatic breast cancer patient progressing under tamoxifen alone. Br J Cancer. 1995;71:854–6.
20. Floreani M, Skaper SD, Facci L, Lipartiti M, Giusti P. Melatonin maintains glutathione homeostasis in kainic acid-exposed rat brain tissues. FASEB J. 1997;11:1309–15.
21. Sainz RM, Mayo JC, Rodriguez C, et al. Melatonin and cell death: differential actions on apoptosis and cancer cells. Cell Mol Life Sci. 2003;60:1407–26.
22. Stephen DS, Biancamaria A, Laura F, Davide F, Pietro G. Melatonin prevents the delayed death of hippocampal neurons by enhanced excitatory neurotransmission and the nitridergic pathway. FASEB J. 1998;12:725–31.
23. Pang SF, Tsang CW, Hong GX, Yip PC, Tang PL, Brown GM. Fluctuation of blood melatonin concentrations with age: result of changes in pineal melatonin secretion, body growth, and aging. J Pineal Res. 1990;8:179–92.
24. Hogan MV, El-Sherif Y, Wieraszko A. The modulation of neuronal activity by melatonin: in vitro studies on mouse hippocampal slices. J Pineal Res. 2001;309:87–96.
25. El-Sherif Y, Hogan MV, Tesoriero J, Wieraszko A. Factors regulating the influence of melatonin on hippocampal evoked potentials: comparative studies on different strains of mice. Brain Res. 2002;945:191–201.
26. Dubocovich ML, Hudson RL, Sumaya IC, Masana MI, Manna E. Effect of MT1 melatonin receptor deletion on melatonin mediated phase shift of circadian rhythms in the C57BL/6 mouse. J Pineal Res. 2005;39:113–20.
27. Dubocovich ML. Melatonin receptors: role on sleep and circadian rhythm regulation. Sleep Med. 2007;8(3):34–42.
28. Benitez-King G, Huerto-Delgadillo L, Anton-Tay F. Binding of 3H-melatonin to calmodulin. Life Sci. 1993;53:201–7.
29. Benitez-King G, Hernandez ME, Tovar R, Ramirez G. Melatonin activates PKC-alpha but not PKC-epsilon in N1E-115 cells. Neurochem Int. 2001;39:95–102.
30. Soto-Vega E, Meza I, Ramirez-Rodriguez G, Benitez-King G. Melatonin stimulates calmodulin phosphorylation by protein kinase C. J Pineal Res. 2004;37:98–106.
31. Reiter RJ. The melatonin rhythm: both a clock and a calendar. Experientia. 1993;49:654–64.
32. Dawson D, Armstrong SM. Chronobiotics–drugs that shift rhythms. Pharmacol Ther. 1996;69:15–36.
33. Kunz D. Chronobiotic protocol and circadian sleep propensity index: new tools for clinical routine and research on melatonin sleep. Pharmacopsychiatry. 2004;37:139–46.
34. Hardeland R, Pandi-Perumal SR, Cardinali DP. Molecules in focus–melatonin. Int J Biochem Cell Biol. 2006;38:313–6.
35. Esquifino AI, Pandi-Perumal SR, Cardinali DP. Circadian organization of the immune response: a role for melatonin. Clin Appl Immunol Rev. 2004;4:423–33.
36. Guerrero JM, Reiter RJ. Melatonin-immune system relationships. Curr Top Med Chem. 2002;2:167–79.
37. Monti JM, Alvarino F, Cardinali DP, Savio I, Pintos A. Polysomnographic study of the effect of melatonin on sleep in elderly patients with chronic primary insomnia. Arch Gerontol Geriatr. 1999;28:85–98.
38. Doolen S, Krause DN, Dubocovich ML, Duckles SP. Melatonin mediates two distinct responses in vascular smooth muscle. Eur J Pharmacol. 1998;345:67–9.
39. Scheer FA, Van Montfrans GA, van Someren EJ, Mairuhu G, Buijs RM. Daily nighttime melatonin reduces blood pressure in male patients with essential hypertension. Hypertension. 2004;43:192–7.
40. Blask DE, Sauer LA, Dauchy C. Melatonin as a chronobiotic/anticancer agent: cellular, biochemical, and molecular mechanisms of action and their implications for circadian-based cancer therapy. Curr Top Med Chem. 2002;2:113–32.

41. Srinivasan V. Psychoactive drugs, pineal gland and affective disorders. Prog Neuropsycopharmacol Biol Psychiatry. 1989;13:653–64.
42. Srinivasan V. The pineal gland, its physiological and pharmacological role. Indian J Physiol Pharmacol. 1989;33:263–72.
43. Srinivasan V. Melatonin, biological rhythm disorders and phototherapy. Indian J Physiol Pharmacol. 1997;41:309–28.
44. Wiechmann AF. Melatonin parallels in pineal gland and retina. Exp Eye Res. 1986;42:507–27.
45. Marchiafava PL, Longoni B. Melatonin as an antioxidant in retinal photoreceptors. J Pineal Res. 1999;26:184–9.
46. Liang FQ, Green L, Wang C, Alssadi R, Godley BF. Melatonin protects human retinal pigment epithelial cells against oxidative stress. Exp Eye Res. 2004;78:1069–75.
47. Uchida K, Okamoto N, Ohara K, Morita Y. Daily rhythm of serum melatonin in patients with dementia of degenerative type. Brain Res. 1996;717: 154–9.
48. Mesulam MM. Neuroplasticity failure in Alzheimer's disease: bridging the gap between plaques and tangles. Neuron. 1999;24(3):521–9.
49. Vassar R, Bennett BD, Babu-Khan S, Kahn S, Mendiaz EA, Denis P. β-Secretase cleavage of Alzheimer's amyloid precursor protein by the transmembrane aspartic protease BACE. Science. 1999;286(5440):735–41.
50. Pappolla MA, Chyan YJ, Omar RA, Hsiao K, Perry G, Smith MA, Bozner P. Evidence of oxidative stress and in vivo neurotoxicity of beta-amyloid in a transgenic mouse model of Alzheimer's disease: a chronic oxidative paradigm for testing antioxidant therapies in vivo. Am J Pathol. 1998;152:871–7.
51. Blanchard B, Pompon D, Ducrocq C. Nitrosation of melatonin by nitric oxide and peroxynitrite. J Pineal Res. 2000;29:184–92.
52. Pappolla MA, Chyan Y-J, Poeggeler B, Frangione B, Wilson G, Ghiso J, Reiter RJ. An assessment of the antioxidant antiamyloidogenic properties of melatonin: implications for Alzheimer's disease. J Neural Transm. 2000;107:203–31.
53. Ferrari E, Arcaini A, Gornati R, Pelanconi L, Cravello L, Fioravanti M, Solerte SB, Magri F. Pineal and pituitary-adrenocortical function in physiological aging and in senile dementia. Exp Gerontol. 2000;35:1239–50.
54. Cardinali DP, Brusco LI, Liberczuk C, Furio AM. The use of melatonin in Alzheimer's disease. Neuro Endocrinol Lett. 2002;23:20–3.
55. Srinivasan V, Pandi-Perumal SR, Maestroni GJM, Esquifino AI, Hardeland R, Cardinali DP. Role of melatonin in neurodegenerative diseases. Neurotox Res. 2005;7:293–318.
56. Magri F, Locatelli M, Balza G, et al. Changes in endocrine circadian rhythms as marker of physiological and pathological brain aging. Chronobiol Int. 1997;14:385–96.
57. Skene DJ, Swaab DF. Melatonin rhythmicity: effects of age and Alzheimer's disease. Exp Gerontol. 2003;38:199–206.
58. Beal MF. Mitochondria, free radicals and neurodegeneration. Curr Opin Neurol. 1996;6:661–6.
59. Skene DJ, Viven-Roels B, Sparks Hunsaker JC, et al. Daily variation in the concentration of melatonin and 5-methoxytryptophol in the human pineal gland: effect of age and Alzheimer's disease. Brain Res. 1990;528:170–4.
60. Bordet R, Devos D, Brique S, et al. Study of circadian melatonin secretion pattern at different stages of Parkinson's disease. Clin Neuropharmacol. 2003;26:65–72.
61. Poeggeler B. Melatonin, ageing and age-related diseases: perspectives for prevention, intervention and therapy. Endocrine. 2005;27:201–12.
62. Gupta YK, Gupta M, Kohli K. Neuroprotective role of melatonin in oxidative stress vulnerable brain. Indian J Physiol Pharmacol. 2003;47:373–86.
63. Lezoualc'h F, Skutella T, Widmann M, et al. Melatonin prevents oxidative stress-induced cell death in hippocampal cells. Neuroreport. 1996;7:2071–7.
64. Skaper SD, Ancona B, Facci L, et al. Melatonin prevents the delayed death of hippocampal neurons induced by enhanced excitatory neurotransmission and the nitridergic pathway. FASEB J. 1998;12: 725–31.
65. Giusti P, Franceschini D, Petrone M, et al. In vitro and in vivo protection against kainate-induced excitotoxicity by melatonin. J Pineal Res. 1996;20: 226–31.
66. Tan DX, Manchester LC, Reiter RJ, et al. Melatonin protects hippocampal neurons in vivo against kainic acid-induced damage in mice. J Neurosci Res. 1998;54:382–9.
67. Franceschini D, Skaper SD, Floreani M, et al. Further evidences for neuroprotective effects of melatonin. Adv Exp Med Biol. 1999;467:207–15.
68. Cagnoli CM, Atabay C, Kharlamova E, et al. Melatonin protects neurons from singlet oxygen-induced apoptosis. J Pineal Res. 1995;18:222–6.
69. Guerrero JM, Reiter RJ, Ortiz GG, et al. Melatonin prevents increases in neural nitric oxide and cyclic GMP production after transient brain ischemia and reperfusion in the Mongolian gerbil (Meriones unguiculatus). J Pineal Res. 1997;23:24–31.
70. Manev H, Uz T, Kharlamov A, et al. Increased brain damage after stroke or excitotoxic seizures in melatonin-deficient rats. FASEB J. 1996;10: 1546–51.
71. Joo JY, Uz T, Manev H. Opposite effects of pinealectomy and melatonin administration on brain damage following cerebral focal ischemia in rat. Restor Neurol Neurosci. 1998;13:185–91.
72. Tang YP, Ma YL, Chao CC, et al. Enhanced glial cell line-derived neurotrophic factor mRNA expression upon (–)-deprenyl and melatonin treatments. J Neurosci Res. 1998;53:593–604.

73. Anhe GF, Caperuto LC, Pereira-Da-Silva M, et al. In vivo activation of insulin receptor tyrosine kinase by melatonin in the rat hypothalamus. J Neurochem. 2004;90:559–66.
74. Henshall DC, Araki T, Schindler CK, et al. Activation of Bcl-2-associated death protein and counter-response of Akt within cell populations during seizure-induced neuronal death. J Neurosci. 2002;22:8458–65.
75. Kim AH, Yano H, Cho H, et al. Akt1 regulates a JNK scaffold during excitotoxic apoptosis. Neuron. 2002;35:697–709.
76. Rodriguez C, Mayo JC, Sainz RM, et al. Regulation of antioxidant enzymes: a significant role for melatonin. J Pineal Res. 2004;36:1–9.
77. Giusti P, Gusella M, Lipartiti M, Milani D, Zhu W, Vicini S, Manev H. Melatonin protects primary cultures of cerebellar granule neurons from kainate but not from N-methyl-D aspartate excitotoxicity. Exp Neurol. 1995;133:39–46.
78. Cho S, Joh TH, Baik HH, Dibinis C, Volpe BT. Melatonin administration protects CA1 hippocampal neurons after transient forebrain ischemia in rats. Brain Res. 1997;755:335–8.
79. Uz T, Giusti P, Franceschini D, Kharlamov A, Manev H. Protective effect of melatonin against hippocampal DNA damage induced by intraperitoneal administration of kainate to rats. Neuroscience. 1996;73:631–6.
80. Mukherjee R, Desai F, Singh S, Gajaria T, Singh PK, Baxi DB, Sharma D, Bhatnagar M, Ramachandran AV. Melatonin protects against alterations in hippocampal cholinergic system, trace metals and oxidative stress induced by gestational and lactational exposure to cadmium. EXCLI J. 2010;9:119–32.
81. Lin AMY, Fang SF, Chao PL, et al. Melatonin attenuates arsenite-induced apoptosis in rat brain: involvement of mitochondrial and ER pathways and aggregation of a-synuclein. J Pineal Res. 2007;43:163–71.
82. Wang X. The antiapoptotic activity of melatonin in neurodegenerative diseases. CNS Neurosci Ther. 2009;15:345–57.
83. Harms C, Lautenschlager M, Bergk A, et al. Melatonin is protective in necrotic but not in caspase-dependent, free radical-independent apoptotic neuronal cell death in primary neuronal cultures. FASEB J. 2000;14:1814–24.
84. Camins A, Sureda FX, Junyent F, et al. An overview of investigational antiapoptotic drugs with potential application for the treatment of neurodegenerative disorders. Expert Opin Investig Drugs. 2010;19:587–604.
85. Guo Y, Wang J, Wang Z, et al. Melatonin protects N2 a against ischemia/reperfusion injury through autophagy enhancement. J Huazhong Univ Sci Technolog Med Sci. 2010;30:1–7.
86. Nopparat C, Porter J, Ebadi M, et al. The mechanism for the neuroprotective effect of melatonin against methamphetamine induced autophagy. J Pineal Res. 2010;49:382–9.
87. Kempermann G, Krebs J, Fabel K. The contribution of failing adult hippocampal neurogenesis to psychiatric disorders. Curr Opin Psychiatry. 2008;21:290–5.
88. Duman RS. Depression: a case of neuronal life and death? Biol Psychiatry. 2004;56:140–5.
89. Sahay A, Hen R. Adult hippocampal neurogenesis in depression. Nat Neurosci. 2007;10:1110–5.
90. Holmes A, Yang RJ, Murphy DL, Crawley JN. Evaluation of antidepressant-related behavioral responses in mice lacking the serotonin transporter. Neuropsychopharmacology. 2002;27:914–23.
91. Mueller AD, Pollock MS, Lieblich SE, Epp JR, Galea LA, Mistlberger RE. Sleep deprivation can inhibit adult hippocampal neurogenesis independent of adrenal stress hormones. Am J Physiol Regul Integr Comp Physiol. 2008;294:1693–703.
92. Moriya T, Horie N, Mitome M, Shinohara K. Melatonin influences the proliferative and differentiative activity of neural stem cells. J Pineal Res. 2007;42:411–8.
93. Kong X, Li X, Cai Z, Yang N, Liu Y, Shu J, et al. Melatonin regulates the viability and differentiation of rat midbrain neural stem cells. Cell Mol Neurobiol. 2008;28:569–79.
94. Collins DR, Davies SN. Melatonin blocks the induction of long term potentiation in an N-methyl-D-aspartate independent manner. Brain Res. 1997;767:162–5.
95. El-Sherif Y, Tesoriero J, Hogan MV, Wieraszko A. Melatonin regulates neuronal plasticity in the hippocampus. J Neurosci Res. 2003;72:454–60.
96. Nonno R, Lucini V, Stankov B, Fraschini F. 2-[125I] Iodomelatonin binding sites in the bovine hippocampus are not sensitive to guanine nucleotides. Neurosci Lett. 1995;194:113–6.
97. Reppert SM, Godson C, Mahle CD, et al. Molecular characterization of a second melatonin receptor expressed in human retina and brain: the mellb melatonin receptor. Proc Natl Acad Sci U S A. 1995;92:8734–8.
98. Mazzuchelli C, Pannacci M, Nonno R, Lucini V, Fraschini F, Stankov BM. The melatonin receptor in the human brain: cloning experiments and distribution studies. Mol Brain Res. 1996;39:117–26.
99. Reppert SM. Melatonin receptors: molecular biology of a new family of G protein-coupled receptors. J Biol Rhythms. 1997;12:528–31.
100. Wan Q, Man H-Y, Liu F, Braunton J, Niznik HB, Pang SF, Brown GM, Wang YT. Differential modulation of GABAA receptor function by Mel1a and Mel1b receptors. Nat Neurosci. 1999; 2:401–3.
101. Nosjean O, Nicolas JP, Klupsch F, Delagrange P, Canet E, Boutin JA. Comparative pharmacological studies of melatonin receptors: MT1, MT2 and MT3/QR2. Tissue distribution of MT3/QR2. Biochem Pharmacol. 2001;61:1369–79.
102. Von Gall C, Stehle JH, Weaver DR. Mammalian melatonin receptors: molecular biology and signal transduction. Cell Tissue Res. 2002;309:151–62.

103. Reppert SM, Weaver DR, Ebisawa T. Cloning and characterization of a mammalian melatonin receptor that mediates reproductive and circadian responses. Neuron. 1994;13:1177–85.
104. Musshoff U, Riewenherm D, Berger E, Fauteck J-D, Speckmann E-J. Melatonin receptors in rat hippocampus: molecular and functional investigations. Hippocampus. 2002;12:165–75.
105. Nadel L. The hippocampus and space revisited. Hippocampus. 1991;1:221–9.
106. Eichenbaum H. The hippocampal system and declarative memory in animals. J Cogn Neurosci. 1992;4:217–31.
107. Zeise ML, Semm P. Melatonin lowers excitability of guinea pig hippocampal neurons in vitro. J Comp Physiol A. 1985;157:23–9.
108. Halliwell B, Gutteridge JM. Free radicals in biology and medicine, vol. 3. Oxford: Oxford University Press; 1999. p. 1–543.
109. Pei Z, Pang SF, Cheung RT. Administration of melatonin after onset of ischemia reduces the volume of cerebral infarction in a rat middle cerebral artery occlusion stroke model. Stroke. 2003;34:770–5.
110. Jain A. In vitro and In vivo study of neuroprotective properties of melatonin. PhD thesis. Udaipur: Mohanlal Sukhadia University; 2009.
111. Reiter RJ, Manda K. Melatonin maintains adult hippocampal neurogenesis and cognitive functions after irradiation. Prog Neurobiol. 2010;90(1):60–8.
112. Cheeseman KH, Slater TF. An introduction to free radical biochemistry. Br Med Bull. 1993;49(3): 481–93.
113. Marklund SL, Westman NG, Lundgren E, Roos G. Copper-and zinc-containing superoxide dismutase, manganese-containing superoxide dismutase, catalase, and glutathione peroxidase in normal and neoplastic human cell lines and normal human tissues. Cancer Res. 1982;42(5):1955–61.
114. Martilla RJ, Roytta M, Lorentz H, Rinne UK. Oxygen toxicity protecting enzymes in human brain. J Neural Transm. 1988;74:87–90.
115. Benzi G, Moretti A. Are reactive oxygen species involved in Alzheimer's disease? Neurobiol Aging. 1995;16(4):661–74.
116. Joseph JA, Villalobos-Molina R, Yamagami K, Roth GS, Kelly J. Age-specific alterations in muscarinic stimulation of K(+)-evoked dopamine release from striatal slices by cholesterol and S-adenosyl-L-methionine. Brain Res. 1995;673(2): 185–93.
117. Bhatnagar M, Sharma D, Salvi M. Neuroprotective effects of Withania somnifera dunal. A possible mechanism. Neurochem Res. 2009;34(11): 1975–83.
118. Das A, McDowell M, Pava MJ, Smith JA, Reiter RJ, Woodward JJ, Varma AK, Ray SK, Banik NL. The inhibition of apoptosis by melatonin in VSC4.1 motoneurons exposed to oxidative stress, glutamate excitotoxicity, or TNF-α toxicity involves membrane melatonin receptors. J Pineal Res. 2010;48(2):157–69.
119. Kim JE, Choi HC, Song HK, Jo SM, Kim DS, Choi SY, Kang TC. Levetiracetam inhibits interleukin-1β inflammatory responses in the hippocampus and piriform cortex of epileptic rats. Neurosci Lett. 2010;471(2):94–9.
120. Chen JC, Ng CJ, Chiu TF, et al. Altered neutrophil apoptosis activity is reversed by melatonin in liver ischemia–reperfusion. J Pineal Res. 2003;34: 260–4.
121. Bardgett ME, Henry JD. Locomotor activity and accumbens Fos expression driven by ventral hippocampal stimulation require D1 and D2 receptors. Neuroscience. 1999;94(1):59.
122. Culmsee C, Bondada S, Mattson MP. Hippocampal neurons of mice deficient in DNA-dependent protein kinase exhibit increased vulnerability to DNA damage, oxidative stress and excitotoxicity. Mol Brain Res. 2001;87(2):257–62.
123. Suzuki WA, Clayton NS. The hippocampus and memory: a comparative and ethological perspective. Curr Opin Neurobiol. 2000;10(6):768–73.
124. Zafra F, Castrén E, Thoenen H, Lindholm D. Interplay between glutamate and γ-aminobutyric acid transmitter systems in the regulation of brain-derived neurotrophic factor and nerve growth factor synthesis in hippocampal neurons. Proc Natl Acad Sci U S A. 1991;88:10037–41.
125. Akhlaq AF, Wei Y, Xin-Rong L, Barry H, Llyod AH. Neurochemical consequences of kainate-induced toxicity in brain: involvement of arachidonic acid release and prevention of toxicity by phospholipase A2 inhibitors. Brain Res. 2001; 38:61–78.
126. Benesova P, Langmeier M, Betka J, Trojan S. Long-lasting changes in the density of nitrergic neurons following kainic acid administration and chronic hypoxia. Physiol Res. 2005;54:565–71.
127. White BC, Sullivan JM, Degracia DJ, Oneil BJ, Neumar RW, Grossman LI, Rafols JA, Krause GS. Brain ischemia and reperfusion: molecular mechanisms of neuronal injury. J Neurol Sci. 2000; 179:1–33.
128. Montecot C, Borredon J, Seylaz J, Pinard E. Nitric oxide of neuronal origin is involved in cerebral blood flow increase during seizures induced by kainate. J Cereb Blood Flow Metab. 1997; 17:94–9.
129. Benesova P, Langmeier M, Betka J, Trojan S. Changes in the number of nitrergic neurons following kainic acid administration and repeated long-term hypoxia. Physiol Res. 2004;53:343–9.
130. Jain A, Bhatnagar M. Melatonin–a "magic biomolecule". Ann Neurosci. 2010;14(4):108–14.
131. Tapias V, Escames G, López LC, López A, Camacho E, Carrión MD, Entrena A, Gallo MA, Espinosa A, Acuna-Castroviejo D. Melatonin and its brain metabolite N(1)-acetyl-5-methoxykynuramine prevent mitochondrial nitric oxide synthase induction in parkinsonian mice. J Neurosci Res. 2009;13: 3002–10.

132. Chung SY, Han SH. Melatonin attenuates kainic acid-induced hippocampal neurodegeneration and oxidative stress through microglial inhibition. J Pineal Res. 2003;34:95–102.
133. Moreno N, López JM, Sánchez-Camacho C, González A. Development of NADPH-diaphorase/ nitric oxide synthase in the brain of the urodele amphibian Pleurodeles waltl. J Chem Neuroanat. 2002;23:105–21.
134. Ben-Ari Y, Cossart R. Kainate, a double agent that generates seizures: two decades of progress. Trends Neurosci. 2000;23:580–7.
135. Langmeier MJ, Folbergrova J, Haugvicova R, Riljak V. Neuronal cell death in hippocampus induced by homocysteic acid in immature rats. Epilepsia. 2003; 44:299–304.
136. Wojtal K, Gniatkowska-Nowakowska A, Czuczwar SJ. Is nitric oxide involved in the anticonvulsant action of antiepileptic drugs? Pol J Pharmacol. 2003;55:535–42.
137. Kotler M, Rodriguez C, Sainz RM, Antolin I, Menéndez-Peláez A. Melatonin increases gene expression for antioxidant enzymes in rat brain cortex. J Pineal Res. 1998;24:83–9.
138. Chang HM, Liao WC, Lue JH, Wen CY, Shieh JY. Upregulation of NMDA receptor and neuronal NADPH-d/NOS expression in the nodose ganglion of acute hypoxic rats. J Chem Neuroanat. 2003;25:137–47.
139. Tan DX, Manchester LC, Sainz RM, Mayo JC, Alvares FL, Reiter RJ. Antioxidant strategies in protection against neurodegenerative disorders. Curr Opin Ther Patents. 2003;13:1513–43.

26 Jet Lag: Use of Melatonin and Melatonergic Drugs

V. Srinivasan, Jarnail Singh, Amnon Brzezinski, Rahimah Zakaria, Samuel D. Shillcutt, and Gregory M. Brown

Abstract

Jet lag comprises a constellation of symptoms that occurs as a result of disruptions of entrainment associated with time zone transitions. The jet lag symptoms include daytime fatigue, impaired alertness, insomnia, loss of appetite, poor psychomotor coordination, reduced cognitive skills, and depressed mood. The severity of jet lag symptoms depends on the number of time zones crossed as well as the direction of travel. Eastbound travel tends to cause difficulties in falling asleep, whereas westbound travel interferes with sleep maintenance. Clinical studies also indicate that jet lag can exacerbate existing affective disorders. It has been suggested that dysregulation of melatonin secretion and occurrence of circadian rhythm disturbances may be the common links which underlie jet lag and affective disorders. Melatonin has proven to be highly effective for treating the range of symptoms that accompany transmeridian air travel largely because of its regulatory effects on the circadian system. The therapeutic

V. Srinivasan, MSc, PhD, MAMS (✉)
Sri Sathya Sai Medical Educational and Research Foundation, An International Medical Sciences Research Study Center, Prasanthi Nilayam, 40-Kovai Thirunagar Extn, Goldwins, Coimbatore, TN 641014, India

National Health Service, Department of Mental Health, Psychiatric Service of Diagnosis and Treatment, Hospital "G. Mazzini", ASL 4, Teramo, Italy

Department of Neuroscience and Imaging, University "G.D' Annunzio", Chieti, 66013, Italy
e-mail: sainivasan@yahoo.com, venkataramanujamsrinivasan6@gmail.com

J. Singh, MBBS, Dip Av Med, MSc(OM), FAMS
Department of Civil Aviation Medical Board, Civil Aviation Authority of Singapore, Singapore Changi Airport, 1, Singapore, Singapore 918141, Singapore
e-mail: jarnail_singh@caas.gov.sg

A. Brzezinski, MD
Department of Obstetrics and Gynecology, Hadassah Hebrew-University Medical Center, Ein-Kerem, Jerusalem 91120, Israel
e-mail: amnonbrz@gmail.com

R. Zakaria, MBBS, MSc, PhD (Physiology)
Department of Physiology, School of Medical Sciences, Universiti Sains Malaysia, Kubang Kerian, Kelantan 16150, Malaysia
e-mail: rahimah@kck.usm.my

S.D. Shillcutt, PharmD, PhD
Department of Psychiatry and Behavioral Science, Mercer University School of Medicine, 655 First Street, Macon, GA 31201, USA
e-mail: shillcutt_s@mercer.edu

G.M. Brown, BA, MD, PhD, FRCPC, FRSC
Department of Psychiatry, Faculty of Medicine, University of Toronto, Centre for Addiction and Mental Health, 250, College Street, Toronto, ON MST 1R8, Canada
e-mail: gregory.brown@camh.ca

V. Srinivasan et al. (eds.), *Melatonin and Melatonergic Drugs in Clinical Practice*,
DOI 10.1007/978-81-322-0825-9_26, © Springer India 2014

values of melatonin and its agonists such as ramelteon in reducing the jet lag symptoms and use of the melatonergic antidepressant, agomelatine, for jet lag-associated depressive disorders are discussed in this chapter.

Keywords
Melatonin • Ramelteon • Jet lag • Time zone transitions • Insomnia

Introduction

The cyclical nature of geophysical variations in the solar day as well as seasonal changes of the environmental day/night cycle is manifested in all living organisms. Adaptation to these changes has evolved to include regulation by both an endogenous mechanism known as the "biological clock" and an exogenous synchronizing component, the environmental *zeitgeber* [1]. The circadian periodicity, which is regulated by the suprachiasmatic nucleus (SCN) of the hypothalamus, the main "the biological clock," is approximately 24.2 h. This periodicity is synchronized to exactly 24.0 h by the external light/dark (LD) cycle acting through retinal-hypothalamic links [2, 3]. Desynchronization of these circadian rhythms occurs under various conditions of environmental insult giving rise to different kinds of circadian rhythm sleep disorders (CRSD) [4]. Major CRSD include delayed sleep-phase syndrome, advanced sleep-phase syndrome, non-24-h sleep-wake rhythm disorder, free-running sleep disorder, jet lag, and shift work [5]. These CRSD have a major impact on the health, social life, and work performance (often negative) of individuals [6, 7].

Jet lag comprises a constellation of symptoms that occurs as a result of disruptions of entrainment associated with time zone transitions [7, 8]. These symptoms consist of daytime fatigue, impaired alertness, insomnia, loss of appetite, poor psychomotor coordination, reduced cognitive skills, and depressed mood. The severity of jet lag symptoms depends on the number of time zones crossed as well as the direction of travel. Eastbound travel tends to cause difficulties in falling asleep, whereas westbound travel interferes with sleep maintenance [9].

The disruptive effects of jet lag have been documented at the molecular level of clock genes present in the SCN and peripheral tissues [1]. Eastbound travel causes phase advances in the body's circadian rhythms, while westbound flight induces phase delays in circadian rhythms. As a consequence jet travelers are forced to synchronize their bodily rhythms; synchronization occurs at a speed of approximately 1.5 h a day after westward flights and approximately 1 h a day after eastward flight irrespective of whether their travel occurs during daytime or night [7, 10, 11]. Regardless of the direction of air travel, there is also travel fatigue due to factors such as the cramped seats, altered feeding schedule, poor air quality, and inability to sleep [12, 13]. These factors aggravate the symptoms of jet lag.

Circadian Rhythm Disturbances in Jet Lag

Synchronization of circadian rhythms, particularly the sleep-wake rhythm, to environmental LD cycles is essential for maintaining man's normal physical and mental health [1]. After time zone transitions, bodily rhythms shift out of phase with local environmental light. The resulting internal desynchronization is largely responsible for the general malaise, sleep disturbances, loss of mental efficiency, irritability, anxiety, and fatigue that are encountered during the first week after transmeridian flight. In as much as the endogenous circadian system is slow to adapt to new time cues, a host of physiological and behavioral problems persist until the correct phase relationship is reestablished between bodily rhythms and external *zeitgebers* [10, 11]. A complicating factor is that each of the body's multiple functions have their own unique circadian rhythms. Furthermore, these functions have separate time requirements for normalizing their phase relationships, not only with other internal rhythms but also with the LD cycles of the environment. The complexity of this dynamic interaction means that the entire process can be impacted by even small physiological changes within the individual, and consequently there is a considerable variability in the time period that each jet traveler requires for full circadian adjustment to local conditions. Under normal conditions, the various circadian rhythms in the body are synchronized with each other and with external LD cycle [14]. When normal human beings are deprived of *zeitgeber* (time givers), some circadian rhythms, e.g., rest-activity cycle, lengthen to nearly 45 h, whereas the period of temperature cycles, REM sleep, and cortisol secretion remain 25 h. This results in "internal desynchronization." This internal desynchronization occurs in some persons travelling across time zones and also in shift workers [15]. Variability occurs in the time period that each jet traveler requires for full circadian adjustment of their circadian rhythms with each other as well as those with the external LD cycle of local conditions. Adaptation to time zone transitions is particularly difficult in the elderly. In the elderly, temporal organization of physiological processes is deficient, and consequently this age group is especially at risk for extended internal desynchronization [16].

Physiological and Behavioral Symptoms of Jet Lag

A comparison has been made of effects of jet lag on several physiological and psychological variables in a 2-year collaborative field study of Spanish pilots flying the routes from Madrid to Mexico City (−7 time zones) or from Madrid to Tokyo (+8 time zones) [17]. Pilots' activities, temperatures, and heart rates were recorded with telemetry, and subjective time estimates of short, intermediate, and long intervals were recorded along with other psychological variables such as anxiety, fatigue, and performance. Urinary 6-sulphatoxymelatonin and cortisol excretion were also measured [18]. Activity/rest and heart rate rhythms, which are hypothesized to be linked to weak or exogenous oscillators, became rapidly synchronized while temperature or 6-sulphatoxymelatonin excretion rhythms, which are regulated by the biological clock, showed more rigid responses after the phase shift [19]. In young (less than 50 years) and old pilots (more than 50 years), the activity/rest rhythm rapidly adjusted to the new time schedule, whereas the acrophase of the temperature rhythm tended to remain close to the initial schedule. This desynchronization was evident until the return flight (day 5) and persisted at least 1 day after arrival in Madrid. In the case of Madrid-Tokyo flights, there was an abrupt phase advance of the activity/rest rhythm coincident with the light/dark *zeitgeber* phase shift during the first day, whereas no apparent phase shift in the temperature rhythm was observed. On the second day in Tokyo, a phase advance in the temperature rhythm occurred. The return flight to Madrid induced rapid re-entrainment of both rhythms. Among the group of older pilots, however, the temperature rhythms showed no evidence of entrainment on reaching Tokyo or following the return flight to Madrid [17]. Changes in urinary 6-sulphatoxymelatonin and cortisol excretion were consistent with temperature regulation [18].

Sleep Disturbances in Jet Lag

Both subjective and objective sleep recording studies have shown that poor sleep is a characteristic feature of rapid time zone transitions. Sleep fragmentation, premature awakenings, difficulty in initiation of sleep, and decrements in performance are the commonest features of jet lag [6–8, 10, 11]. Effects of transmeridian travel on various sleep parameters such as total sleep time, sleep onset latency, and sleep offset were evaluated in a group of academicians who travelled from Japan to the USA and Canada and back [20]. A significant decrease in total sleep time was noted on the second post-travel day following eastward travel. After the decrease, however, the total sleep time increased and then decreased again before returning to pretravel baseline. No significant variation in total sleep time was noted among westward travelers. The findings are consistent with those of earlier reports showing that the times of sleep onset and offset at the point of destination were affected by direction of travel. Eastward flight produced earlier times of sleep onset (0.5 h) and sleep offset (1.5 h) after trips, and the effect lasted for 2 days. Conversely westward flights delayed the times of sleep onset and offset approximately by 1 h till the fifth post-travel day. No effect on the quality or the length of sleep was noted [13, 21, 22]. The reduction in daytime activity seen following international air travel is linked to a restriction of the length of nocturnal sleep prior to arrival at the new destination [23]. Several studies have reported on the effects of simulated and real jet lag on sleep-wake problems [24–27].

Jet Lag and Athletic Performance

It has been shown that elite athletes travelling to the west or east over six to eight time zones demonstrate reduced grip strength and poor performance in training sessions lasting up to several days after the flight [28]. Decreases in daily profiles of grip strength were also reported for a group of Olympic athletes and sedentary people who travelled eastward over ten time zones [29]. In addition to poor athletic performance, sleep loss and mood disturbances also have been reported following rapid travel over several time zones [28, 30].

Use of Melatonin and Its Analogs in Jet Lag

A number of pharmacological interventions have been tried to minimize the effects of jet lag. Drugs such as modafinil, dextroamphetamine sulfate, and caffeine have been tried as techniques for combating the fatigue and reduced alertness associated with jet lag. Of these both slow-release and fast-release caffeine have been found effective [26, 31, 32]. As noted below, several studies have also shown that exogenously administered melatonin is effective for alleviating jet lag symptoms both by causing sleep propensity and by regulating timing of the sleep-wake cycle.

Melatonin in Jet Lag

In the earlier discussion of jet lag symptoms, it was noted that transmeridian travel affects the sleep, circadian rhythms, and daytime activity of travelers, effects which often take several days to resynchronize to local environmental conditions. The time required for adaptation is generally determined by the size of the phase shift and *zeitgeber* strength. This approximates to an adaptive shift of 1–1.5 h per day, with eastbound flight causing a greater prolongation of symptoms when compared to westbound flights [33, 34].

Melatonin administration has been shown to shift circadian rhythms in humans [35–37]. This effect is a key factor in melatonin's actions in reducing jet lag symptoms, the therapeutic value of which has now been demonstrated in numerous studies [26, 38–45]. In the first placebo-controlled clinical trial, melatonin (5 mg dose) was administered in the early evening (18:00 h) 3 days prior to flight and for 4 days (postflight) at 23:00 h to passengers travelling east over 8 time zones [38]. Melatonin's superiority over the placebo substance was shown by both subjective measures of jet lag, self-recorded sleep parameters, mood ratings, as well as objective measures such as melatonin and cortisol rhythms, which adapted more rapidly in the melatonin-treated group than in the placebo-controlled group. The same investigators later carried out a similar larger sample study consisting of 52 passengers who flew eastbound across 8 time zones (from the UK to Australia). Melatonin in 5 mg doses was given 2 days prior to departure and for 4 days following their arrival at the destination point. Significant reductions in jet lag symptoms were reported following melatonin ingestion [46]. Melatonin administration was also found to be of benefit to aircrew members whose jet lag symptoms were significantly reduced following the therapeutic regimen [39]. A meta-analysis of ten studies using melatonin to alleviate jet lag symptoms found that melatonin taken at bedtime (22:00 h) at the destination of the flight effectively decreased the symptoms of jet lag [47]. The dose of melatonin varied from 0.5 to 5.0 mg/ day.

In a study of the effects of melatonin plus other interventions on jet lag, sedentary volunteers, 75 subjects on an eastbound flight from Sydney to Buenos Aires and 49 subjects on a westbound flight from Buenos Aires to Sydney both by a transpolar route, were selected for investigation [48]. Passengers on the eastbound flight received 3 mg of melatonin daily 30 min before their expected bedtime at Sydney, beginning on the day of the flight and continuing throughout the period of their trip. All subjects were advised to perform their normal routine and to walk outdoors for at least 30 min at two restricted times of the day. Passengers on the westbound flight took 3 mg melatonin on the day of their flight to Buenos Aires at the expected sleeping time at Buenos Aires and continued it for 8 days in Buenos Aires. On reaching Buenos Aires all volunteers were advised to perform their normal routines and to walk outdoors for at least 30 min at the same two restricted periods of the day as in Sydney. Subjects were also advised to maintain sleep diaries throughout the period of study. The sleep log diaries included the evaluation of sleep quality, morning freshness, and daily alertness on a visual analog scale [48]. The mean resynchronization rate was 2.27 ± 1.1 days during the eastbound flight and 2.54 ± 1.3 days for the westbound flight. These findings compared favorably to the expected minimal resynchronization rate after 13 h of flight without any treatment, which is 7 days, thus supporting the conclusion that jet lag symptoms can be significantly reduced by the carefully timed application of melatonin, light exposure, and physical activity.

In another study the combined use of slow release caffeine and melatonin improved several jet lag symptoms during an eastbound flight [26]. For travel of 11–13 h, whether eastbound or westbound, available data from limited field studies indicate that a combination of melatonin, exposure to outdoor light, and exercise has a potent ameliorative effect on jet lag symptoms [49]. Since there is very little information on the relative merits of different melatonin preparations for use on the alleviation of jetlag, a recent study undertaken by Prof. Paul's group who evaluated the efficacy of three melatonin preparations, 3 mg regular release (RR), 3 mg sustained release (SR), and 3 mg sugar-sustained release, was evaluated for circadian phase advance or circadian phase delay in two separate studies [36]. Thirteen normal healthy male subjects with age range from 26 to 53 years (37.3 ± 8.9 years) were chosen for experiment 1 (circadian phase advance group), and nine normal healthy male subjects with age range 26–54 years (40.7 ± 10.5 years) were include in experiment 2 (circadian phase delay group). In both studies melatonin administration induced significant phase changes. No difference in phase-shifting efficacy was observed between slow- and fast-release preparations. The mean phase shifts noted in experiment 1 were: 1.08 ± 0.16 h advance for RR formulation, a 1.01 ± 0.20 h advance for the SR formulation, and a 0.95 ± 0.20 h advance for the SSR formulation. The phase advances induced with RR ($P < 0.015$) and the SR ($P < 0.036$) formulations were significantly larger than for the placebo conditions. However, there were no significant differences among melatonin formulations. In experiment 2 conducted on nine subjects, it was noted that RR formulation induced phase delay of 0.75 ± 0.30 h relative to placebo ($P < 0.36$). Slow-release preparation was not recommended for inducing phase delay. Based on this study the authors concluded that melatonin is effective for reducing circadian misalignment for both eastward travel and westward travel [36].

Analysis of the evidence reviewed above indicates that oral administration of melatonin is the best pharmacological treatment currently available for reducing the symptoms of jet lag. Hence we conclude that strategically timed administration of melatonin is helpful for readjusting the body clock during rapid time zone transitions and could help millions of air travelers who suffer from jet lag symptoms.

Potential Use of Melatonin Agonists in Jet Lag

Ramelteon (Rozerem™), a MT_1/MT_2 melatonin receptor agonist, has been shown in randomized double-blind placebo-controlled trials to be effective for treating insomnia [50–52]. It also has been shown to accelerate re-entrainment of circadian rhythms after an 8-h phase advance of the LD cycle in rodents [53]. Compared to melatonin, ramelteon has an affinity for MT_1 and MT_2 melatonin receptors which is 3–16 times greater and additionally has a longer half-life [54]. In addition to efficacy for treating insomnia, its safety for treating chronic insomnia has been shown in various studies [55–58].

Ramelteon has been shown to be effective as a phase-shifting agent in humans. In the first study of its effectiveness for treating CRSD, ramelteon was administered at doses of 1, 2, 4, and 8 mg to 75 affected adult subjects (18–45 years) for 6 days [59]. Ramelteon's significant promotion of phase advance shifts in the target subjects demonstrated its efficacy for treating CRSD. A recent placebo-controlled study included 110 healthy adults with a history of jet lag sleep disturbances and flying eastward across five time zones from Hawaii to the east coast of the USA [60]. Ramelteon (1–8 mg) was administered 5 min before bedtime (local time) for four nights. Sleep parameters were measured using polysomnography on nights 2, 3, and 4 while next-day residual effects were assessed using psychomotor and memory function tests. Compared to placebo, there was a significant decrease in mean latency to persistent sleep on nights 2–4 with ramelteon 1 mg ($n=29$), $P=0.030$. There was a trend towards reduction in mean latency to persistent sleep (LPS) with 4 and 8 mg, but no significant differences were observed with ramelteon vs. placebo. But on individual nights, significant reductions in LPS were detected at night 4 for ramelteon 8 mg group ($P=0.025$) compared to placebo. In the subset participants kept in dim light, there was significant reduction in mean LPS for nights 2–4 in the ramelteon 1 mg group ($n=10$; $P=0.014$) and trend towards reduction in the ramelteon 4 and 8 mg group ($n=8$, $P=0.070$; $n=7$, $P=0.082$, respectively). On individual nights significant reductions in LPS were detected at night 2 and 3 for ramelteon 1 mg group ($P=0.040$ and $P=0.010$, respectively). For ramelteon 4 mg group, significant reduction in LPS at night 3 was noted as compared to placebo ($P=0.049$). A trend towards reduction in LPS at night 4 in the ramelteon 1 and 8 mg was noted compared to placebo ($P=0.062$ and $P=0.093$, respectively). For those participants kept in natural light, there were no significant reductions in mean LPS for any ramelteon group compared to placebo. Quality of sleep was significantly improved in the dim light setting on day 4 in the ramelteon 8 mg group ($P=0.037$). In ramelteon 4 mg group, trend towards improvement in quality of sleep was noted on day 4 ($P=0.090$) and day 5 ($P=0.078$). On measures of next-day alertness, participants of the subset group kept in dim light showed improvement in the ramelteon 4 mg group on day 4 ($P=0.080$). Ability to concentrate also showed a trend towards improvement in the ramelteon 4 mg group in the dim light setting on day 5 ($P=0.061$). Compared to placebo there were significant improvements in daytime ability with ramelteon 4 mg on day 4 ($P=0.022$) and day 5 ($P=0.040$). There were no significant differences between any of the ramelteon dose groups and placebo on the DSST or delayed memory recall test. On day 4, participants in the ramelteon 1, 4, and 8 mg groups performed significantly worse on the immediate memory recall test compared to placebo. From this study, the authors have concluded that with 1 mg dose of ramelteon taken before bedtime for four nights, there were significant reductions in mean LPS on night 2–4 relative to placebo in healthy adults [60]. Ramelteon 4 and 8 mg also reduced mean LPS but did not reach significance compared to placebo. This lack of significant reductions in higher doses might be due to smaller sample size used for study ($n=27$ for each ramelteon group) [60]. Ramelteon 4 mg reduced some of the daytime symptoms of jet lag after a 5-h eastward flight in healthy adults. There were no significant melatonin phase shifts in any of ramelteon groups studied. Future studies on large samples with more than 8-h phase shifts of jet travel will be able to prove the efficacy of ramelteon in different doses in improving sleep quality and daytime performance and alertness in healthy adults. However, this study certainly points out the beneficial effects of ramelteon in jet lag. In view of its circadian phase-shifting effects, ramelteon can be proposed as a potential therapy for inducing rapid resynchronization following time zone transition of jet travelers [60].

Vanda Pharmaceutical has completed phase 2 and 3 studies on the melatonin MT_1/MT_2 agonist tasimelteon, and a randomized controlled trial for transient insomnia after sleep-time shift was recently published [61]. Tasimelteon was effective in reducing sleep onset latency and in resetting the circadian melatonin rhythm, which indicated its potential suitability as treatment for jet lag, shift work, and other circadian rhythm sleep disorders [61]. The drug is well tolerated, does not induce impairment of next-day functioning or dependence, and seems to be safe in short-term treatment. Potential use of melatonin in jet lag is summarized in Table 26.1.

Jet Lag, Depression, and the Possible Role of Agomelatine

As noted above jet lag symptoms are not exclusively physical. Jet airline passengers who have travelled both eastward and westward also frequently report that they have experienced depressive symptoms [62–64]. Over a 6-year period, Katz and coworkers studied 152 long-distance travelers who had been hospitalized in the Kfar Shaul Mental Health Center in Jerusalem, for psychiatric complaints [64]. The patients were divided into groups based upon the number of time zones crossed. The direction of flight was mainly eastbound. Possible links between jet lag and major depressive disorder or psychotic disorder were evaluated based upon the following criteria: (a) absence of major mental problems before the flight or good remission of existing disorders 1 year or more before the commencement of flight and (b) the appearance of major affective syndromes or psychotic syndromes during first 7 days after landing. Although the number of first major affective episodes or psychotic syndromes associated with jet lag was found to be similar among groups, the number of relapses occurring conjointly with jet lag was found to be significantly higher in people crossing seven or more time zones [63]. In earlier studies depression was noted in passengers with westbound flights and mania with eastbound flights [62, 63]. It has been suggested that the transient desynchronization seen in jet travelers can trigger affective disorders [65].

The hypothesis that various subtypes of affective disorders might be the result of rhythm failures (i.e., that they were linked to "free-running rhythms") was first proposed by Halberg et al. [66]. A "free-running rhythm" refers to the genetically determined internal rhythm that a healthy individual displays when isolated from all external time cues. When dissociated from these external cues, the individually generated rhythm varies somewhat from the normal daily pattern (humans usually showing periods longer than 24 h). A rhythm is said to be "phase advanced" when its peak occurs earlier than its normal pattern and is said to be "phase delayed" when it occurs later.

It has been suggested that internal phase angle disturbances, desynchronizations among various endogenous rhythms, i.e., when these rhythms go in and out of phase with each other, may lie at the heart of depressive disorders [67, 68]. The correction of the phase angle disturbances between sleep-wake cycles and circadian rhythms could thus remove the symptoms of depressive illness triggered by any factor including time zone transitions.

In addition to the circadian rhythm disturbances, sleep disturbances also constitute the major feature encountered during rapid time zone transitions [20, 49]. Evidence from epidemiological and electroencephalographic studies additionally implicates sleep disturbances as key factors in the pathogenesis of depressive illness [69]. Other evidence consistent with the circadian disruption hypothesis of depression comes from the observation that more than 80 % of depressed patients have complaints of sleep disturbances

Table 26.1 Potential use of melatonin in jet lag

Time zones	Dose (mg)	Number of days preflight	Time preflight	Time on flight day	Time at destination	Number of days	Results (comments)	Reference
8	5	2	18:00 h	18:00 h	22:00–24:00 h	4	VAS jet lag improved	[15]
	8	None	None	17:00–18:00 h	22:00–23:00 h	3	VAS and sleepiness improved	[40]
12	5	None	07:00–08:00 h	05:00 h	22:00–24:00 h	5	Worse than placebo trend to improve (preflight rhythms disordered)	[39]
			None	05:00 h	22:00–24:00 h	5		
6	5 or 0.5	None	None	Bedtime shifting schedule	Prebed	4	No effect (shifted bedtime 1 h earlier daily, timing of melatonin poor)	[42]
10	5	None	None	09:00–10:00 h	22:00–23:00 h	4	No difference from placebo (irregular activity after arrival, inappropriate timing of melatonin)	[44]
12	3	None	None	11:00 h	23:00 h	6	Sleep and wakefulness resynchronized in 2.13 days (2–3 h daily blocks of exercise outdoors at destination. No placebo control)	[37]
7	5 SR caffeine 300	None	17:00 h	16:00 h	23:00 h 08:00 h	3 5	Improved recovery of sleep. Less daytime sleepiness (caffeine affected sleep quality)	[26]
13	3	None	None	10:00 h	Prebed	7	Sleep and wakefulness resynchronized in 2.27 days (20–30 min daily blocks of exercise outdoors at destination. No placebo control)	[48]
11	3	None	None	13:00 h	Prebed	8	Sleep and wakefulness resynchronized in 2.54 days (20–30 min daily blocks of exercise outdoors at destination. No placebo control)	[48]

and demonstrate a variety of polysomnographic abnormalities and further that antidepressant therapies that also improve sleep efficiency are especially effective in reducing depressive symptomatology [70–73]. Moreover, detailed analyses have shown that currently used antidepressants such as selective serotonin reuptake inhibitors exert adverse effects on sleep and that the antidepressant effect may be counteracted by their effects on sleep [74, 75]. Hence an ideal antidepressant should improve sleep efficiency and reduce depressive symptomatology.

Recently, the melatonergic antidepressant agomelatine has been introduced. Agomelatine is a novel antidepressant that acts simultaneously as an MT_1/MT_2 receptor agonist and as a $5HT_{2c}$ receptor antagonist [76, 77]. This dual mechanism of action is unique and is the basis for its antidepressant efficacy and for mitigating sleep-wakefulness rhythm disturbances. The effectiveness of agomelatine in improving sleep quality and reducing depressive symptoms has been demonstrated in number of clinical trials [78–81].

It has been proposed that the dysregulation of melatonin secretion underlies various circadian rhythm sleep disorders and depression [82]. A number of clinical studies have reported that melatonin secretion is disturbed in depressives [83–91]. These results would suggest that melatonin administration might be a useful strategy for mood disorders.

However treatment of depressive disorders with exogenous melatonin alone has not been successful. Nevertheless the introduction of the combined action antidepressant agomelatine, which, as noted above, affects both melatonergic and serotonergic receptors, provides a new possibility for the treatment of mood disorders. The chronobiotic action of agomelatine was clinically evaluated in a study conducted in healthy older men. Administration of agomelatine (50 mg) or placebo to eight healthy older adults for a period of 15 days revealed that agomelatine caused phase advance of an average of 2 h in the temperature profile as well as in the temporal organization of cortisol secretion [92]. These findings suggest that agomelatine is useful as a chronobiotic agent.

Further evidence for agomelatine's usefulness as a treatment for chronobiological disorders emerged from its application in the treatment of seasonal affective disorder (SAD). In chronobiological studies on human subjects, core body temperature and melatonin levels have been used as markers for assessing circadian phase position. Phase delay of the circadian pacemaker relative to the timing of the habitual sleep-wake cycle is considered as one of the major contributing factors in the pathophysiology of SAD [93]. Agomelatine (25 mg/day administered in the evening) was used to treat 37 acutely depressed SAD patients for a period of 14 weeks, with treatment outcome being assessed by the SIGH-SAD scale and *Circascreen*, a self-rating scale for the assessment of sleep and circadian rhythm disturbances [94]. Agomelatine treatment caused a significant decrease in SAD symptoms starting from 2 weeks onward.

Conclusion

Jet lag symptoms include daytime fatigue, circadian rhythm sleep disturbances, impaired alertness, and many other minor conditions such as gastrointestinal disturbances, hormonal imbalances, and menstrual irregularities. In addition to these well-documented effects of jet lag, intercontinental air travel also exacerbates preexisting affective disorders and can produce severe symptoms in at risk individuals, i.e., those with a history of major depressive disorders.

Although only a few studies have specifically explored the potential linkage between jet lag and major psychiatric disturbance, the frequency of its reported occurrence strongly suggests that this association merits further investigation. Accumulating evidence shows that jet lag can be managed by a combined treatment programs which include good sleep hygiene; adherence to work-rest schedules in accordance with circadian rhythm principles; the strategically timed use of the well-known chronobiotic, namely, melatonin; and limited and carefully timed exposure to environmental light. The melatonergic agonists ramelteon and tasimelteon, which have strong affinity for MT_1

and MT_2 melatonin receptors, and, compared to melatonin, have a longer duration of its action, can be more effective than melatonin alone in reducing the symptoms of jet lag.

Taken together, the research evidence showing the close linkage between jet lag and a number of symptoms such as disturbed sleep and transient disturbances to mood points out the importance of applying a program of combined therapies for treating the constellation of complaints which are often reported by jet travelers. In particular, when clinicians need to treat patients who have recently crossed a number of time zones and who additionally have symptoms of dysphoria or depression, an antidepressant having both chronobiotic and sleep-promoting properties appears justified as a first-line choice for therapy. In this regard, the newly introduced melatonergic antidepressant agomelatine may well be the best choice for jet lag-associated depressive disorders.

References

1. Kyriacou CP, Hastings MH. Circadian clocks: genes, sleep, and cognition. Trends Cogn Sci. 2010;16(6):259–67.
2. Moore RY, Speh JC, Leak RK. Suprachiasmatic nucleus organization. Cell Tissue Res. 2002;309:89–98.
3. Morin LP, Allen CN. The circadian visual system, 2005. Brain Res Brain Res Rev. 2006;51:1–60.
4. Pandi-Perumal SR, Trakht I, Spence DW, Srinivasan V, Dagan Y, Cardinali DP. The roles of melatonin and light in the pathophysiology and treatment of circadian rhythm sleep disorders. Nat Clin Pract Neurol. 2008;4(8):436–47.
5. Zee PC, Manthena P. The brain's master circadian clock: implications and opportunities for therapy of sleep disorders. Sleep Med Rev. 2007;11:59–70.
6. Samuels C. Sleep, recovery, and performance: the new frontier in high-performance athletics. Phys Med Rehabil Clin N Am. 2009;20:149–59.
7. Sack RL. Clinical practice. Jet lag. N Engl J Med. 2010;362:440–7.
8. Waterhouse J, Reilly T. Managing jet lag. Sleep Med Rev. 2009;13:247–8.
9. Fahey CD, Zee PC. Circadian rhythm sleep disorders and phototherapy. Psychiatr Clin North Am. 2006;29:989–1007.
10. Arendt J. Managing jet lag: some of the problems and possible new solutions. Sleep Med Rev. 2009;13:249–56.
11. Auger RR, Morgenthaler TI. Jet lag and other sleep disorders relevant to the traveler. Travel Med Infect Dis. 2009;7:60–8.
12. Reilly T, Atkinson G, Waterhouse J. Travel fatigue and jet-lag. J Sports Sci. 1997;15:365–9.
13. Nicholson AN. Intercontinental air travel: the cabin atmosphere and circadian realignment. Travel Med Infect Dis. 2009;7:57–9.
14. Aschoff J. Response curves in circadian periodicity. In: Aschoff J, editor. Circadian clocks. Amsterdam: North-Holland; 1965. p. 95–111.
15. Arendt J, Marks V. Physiological changes underlying jet lag. Br Med J (Clin Res Ed). 1982;284(6310):144–6.
16. Monk TH. Aging human circadian rhythms: conventional wisdom may not always be right. J Biol Rhythms. 2005;20:366–74.
17. Ariznavarreta C, Cardinali DP, Villanua M, Granados B, Martín M, Chiesa JJ, et al. Circadian rhythms in airline pilots submitted to long-haul transmeridian flights. Aviat Space Environ Med. 2002;73:445–55.
18. Tresguerres J, Ariznavarreta C, Granados B, Martín M, Villanúa MA, Golombek DA, et al. Circadian urinary 6-sulphatoxymelatonin, cortisol excretion and locomotor activity in airline pilots during transmeridian flights. J Pineal Res. 2001;31:16–22.
19. Shanahan TL, Czeisler CA. Physiological effects of light on the human circadian pacemaker. Semin Perinatol. 2000;24:299–320.
20. Takahashi T, Sasaki M, Itoh H, Yamadera W, Ozone M, Obuchi K, et al. Melatonin alleviates jet lag symptoms caused by an 11-hour eastward flight. Psychiatry Clin Neurosci. 2002;56:301–2.
21. Nicholson AN. Sleep and intercontinental flights. Travel Med Infect Dis. 2006;4:336–9.
22. Lowden A, Akerstedt T, Wibom R. Suppression of sleepiness and melatonin by bright light exposure during breaks in night work. J Sleep Res. 2004;13:37–43.
23. Roehrs T, Turner L, Roth T. Effects of sleep loss on waking actigraphy. Sleep. 2000;23:793–7.
24. Wegmann HM, Gundel A, Naumann M, Samel A, Schwartz E, Vejvoda M. Sleep, sleepiness, and circadian rhythmicity in aircrews operating on transatlantic routes. Aviat Space Environ Med. 1986;57:B53–64.
25. Samel A, Wegmann HM, Vejvoda M. Jet lag and sleepiness in aircrew. J Sleep Res. 1995;4:30–6.
26. Beaumont M, Batejat D, Pierard C, Van Beers P, Denis JB, Coste O, et al. Caffeine or melatonin effects on sleep and sleepiness after rapid eastward transmeridian travel. J Appl Physiol. 2004;96:50–8.
27. Sack RL. The pathophysiology of jet lag. Travel Med Infect Dis. 2009;7:102–10.
28. Lemmer B, Kern RI, Nold G, Lohrer H. Jet lag in athletes after eastward and westward time-zone transition. Chronobiol Int. 2002;19:743–64.
29. Steenland K, Deddens JA. Effect of travel and rest on performance of professional basketball players. Sleep. 1997;20:366–9.
30. Waterhouse J, Edwards B, Nevill A, Carvalho S, Atkinson G, Buckley P, et al. Identifying some determinants of "jet lag" and its symptoms: a study

of athletes and other travellers. Br J Sports Med. 2002;36:54–60.
31. Schwartz JR. Pharmacologic management of daytime sleepiness. J Clin Psychiatry. 2004;65 Suppl 16:46–9.
32. Caldwell JA. Fatigue in aviation. Travel Med Infect Dis. 2005;3:85–96.
33. Gherardin T. Jet lag. A problem for 'long haul' travellers. Aust Fam Physician. 1999;28:833.
34. Arendt J. Jet-lag. Lancet. 1998;351:293–4.
35. Kennaway DJ, Wright H. Melatonin and circadian rhythms. Curr Top Med Chem. 2002;2:199–209.
36. Paul MA, Miller JC, Gray GW, Love RJ, Lieberman HR, Arendt J. Melatonin treatment for eastward and westward travel preparation. Psychopharmacology (Berl). 2010;208:377–86.
37. Cardinali DP, Bortman GP, Liotta G, Pérez Lloret S, Albornoz LE, Cutrera RA, et al. A multifactorial approach employing melatonin to accelerate resynchronization of sleep-wake cycle after a 12 time-zone westerly transmeridian flight in elite soccer athletes. J Pineal Res. 2002;32:41–6.
38. Arendt J, Aldhous M, Marks V. Alleviation of jet lag by melatonin: preliminary results of controlled double blind trial. Br Med J (Clin Res Ed). 1986;292:1170.
39. Petrie K, Dawson AG, Thompson L, Brook R. A double-blind trial of melatonin as a treatment for jet lag in international cabin crew. Biol Psychiatry. 1993;33:526–30.
40. Claustrat B, Brun J, David M, Sassolas G, Chazot G. Melatonin and jet lag: confirmatory result using a simplified protocol. Biol Psychiatry. 1992;32:705–11.
41. Lino A, Silvy S, Condorelli L, Rusconi AC. Melatonin and jet lag: treatment schedule. Biol Psychiatry. 1993;34:587.
42. Spitzer RL, Terman M, Williams JB, Terman JS, Malt UF, Singer F, et al. Jet lag: clinical features, validation of a new syndrome-specific scale, and lack of response to melatonin in a randomized, double-blind trial. Am J Psychiatry. 1999;156:1392–6.
43. Samel A. Melatonin and jet-lag. Eur J Med Res. 1999;4:385–8.
44. Edwards BJ, Atkinson G, Waterhouse J, Reilly T, Godfrey R, Budgett R. Use of melatonin in recovery from jet-lag following an eastward flight across 10 time-zones. Ergonomics. 2000;43:1501–13.
45. Revell VL, Burgess HJ, Gazda CJ, Smith MR, Fogg LF, Eastman CI. Advancing human circadian rhythms with afternoon melatonin and morning intermittent bright light. J Clin Endocrinol Metab. 2006;91:54–9.
46. Arendt J, Skene DJ, Middleton B, Lockley SW, Deacon S. Efficacy of melatonin treatment in jet lag, shift work, and blindness. J Biol Rhythms. 1997;12:604–17.
47. Herxheimer A, Petrie KJ. Melatonin for the prevention and treatment of jet lag. Cochrane Database Syst Rev. 2002;(2):CD001520.
48. Cardinali DP, Furio AM, Reyes MP, Brusco LI. The use of chronobiotics in the resynchronization of the sleep/wake cycle. Cancer Causes Control. 2006;17(4):601–9.
49. Brown GM, Pandi-Perumal SR, Trakht I, Cardinali DP. Melatonin and its relevance to jet lag. Travel Med Infect Dis. 2009;7:69–81.
50. Bellon A. Searching for new options for treating insomnia: are melatonin and ramelteon beneficial? J Psychiatr Pract. 2006;12:229–43.
51. Dobkin RD, Menza M, Bienfait KL, Allen LA, Marin H, Gara MA. Ramelteon for the treatment of insomnia in menopausal women. Menopause Int. 2009;15:13–8.
52. Gross PK, Nourse R, Wasser TE. Ramelteon for insomnia symptoms in a community sample of adults with generalized anxiety disorder: an open label study. J Clin Sleep Med. 2009;5:28–33.
53. Hirai K, Kita M, Ohta H, Nishikawa H, Fujiwara Y, Ohkawa S, Miyamoto M. Ramelteon (TAK-375) accelerates reentrainment of circadian rhythm after a phase advance of the light–dark cycle in rats. J Biol Rhythms. 2005;20:27–37.
54. Kato K, Hirai K, Nishiyama K, Uchikawa O, Fukatsu K, Ohkawa S, et al. Neurochemical properties of ramelteon (TAK-375), a selective MT1/MT2 receptor agonist. Neuropharmacology. 2005;48:301–10.
55. Erman M, Seiden D, Zammit G, Sainati S, Zhang J. An efficacy, safety, and dose–response study of Ramelteon in patients with chronic primary insomnia. Sleep Med. 2006;7(1):17–24.
56. Roth T, Seiden D, Wang-Weigand S, Zhang J. A 2-night, 3-period, crossover study of ramelteon's efficacy and safety in older adults with chronic insomnia. Curr Med Res Opin. 2007;23:1005–14.
57. Zammit G, Erman M, Wang-Weigand S, Sainati S, Zhang J, Roth T. Evaluation of the efficacy and safety of ramelteon in subjects with chronic insomnia. J Clin Sleep Med. 2007;3:495–504.
58. Mini L, Wang-Weigand S, Zhang J. Ramelteon 8 mg/d versus placebo in patients with chronic insomnia: post hoc analysis of a 5-week trial using 50% or greater reduction in latency to persistent sleep as a measure of treatment effect. Clin Ther. 2008;30:1316–23.
59. Richardson GS, Zee PC, Wang-Weigand S, Rodriguez L, Peng X. Circadian phase-shifting effects of repeated ramelteon administration in healthy adults. J Clin Sleep Med. 2008;4:456–61.
60. Zee PC, Wang-Weigand S, Wright Jr KP, Peng X, Roth T. Effects of ramelteon on insomnia symptoms induced by rapid, eastward travel. Sleep Med. 2010;11:525–33.
61. Rajaratnam SM, Polymeropoulos MH, Fisher DM, Roth T, Scott C, Birznieks G, Klerman EB. Melatonin agonist tasimelteon (VEC-162) for transient insomnia after sleep-time shift: two randomised controlled multicentre trials. Lancet. 2009;373:482–91.
62. Jauhar P, Weller MP. Psychiatric morbidity and time zone changes: a study of patients from Heathrow airport. Br J Psychiatry. 1982;140:231–5.
63. Young DM. Psychiatric morbidity in travelers to Honolulu, Hawaii. Compr Psychiatry. 1995;36:224–8.
64. Katz G, Knobler HY, Laibel Z, Strauss Z, Durst R. Time zone change and major psychiatric morbidity: the results of a 6-year study in Jerusalem. Compr Psychiatry. 2002;43:37–40.

65. Srinivasan V, Spence DW, Pandi-Perumal SR, Trakht I, Cardinali DP. Jet lag: therapeutic use of melatonin and possible application of melatonin analogues. Travel Med Infect Dis. 2008;6(1):17–28.
66. Halberg F, Vestergaard P, Sakai M. Rhythmometry on urinary 17-ketosteroid excretion by healthy men and women and patients with chronic schizophrenia; possible chronopathology in depressive illness. Arch Anat Histol Embryol. 1968;51:299–311.
67. Wehr TA, Wirz-Justice A. Circadian rhythm mechanisms in affective illness and in antidepressant drug action. Pharmacopsychiatria. 1982;15:31–9.
68. Healy D, Waterhouse JM. The circadian system and the therapeutics of the affective disorders. Pharmacol Ther. 1995;65:241–63.
69. Lustberg L, Reynolds CF. Depression and insomnia: questions of cause and effect. Sleep Med Rev. 2000;4:253–62.
70. Reynolds 3rd CF, Monk TH, Hoch CC, Jennings JR, Buysse DJ, Houck PR, et al. Electroencephalographic sleep in the healthy "old old": a comparison with the "young old" in visually scored and automated measures. J Gerontol. 1991;46:M39–46.
71. Bunney JN, Potkin SG. Circadian abnormalities, molecular clock genes and chronobiological treatments in depression. Br Med Bull. 2008;86:23–32.
72. Quera-Salva MA, Lemoine P, Guilleminault C. Impact of the novel antidepressant agomelatine on disturbed sleep-wake cycles in depressed patients. Hum Psychopharmacol. 2010;25:222–9.
73. Riemann D, Berger M, Voderholzer U. Sleep and depression – results from psychobiological studies: an overview. Biol Psychol. 2001;57:67–103.
74. Lam RW. Sleep disturbances and depression: a challenge for antidepressants. Int Clin Psychopharmacol. 2006;21 Suppl 1:S25–9.
75. Moltzen EK, Bang-Andersen B. Serotonin reuptake inhibitors: the corner stone in treatment of depression for half a century – a medicinal chemistry survey. Curr Top Med Chem. 2006;6:1801–23.
76. Yous S, Andrieux J, Howell HE, Morgan PJ, Renard P, Pfeiffer B, et al. Novel naphthalenic ligands with high affinity for the melatonin receptor. J Med Chem. 1992;35:1484–6.
77. Millan MJ, Gobert A, Lejeune F, Dekeyne A, Newman-Tancredi A, Pasteau V, et al. The novel melatonin agonist agomelatine (S20098) is an antagonist at 5-hydroxytryptamine2C receptors, blockade of which enhances the activity of frontocortical dopaminergic and adrenergic pathways. J Pharmacol Exp Ther. 2003;306:954–64.
78. Loo H, Hale A, D'haenen H. Determination of the dose of agomelatine, a melatoninergic agonist and selective 5-HT(2C) antagonist, in the treatment of major depressive disorder: a placebo-controlled dose range study. Int Clin Psychopharmacol. 2002;17:239–47.
79. Kennedy SH, Emsley R. Placebo-controlled trial of agomelatine in the treatment of major depressive disorder. Eur Neuropsychopharmacol. 2006;16:93–100.
80. Montgomery SA. Major depressive disorders: clinical efficacy and tolerability of agomelatine, a new melatonergic agonist. Eur Neuropsychopharmacol. 2006;16 Suppl 5:S633–8.
81. Kupfer DJ. Depression and associated sleep disturbances: patient benefits with agomelatine. Eur Neuropsychopharmacol. 2006;16 Suppl 5:S639–43.
82. Srinivasan V, Smits M, Spence W, Lowe AD, Kayumov L, Pandi-Perumal SR, et al. Melatonin in mood disorders. World J Biol Psychiatry. 2006;7(3):138–51.
83. Branchey L, Weinberg U, Branchey M, Linkowski P, Mendlewicz J. Simultaneous study of 24-hour patterns of melatonin and cortisol secretion in depressed patients. Neuropsychobiology. 1982;8:225–32.
84. Claustrat B, Chazot G, Brun J, Jordan D, Sassolas G. A chronobiological study of melatonin and cortisol secretion in depressed subjects: plasma melatonin, a biochemical marker in major depression. Biol Psychiatry. 1984;19:1215–28.
85. Nair NP, Hariharasubramanian N, Pilapil C. Circadian rhythm of plasma melatonin in endogenous depression. Prog Neuropsychopharmacol Biol Psychiatry. 1984;8:715–8.
86. Beck-Friis J, Kjellman BF, Aperia B, Undén F, von Rosen D, Ljunggren JG, et al. Serum melatonin in relation to clinical variables in patients with major depressive disorder and a hypothesis of a low melatonin syndrome. Acta Psychiatr Scand. 1985;71:319–30.
87. Wehr TA, Sack DA, Rosenthal NE. Antidepressant effects of sleep deprivation and phototherapy. Acta Psychiatr Belg. 1985;85:593–602.
88. Rubin RT, Heist EK, McGeoy SS, Hanada K, Lesser IM. Neuroendocrine aspects of primary endogenous depression. XI. Serum melatonin measures in patients and matched control subjects. Arch Gen Psychiatry. 1992;49:558–67.
89. Sekula LK, Lucke JF, Heist EK, Czambel RK, Rubin RT. Neuroendocrine aspects of primary endogenous depression. XV: mathematical modeling of nocturnal melatonin secretion in major depressives and normal controls. Psychiatry Res. 1997;69:143–53.
90. Crasson M, Kjiri S, Colin A, Kjiri K, L'Hermite-Baleriaux M, Ansseau M, et al. Serum melatonin and urinary 6-sulfatoxymelatonin in major depression. Psychoneuroendocrinology. 2004;29:1–12.
91. Tuunainen A, Kripke DF, Elliott JA, Assmus JD, Rex KM, Klauber MR, et al. Depression and endogenous melatonin in postmenopausal women. J Affect Disord. 2002;69:149–58.
92. Leproult R, Van Onderbergen A, L'hermite-Baleriaux M, Van Cauter E, Copinschi G. Phase-shifts of 24-h rhythms of hormonal release and body temperature following early evening administration of the melatonin agonist agomelatine in healthy older men. Clin Endocrinol (Oxf). 2005;63:298–304.
93. Koorengevel KM, Beersma DG, den Boer JA, van den Hoofdakker RH. A forced desynchrony study of circadian pacemaker characteristics in seasonal affective disorder. J Biol Rhythms. 2002;17:463–75.
94. Pjrek E, Winkler D, Konstantinidis A, Willeit M, Praschak-Rieder N, Kasper S. Agomelatine in the treatment of seasonal affective disorder. Psychopharmacology (Berl). 2007;190:575–9.

Sleep, Melatonin, and Circadian Rhythmicity in Attention Deficit Hyperactivity Disorder

27

Mark A. Snitselaar and Marcel G. Smits

Abstract

Sleep problems are very common in children and adults with ADHD. Chronic sleep onset insomnia in ADHD had been described as a key characteristic of circadian rhythm problems. ADHD patients are more often and more extreme evening chronotypes and more often meet the criteria for delayed sleep-phase disorder (DSPD). DSPD is associated with delayed dim-light melatonin onset (DLMO). A delayed DLMO was found in both children and adult ADHD patients with sleep onset insomnia. Besides ADHD that influences the circadian rhythmicity, also medication used to treat ADHD seems to disturb the circadian rhythm.

Evening preference is associated with inattention and impulsivity-hyperactivity, while morningness is associated with better memory functioning. Vice versa, high scores in ADHD symptoms are associated with lower morningness and higher eveningness. This suggests that treatment with melatonin in the evening or light therapy in the morning, which results in greater morningness, could decrease ADHD symptoms.

Keywords

ADHD • Attention deficit hyperactivity disorder • Sleep • Melatonin • Circadian rhythmicity • Delayed sleep-phase disorder

Introduction

Chronic impaired sleep quality negatively influences daily functioning. This especially applies patients with attention deficit hyperactivity disorder (ADHD). It is long time presumed that the ADHD behavior during the day is the main cause of impaired sleep quality. One of the explanations was that the busy brain activity during the day prevented optimal sleep quality at night.

M.A. Snitselaar, MD, MSc (✉)
Department of Mental Health Care, Pro Persona, Willy Brandtlaan 20, Ede 6716 RR, The Netherlands
e-mail: m.snitselaar@propersona.nl

M.G. Smits, MD, PhD
Department of Neurology and Sleep-Wake Disorders, Gelderse Vallei Hospital Ede, Willy Brandtlaan 10, Ede 6716 RP, The Netherlands
e-mail: smitsm@zgv.nl

V. Srinivasan et al. (eds.), *Melatonin and Melatonergic Drugs in Clinical Practice*, DOI 10.1007/978-81-322-0825-9_27, © Springer India 2014

However, there is increasing evidence that the main cause of impaired sleep quality in ADHD patients is a delayed sleep-phase disorder (DSPD). Furthermore, several psychiatrists report that ADHD behavior can be treated much more successfully when the DSPD is treated.

This chapter summarizes the present knowledge.

Delayed Sleep-Phase Disorder

The DSPD was first described by Weizmann in 1981 [1]. The major symptoms are extreme difficulty to initiate sleep at a conventional hour of the night and great difficulty to wake up on time for school or work. This delayed sleep-wake rhythm offered to be associated with a delayed 24-h melatonin rhythm.

DSPD can be caused by extrinsic factors, i.e., disturbance of sleep-wake rhythm by trauma, shift work, and jetlag [2–4], or by intrinsic factors such as gene polymorphisms [5, 6].

Treatment of the DSPD is based on three pillars: (1) regular lifestyle with strengthening of time cues, such as strict bed-in and bed-out times, and strict eating times, and movement/sport; (2) bright light during the day; and (3) melatonin at the right time and in the right dose.

Treatment with Melatonin

Melatonin is a chronobiotic drug which makes it possible to shift sleep-wake rhythms in the desired direction when it is administered at the right time and in the right dose.

The time at which melatonin should be administered depends of the time the endogenous melatonin rhythm starts to rise in dim light, the so-called dim-light melatonin onset (DLMO). When melatonin is administered 5 h before DLMO, the endogenous melatonin rhythm and the sleep-wake rhythm which is associated with it advance most powerfully. When melatonin is administered 10 h after the DLMO, the sleep-wake rhythm delays most powerfully [7]. In patients with sleep disorders, it is not possible to predict the DLMO, e.g., by knowing sleep onset time. It has been shown that the DLMO does not correlate clinically reliably with sleep onset recorded in a diary measured using polysomnography [8]. It is not advisable to start treatment with melatonin before knowing DLMO, as several observations suggest that it may take 2–3 months after stopping melatonin treatment before the original melatonin rhythm is reached again and properly timed melatonin treatment can start [8, 9].

As to the optimal dose, it is important to be aware of the possibility of slow melatonin metabolization. When the dose of melatonin is too high, the exogenous melatonin taken the day before may still be present when the next dose is administered. Consequently melatonin heaps up, and circadian rhythmicity disappears. Melatonin treatment will then be not effective anymore.

Heaping up of melatonin may occur when the dose is too high. Recently it was suggested that heaping up also may occur when melatonin is metabolized very slowly, possibly due to a polymorphism of the CYP1A2 gene [10].

Melatonin and ADHD in Children

Sleep problems are very common in children, adolescents, and adults with ADHD; sleep problems are reported in 50 % of the children and 80 % of the adults with ADHD [11]. In children with ADHD, chronic sleep onset insomnia (SOI) has been described as a key characteristic of circadian rhythm problems [12]. This rhythm is believed to be closely associated with the sleep-wake cycle and the melatonin concentration in body fluids which is high at night and low during daytime [13]. DLMO is now acknowledged as the best marker for clinical phase position in humans [14].

In medication naïve children with ADHD and SOI, the DLMO was 45 min delayed compared to patients without SOI [15]. This was associated with difficulty falling asleep (increased sleep latency), later wake-up time, and a 17-min shorter total sleep time [15]. The shorter total sleep time despite the later waking-up time suggests a shorter melatonin signal. Because van der

Heijden et al. [15] only measured a partial melatonin curve (between 18:00 h and 23:00 h), no data were available about the length of the melatonin signal, and the shortened melatonin curve is hypothetical.

Novakova et al. [16] investigated salivary melatonin during 24 h in 34 children with ADHD between 6 and 12 years of age who were never treated pharmacologically for their ADHD. No differentiation between patients with and without SOI was made. They found changes in nighttime melatonin signal in children with ADHD. The melatonin profiles more frequently exhibit two nighttime peaks. Also a shortened nighttime melatonin signal was found compared to controls due to an earlier melatonin decline, namely, at 6:00 h. The mean of the maximum nighttime melatonin levels showed no significant difference in children with ADHD compared to healthy controls. Also the number of subjects exhibiting an elevated melatonin daytime level was almost the same in children with ADHD and healthy controls [16].

In conclusion, ADHD in children is associated with disturbed melatonin profiles like two nighttime peaks in patients without differentiating between SOI and non-SOI and delayed DLMO in children with ADHD and SOI. Although both studies [15, 16] found clues for a shortened nighttime melatonin signal, in the study of van der Heijden et al. [15], it was due to a later start of the melatonin signal (in patients with SOI), while in the study of Novakova et al. [16], it was due to an earlier melatonin decline. Possibly, the shortened melatonin signal is independent of sleep onset.

Besides ADHD that influences the circadian rhythmicity, also medication used to treat ADHD seems to disturb the circadian rhythm. Two studies report on the effect of medication on the circadian rhythm [17, 18]. Methylphenidate treatment caused a reduction in relative circadian amplitude and a phase delay in the timing of the daily rhythm in children with ADHD [17]. In this study actigraphic parameters were used to measure circadian rhythmicity, but the melatonin signal was not assessed. O'Keeffe et al. [18] reported that atomoxetine, a noradrenalin reuptake inhibitor, licensed for the treatment of ADHD, can alter circadian rhythmicity in mice. They suggest that part of the therapeutic profile of atomoxetine may be through circadian rhythm modulation.

Further studies into the effect of ADHD medication on the melatonin curve are needed to do final statements.

Circadian Rhythmicity, Melatonin, and ADHD in Adults

Various studies showed that ADHD-like symptoms in the adult general population are related to circadian preference and vice versa. Evening preference (eveningness) is associated with inattention and impulsivity-hyperactivity [19], while morningness is associated with better memory functioning, better social relationships, higher self-esteem, and more self-confidence [20]. Vice versa, high scores in ADHD symptoms are associated with lower morningness and higher eveningness [19, 21]. Adults diagnosed ADHD are more often evening chronotypes and more extreme evening chronotypes than healthy controls [22]; 40.7 % could be designated as evening type [22, 23]. They report later midsleep on free days corrected for sleep debt on workdays (MSFsc), a standardized measure for chronotype classification [24, 25]. Van Veen et al. [26] investigated the DLMO in adult ADHD and found an 83-min delayed DLMO in ADHD patients with SOI compared to healthy controls. ADHD patients with SOI showed a 75-min delayed DLMO in comparison to patients without SOI. Because increased sleep onset latency is common in ADHD, independently of subjective sleep onset insomnia and later DLMO, wake-up time seems to be a better discriminating parameter for DSPD than later sleep onset [27].

As in children, stimulant treatment of adult ADHD patients seems to result in a phase delay. The onset of the five least active hours, measured with actigraphy, was 18 min later in adult ADHD patients treated with stimulants compared to patients receiving placebo [28]. Treating ADHD patients with light therapy increased morningness, which was correlated with decrease of ADHD symptoms [29].

Besides stimulants, antidepressants (tricyclic antidepressants and bupropion) have been reported to have some benefits in adult ADHD [30]. Agomelatine has affinities to MT1 and MT2 which are responsible for the circadian rhythm. Agomelatine might improve ADHD symptoms by restoring the disturbed circadian rhythm, which is associated with ADHD symptoms as inattention and sleeping problems [19, 21]. Ten ADHD patients ranging in age from 17 to 19 years were included in an open trial [31]. Five received agomelatine 25 mg daily and five placebo. Patients receiving agomelatine reported a significant improvement in functioning and significantly fewer ADHD symptoms as restlessness, frustration, excessive energy, and inattention. Although further randomized controlled trials are needed to prove the benefits of agomelatine in ADHD patients, the effect on circadian rhythm of agomelatine might be the underlying mechanism.

Melatonin Treatment in ADHD and Insomnia

Treating sleep onset insomnia in children with ADHD by melatonin is effective on the short and long term. Four weeks' melatonin treatment in children with ADHD, not receiving stimulants, resulted in a 27-min earlier sleep onset and an increased total sleep time of almost 20 min compared to placebo. Furthermore, a decrease in sleep latency, increase in sleep efficiency, and decrease of nocturnal restlessness were shown. The decrease in sleep latency was found objectively, measured with actigraphy, and subjectively as difficulty falling asleep decreased in the children treated with melatonin. They showed a 45-min earlier DLMO. Greater disturbances of the DLMO pretreatment were related to improvements in sleep onset after melatonin treatment. There were no differences in side effects between melatonin and placebo [32]. In long-term treatment, melatonin remains an effective and safe therapy in children with ADHD and chronic sleep onset insomnia. In a follow-up study of 3.7 years, no serious adverse events were reported, and in 92 % of the children, discontinuation of melatonin resulted in a delay of sleep onset [9].

Also in children with ADHD and sleep onset insomnia treated with stimulants, melatonin treatment showed significant reduction in initial insomnia of 16 min relative to placebo [33]. In a double-blind, placebo-controlled crossover trial with ADHD patients who did not respond to sleep hygiene training, insomnia was significantly reduced compared to placebo treatment, measured with subjective sleep log and actigraphy.

Next to the positive effects of melatonin on sleep in children with ADHD and sleep onset insomnia, it is also effective in treating stimulant-induced sleep onset insomnia. In a small open-label study, 24 children with ADHD, treated with methylphenidate with resulting new-onset insomnia, were treated with 3 mg melatonin. Immediately after the start of melatonin treatment, the subjects fell significantly earlier asleep, varying between 15 and 240 min with a mean value of 135 min. The long-term effect after 3 months was comparable with the immediate effect after 1 week [34].

Conclusion

Both in children and adults, ADHD is associated with insomnia, often due to a delayed circadian rhythm and a later DLMO. Clinicians should be aware of DSPD in ADHD. Since eveningness is associated with ADHD-like symptoms, a comorbid DSPD in ADHD patients can increase symptoms of inattention and hyperactivity/impulsivity. Treating ADHD with stimulants can lead to further delay of the circadian rhythm, resulting in greater eveningness. Although eveningness is associated with more severe ADHD symptoms, it seems important, especially in patients who do not respond to stimulants, to look at the chronotype. Hypothetically, the shift to greater eveningness due to stimulants can nullify the positive effect of the medication on ADHD symptoms. Although the benefits of stimulants in ADHD are not due to positive effects on the circadian rhythm, other medication as atomoxetine and agomelatine may have positive effects on ADHD due to a shift to greater morningness.

Treating insomnia due to DSPD with melatonin is proven to be effective and safe in children with ADHD. In adults however no valid data are available. However, clinical experience with melatonin for adult ADHD patients, with insomnia and late DLMO, is positive.

In the outpatient clinic of the Centre for Sleep-Wake Disorders and Chronobiology of Hospital Gelderse Vallei in Ede (the Netherlands), many adult ADHD patients with a delayed sleep-phase disorder are treated with melatonin. Melatonin is administered 5 h before DLMO, but not earlier than 19:00 h. The daily dose is started with 1 mg; when within 2 weeks of effect is seen, the dose is increased every 2 weeks with 1 mg until the patient feels effect. Maximum dose is 5 mg.

The effect of melatonin treatment on ADHD symptoms, however, is not clear. Melatonin could have a positive effect on ADHD symptoms as melatonin can influence the circadian rhythm: evening preference can be shifted to morning preference, and shifting to greater morningness is associated with decrease of ADHD symptoms. Light therapy was investigated in adult ADHD in one study [29]. In this study light therapy resulted in greater morningness and decrease of ADHD symptoms.

Further research is needed to elucidate whether chronotherapy by means of melatonin treatment, light therapy, or agomelatine can be an alternative for stimulant treatment in ADHD patients.

References

1. Weitzman ED, Czeisler CA, Coleman RM, Spielman AJ, Zimmerman JC, Dement W, Richardson G, Pollak CP. Delayed sleep phase syndrome. A chronobiological disorder with sleep-onset insomnia. Arch Gen Psychiatry. 1981;38:737–46.
2. Smits MG. Whiplash injury may deregulate the biological clock. J Neurol Neurosurg Psychiatry. 2005;76:1044.
3. Arendt J, Skene DJ. Melatonin as a chronobiotic. Sleep Med Rev. 2005;9:25–39.
4. Srinivasan V, Spence DW, Pandi-Perumal SR, Trakht I, Cardinali DP. Jet lag: therapeutic use of melatonin and possible application of melatonin analogs. Travel Med Infect Dis. 2008;6:17–28.
5. Archer SN, Robilliard DL, Skene DJ, Smits M, Williams A, Arendt J, Von Schantz M. A length polymorphism in the circadian clock gene Per3 is linked to delayed sleep phase syndrome and extreme diurnal preference. Sleep. 2003;26:413–5.
6. Robilliard DL, Archer SN, Arendt J, Lockley SW, Hack LM, English J, Leger D, Smits MG, Williams A, Skene DJ, Von Schantz M. The 3111 clock gene polymorphism is not associated with sleep and circadian rhythmicity in phenotypically characterized human subjects. J Sleep Res. 2002;11:305–12.
7. Pandi-Perumal SR, Smits M, Spence W, Srinivasan V, Cardinali DP, Lowe AD, Kayumov L. Dim light melatonin onset (DLMO): a tool for the analysis of circadian phase in human sleep and chronobiological disorders. Prog Neuropsychopharmacol Biol Psychiatry. 2007;31:1–11.
8. Keijzer H, Smits MG, Peeters T, Looman CW, Endenburg SC, Gunnewiek JM. Evaluation of salivary melatonin measurements for Dim Light Melatonin Onset calculations in patients with possible sleep-wake rhythm disorders. Clin Chim Acta. 2011;412:1616–20.
9. Hoebert M, Van der Heijden KB, van Geijlswijk IM, Smits MG. Long-term follow-up of melatonin treatment in children with ADHD and chronic sleep onset insomnia. J Pineal Res. 2009;47:1–7.
10. Braam W, van Geijlswijk I, Keijzer H, Smits MG, Didden R, Curfs LM. Loss of response to melatonin treatment is associated with slow melatonin metabolism. J Intellect Disabil Res. 2010;54:547–55.
11. Konofal E, Lecendreux M, Cortese S. Sleep and ADHD. Sleep Med. 2010;11:652–8.
12. Walters AS, Silvestri R, Zucconi M, Chandrashekariah R, Konofal E. Review of the possible relationship and hypothetical links between attention deficit hyperactivity disorder (ADHD) and the simple sleep related movement disorders, parasomnias, hypersomnias, and circadian rhythm disorders. J Clin Sleep Med. 2008;4:591–600.
13. Arendt J. Melatonin, circadian rhythms, and sleep. N Engl J Med. 2000;343:1114–6.
14. Klerman EB, Gershengorn HB, Duffy JF, Kronauer RE. Comparisons of the variability of three markers of the human circadian pacemaker. J Biol Rhythms. 2002;17:181–93.
15. van der Heijden KB, Smits MG, van Someren EJ, Gunning WB. Idiopathic chronic sleep onset insomnia in attention-deficit/hyperactivity disorder: a circadian rhythm sleep disorder. Chronobiol Int. 2005;22:559–70.
16. Novakova M, Paclt I, Ptacek R, Kuzelova H, Hajek I, Sumova A. Salivary melatonin rhythm as a marker of the circadian system in healthy children and those with attention-deficit/hyperactivity disorder. Chronobiol Int. 2011;28:630–7.
17. Ironside S, Davidson F, Corkum P. Circadian motor activity affected by stimulant medication in children with attention-deficit/hyperactivity disorder. J Sleep Res. 2010;19:546–51.
18. O'Keeffe SM, Thome J, Coogan AN. The noradrenaline reuptake inhibitor atomoxetine phase-shifts

the circadian clock in mice. Neuroscience. 2012;201: 219–30.
19. Bae SM, Park JE, Lee YJ, Cho IH, Kim JH, Koh SH, Kim SJ, Cho SJ. Gender difference in the association between adult attention deficit hyperactivity disorder symptoms and morningness-eveningness. Psychiatry Clin Neurosci. 2010;64:649–51.
20. Gruber R, Oiveri T, Tong E. Chronotype preference in association with memory, self concept, and social functioning in healthy men. Sleep. 2009;32: A54–5.
21. Caci H, Robert P, Boyer P. Novelty seekers and impulsive subjects are low in morningness. Eur Psychiatry. 2004;19:79–84.
22. Baird AL, Coogan AN, Siddiqui A, Donev RM, Thome J. Adult attention-deficit hyperactivity disorder is associated with alterations in circadian rhythms at the behavioural, endocrine and molecular levels. Mol Psychiatry. 2012;17(10):988–95.
23. Rybak YE, McNeely HE, Mackenzie BE, Jain UR, Levitan RD. Seasonality and circadian preference in adult attention-deficit/hyperactivity disorder: clinical and neuropsychological correlates. Compr Psychiatry. 2007;48:562–71.
24. Bijlenga D, van der Heijden KB, Breuk M, van Someren EJ, Lie ME, Boonstra AM, Swaab HJ, Kooij JJ. Associations between sleep characteristics, seasonal depressive symptoms, lifestyle, and ADHD symptoms in adults. J Atten Disord. 2013;17(3):261–75.
25. Roenneberg T, Kuehnle T, Pramstaller PP, Ricken J, Havel M, Guth A, Merrow M. A marker for the end of adolescence. Curr Biol. 2004;14:R1038–9.
26. Van Veen MM, Kooij JJ, Boonstra AM, Gordijn MC, Van Someren EJ. Delayed circadian rhythm in adults with attention-deficit/hyperactivity disorder and chronic sleep-onset insomnia. Biol Psychiatry. 2010;67:1091–6.
27. Snitselaar MA, Smits MG, van der Heijden KB, Spijker J. Sleep and circadian rhythmicity in adult ADHD and the effect of stimulants: a review of the current literature. J Atten Disord. 2013.
28. Boonstra AM, Kooij JJ, Oosterlaan J, Sergeant JA, Buitelaar JK, van Someren EJ. Hyperactive night and day? Actigraphy studies in adult ADHD: a baseline comparison and the effect of methylphenidate. Sleep. 2007;30:433–42.
29. Rybak YE, McNeely HE, Mackenzie BE, Jain UR, Levitan RD. An open trial of light therapy in adult attention-deficit/hyperactivity disorder. J Clin Psychiatry. 2006;67:1527–35.
30. Faraone SV, Glatt SJ. A comparison of the efficacy of medications for adult attention-deficit/hyperactivity disorder using meta-analysis of effect sizes. J Clin Psychiatry. 2010;71:754–63.
31. Niederhofer H. Treating ADHD with agomelatine. J Atten Disord. 2012;16:346–8.
32. van der Heijden KB, Smits MG, van Someren EJ, Ridderinkhof KR, Gunning WB. Effect of melatonin on sleep, behavior, and cognition in ADHD and chronic sleep-onset insomnia. J Am Acad Child Adolesc Psychiatry. 2007;46:233–41.
33. Weiss MD, Wasdell MB, Bomben MM, Rea KJ, Freeman RD. Sleep hygiene and melatonin treatment for children and adolescents with ADHD and initial insomnia. J Am Acad Child Adolesc Psychiatry. 2006;45:512–9.
34. Tjon Pian Gi CV, Broeren JP, Starreveld JS, Versteegh FG. Melatonin for treatment of sleeping disorders in children with attention deficit/hyperactivity disorder: a preliminary open label study. Eur J Pediatr. 2003;162:554–5.

Melatonergic Drugs and Their Therapeutic Use in Nasal Polyposis

28

Vural Fidan and Onder Karaaslan

Abstract

Nasal polyposis is a common, chronic, and inflammatory disease of the mucous membranes of the nose and paranasal sinuses. The overall prevalence of rate ranges from 1 to 4 %. This chronic condition is characterized by edematous aggregates of inflamed mucosa prolapsing into the nose. The formation of nasal polyposis may lead to nasal airway obstruction, loss of smell, headache, increased secretion, and also a reduced quality of life.

Keywords

Polyposis • Asthma • Cortisol • Circadian rhythm • Inflammation • Nasal mucosa • Paranasal sinus

Introduction

Nasal polyposis is a common, chronic, and inflammatory disease of the mucous membranes of the nose and paranasal sinuses [1]. The overall prevalence of rate ranges from 1 to 4 % [1]. This chronic condition is characterized by edematous aggregates of inflamed mucosa prolapsing into the nose. The formation of nasal polyposis may lead to nasal airway obstruction, loss of smell, headache, increased secretion, and also a reduced quality of life [2].

The exact pathogenesis of nasal polyposis is still unknown. The development of polyposis has been linked to chronic inflammation, autonomic nervous system dysfunction, and also genetic predisposition [1, 3]. Most of the proposed theories consider nasal polyps to be the ultimate manifestation of chronic inflammation; thus, conditions leading to chronic inflammation in the nasal cavity can lead to nasal polyps [4].

Extensive nasal polyposis (ENP) is described as the protrusion of benign polyps into the nasal

V. Fidan, MD (✉)
Department of Otorhinolaryngology, Yunusemre Government Hospital, Uluonder District, Salih Bozok Street No: 23, Eskissehir 26100, Turkey
e-mail: vuralf@mynet.com

O. Karaaslan, MD, FEBOPRAS
Plastic, Aesthetic and Reconstructive Surgery Department, Izmir Katip Celebi University, Ataturk Training and Research Hospital, Polat Street, Karabaglar, Izmir 35360, Turkey
e-mail: drokaraaslan@yahoo.com

V. Srinivasan et al. (eds.), *Melatonin and Melatonergic Drugs in Clinical Practice*, DOI 10.1007/978-81-322-0825-9_28, © Springer India 2014

passages, and many mechanisms have been proposed for the development of these lesions [5, 6]. This condition is not a single disease entity; it is a multifactorial disease usually associated with asthma or other respiratory diseases such as cystic fibrosis, primary ciliary dyskinesia, and aspirin sensitivity [1]. Sleep impairment is one of the significant problems for patients with ENP [7] and has multiple influences on endocrine and metabolic function. Especially, sleep impairment is accompanied by a damaged circadian rhythm, which affects cortisol and melatonin secretion [8].

Melatonin

Circulating melatonin is secreted by the pineal gland excessively at night in all mammals, and it regulates a variety of important central and peripheral functions related to its cyclic secretion [9]. Within recent years, many investigators have implicated the pineal gland and melatonin in the processes of both aging and age-related diseases [10]. These theories stem from the importance of melatonin in a number of biological functions, and the fact that melatonin production in the organism is gradually lost throughout life, such that in very old individuals of any species, the circadian melatonin rhythm is discernible. In most species, from algae to humans, where it has been investigated, melatonin has been shown to exhibit a strong circadian rhythm in production and secretion, with high levels of the indole always being associated with the dark period of the light/dark cycle [11]. In addition, melatonin has also an important role in the antioxidative defense systems and the anti-inflammatory cascade [12]. In humans, the circadian rhythm of melatonin level is synchronized with the hours of sleep [10]. Measurements of melatonin in body fluids in elderly patients have convincingly demonstrated an age-related impairment of nocturnal pineal melatonin synthesis [10].

During the last two decades, much attention has centered on melatonin (5-methoxy-*N-acetyltryptamine*), one of the secretory products of the diffuse neuroendocrine system [12, 13]. A considerable amount of evidence has demonstrated that melatonin enhances immune function, both at central and at peripheral levels [12]. Melatonin has been shown to enhance interleukin-2 (IL-2) production and T-helper cell activity and also to exert a modulatory effect on lymphocyte proliferation. Indirectly, the increased IL-2 production and T-helper cell activity lead to increased antibody production in response to melatonin. Melatonin also regulates natural killer (NK) cell cytotoxicity, antibody production, lymphocyte interferon-gamma (IFN-γ) production, and T-helper-2 function [13].

Cortisol is another hormone that also demonstrates a circadian rhythm like melatonin. It has a typical circadian pattern with elevated levels in the early morning [14]. Cortisol levels are tightly regulated by the hippocampus and hypothalamic-pituitary-adrenal network. Interestingly, it was clearly documented that there is a significant positive correlation between the plasma-serum and salivary levels of melatonin and cortisol [15].

The daily cyclicity and seasonal cyclicity of immune roles are temporally with other physiological and behavioral processes, and all of them are regulated and coordinated with daily and seasonal changes of the external environment by the neuroendocrine homeostatic system [16]. Barriga et al. examined the possible physiological connection between the melatonin and corticosterone relationship in the immune system in basal situation and also under stress, but they found that melatonin takes no part in that type of situations following stress [16].

Melatonin Deficiency and Dysfunction

Decreased levels of melatonin levels are observed in multiple diseases, such as dementia, some mood disturbances, severe pain, cancer, and diabetes mellitus type II [17]. Melatonin dysfunction is usually related to deviations in amplitudes, phasing, and coupling of circadian rhythms [18].

A frequent complaint of insufficient melatonin signaling is sleep disturbances. It is necessary to distinguish between symptoms that are curable by short melatonergic actions and others that require extended actions during night. Melatonin immediate release is already effective, at moderate doses, for reducing difficulties of falling asleep or improving symptoms associated with poorly coupled circadian rhythms, including seasonal affective and bipolar disorders. For purposes of melatonin replacement therapy based on longer-lasting melatonergic actions, melatonin prolonged release and synthetic agonists have been developed [17, 18]. Therapies with melatonin or synthetic melatonergic drugs have to consider that these agents do act not only on the suprachiasmatic nucleus but also on numerous organs and cells in which melatonin receptors are also expressed [17].

The Relationship Between Melatonin and Extensive Nasal Polyposis: Is It Possible?

Sleep impairment is an important problem for patients who have inflammatory disorders of the upper airway tract, such as allergic rhinitis, rhinosinusitis, or nasal polyposis [9]. Several previous studies of melatonin and cortisol levels in inflammatory diseases have been published [9]. We designed a clinical trial which was one of the firsts to report disturbed salivary melatonin and cortisol levels in patients with extensive nasal polyposis. Papers describing lower melatonin levels in inflammatory patients can be found in the published literature [19, 20]. In our study, we observed overall lower levels of salivary melatonin in ENP patients, but rhythmicity was seen in all subjects similar to the previously published papers [19, 20]. The underlying mechanism causing the decline of melatonin in ENP patients is still unknown. This decrease may be associated with sleep impairment, but it could also be associated with inflammation. Some investigators have suggested that the decline in the melatonin levels might be either due to the direct inhibitory effect of cortisone on pinealocytes or because melatonin is more rapidly metabolized during the stress caused by disease [16]. In our study, we found that salivary cortisol levels were lower in patients with ENP compared to healthy subjects, and we know that chronic inflammation is present in patients with ENP. Some researchers have also detected lower cortisol levels among patients with inflammatory diseases [19–21].

Chronic inflammation may be seen in an atopic disease, and chronic inflammation may be associated with a lower response of the hypothalamic-pituitary axis, as different proinflammatory cytokines inhibit the ACTH-induced production of cortisol [22, 23]. In a mouse model of asthma, Silverman et al. showed that the increased airway inflammation was associated with decreased corticosterone levels [24]. Lower basal cortisol levels may contribute to a lack of suppression of airway inflammation and thus increased sinonasal inflammation, which leads to nasal polyposis. In ENP, the expression of the disease can be linked to endogenous cortisol levels, but it is unknown whether reduced basal cortisol levels are present before the onset of disease or if they are a result of the supposed chronic stress in ENP.

We also identified that the acrophase was significantly delayed in the ENP patients. Similar to our result, other researchers have found that acrophase occurs later in inflammatory patients [25]. This delay can be explained by sleep disturbance. According to our results, cortisol levels were disturbed in both the quantitative evaluation and the cyclic pattern in patients with ENP. Since cortisol is anti-inflammatory, the decrease in this parameter could worsen the inflammatory process in the nose as well as the whole body.

Conclusion

In summary, it is important to remember that extensive nasal polyposis is a multifactorial disease, and there is no a single strategy to handle with it. However, inflammation still remains the central major factor in patients. It was quantitatively shown that the circadian rhythms of melatonin and cortisol are disrupted in patients with extensive nasal polyposis. These promising results may take a place in clinical practice, and melatonin may be a new therapeutic target in the future for the patients with nasal polyposis. Melatoninergic drugs might be beneficial in the therapy of nasal polyposis like corticosteroids.

References

1. Pawankar R. Nasal polyposis: an update: editorial review. Curr Opin Allergy Clin Immunol. 2003;3(1):1–6.
2. Bachert C, Van Bruaene N, Toskala E, Zhang N, Olze H, Scadding G, Van Drunen CM, Mullol J, Cardell L, Gevaert P, Van Zele T, Claeys S, Halldén C, Kostamo K, Foerster U, Kowalski M, Bieniek K, Olszewska-Ziaber A, Nizankowska-Mogilnicka E, Szczeklik A, Swierczynska M, Arcimowicz M, Lund V, Fokkens W, Zuberbier T, Akdis C, Canonica G, Van Cauwenberge P, Burney P, Bousquet J. Important research questions in allergy and related diseases: 3-chronic rhinosinusitis and nasal polyposis – a GALEN study. Allergy. 2009;64(4):520–33.
3. Dalziel K, Stein K, Round A, Garside R, Royle P. Systematic review of endoscopic sinus surgery for nasal polyps. Health Technol Assess. 2003;7(17):iii,1–159.
4. Stammberger H. Surgical treatment of nasal polyps: past, present, and future. Allergy. 1999;54 Suppl 53:7–11.
5. Norlander T, Brönnegård M, Stierna P. The relationship of nasal polyps, infection, and inflammation. Am J Rhinol. 1999;13(5):349–55.
6. Pácová H, Kucera T, Astl J, Martínek J. Detection of beta-defensins and NOS in healthy and pathological nasal mucosa. Biomed Pap Med Fac Univ Palacky Olomouc Czech Repub. 2004;148(2):239–40.
7. Craig TJ, Ferguson BJ, Krouse JH. Sleep impairment in allergic rhinitis, rhinosinusitis, and nasal polyposis. Am J Otolaryngol. 2008;29(3):209–17.
8. Copinschi G. Metabolic and endocrine effects of sleep deprivation. Essent Psychopharmacol. 2005;6(6):341–7.
9. Fidan V, Alp HH, Kalkandelen S, Cingi C. Melatonin and cortisol rhythm in patients with extensive nasal polyposis. Am J Otolaryngol. 2013;34(1):61–4.
10. Cardinali DP, Srinivasan V, Brzezinski A, Brown GM. Melatonin and its analogs in insomnia and depression. J Pineal Res. 2012;52(4):365–75.
11. Reiter RJ. The pineal gland and melatonin in relation to aging: a summary of the theories and of the data. Exp Gerontol. 1995;30(3–4):199–212.
12. Pierpaoli W, Maestroni GJ. Melatonin: a principal neuroimmunoregulatory and anti-stress hormone: its anti-aging effects. Immunol Lett. 1987;16(3–4):355–61.
13. Martins Jr E, Ligeiro de Oliveira AP, Fialho de Araujo AM, Tavares de Lima W, Cipolla-Neto J, Costa Rosa LF. Melatonin modulates allergic lung inflammation. J Pineal Res. 2001;31(4):363–9.
14. Beyer HS, Matta SG, Sharp BM. Regulation of the messenger ribonucleic acid for corticotropin-releasing factor in the paraventricular nucleus and other brain sites of the rat. Endocrinology. 1988;123(4):2117–23.
15. Jensen MA, Hansen AM, Abrahamsson P, Nørgaard AW. Development and evaluation of a liquid chromatography tandem mass spectrometry method for simultaneous determination of salivary melatonin, cortisol and testosterone. J Chromatogr B Analyt Technol Biomed Life Sci. 2011;879(25):2527–32.
16. Barriga C, Martín MI, Tabla R, Ortega E, Rodríguez AB. Circadian rhythm of melatonin, corticosterone and phagocytosis: effect of stress. J Pineal Res. 2001;30(3):180–7.
17. Hardeland R. Neurobiology, pathophysiology, and treatment of melatonin deficiency and dysfunction. Sci World J. 2012;2012:640389. doi:10.1100/2012/640389.
18. Hardeland R. Melatonin in aging and disease -multiple consequences of reduced secretion, options and limits of treatment. Aging Dis. 2012;3(2):194–225.
19. Kos-Kudla B, Ostrowska Z, Marek B, et al. Diurnal rhythm of serum melatonin, ACTH and cortisol in asthma patients with long term glucocorticoid treatment. Endocr Regul. 1997;31:47–54.
20. Fei GH, Liu RY, Zhang ZH, et al. Alterations in circadian rhythms of melatonin and cortisol in patients with bronchial asthma. Acta Pharmacol Sin. 2004;25:651–6.
21. Bakkeheim E, Mowinckel P, Carlsen KH, et al. Reduced basal salivary cortisol in children with asthma and allergic rhinitis. Acta Paediatr. 2010;99:1705–11.
22. Calcagni E, Elenkov I. Stress system activity, innate and T helper cytokines, and susceptibility to immune-related diseases. Ann N Y Acad Sci. 2006;1069:62–76.
23. Tsigos C, Chrousos GP. Hypothalamic–pituitary–adrenal axis, neuroendocrine factors and stress. J Psychosom Res. 2002;53:865–71.
24. Silverman ES, Breault DT, Vallone J, et al. Corticotropin-releasing hormone deficiency increases allergen-induced airway inflammation in a mouse model of asthma. J Allergy Clin Immunol. 2004;114:747–54.
25. Haen E, Hauck R, Emslander HP, et al. Nocturnal asthma. Beta 2-adrenoceptors on peripheral mononuclear leukocytes, cAMP- and cortisol-plasma concentrations. Chest. 1991;100:1239–45.

Protective Effects of Exogenous Melatonin Against Methotrexate-Induced Intestinal Injury

29

Premila Abraham and Bina Isaac

Abstract

Methotrexate is widely used as a chemotherapeutic agent for leukemia and other malignancies. The efficacy of this drug is often limited by mucositis and intestinal injury, which are the major causes of morbidity in children and adults. We investigated whether melatonin, a powerful antioxidant, could have a protective effect. The rats were pretreated with melatonin (20 and 40 mg/kg body weight) daily 1 h before the MTX (7 mg/kg body weight) administration for three consecutive days. After the final dose of MTX, the rats were sacrificed, and the small intestine was used for light microscopy and biochemical assays. Intestinal homogenates were used for assay of oxidative stress parameters malondialdehyde and protein carbonyl content and myeloperoxidase activity, a marker of neutrophil infiltration, as well as for the activities of the antioxidant enzymes. Pretreatment with melatonin had a dose-dependent protective effect on MTX-induced alterations in small intestinal morphology. Morphology was saved to some extent with 20 mg melatonin pretreatment, and near-normal morphology was achieved with 40 mg melatonin pretreatment. Biochemically, pretreatment with melatonin significantly attenuated MTX-induced oxidative stress and restored the activities of the antioxidant enzymes. The results of the present study demonstrate that supplementation by exogenous melatonin significantly reduces MTX-induced small intestinal damage, indicating that it may be beneficial in ameliorating MTX-induced enteritis in humans.

Keywords

Methotrexate • Melatonin • Small intestinal damage • Oxidative stress • Rat

P. Abraham, PhD (✉)
Department of Biochemistry, Christian Medical College and Hospital, CMC College Campus, Bagayam, Vellore, TN 632002, India
e-mail: premilaabraham@cmcvellore.ac.in

B. Isaac, MS
Department of Anatomy, Christian Medical College and Hospital, CMC College Campus, Bagayam, Vellore, TN 632002, India
e-mail: isaac_bina@yahoo.co.in

V. Srinivasan et al. (eds.), *Melatonin and Melatonergic Drugs in Clinical Practice*,
DOI 10.1007/978-81-322-0825-9_29, © Springer India 2014

Introduction

Methotrexate (MTX) is used widely as chemotherapeutic agent in the treatment of malignancies and various inflammatory diseases, such as psoriasis, rheumatoid arthritis, and inflammatory bowel disease [1]. However, the usage of this drug is often limited by severe side effects and toxic sequelae. One of the major toxic effects of MTX is intestinal injury and mucositis. The small intestinal damage induced by MTX treatment results in malabsorption and diarrhea disturbing the cancer chemotherapy of patients [2, 3].

Reactive oxygen species (ROS) is reported to play an important role in the pathogenesis of MTX-induced intestinal damage [4–8]. Miyazono et al. [4] reported that increased oxidative stress and MPO activity (marker of neutrophil infiltration/inflammation) contribute to MTX-induced small intestinal damage. They have also shown that the ROS production precedes an increase in myeloperoxidase activity, suggesting neutrophil infiltration. MTX administration has been shown to increase cytosolic peroxide and decrease cellular levels of the antioxidant glutathione [5]. Huang et al. [6] demonstrated that MTX-induced intestinal injury is ROS dependent. Maeda et al. [7] have shown that MTX-induced ROS generation and lipid peroxidation are responsible for enhanced paracellular permeability of the small intestines. In addition, we previously demonstrated an increase of MDA and protein carbonyl content, the measures of oxidative damage to lipids and proteins, respectively, and myeloperoxidase (MPO) activity in the small intestine of methotrexate (MTX)-treated rats [8]. Studies have shown that the administration of antioxidants such as *N*-acetyl cysteine [9], vitamin A [10], garlic extract [11], and, most recently, lipoic acid [12] prevent MTX-induced damage in animal models.

Melatonin [MT] has been shown to have free radical scavenging actions at both physiological and pharmacological concentrations. A number of studies have shown that melatonin is significantly better than the classic antioxidants in resisting free radical-induced molecular destruction. In vivo studies have shown that melatonin was more effective than vitamin E [13], vitamin C [14], β-carotene [15], and superior to garlic oil [16]. In addition, several evidences suggest that the gut mucosa barrier tissue is a target for melatonin's protective effects [17–22]. Melatonin has been shown to be gastroprotective, and its action has been attributed to scavenging of free radicals and to its ability to attenuate lipid membrane peroxidation, neutrophil-induced infiltration, and cytotoxicity caused by mucosal irritants [23–25]. Evidence exists for de novo melatonin synthesis and high tissue melatonin levels in the gut [21, 22]. Melatonin levels in the gut have been shown to be independent of pineal production, since in rats pinealectomy had no influence on gut melatonin concentrations [18]. Interestingly, at any time of the day or night, the gut contains at least 400 times more melatonin than the pineal gland, once again emphasizing the functional importance of melatonin in the gut [26]. Studies have shown that melatonin is synthesized by gut enterochromaffin cells, where it acts in a paracrine fashion by binding to MT2 receptors in the gut tissue as an antioxidant/anti-inflammatory agent [27]. The major function of locally produced MT in GIT is to help it in coping with the stressors such as oxidants and inflammatory agents and various irritants present in the digested food [28–30].

The abovementioned findings prompted us to study whether melatonin pretreatment protects against MTX-induced small intestinal injury. In the present study, we have demonstrated that melatonin pretreatment attenuates MTX-induced oxidative stress and small intestinal damage in a dose-dependent manner, indicating that it may be beneficial in ameliorating MTX-induced enteritis in humans.

Methods

Dosage and route of administration of methotrexate were determined from those described in literature as causing consistent intestinal injury in normal rats [31]. After administration of methotrexate, the rats present with histological evidence of drug-induced small intestinal enteropathy and villus atrophy as seen in humans. The dose of melatonin was decided based on a recent study reported by Ucar et al. [32]. The study was approved by the institution's animal ethics committee (IAEC).

Adult male Wistar rats (200–225 g) were divided into six groups and treated as follows:

Group I: The rats in this group ($n=6$) received the vehicle alone intraperitoneally for 3 days.

Group II: The rats in this group ($n=6$) received 20 mg of melatonin/kg body weight intraperitoneally for 3 days.

Group III: The rats in this group ($n=6$) received 40 mg of melatonin/kg body weight intraperitoneally for 3 days.

Group IV: The rats in this group ($n=8$) received three consecutive daily intraperitoneal injections of methotrexate at the dose 7 mg/kg body weight.

Group V: The rats in this group ($n=8$) received 20 mg of melatonin/kg body weight 1 h prior to MTX administration intraperitoneally for three consecutive days.

Group VI: The rats in this group ($n=8$) received 40 mg of melatonin/kg body weight 1 h prior to MTX administration intraperitoneally for three consecutive days.

The rats were sacrificed 24 h after the final dose of methotrexate/vehicle.

Tissue Procurement

Rats were weighed, anesthetized with halothane, and then killed by cervical dislocation. The entire length of the small intestine was removed and flushed with cold phosphate-buffered saline and weighed. The small intestine was divided into duodenum, jejunum, and ileum and used for biochemical analysis as well as for histological assessment of injury.

Histology (Light Microscopy)

For light microscopic studies a portion of the tissue was fixed in 10 % buffered formaldehyde and paraffin embedded. Four micron serial sections were cut and stained with hematoxylin and eosin.

Mucosal injury, inflammation, and hyperemia/hemorrhage were assessed and graded from one to five in a blinded manner using the histological injury scale as defined by Chiu et al. [33].

Briefly, the mucosal damage was graded from one to five according to the following criteria: grade 0, normal mucosal villi; grade 1, development of subepithelial Gruenhagen's space at the apex of the villus, often with capillary congestion; grade 2, extension of the subepithelial space with moderate lifting of the epithelial layer from the lamina propria; grade 3, massive epithelial lifting down the sides of villi, possibly with a few denuded tips; grade 4, denuded villi with lamina propria and dilated capillaries exposed, possibly with increased cellularity of lamina propria; and grade 5, digestion and disintegration of the lamina propria, hemorrhage, and ulceration.

Biochemical Assays

The mucosa was scraped off from the remaining part of the small intestine using glass slide, weighed, homogenized in appropriate buffers, and used for the biochemical assays including malondialdehyde level, protein carbonyl content, protein content, myeloperoxidase activity and the activities of antioxidant enzymes, superoxide dismutase, glutathione peroxidase, glutathione reductase, glutathione S-transferase, and catalase by methods as described in detail earlier [34].

Statistical analysis

The data represent mean value ± SD. Means of three groups were compared by ANOVA. Student's t test with Bonferroni correction was used to compare individual means in the case of a significant F.

Results

Effect of Pretreatment of Melatonin on MTX-Induced Light Microscopic Changes in the Small Intestine

Light microscopic examination of the parts of small intestine in vehicle-treated rats showed normal morphology with sharp villi, long crypts, intact lining epithelium with normal mucus secreting cells, normal vasculature, and normal cellularity lamina propria (Fig. 29.1a–c). The administration of 40 mg melatonin alone caused slight alteration in mucosal morphology especially in jejunum. The tips of the villi were mildly blunted, but those of the crypts appeared normal (Fig. 29.1d–f).

The administration of MTX alone caused damage to the architecture of the small intestine (Fig. 29.2a–c). The villi were distorted and blunted in the duodenum (Fig. 29.2a), atrophied and focally absent in the jejunum (Fig. 29.2b), and aborted, flattened, and fused in the ileum (Fig. 29.2c). The crypt abscesses were found in all the three segments of the small intestine, suggesting an inflammatory response. The mucosal thickness was reduced and was accompanied by decreased villus/crypt ratio. There was acute transmural inflammatory infiltrate in the mucosa, submucosa, and the muscularis layers.

Pretreatment with 20 mg/kg melatonin did show some recovery from MTX-induced small intestinal damage (images not shown).

Pretreatment with 40 mg/kg melatonin before the administration of MTX almost restored the morphology of the small intestines (Fig. 29.2d–f).

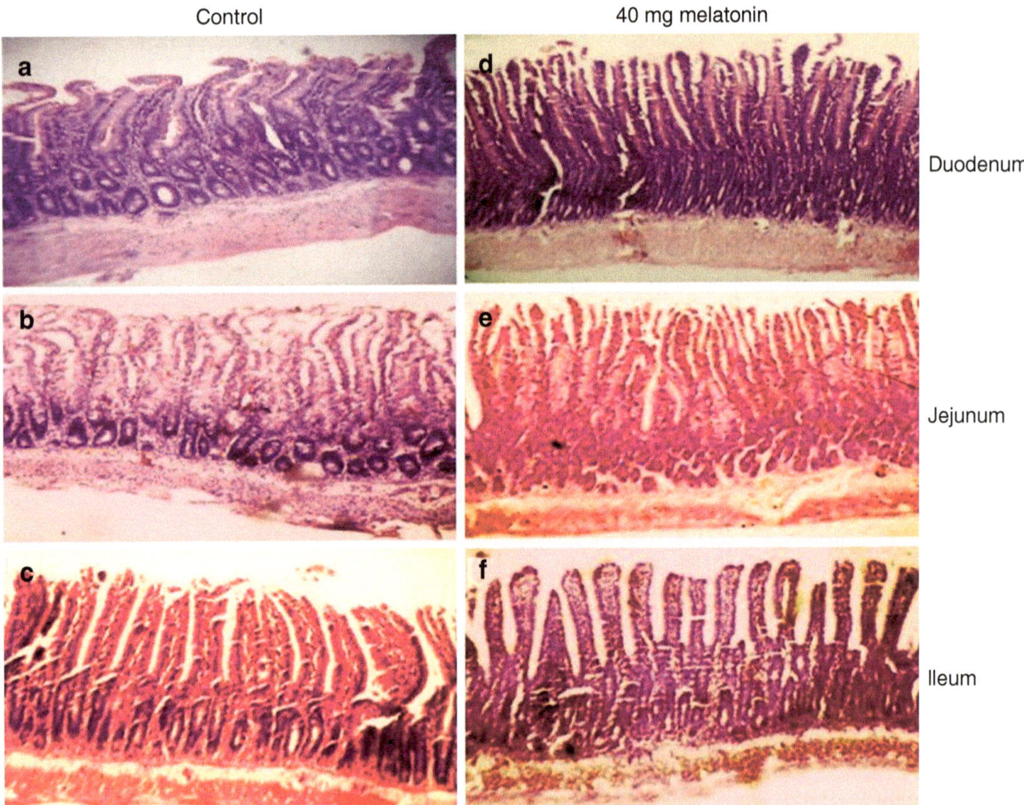

Fig. 29.1 Histology of the duodenum, jejunum, and ileum of control (**a**–**c**) 40×. The small intestines showed normal morphology with sharp villi, long crypts, intact lining epithelium with normal mucus secreting cells, normal vasculature, and normal lamina propria. Histology of duodenum, jejunum, and ileum of rats treated with 40 mg/kg body wt. melatonin alone (**d**–**f**), magnification 40×. The crypts were normal, but the villi were slightly blunted

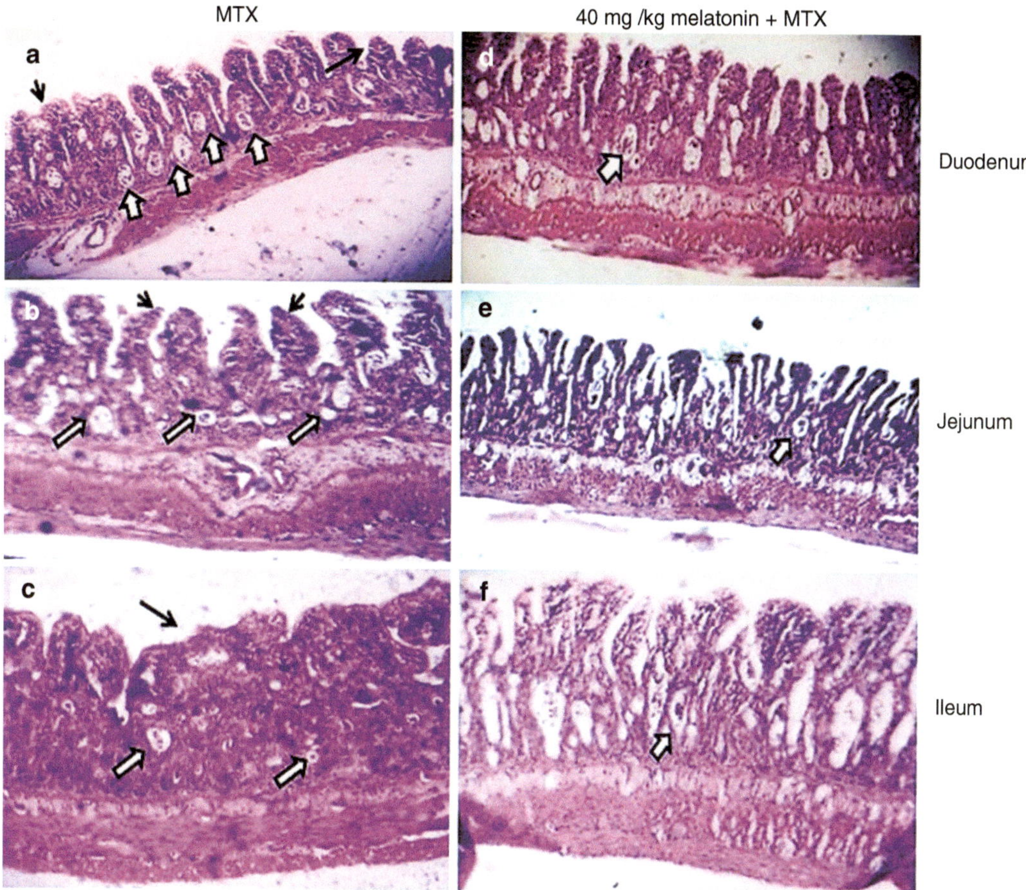

Fig. 29.2 Effect of MTX and melatonin (40 mg/kg) pretreatment on the small intestine of rat. 40×. Figures (**a**–**c**) represent duodenum, jejunum, and ileum of MTX-treated rats, respectively. The villi were shortened in the duodenum (**a**), distorted in the jejunum (**b**), and aborted, flattened, blunted, and fused in the ileum (**c**). Figures (**d**–**f**) represent the duodenum, jejunum, and ileum of melatonin (40 mg/kg)-pretreated rats, respectively. *Black arrow* indicates the villi and the *white arrow* indicates the crypt abscess

The damage to the mucosa and the severity of inflammatory response was less as compared to the MTX-treated rats. There was less damage to the villi and less crypt abscess in the small intestines of melatonin-pretreated rats. The villi/crypt ratio was more, and the inflammatory infiltrate of the mucosa and muscularis propria was less as compared to the MTX-treated rat. The order of recovery with 40 mg/kg melatonin pretreatment was jejunum > duodenum > ileum. In conclusion, pretreatment with 40 mg/kg melatonin significantly protects the small intestine from the deleterious effects of MTX.

Effect of Melatonin Pretreatment on MTX-Induced Changes in Parameters of Oxidative Stress

MTX treatment resulted in increased oxidative stress as indicated by elevated malondialdehyde level and protein carbonyl content in the small intestines. It also resulted in significant decrease in the activities of the antioxidant enzymes, superoxide dismutase, glutathione reductase, catalase, and glutathione S-transferase. A significant increase in MPO activity, marker of neutrophil infiltration, was observed in the small intestines of MTX-treated rats.

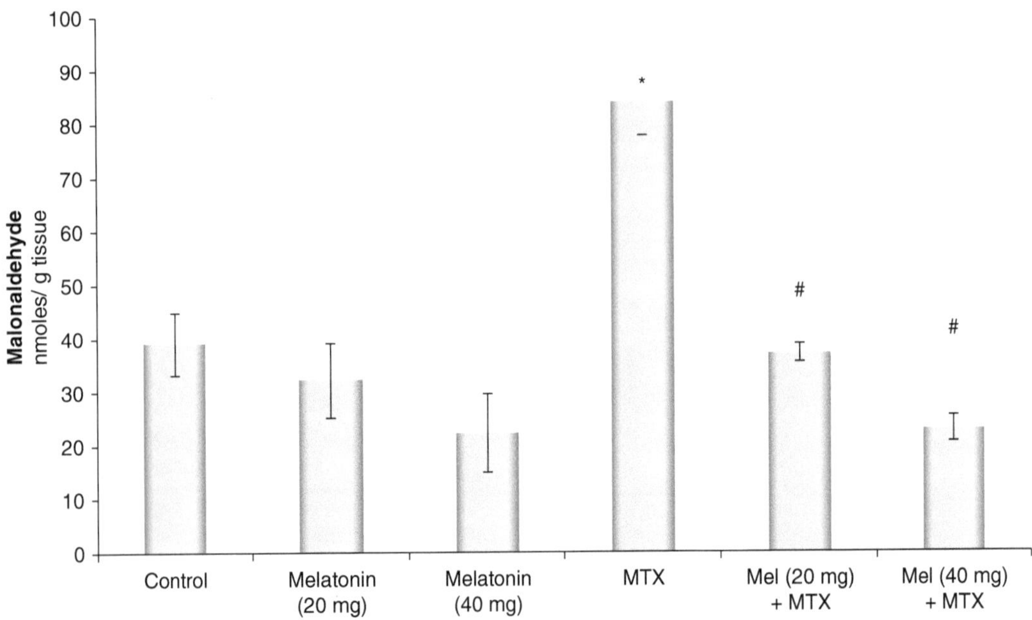

Fig. 29.3 Malondialdehyde levels in the small intestines of control rats and experimental rats with melatonin (20 and 40 mg) treatment, MTX treatment, and melatonin pretreatment groups. Data represent mean ± SD, $n=6$ in each group, * $p<0.01$ as compared with control group; # $p<0.01$ as compared with MTX group

Pretreatment with 40 mg/kg melatonin completely attenuated MTX-induced elevation in the levels of MDA and protein carbonyl content in the small intestines, confirming the antioxidant role of MT (Figs. 29.3 and 29.4).

Pretreatment with melatonin restored the activities of many antioxidant enzymes. Melatonin at 40 mg/kg completely restored the activity of superoxide dismutase (Fig. 29.5). Melatonin pretreatment partially but significantly restored the activity of glutathione reductase in a dose-dependent manner (Fig. 29.6). Pretreatment with 20 mg/kg body wt. melatonin significantly attenuated MTX-induced elevation in the activity of GPO, but 40 mg dose had no effect (Fig. 29.7). However, melatonin pretreatment had no significant effect on MTX-induced alterations in the activities of catalase and glutathione S-transferase (Figs. 29.8 and 29.9). Surprisingly, melatonin pretreatment had no effect on MTX-induced increased myeloperoxidase activity (Fig. 29.10).

The administration of melatonin alone (20 or 40 mg/kg body wt.) increased the activities of the antioxidant enzymes and decreased MDA levels in the small intestines as compared with control, but the results were not statistically significant.

Discussion

Methotrexate, a structural analogue of folic acid, is widely used as a chemotherapeutic agent for cancer treatment. It is also used in the treatment of various inflammatory diseases, such as psoriasis, rheumatoid arthritis, and inflammatory bowel disease [1]. Mucositis, intestinal injury, diarrhea, and malabsorption are serious side effects and major causes of MTX-related morbidity in children and adults. The damage to the gastrointestinal (GI) epithelium after MTX chemotherapy includes villus shortening and fusion, epithelial atrophy, crypt loss, inflammatory infiltrate in the lamina propria, goblet cell depletion, and loss of mucosal integrity [2, 3]. Accordingly, in the present study, most of these features were observed in the small intestines of MTX-treated rats.

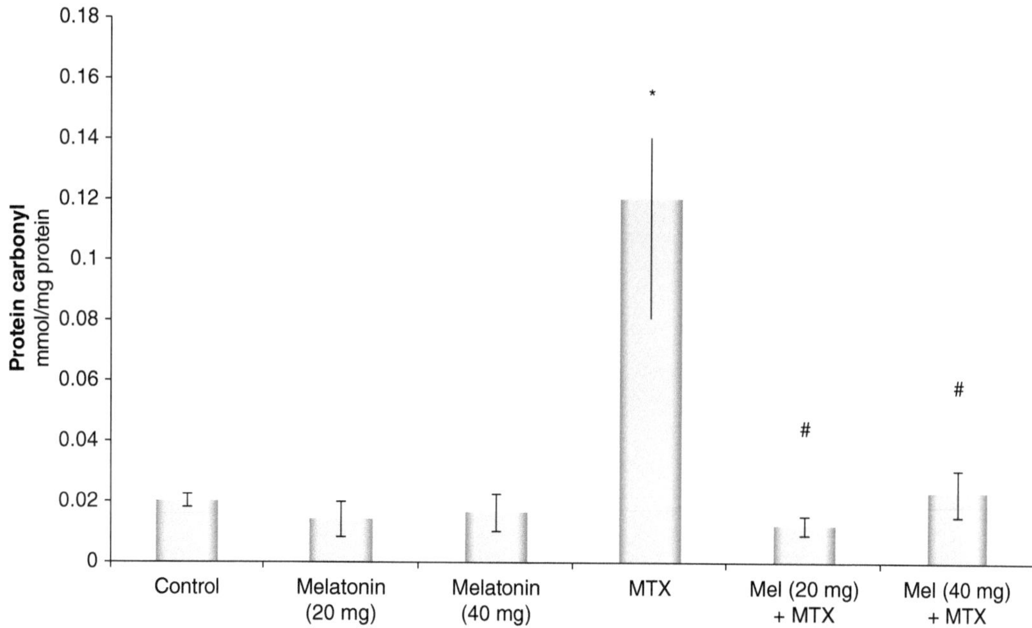

Fig. 29.4 Protein carbonyl content in the small intestines of control rats and experimental rats with melatonin (20 and 40 mg) treatment, MTX treatment, and melatonin pretreatment groups. Data represent mean ± SD, $n=6$ in each group, * $p<0.01$ as compared with control group; # $p<0.01$ as compared with MTX group

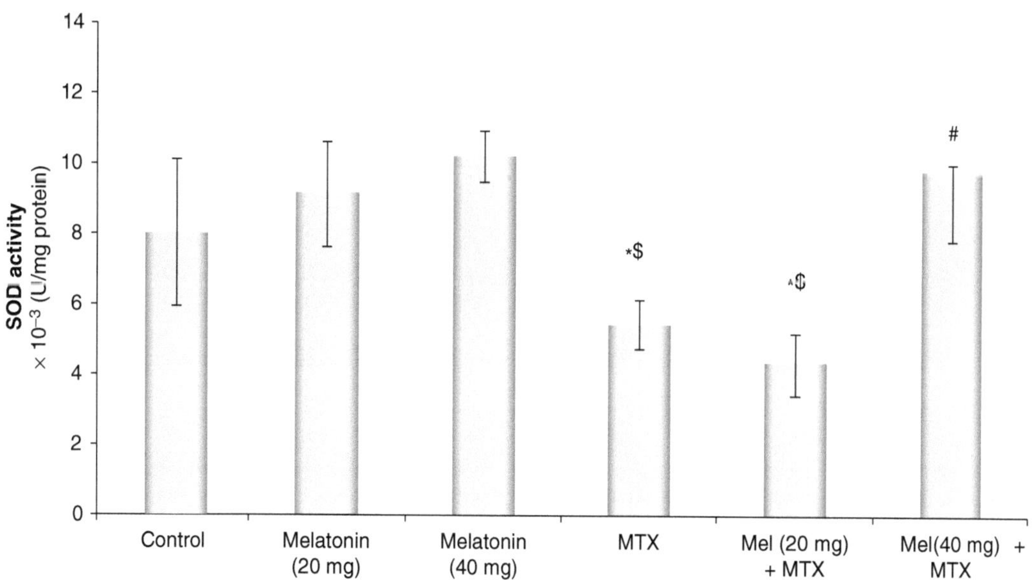

Fig. 29.5 Superoxide dismutase activity in the small intestines of control rats and experimental rats with melatonin (20 and 40 mg) treatment, MTX treatment, and melatonin pretreatment groups. Data represent mean ± SD, $n=6$ in each group, * $p<0.05$ as compared with control group; # $p<0.01$ as compared with MTX group; $ $p<0.05$ as compared to melatonin groups

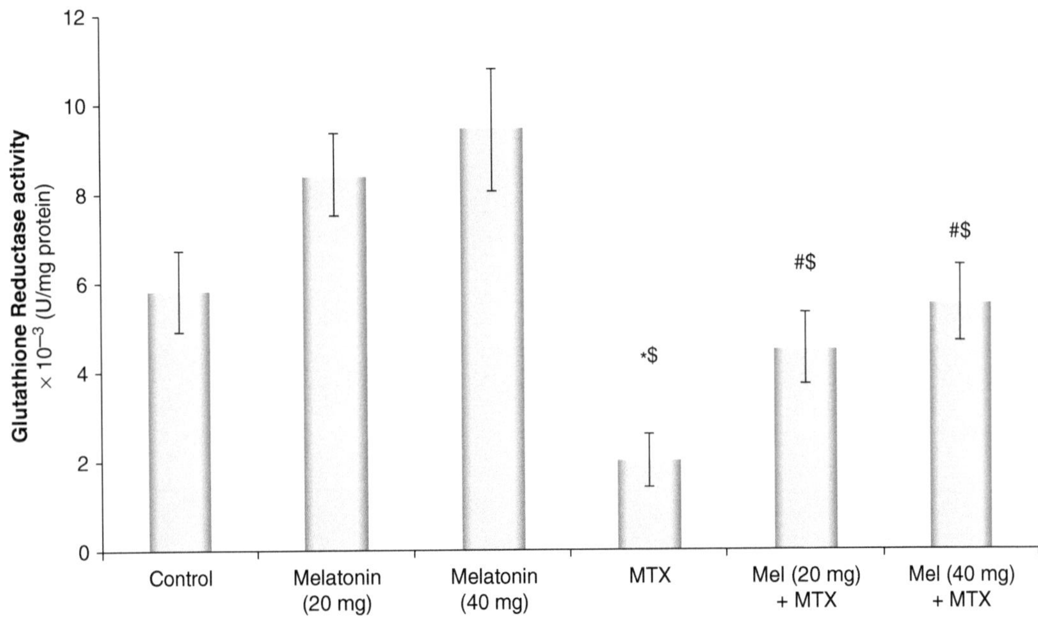

Fig. 29.6 Glutathione reductase activity in the small intestines of control rats and experimental rats with melatonin (20 and 40 mg) treatment, MTX treatment, and melatonin pretreatment groups. Data represent mean ± SD, $n = 6$ in each group, * $p < 0.01$ as compared with control group; # $p < 0.05$ as compared with MTX group. $ $p < 0.05$ as compared with melatonin group

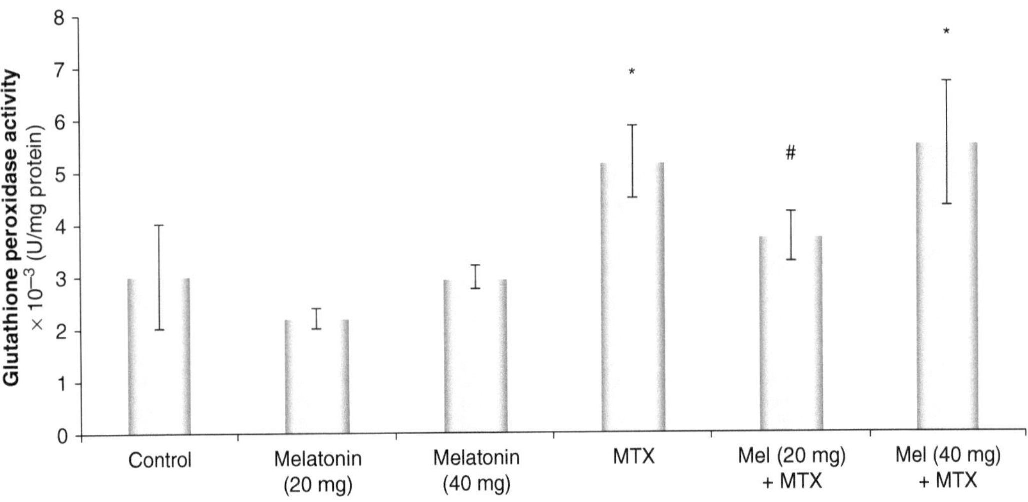

Fig. 29.7 Glutathione peroxidase activity in the small intestines of control rats and experimental rats with melatonin (20 and 40 mg) treatment, MTX treatment, and melatonin pretreatment groups. Data represent mean ± SD, $n = 6$ in each group, * $p < 0.05$ as compared with control group; # $p < 0.05$ as compared with MTX group

Although pretreatment with 20 mg/kg melatonin showed some recovery from MTX-induced small intestinal damage, 40 mg/kg body wt. melatonin showed almost complete recovery from damage. The villi/crypt ratio was more, and the inflammatory infiltrate of the mucosa and muscularis propria was less as compared to the MTX-treated rat.

In agreement to those reported by us [8] and others [4–7], MTX treatment resulted in

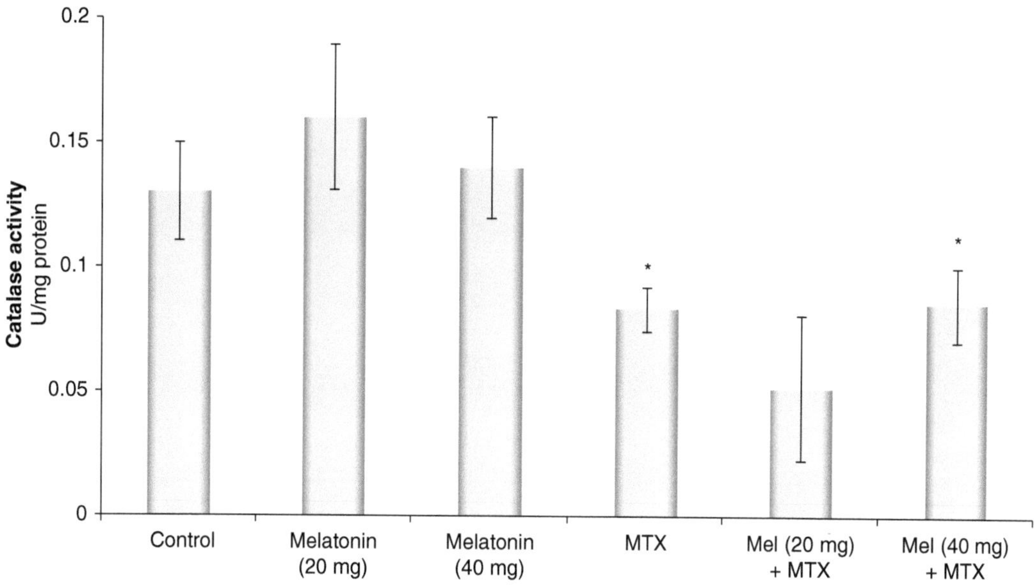

Fig. 29.8 Catalase activity in the small intestines of control rats and experimental rats with melatonin (20 and 40 mg) treatment, MTX treatment, and melatonin pretreatment groups. Data represent mean ± SD, $n = 6$ in each group, * $p < 0.05$ as compared with control group

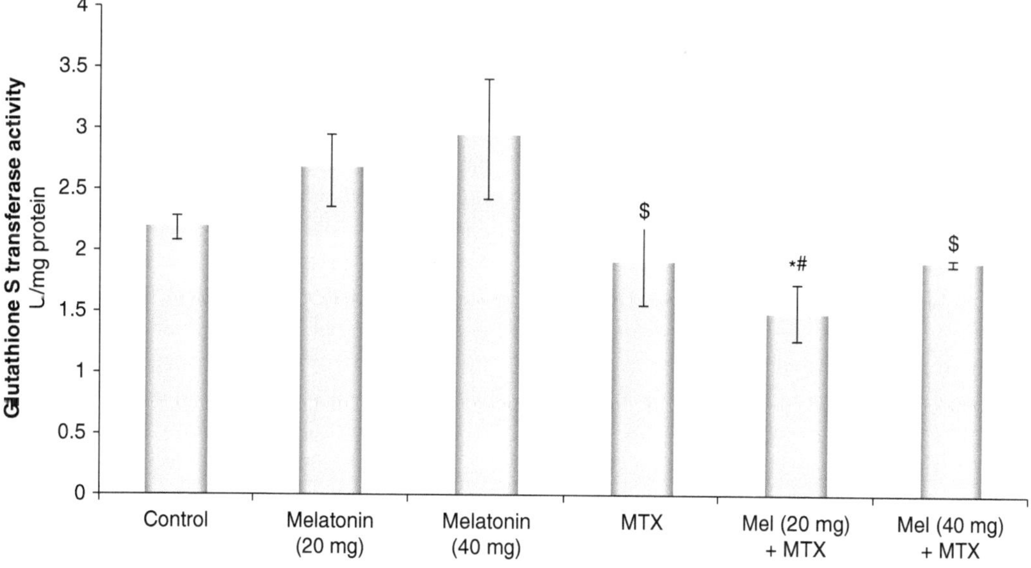

Fig. 29.9 Glutathione S-transferase activity in the small intestines of control rats and experimental rats with melatonin (20 and 40 mg) treatment, MTX treatment, and melatonin pretreatment groups. Data represent mean ± SD, $n = 6$ in each group, * $p < 0.05$ as compared to control group; $ $p < 0.05$ as compared with 40 mg melatonin group; # $p < 0.05$ as compared with both melatonin groups

increased oxidative stress in the small intestines as evidenced by elevated MDA levels and protein carbonyl content. There was decreased activities of important antioxidant enzymes as well as increase in MPO activity, a marker of neutrophil infiltration. All these studies provide evidence for important role for ROS in MTX-induced small intestinal damage.

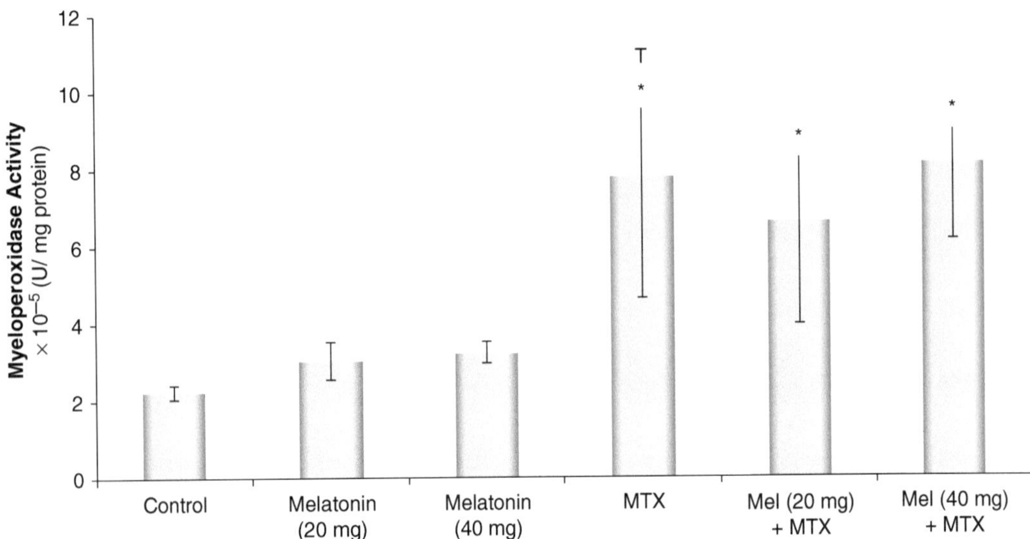

Fig. 29.10 Myeloperoxidase activity in the small intestines of control rats and experimental rats with melatonin (20 and 40 mg) treatment, MTX treatment, and melatonin pretreatment groups. Data represent mean ± SD, $n=6$ in each group, * $p<0.01$ as compared with control and melatonin groups

In the present study, the protective effect of MT on MTX-induced small intestinal damage involved attenuation of oxidative stress. MT pretreatment attenuated MTX-induced increased MDA level and protein carbonyl content and restored the activities of important antioxidant enzymes such as superoxide dismutase and glutathione reductase. Besides, melatonin pretreatment ameliorated MTX-induced small intestinal damage in a dose-dependent manner. This finding suggests that melatonin protects against MTX-induced small intestinal damage by acting as an antioxidant. Melatonin is a versatile antioxidant and acts in different ways. It is a major scavenger of free radicals [34, 35]. It also supports several intracellular enzymatic antioxidant enzymes, including SOD and glutathione peroxidase (GPO) [36]. Melatonin has been shown to influence both enzyme activity and cellular mRNA levels for SOD and GPO under physiological conditions and during elevated oxidative stress [36]. Melatonin preserves or even increases the content of GSH in tissues. Melatonin has been shown to induce the activity of γ-glutamylcysteine synthetase, thereby stimulating the production of glutathione (GSH) [37]. Accordingly, Jahovic et al. [31] have shown that MT pretreatment reverses MTX-induced depletion of GSH in the intestines, liver, and kidney of rats. Melatonin has many advantages over the other antioxidants. One advantage is that melatonin has a sparing effect on GSH as it sacrifices itself and does not participate in redox cycling after scavenging free radicals, as other antioxidants such as vitamins E and C do by consuming GSH. Therefore, melatonin is classified as a suicidal or terminal antioxidant [38]. Another advantage of melatonin is that it also stabilizes lipid membranes and defends them from peroxidation, particularly due to its high lipophilicity and easy entrance into the cells to protect their subcellular compartments [39].

Unlike other antioxidants is believed to lack of pro-oxidant activity [40]. Its lack of toxicity and the ease with which melatonin crosses morphophysiological barriers and enters subcellular compartments are essential features of this antioxidant. Thus, melatonin appears to be superior to other cellular antioxidants.

It is important to mention that the gastrointestinal tract of vertebrate species is a rich source of extrapineal melatonin. The concentration of melatonin in the gastrointestinal tissues exceeds blood levels by 10–100 times, and there is at least 400 times more melatonin in the gastrointestinal tract than in the pineal gland. The gastrointestinal tract contributes significantly to circulating concentrations of melatonin, especially during the daytime, and melatonin may serve as an endocrine, paracrine, or autocrine hormone influencing the regeneration and function of epithelium, enhancing the immune system of the gut, and reducing the tone of gastrointestinal muscles [41, 42]. There is strong evidence that GIT mucosa, particularly that of duodenal cluster unit (stomach, duodenum, and hepatobiliary system), exhibits high biosynthetic activity for MT. The highest content of MT was recorded in the gastric, duodenal, jejunal, and ileal mucosa and somewhat less in the liver [26, 27]. Melatonin receptors have been identified in different parts of the gut, suggesting its role in gut physiology. The main receptor in the GIT for melatonin is the MT2 receptor [27]. The major function of locally produced MT in GIT is to help it cope with the stressors such as oxidants and inflammatory agents and various irritants present in the digested food [28–30].

As mentioned earlier, studies have shown that melatonin is synthesized by gut enterochromaffin cells, where it acts in a paracrine fashion by binding to MT2 receptors in the gut tissue as an antioxidant/anti- inflammatory agent and gets absorbed through mesenteric circulation, to be passed on through the hepatic portal circulation to the liver, where it gets recycled through bile or catabolized and excreted through the kidneys [28–30, 41, 42]. Several recent reports indicating an anti-inflammatory/antioxidant role for melatonin as well as data linking extrapineal melatonin imbalance to gut pathophysiology have been reported [43–45]. These studies prove the antioxidant role for melatonin under physiological conditions.

In an earlier study, we have shown that MTX administration results in increased neutrophil infiltration as well as increased activity of MPO in small intestines of rats [8]. This finding is in agreement with those reported earlier [4, 46–48]. MPO is released by activated neutrophils and is a biomarker for inflammation. MPO, an enzyme linked to both inflammation and oxidative stress, catalyzes the production of hypochlorous acid and a range of other highly reactive species, which, by killing pathogens, play a protective role in the innate immune response.

Melatonin is reported to possess anti-inflammatory properties [49]. Galijasevic et al. [50] identified melatonin as a potent inhibitor of MPO. They showed that, at physiological and supraphysiological concentrations, melatonin interferes with the catalytic activity of MPO by multiple pathways that includes switching the activity of MPO from peroxidation to catalase-like activity and conversion of MPO to an inactive form. Other than inhibition of MPO, melatonin may also reduce the activity of MPO by two other mechanisms. First, it is a potent scavenger of reactive oxygen species and may thereby limit the production of hydrogen peroxide, the co-substrate of MPO [34]. Second, the anti-inflammatory properties of melatonin may reduce infiltration by MPO-secreting leukocytes.

In the present study however, the protective effect of melatonin on MTX-induced small intestinal damage was mediated by attenuation of oxidative stress and not MPO activity. One possible explanation for this observation is that in "in vivo" conditions, MT administration scavenges hydrogen peroxide, the co-substrate for MPO, thereby resulting in decreased activity of MPO. However, in "ex vivo" conditions, this cannot be demonstrated as the substrate (H_2O_2) is provided in the incubation medium. The decrease in MPO activity in response to MT treatment despite the provision of the substrate H_2O_2 as reported in other studies may be due to the direct inactivation of the enzyme by MT as suggested by Galijasevic et al. [50].

In our study, although the administration of melatonin had no significant inhibitory effect on MPO activity, it attenuated MTX-induced crypt abscess formation in the small intestines. This could be explained based on the fact that the inhibition of MPO activity is not the only mechanism by which melatonin ameliorates inflammation, it can also act by blocking transcriptional factors (NFkB) and TNF-α [42, 51]. In addition, studies have shown that COX-2 and iNOS, the mediators of inflammation, are molecular targets for melatonin and its metabolites [52].

There are studies that show that melatonin may not exert its anti-inflammatory effect by inhibiting neutrophil infiltration. Exogenous melatonin has been shown to preserve renal functional status following I/R-induced injury by increasing glutathione and reducing lipid peroxidation, without any apparent effect on neutrophil infiltration [53]. Alarcon et al. [54] have shown that pretreatment with melatonin inhibits indomethacin-induced gastric ulceration and was not associated with a reduction in neutrophil infiltration. These authors have suggested that the protection afforded by melatonin against indomethacin-induced gastric injury may involve mechanisms other than inhibition of neutrophil infiltration.

Melatonin has been shown to prevent ulcerations of gastrointestinal mucosa by an antioxidant action, reduction of secretion of hydrochloric acid, stimulation of the immune system, fostering epithelial regeneration, and increasing microcirculation [41, 55, 56].

Melatonin is proven to be nontoxic to humans and animals when administered in both physiological and pharmacological amounts to humans and animals [40, 57]. Melatonin is easily synthesized in a pharmacologically pure form and is inexpensive and affordable. Besides, as melatonin is an endogenous antioxidant, the chances of it to produce side effects may be lesser than the exogenous antioxidants.

Beneficial antioxidant effects of melatonin have been recently shown in clinical settings for several chronic diseases, including patients with rheumatoid arthritis [58], elderly patients with primary essential hypertension [59], and females with infertility [60].

Thus, supplementation with melatonin as an adjuvant therapy may be promising in alleviating the gastrointestinal side effects of methotrexate. However, it should be borne in mind that pharmacological doses and not physiological dose of melatonin protect against oxidative stress and organ injury. Melatonin plays an important role in the regulation of various body functions including circadian rhythms, blood pressure, seasonal reproduction, and immunity [61]. Besides, recent studies have demonstrated that melatonin can act as a pro-oxidant at high concentrations [62], although earlier studies have reported that melatonin in pharmacological doses is nontoxic to humans [57]. Therefore, before administering melatonin to humans, the side effects of long-term intake of melatonin need to be verified.

Acknowledgements The authors acknowledge the Council for Scientific and Industrial Research (CSIR), New Delhi, for the financial support for the study and Mr. Viswa Kalyan Kolli, research fellow, for carrying out the biochemical studies.

References

1. da Fonseca MA, Casamassimo P. Old drugs, new uses. Pediatr Dent. 2011;33:67–74. Review.
2. Maiguma T, Hayashi Y, Ueshima S, Kaji H, Egawa T, Chayama K. Relationship between oral mucositis and high-dose methotrexate therapy in pediatric acute lymphoblastic leukemia. Int J Clin Pharmacol Ther. 2008;46:584–90.
3. Ishaq M, Muhammad JS, Hameed K, Mirza AI. Leflunomide or methotrexate? Comparison of clinical efficacy and safety in low socio-economic rheumatoid arthritis patients. Mod Rheumatol. 2011;21:375–80.
4. Miyazono Y, Gao F, Horie T. Oxidative stress contributes to methotrexate-induced small intestinal toxicity in rats. Scand J Gastroenterol. 2004;39:1119–27.
5. Phillips DC, Woollard KJ, Griffiths HR. The anti-inflammatory actions of methotrexate are critically dependent upon the production of reactive oxygen species. Br J Pharmacol. 2003;138:501–11.
6. Huang CC, Hsu PC, Hung YC, Liao YF, Liu CC, Hour CT. Ornithine decarboxylase prevents methotrexate-induced apoptosis by reducing intracellular reactive oxygen species production. Apoptosis. 2005;10:895–907.
7. Maeda T, Miyazono Y, Ito K, Hamada K, Sekine S, Horie T. Oxidative stress and enhanced paracellular permeability in the small intestine of methotrexate-treated rats. Cancer Chemother Pharmacol. 2010;65:1117–23.
8. Kolli VK, Abraham P, Isaac B. Alteration in antioxidant defense mechanisms in the small intestines of methotrexate treated rat may contribute to its gastrointestinal toxicity. Cancer Ther. 2007;5:501–10.
9. Ciralik H, Bulbuloglu E, Cetinkaya A, Kurutas EB, Celik M, Polat A. Effects of N-acetylcysteine on methotrexate-induced small intestinal damage in rats. Mt Sinai J Med. 2006;73:1086–92.
10. Yuncu M, Eralp A, Koruk M, Sari I, Bagci C, Inaloz S. Effect of vitamin A against methotrexate-induced damage to the small intestine in rats. Med Princ Pract. 2004;13:346–52.
11. Yüncü M, Eralp A, Celik A. Effect of aged garlic extract against methotrexate-induced damage to the small intestine in rats. Phytother Res. 2006;20:504–10.

12. Somi MH, Hajipour B, Abad GD, Hemmati MR, Ghabili K, Khodadadi A, Vatankhah AM. Protective role of lipoic acid on methotrexate induced intestinal damage in rabbit model. Indian J Gastroenterol. 2011;30:38–40.
13. Baydas G, Canatan H, Turkoglu A. Comparative analysis of the protective effects of melatonin and vitamin E on streptozocin-induced diabetes mellitus. J Pineal Res. 2002;32:225–30.
14. Gultekin F, Delibas N, Yasar S, Kilinc I. In vivo changes in antioxidant systems and protective role of melatonin and a combination of vitamin C and vitamin E on oxidative damage in erythrocytes induced by chlorpyrifos-ethyl in rats. Arch Toxicol. 2001;75:88–96.
15. Hsu C, Han B, Liu M, Yeh C, Casida JE. Phosphine-induced oxidative damage in rats: attenuation by melatonin. Free Radic Biol Med. 2000;28:636–42.
16. Anwar MM, Meki AR. Oxidative stress in streptozotocin-induced diabetic rats: effects of garlic oil and melatonin. Comp Biochem Physiol A Mol Integr Physiol. 2003;135:539–47.
17. Reiter RJ, Tan DX, Mayo JC. Neurally-mediated and neurally-independent beneficial actions of melatonin in the gastrointestinal tract. J Physiol Pharmacol. 2003;54 Suppl 4:113–25.
18. Sewerynek E, Reiter RJ, Melchiorri D. Oxidative damage in the liver induced by ischemia-reperfusion: protection by melatonin. Hepatogastroenterology. 1996;43:898–905.
19. Messner M, Huether G, Lorf T. Presence of melatonin in the human hepatobiliary-gastrointestinal tract. Life Sci. 2001;69:543–51.
20. Konturek SJ, Konturek PC, Brzozowska I. Localization and biological activities of melatonin in intact and diseased gastrointestinal tract (GIT). J Physiol Pharmacol. 2007;58:381–405.
21. Huether G. The contribution of extrapineal sites of melatonin synthesis to circulating melatonin levels in higher vertebrates. Experientia. 1993;49:665–70.
22. Stefulj J, Hörtner M, Ghosh M. Gene expression of the key enzymes of melatonin synthesis in extrapineal tissues of the rat. J Pineal Res. 2001;30:243–7.
23. Bubenik GA, Pang SF, Cockshut JR. Circadian variation of portal, arterial and venous blood levels of melatonin in pigs and its relationship to food intake and sleep. J Pineal Res. 2000;28:9–15.
24. Reiter RJ, Tan DX. What constitutes a physiological concentration of melatonin? J Pineal Res. 2003;34:79–80.
25. Tan DX, Manchester LC, Reiter RJ, et al. High physiological levels in the bile of mammals. Life Sci. 1999;65:2523–9.
26. Kvetnoy IM, Ingel IE, Kvetnaia TV, Malinovskaya NK, Rapoport SI, Raikhlin NT, Trofimov AV, Yuzhakov VV. Gastrointestinal melatonin: cellular identification and biological role. Neuro Endocrinol Lett. 2002;23:121–32.
27. Lee PPN, Pang SF. Melatonin and its receptors in the gastrointestinal tract. Biol Signals. 1993;2:181–93.
28. Pandi-Perumal SR, Srinivasan V, Maestroni GJM, Cardinali DP, Poeggeler B, Hardeland R. Melatonin nature is most versatile biological signal? FEBS J. 2006;273:2813–38.
29. Tan DX, Manchester LC, Reiter RJ. A novel melatonin metabolite, cyclic 3-hydroxymelatonin: a biomarker of in vivo hydroxyl radical generation. Biochem Biophys Res Commun. 1998;253:614–20.
30. Hirata F, Hayaishi O, Tokuyama T, Seno S. In vitro and in vivo formation of two new metabolites of melatonin. J Biol Chem. 1974;249:1311–3.
31. Jahovic N, Cevik H, Sehirli AO. Melatonin prevents methotrexate induced hepatorenal oxidative injury in rats. J Pineal Res. 2003;34:282–7.
32. Ucar M, Korkmaz A, Reiter RJ. Melatonin alleviates lung damage induced by the chemical warfare agent nitrogen mustard. Toxicol Lett. 2007;173:124–31.
33. Chiu CJ, McArdle AH, Brown R, Scott HJ, Gurd FN. Intestinal mucosal lesion in low-flow states. I. A morphological, hemodynamic, and metabolic reappraisal. Arch Surg. 1970;101:478–83.
34. Reiter RJ, Tan DX, Maldonado MD. Melatonin as an antioxidant: physiology versus pharmacology. J Pineal Res. 2005;39:215–6.
35. Reiter RJ, Tan DX, Terron MP, Flores LJ, Czarnocki Z. Melatonin and its metabolites: new findings regarding their production and their radical scavenging actions. Acta Biochim Pol. 2007;54:1–9.
36. Rodriguez C. Regulation of antioxidant enzymes: a significant role for melatonin. J Pineal Res. 2004;36:1–9.
37. Winiarska K, Fraczyk T, Malinska D, Drozak J, Bryla J. Melatonin attenuates diabetes induced oxidative stress in rabbits. J Pineal Res. 2006;40:168–76.
38. Tan DX. Chemical and physical properties and potential mechanisms: melatonin as a broad spectrum antioxidant and free radical scavenger. Curr Top Med Chem. 2002;2:181–97.
39. Costa EJX, Lopes RH, Lamy-Freund MT. Solubility of pure bilayers to melatonin. J Pineal Res. 1995;19:123–6.
40. Seabra ML, Bignotto M, Pinto Jr LR, Tufik S. Randomized, double-blind clinical trial, controlled with placebo, of the toxicology of chronic melatonin treatment. J Pineal Res. 2000;29:193–200.
41. Aydin M, Canpolat S, Kuloğlu T, Yasar A, Colakoglu N, Kelestimur H. Effects of pinealectomy and exogenous melatonin on ghrelin and peptide YY in gastrointestinal system and neuropeptide Y in hypothalamic arcuate nucleus: immunohistochemical studies in male rats. Regul Pept. 2008;146:197–203.
42. Reiter RJ. Melatonin: clinical relevance. Best Pract Res Clin Endocrinol Metab. 2003;17:273–85.
43. Freeman SL, Hossain M, MacNaughton WK. Radiation-induced acute intestinal inflammation differs following total-body versus abdominopelvic irradiation in the ferret. Int J Radiat Biol. 2001;77:389–95.
44. Sener G, Jahovic N, Tosun O, Atasoy BM, Yegen BC. Melatonin ameliorates ionizing radiation-induced oxidative organ damage in rats. Life Sci. 2003;74:563–72.

45. Al-Ghoul WM, Abu-Shaqra S, Park BG, Fazal N. Melatonin plays a protective role in postburn rodent gut pathophysiology. Int J Biol Sci. 2010;6:282–93.
46. Gao F, Ueda S, Horie T. Effect of a synthetic analog of prostaglandin E1 on the intestinal mucosa of methotrexate-treated rats. Anticancer Res. 2001;21(3B):1913–7.
47. Sener G, Ekşioğlu-Demiralp E, Cetiner M, Ercan F, Yeğen BC. Beta-glucan ameliorates methotrexate-induced oxidative organ injury via its antioxidant and immunomodulatory effects. Eur J Pharmacol. 2006;542:170–8.
48. Sener G, Ekşioğlu-Demiralp E, Cetiner M, Ercan F, Sirvanci S, Gedik N, Yeğen BC. L-Carnitine ameliorates methotrexate-induced oxidative organ injury and inhibits leukocyte death. Cell Biol Toxicol. 2006;22:47–60.
49. Konturek SJ, Konturek PC, Brzozowski T. Melatonin in gastroprotection against stress-induced acute gastric lesions and in healing of chronic gastric ulcers. J Physiol Pharmacol. 2006;57 Suppl 5:51–66. Review.
50. Galijasevic S, Abdulhamid I, Abu-Soud HM. Melatonin is a potent inhibitor for myeloperoxidase. Biochemistry. 2008;47:2668–77.
51. Li JH. Melatonin reduces inflammatory injury through inhibiting NF-kappaB activation in rats with colitis. Mediators Inflamm. 2005;2005:185–93.
52. Mayo JC, Sainz RM, Tan DX, Hardeland R, Leon J, Rodriguez C, Reiter RJ. Anti-inflammatory actions of melatonin and its metabolites, N1-acetyl-N2-formyl-5-methoxy-kynuramine (AFMK) and N1-acetyl-5-methoxykynuramine (AMK), in macrophages. J Neuroimmunol. 2005;165:139–49.
53. Rodríguez-Reynoso S, Leal C, Portilla-de Buen E, Castillo JC, Ramos-Solano F. Melatonin ameliorates renal ischemia/reperfusion injury. J Surg Res. 2004;116:242–7.
54. Alarcón de la Lastra C, Motilva V, Martín MJ, Nieto A, Barranco MD, Cabeza J, Herrerías JM. Protective effect of melatonin on indomethacin-induced gastric injury in rats. J Pineal Res. 1999;26:101–7.
55. Cuzzocrea S, Mazzon E, Serraino I, Lepore V, Terranova ML, Ciccolo A. Melatonin reduces dinitrobenzene sulfonic acid-induced colitis. J Pineal Res. 2001;30:1–12.
56. Konturek PC, Konturek SJ, Brzozowski T, Dembinski A, Zembala M, Mytar B, Hahn EG. Gastroprotective activity of melatonin and its precursor, L-tryptophan, against stress-induced and ischaemia-induced lesions is mediated by scavenge of oxygen radicals. Scand J Gastroenterol. 1997;32:433–8.
57. Reiter RJ. Oxidative processes and antioxidative defense mechanisms in the aging brain. FASEB J. 1995;9:526–33.
58. Forrest CM, Mackay GM, Stoy N, Stone TW, Darlington LG. Inflammatory status and kynurenine metabolism in rheumatoid arthritis treated with melatonin. Br J Clin Pharmacol. 2007;64:517–26.
59. Kedziora-Kornatowska K. Antioxidative effects of melatonin administration in elderly primary essential hypertension patients. J Pineal Res. 2008;45:312–7.
60. Tamura H. Oxidative stress impairs oocyte quality and melatonin protects oocytes from free radical damage and improves fertilization rate. J Pineal Res. 2008;44:280–7.
61. Brzezinski A. Melatonin in humans. N Engl J Med. 1997;336:186–95.
62. Kadoma Y, Fujisawa S. Radical-scavenging activity of melatonin, either alone or in combination with vitamin E, ascorbate or 2-mercaptoethanol as co-antioxidants, using the induction period method. In Vivo. 2011;25:49–53.